*Hansten and Horn's*
# Managing Clinically Important Drug Interactions

Philip D. Hansten, Pharm.D.
University of Washington, Seattle

John R. Horn, Pharm.D.
University of Washington, Seattle

**Editors**

Mary Anne Koda-Kimble, Pharm.D.
Professor, Chairwoman
Division of Clinical Pharmacy
University of California, San Francisco

Lloyd Y. Young, Pharm.D.
Professor, Director, Assistant Dean
University of Texas at El Paso/Austin

Applied Therapeutics, Inc.
Vancouver, WA

# Other Publications by Applied Therapeutics, Inc.

**Hansten and Horn's Drug Interactions Analysis and Management**
by Philip D. Hansten and John R. Horn
ISSN 1092-048X

**Applied Therapeutics: The Clinical Use of Drugs, 6th edition**
edited by Lloyd Y. Young and Mary Anne Koda-Kimble
ISBN 0-915486-23-7

**Basic Clinical Pharmacokinetics, 3rd edition**
by Michael E. Winter
ISBN 0-915486-22-9

**A Short Course in Clinical Pharmacokinetics**
by Dennis A. Noe
ISBN 0-915486-19-9

**Handbook of Applied Therapeutics, 6th edition**
by Lloyd Y. Young, Mary Anne Koda-Kimble, B. Joseph Guglielmo, and Wayne A. Kradjan
ISBN 0-915486-24-5

**Applied Pharmacokinetics: Principles of Therapeutic Drug Monitoring, 3rd edition**
edited by William E. Evans, Jerome J. Schentag, and William J. Jusko
ISBN 0-915486-15-6

**Applied Drug Information: Strategies for Information Management**
Edited by Mirta Millares, Pharm.D., FCSHP
ISBN 0-915486-28-8

**Physical Assessment: A Guide for Evaluating Drug Therapy**
by R. Leon Longe and Jon C. Calvert
ISBN 0-915486-20-2

**Clinical Clerkship Manual**
edited by Larry E. Boh
ISBN 0-915486-17-2

**Ethical Issues in Pharmacy**
edited by Bruce Weinstein
ISBN 0-915486-25-3

To order your complete copy of **Hansten and Horn's Drug Interactions Analysis and Management**, contact:

Applied Therapeutics, Inc.
P.O. Box 5077
Vancouver, WA 98668-5077
Phone: (360) 253-7123
FAX: (360) 253-8475

ISBN 0-915486-30-x

First Printing July 1998

## Table of Contents

For a more complete listing of known and potential drug interactions order your copy of **Hansten and Horn's Drug Interactions Analysis and Management** today.

For more information, call 1-800-345-0247.

# Notice to Reader

Drug therapy information is constantly evolving. Our ever changing knowledge and experience with drugs, and the continual development of new drugs, necessitate changes in treatment and drug therapy. The editors, authors, and publisher of **Hansten and Horn's Managing Clinically Important Drug Interactions** have made diligent efforts to provide information within this work that is consistent with applicable pharmaceutical standards existing at the time of the copyright date, or the date of the particular section of the work, whichever is most recent. *It remains the responsibility of every practitioner to evaluate the appropriateness of a particular opinion or therapy in the context of the actual clinical situation and with due consideration for any new developments in the field.* Although the recommendations for managing drug interactions are consistent with the standards and responsible literature existing as of the date of the copyright, or the date of the particular section of the work, whichever is most recent, readers should consult several appropriate information sources when dealing with new or unfamiliar drugs.

At one time, it was possible (albeit with considerable effort) for the individual practitioner to commit to memory virtually all drug interactions of potential clinical importance. Today, due to a more than eightfold increase in the number of known drug interactions, few practitioners have the time or inclination to remember them all. In addition to the discovery of many new drug interactions over the past 20 years, there have also been major advances in the understanding of drug interaction mechanisms and of pharmacokinetic principles of drug interactions. The influence of genetics on interactions is beginning to be studied. Still generally lacking, however, are studies identifying the types of patients who are predisposed to adverse effects of particular drug interactions, and studies of the clinical characteristics (e.g., time course and dose dependency of drug interactions). Also badly needed are well conceived pharmacoepidemiologic studies on the incidence of adverse drug interactions in patients exposed to interacting drugs.

The reader is urged to review the "Instructions to Users," which describe the criteria used to assign the clinical significance ratings. In an effort to maintain clinical relevance, human studies are cited almost exclusively, and all statements refer to humans unless specifically stated otherwise.

To keep the discussion as concise as possible, a basic understanding of pharmacologic and physiologic principles has been assumed.

# Introduction

Hansten and Horn's Managing Clinically Important Drug Interactions is intended to provide the user with a brief description of drug interactions selected on the basis of their potential to alter patient outcomes. The interactions included herein were selected from Hansten and Horn's Drug Interactions Analysis and Management. It is not intended to be an inclusive listing of all known or potential drug interactions nor is it intended to be a substitute for a more complete reference such as Drug Interactions Analysis and Management.

Each interaction is assigned a significance class rating, based primarily on the management options one should consider. Interactions included in this book are assigned to one of three classes. This classification system was originally developed by the Drug Interaction Foundation. Only drug interactions rated as Class 1, 2, or 3 are included in this book.

For each interaction, a brief monograph is presented that includes the following sections.

Summary provides a concise description of the potential outcome of the interaction and its clinical significance.

Risk Factors describe patient specific factors that have been identified as contributing to the magnitude or severity of the interaction.

Obvious factors that apply universally are not listed. For example, virtually all drug interactions are dose dependent, or more precisely dependent on the concentration of the precipitant drug at the site of the interaction. The larger the dose or the higher the concentration of the pre-

cipitant drug, the greater the magnitude of the interaction and the larger the risk that an adverse outcome may result. If the literature provides specific data on dose- or concentration-effect relationships, they are included here. Included in risk factors, if available, in addition to information on dosage regiments of the interacting drugs, are data on the effects of age, concurrent diseases, diet/food, gender, route of administration, order of drug administration, other drugs, time of day, and pharmacogenetics. The risk factors section is limited to documented risk factors. Risk factors for most interactions have not been identified and in those cases the phrase, "No specific risk factors known," will appear.

Related Drugs cites examples of closely related agents that would be expected to interact in a similar manner as the monograph agents. Related drugs usually are confined to the chemical class as those in the monograph that have similar pharmacokinetic or pharmacodynamic interaction potential. This listing aids in selecting alternative therapy by noting those drugs that should be eliminated from consideration as alternatives. Prediction of potential interactions that are as yet undocumented is simplified by consulting this section. When specific data are available, related drugs also appear in individual monographs. Please consult the Index.

Management Options are placed into three classifications that assist the reader in eliminating or minimizing the risk to the patient. Each drug interaction in the Index identifies the management class (as shown in the shaded Significance Classification box) to which it has been assigned.

*Class 1 Interactions.* Avoid administration of the drug combination. The drugs listed as class one interactions should not be administered together. The risk of adverse patient outcome precludes the concomitant administration of the drugs.

*Class 2 Interactions* should be avoided unless it is determined that the benefit of coadministration of the drugs outweighs the risk to the patient. The use of an alternative to one of the interacting drugs is recommended when appropriate. Patients should be monitored carefully if the drugs are coadministered.

*Class 3 Interactions.* Several potential management options are available for class 3 Interactions. When an alternative agent should be considered, examples of documented noninteracting drugs are provided. Changes in drug dosage or route of administration that can circumvent or minimize the potential interaction are suggested. Again, patient monitoring is suggested in case the interacting drugs are administered.

**References** will not be an attempt to be all inclusive but will contain pertinent citations that provide meaningful insight for the interaction.

**Monographs** are listed alphabetically and both interacting drugs are placed in the Index. All drugs are listed by generic name and not pharmacological class except combination products like antacids which are listed under Antacids as well as by brand name. The few exceptions are, from the standpoint of drug interactions, homogeneous (e.g., thyroid, oral contraceptives, and thiazides) where interactions apply equally to all members of the class.

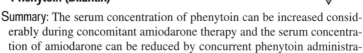

### Amiodarone (Cordarone)

### Phenytoin (Dilantin)

Summary: The serum concentration of phenytoin can be increased considerably during concomitant amiodarone therapy and the serum concentration of amiodarone can be reduced by concurrent phenytoin administration.

Risk Factors: No specific risk factors known.

Related Drugs: **Mephenytoin (Mesantoin)** has been reported not to interact with amiodarone.

Management Options:
- *Monitor.* Patients being treated with phenytoin should have their phenytoin serum concentrations monitored carefully when amiodarone is added to or removed from their drug regimen. This drug interaction may take several weeks to become fully apparent. In addition, patients taking amiodarone should be monitored for reduced antiarrhythmic efficacy, and amiodarone serum concentrations should be monitored if phenytoin is added to their drug regimen.

References:

1. Gore JM et al. Interaction of amiodarone and diphenylhydantoin. Am J Cardiol. 1984;54:1145.
2. MacGovern B et al. Possible interaction between amiodarone and phenytoin. Ann Intern Med. 1984;101:650.
3. Shackleford EJ et al. Amiodarone-phenytoin interaction. Drug Intell Clin Pharm. 1987;21:921.
4. Nolan PE Jr. et al. Pharmacokinetic interaction between intravenous phenytoin and amiodarone in healthy volunteers. Clin Pharmacol Ther. 1989;46:43.
5. Nolan PE et al. Evidence for an effect of phenytoin on the pharmacokinetics of amiodarone. J Clin Pharmacol. 1990;30:1112.
6. Nolan PE et al. Steady-state interaction between amiodarone and phenytoin in normal subjects. Am J Cardiol. 1990;65:1252.

## Significance Classification

1 - **Avoid Combination.** Risk always outweighs benefit.

2 - **Usually Avoid Combination.** Use combination only under special circumstances.

3 - **Minimize Risk.** Take action as necessary to reduce risk.

viii

## *Acknowledgements*

The publisher, Applied Therapeutics Inc., would like to express its appreciation for the efforts of this book's production staff. Their attention to detail, committment, and dedication to excellence helped make this book possible. Thank you to Tami Martin, Nannette Naught, Dianne Ellis, Steve Naught, Barry Espenson, and Cindy Cutburth.

### Acetaminophen (Tylenol)

### Cholestyramine (Questran)

Summary: Cholestyramine markedly reduces plasma acetaminophen concentrations and probably reduces acetaminophen therapeutic response.

Risk Factors: No specific risk factors known.

Related Drugs: **Colestipol (Colestid)** probably would reduce plasma acetaminophen concentrations also, but clinical studies are lacking.

Management Options:
- *Circumvent/Minimize.* Give acetaminophen 2 hr before or 6 hr after cholestyramine.
- *Monitor* for reduced acetaminophen effects if combination is given.

References:
1. Dordoni B et al. Reduction of absorption of paracetamol by activated charcoal and cholestyramine: a possible therapeutic measure. Br Med J. 1973;3:86.

### Acetaminophen (Tylenol)

### Ethanol (Ethyl Alcohol)

Summary: Substantial evidence indicates that chronic, excessive alcohol ingestion increases the toxicity of high therapeutic doses or overdoses of acetaminophen, while preliminary evidence indicates that acute alcohol intoxication protects against acetaminophen overdose toxicity.

Risk Factors:
- *Dosage Regimen.* The increased risk of acetaminophen hepatotoxicity occurs primarily with excessive doses of acetaminophen in the presence of chronic, excessive alcohol ingestion.

Related Drugs: No information available.

Management Options:
- *Circumvent/Minimize.* Patients who chronically ingest large amounts of alcohol (e.g., several drinks a day or more) should be warned to avoid taking large and/or prolonged doses of acetaminophen.
- *Monitor.* When monitoring serum acetaminophen following acute acetaminophen overdose in alcohol abusers, be aware that acetylcysteine may be indicated even if the serum acetaminophen concentration is below the "action line" on the standard nomogram. This is probably due to the ability of alcohol to enhance acetaminophen

## Significance Classification

① - *Avoid Combination.* Risk always outweighs benefit.

② - *Usually Avoid Combination.* Use combination only under special circumstances.

③ - *Minimize Risk.* Take action as necessary to reduce risk.

metabolism. (Some have recommended that the serum acetaminophen threshold for acetylcysteine therapy should be reduced by as
much as 70% in patients who chronically ingest large amounts of
alcohol.)[4]

References:
1. Seifert CF et al. Patterns of acetaminophen use in alcoholic patients. Pharmacotherapy. 1993;13:391.
2. Kumar S et al. Failure of physicians to recognize acetaminophen hepatotoxicity in
chronic alcoholics. Arch Intern Med. 1991;151:1189.
3. Cheung L et al. Acetaminophen treatment nomogram. New Engl J Med. 1994;
330:1907. Letter.
4. McClements BM et al. Management of paracetamol poisoning complicated by
enzyme induction due to alcohol or drugs. Lancet. 1990;1:1526. Letter.

### Acetaminophen (Tylenol)
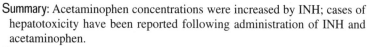
### Isoniazid (INH)

Summary: Acetaminophen concentrations were increased by INH; cases of
hepatotoxicity have been reported following administration of INH and
acetaminophen.
Risk Factors: No specific risk factors known.
Related Drugs: No information available.
Management Options:
- *Circumvent/Minimize.* Until further data are available, it would be
prudent for patients taking INH to limit their consumption of acetaminophen. Aspirin or an NSAID could be used instead of acetaminophen.
- *Monitor.* Until further data are available, patients taking INH and
acetaminophen should be monitored for hepatotoxicity.

References:
1. Moulding TS et al. Acetaminophen, isoniazid, and hepatic toxicity. Ann Intern Med.
1991;114:431.
2. Epstein MM et al. Inhibition of the metabolism of paracetamol by isoniazid. Br J
Clin Pharmacol. 1991;31:139.
3. Zand R et al. Inhibition and induction of cytochrome p450e1-catalyzed oxidation by
isoniazid in humans. Clin Pharmacol Ther. 1993;54:142.

### Acetaminophen (Tylenol)
### Phenobarbital

Summary: Barbiturates may enhance the hepatotoxic potential of overdoses (and possibly large therapeutic doses) of acetaminophen; it is also
possible that barbiturates reduce the therapeutic response to acetaminophen.
Risk Factors:
- *Dosage Regimen.* The danger of hepatotoxicity is primarily with
overdoses or large and/or prolonged use of acetaminophen.

Related Drugs: Enzyme inducers other than phenobarbital [e.g., other barbiturates, **carbamazepine (Tegretol)**, **phenytoin (Dilantin)**, **primidone (Mysoline)**, **rifabutin (Mycobutin)**, and **rifampin (Rifadin)**] may interact similarly.

Management Options:

- *Circumvent/Minimize.* Patients on barbiturate therapy should probably avoid taking large and/or prolonged doses of acetaminophen. With acute acetaminophen overdoses, acetylcysteine may be indicated even if the serum acetaminophen concentration is below the "action line" on the standard nomogram. (Some have recommended that the serum acetaminophen threshold for acetylcysteine therapy should be reduced by as much as 70% in patients who are taking enzyme inducers such as barbiturates.)[1]

- *Monitor* for reduced acetaminophen effect. In patients taking large and/or prolonged doses of acetaminophen watch for evidence of hepatotoxicity.

References:

1. McClements BM et al. Management of paracetamol poisoning complicated by enzyme induction due to alcohol or drugs. Lancet. 1990;1:1526. Letter.
2. Minton NA et al. Fatal paracetamol poisoning in an epileptic. Hum Toxicol. 1988; 7:33.
3. Pessayre E et al. Additive effects of inducers and fasting on acetaminophen hepatotoxicity. Biochem Pharmacol. 1980;29:2219.

## Acetaminophen (Tylenol)

### Phenytoin (Dilantin)

Summary: Phenytoin may enhance the hepatotoxic potential of overdoses (and possibly large therapeutic doses) of acetaminophen; it is also possible that phenytoin reduces the therapeutic response to acetaminophen.

Risk Factors: No specific risk factors known.

Related Drugs: Other enzyme-inducing anticonvulsants such as **carbamazepine (Tegretol)**, **phenobarbital**, and **primidone (Mysoline)** probably also increase acetaminophen hepatotoxicity.

Management Options:

- *Circumvent/Minimize.* Patients on phenytoin therapy should probably avoid taking large and/or prolonged doses of acetaminophen. In cases of acute acetaminophen overdoses, acetylcysteine may be indicated even if the serum acetaminophen concentration is below the "action line" on the standard nomogram. (Some have recommended that the serum acetaminophen threshold for acetylcysteine therapy should be reduced by as much as 70% in patients who are taking enzyme inducers such as phenytoin.)[2]

- *Monitor* for evidence of hepatotoxicity.

References:

1. Neuvonen PJ et al. Antipyretic analgesics in patients on antiepileptic drug therapy. Eur J Clin Pharmacol. 1979;15:263.

2. McClements BM et al. Management of paracetamol poisoning complicated by enzyme induction due to alcohol or drugs. Lancet. 1990;1:1526. Letter.
3. Minton NA et al. Fatal paracetamol poisoning in an epileptic. Hum Toxicol. 1988;7:33.

### Acetaminophen (Tylenol)
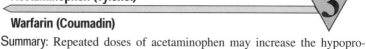

### Warfarin (Coumadin)

**Summary:** Repeated doses of acetaminophen may increase the hypoprothrombinemic response to oral anticoagulants like warfarin in some patients.

**Risk Factors:**

- *Dosage Regimen.* Although the dose relationship is not clearly established, an interaction appears more likely with daily acetaminophen doses of greater than 2 gm/day for a week or more. Maximal effects on the hypoprothrombinemic response have occurred 1–3 weeks after starting acetaminophen.[1-5] Occasional doses of acetaminophen do not appear likely to interact.

**Related Drugs:** Although most data on this interaction involve warfarin, limited clinical information suggests that other oral anticoagulants such as **acenocoumarol** and **phenprocoumon** may interact with acetaminophen as well. Most alternative analgesics (e.g., **aspirin**, nonsteroidal anti-inflammatory drugs) would not be suitable alternatives to acetaminophen in patients receiving oral anticoagulants.

- *Circumvent/Minimize.* Patients receiving warfarin or other oral anticoagulants should be warned to limit their intake of acetaminophen-containing products. Although a "safe" amount cannot be determined with certainty, it would be prudent to limit acetaminophen intake to no more than 2 gm/day for no more than a few days. Aspirin-containing products should not be used as alternatives; acetaminophen lacks the adverse effects of aspirin on the gastric mucosa and platelets, and it is considered safer than aspirin in anticoagulated patients.

- *Monitor.* Patients taking amounts of acetaminophen larger than recommended above should be monitored for enhanced hypoprothrombinemic response and the anticoagulant dose adjusted as needed.

**References:**

1. Antlitz AM et al. Potentiation of oral anticoagulant therapy by acetaminophen. Curr Ther Res. 1968;10:501.

## Significance Classification

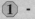 - *Avoid Combination.* Risk always outweighs benefit.

 - *Usually Avoid Combination.* Use combination only under special circumstances.

 - *Minimize Risk.* Take action as necessary to reduce risk.

2. Rubin RN et al. Potentiation of anticoagulant effect of warfarin by acetaminophen (Tylenol). Clin Res. 1984;32:698a. Abstract.
3. Boeijinga JJ et al. Interaction between paracetamol and coumarin anticoagulants. Lancet. 1982;1:506.
4. Antlitz AM et al. A double-blind study of acetaminophen used in conjunction with oral anticoagulant therapy. Curr Ther Res. 1969;11:360.
5. Kaye L. Warfarin and paracetamol. Pharmaceutical J. 1991;246:692.

## Acetazolamide (Diamox)

## Aspirin

**Summary:** Aspirin increases the plasma concentration of acetazolamide, leading to central nervous system (CNS) toxicity.

**Risk Factors:** No specific risk factors known.

**Related Drugs:** Theoretically, salicylates other than aspirin would also interact with acetazolamide. The effect of salicylates on carbonic anhydrase inhibitors other than acetazolamide is not established.

**Management Options:**
- *Avoid Unless Benefit Outweighs Risk.* Concurrent use of salicylates and acetazolamide should be avoided if possible, particularly in patients with renal dysfunction.
- *Monitor.* If the combination is used, monitor the patient carefully for symptoms of CNS toxicity, such as lethargy, confusion, somnolence, tinnitus, and anorexia.

**References:**
1. Hill JB. Experimental salicylate poisoning: observations on effects of altering blood pH on tissue and plasma salicylate concentrations. Pediatrics. 1971;47:658.
2. Anderson CJ et al. Toxicity of combined therapy with carbonic anhydrase inhibitors and aspirin. Am J Ophthalmol. 1978;86:516.

## Acetazolamide (Diamox)

## Phenytoin (Dilantin)

**Summary:** Acetazolamide may increase the risk of osteomalacia in patients receiving anticonvulsants.

**Risk Factors:** No specific risk factors known.

**Related Drugs:** Other carbonic anhydrase inhibitors when prescribed with an anticonvulsant could increase the risk of osteomalacia.

**Management Options:**
- *Monitor.* In patients receiving acetazolamide (or other carbonic anhydrase inhibitors) in addition to an anticonvulsant such as phenytoin, phenobarbital, or primidone, special attention should be given to early detection of osteomalacia. If osteomalacia does occur under these conditions, stopping the acetazolamide and instituting replacement therapy with phosphate or vitamin D may be beneficial.[1,3]

**References:**
1. Matsuda I et al. Renal tubular acidosis and skeletal demineralization in patients on long-term anticonvulsant therapy. J Pediatr. 1975;87:202.

2. Mallette LE. Anticonvulsants, acetazolamide, and osteomalacia. N Engl J Med. 1975;293:668. Letter.
3. Mallette LE. Acetazolamide-accelerated anticonvulsant osteomalacia. Arch Intern Med. 1977;137:1013.

### Acetazolamide (Diamox)

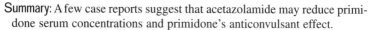

### Primidone (Mysoline)

Summary: A few case reports suggest that acetazolamide may reduce primidone serum concentrations and primidone's anticonvulsant effect.

Risk Factors: No specific risk factors known.

Related Drugs: The effect of other carbonic anhydrase inhibitors on primidone is unknown.

Management Options:
- *Monitor.* It seems unnecessary to avoid the concomitant use of acetazolamide and primidone. However, until this interaction is better described, patients receiving primidone and acetazolamide should be monitored for a decreased primidone effect.

References:
1. Syversen BG et al. Acetazolamide-induced interference with primidone absorption. Arch Neurol. 1977;34:80.

### Acetazolamide (Diamox)

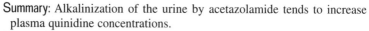

### Quinidine

Summary: Alkalinization of the urine by acetazolamide tends to increase plasma quinidine concentrations.

Risk Factors: No specific risk factors known.

Related Drugs: Other drugs that alkalinize the urine (e.g., **sodium bicarbonate**) would produce similar effects on quinidine serum concentrations. Acetazolamide may increase **quinine** concentrations.

Management Options:
- *Monitor.* Initiation, discontinuation, or a change in dose of acetazolamide in a patient receiving quinidine may necessitate a change in the quinidine dose. Monitor for altered quinidine response of urine pH changes.

References:
1. Knouss RF et al. Variation in quinidine excretion with changing urine pH. Ann Intern Med. 1968;68:1157. Abstract.
2. Gerhardt RE et al. Quinidine excretion in aciduria and alkaluria. Ann Intern Med. 1969;71:927.

### Adenosine (Adenocard)

### Dipyridamole (Persantine)

Summary: Dipyridamole increases the serum concentrations of endogenous and exogenous adenosine, thereby potentiating its pharmacologic effects.

Risk Factors: No specific risk factors known.

Related Drugs: No information available.

Management Options:
- *Circumvent/Minimize.* Patients taking dipyridamole should receive reduced doses of adenosine for the treatment of arrhythmias or diagnostic tests.
- *Monitor.* Be alert for bradycardia and prolonged AV conduction when dipyridamole and adenosine are coadministered. The enhancement of adenosine effects on AV conduction (e.g., bradycardia) by dipyridamole may be reversed by aminophylline.

References:
1. Lerman BB et al. Electrophysiologic effects of dipyridamole on atrioventricular nodal conduction and supraventricular tachycardia. Circulation. 1989;80:1536.
2. German DC et al. Oral dipyridamole increases plasma adenosine levels in human beings. Clin Pharmacol Ther. 1989;45:80.
3. McCollam PL et al. Adenosine-related ventricular asystole. Ann Intern Med. 1993; 118:315. Letter.

### Adenosine (Adenocard)

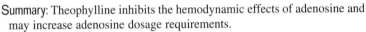

### Theophylline

Summary: Theophylline inhibits the hemodynamic effects of adenosine and may increase adenosine dosage requirements.

Risk Factors: No specific risk factors known.

Related Drugs: *Caffeine* produces similar effects on adenosine hemodynamics.

Management Options:
- *Circumvent/Minimize.* Patients maintained on theophylline may require greater-than-normal doses of adenosine to control arrhythmias.
- *Monitor.* Watch for decreased therapeutic response to adenosine when theophylline is initiated and watch for adenosine toxicity (e.g., bradycardia) when theophylline is discontinued.

References:
1. Smits P et al. Caffeine and theophylline attenuate adenosine-induced vasodilation in humans. Clin Pharmacol Ther. 1990;48:410.
2. Minton NA et al. Pharmacodynamic interactions between infused adenosine and oral theophylline. Hum Exp Toxicol. 1991;10:411.
3. Heller GV et al. Pretreatment with theophylline does not affect adenosine-induced thallium-201 myocardial imaging. Am Heart J. 1993;126:1077.

### Alfentanil (Alfenta)

### Cimetidine (Tagamet)

Summary: Cimetidine appears to substantially increase serum concentrations of alfentanil, but it is not known how often this leads to adverse effects.

Risk Factors: No specific risk factors known.

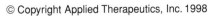

Related Drugs: Preliminary evidence suggests that *ranitidine (Zantac)* does not seem to affect the pharmacokinetics of alfentanil. The effect of *famotidine (Pepcid)* and *nizatidine (Axid)* on alfentanil is not established, but theoretically they would not be expected to interact.

Management Options:

- *Consider Alternative.* Consider using $H_2$-receptor antagonists other than cimetidine.
- *Monitor.* If alfentanil is used in a patient receiving cimetidine, monitor for excessive and/or prolonged alfentanil effect. Adjust alfentanil dose as needed.

References:

1. Keinlen J et al. Pharmacokinetics of alfentanil in patients treated with either cimetidine or ranitidine. Drug Invest. 1993;6:257.

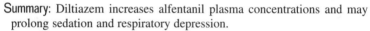

**Alfentanil (Alfenta)**

**Diltiazem (Cardizem)**

Summary: Diltiazem increases alfentanil plasma concentrations and may prolong sedation and respiratory depression.

Risk Factors: No specific risk factors known.

Related Drugs: Diltiazem is likely to affect other analgesics that are metabolized by CYP3A4 including *fentanyl (Sublimaze)* and *sufentanil (Sufenta)*. *Verapamil (Calan)* and *mibefradil (Posicor)* may inhibit the metabolism of alfentanil.

Management Options:

- *Consider Alternative.* The use of a dihydropyridine calcium channel blocker [e.g., amlodipine (Norvasc) or felodipine (Plendil)] would probably avoid the interaction.
- *Monitor.* Patients receiving diltiazem and alfentanil should be monitored for prolonged sedation and respiratory depression.

References:

1. Ahonen J et al. Effect of diltiazem on midazolam and alfentanil disposition in patients undergoing coronary artery bypass grafting. Anesthesiology. 1996;85:1246.

**Alfentanil (Alfenta)**

**Erythromycin**

Summary: Patients taking erythromycin may experience prolonged anesthesia or increased respiratory depression when given alfentanil.

Risk Factors: No specific risk factors known.

Related Drugs: Other macrolides such as *troleandomycin (TAO)* or *clarithromycin (Biaxin)* also may inhibit alfentanil. *Azithromycin (Zithromax)* and *dirithromycin (Dynabac)* would be unlikely to inhibit alfentanil metabolism.

Management Options:

- *Circumvent/Minimize.* Erythromycin has no effect on sufentanil serum concentrations.[3] Consider using azithromycin or dirithromycin with alfentanil.

- *Monitor.* Until further information is available, patients taking erythromycin should be monitored for enhanced effects following usual doses of alfentanil.

References:
1. Bartkowski RR et al. Inhibition of alfentanil metabolism by erythromycin. Clin Pharmacol Ther. 1989;46:99.
2. Barkowski RR et al. Prolonged alfentanil effect following erythromycin administration. Anaesthesiology. 1990;73:566.
3. Barkowski RR et al. Sufentanil disposition. Is it affected by erythromycin? Anesthesiology. 1993;78:260.

### Allopurinol (Zyloprim)

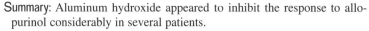

### Antacids

Summary: Aluminum hydroxide appeared to inhibit the response to allopurinol considerably in several patients.

Risk Factors: No specific risk factors known.

Related Drugs: Pending additional information, all aluminum-containing antacids should be considered capable of inhibiting allopurinol absorption. Although little is known regarding **magnesium-** or **calcium-**containing antacids, assume that they also inhibit allopurinol absorption until proven otherwise.

Management Options:
- *Circumvent/Minimize.* Until more information is available, allopurinol should be administered at least 3 hours before or 6 hours after aluminum hydroxide.
- *Monitor.* Patients also should be monitored for reduced allopurinol response. The same precautions would apply to other antacids until information on their effect on allopurinol is available.

References:
1. Weissman I et al. Interaction of aluminum hydroxide and allopurinol in patients on chronic hemodialysis. Ann Intern Med. 1987;107:787. Letter.

### Allopurinol (Zyloprim)

### Azathioprine (Imuran)

Summary: Allopurinol may increase the toxicity of azathioprine; careful dosage adjustment is necessary.

## Significance Classification

 - *Avoid Combination.* Risk always outweighs benefit.

 - *Usually Avoid Combination.* Use combination only under special circumstances.

 - *Minimize Risk.* Take action as necessary to reduce risk.

Risk Factors: No specific risk factors known.

Related Drugs: **Mercaptopurine (Purinethol)** interacts similarly with allopurinol.

Management Options:

- *Avoid Unless Benefit Outweighs Risk.* Several authors have recommended that the azathioprine dose be reduced to one-fourth of the recommended dose when it is used concurrently with allopurinol.
- *Monitor.* Allopurinol and azathioprine should never be given together without meticulous attention to adjusting the dosage of the azathioprine.

References:
1. Anon. Clinicopathologic conference: hypertension and the lupus syndrome. Am J Med. 1970;49:519.
2. Nies AS, Oates JA. Clinicopathologic conference: hypertension and the lupus syndrome revisited. Am J Med. 1971;51:812.

## Allopurinol (Zyloprim)

## Captopril (Capoten)

Summary: Isolated case reports indicate that patients on allopurinol and angiotensin-converting enzyme (ACE) inhibitors such as captopril or enalapril may be predisposed to hypersensitivity reactions including Stevens-Johnson syndrome, anaphylaxis, skin eruptions, fever, and arthralgias, but a causal relationship has not been established.

Risk Factors:

- *Concurrent Diseases.* Impaired renal function has been proposed as a risk factor, but more study is needed.

Related Drugs: It is not known whether ACE inhibitors other than captopril and **enalapril (Vasotec)** would produce similar reactions if combined with allopurinol.

Management Options:

- *Avoid Unless Benefit Outweighs Risk.* Although it is not firmly established that these reactions resulted from the combined effects of ACE inhibitors and allopurinol, the severity of the potential reactions suggests that the combinations generally should be avoided until more information is available.
- *Monitor* patients receiving the combination carefully for hypersensitivity reactions. Prompt discontinuation of the offending drugs is important.

References:
1. Pennell DJ et al. Fatal Stevens-Johnson syndrome in a patient on captopril and allopurinol. Lancet. 1984;1:463.
2. Al-Kawas FH et al. Allopurinol hepatotoxicity. Report of two cases and review of the literature. Ann Intern Med. 1981;95:588.
3. Ahmad S. Allopurinol and enalapril: drug induced anaphylactic coronary spasm and acute myocardial infarction. Chest. 1995;108:586. Letter.

### Allopurinol (Zyloprim)

### Cyclophosphamide (Cytoxan)

Summary: Some evidence indicates that allopurinol increases cyclophosphamide toxicity, but this has not been a consistent finding.

Risk Factors: No specific risk factors known.

Related Drugs: No information available.

Management Options:
- *Monitor.* It has been proposed that the appropriateness of routine prophylactic use of allopurinol in patients receiving cytotoxic drugs be re-evaluated. When it is necessary to give allopurinol and cyclophosphamide concomitantly, one should be alert for evidence of excessive cyclophosphamide effect.

References:
1. Boston Collaborative Drug Surveillance Program. Allopurinol and cytotoxic drugs. Interaction in relation to bone marrow depression. JAMA. 1974;227:1036.
2. Stolbach L et al. Evaluation of bone marrow toxic reaction in patients treated with allopurinol. JAMA. 1982;247:334.
3. Witten J et al. The pharmacokinetics of cyclophosphamide in man after treatment with allopurinol. Acta Pharmacol et Toxicol. 1980;46:392–94. Letter.

### Allopurinol (Zyloprim)

### Cyclosporine (Sandimmune)

Summary: Case reports suggest that allopurinol may increase cyclosporine blood concentrations and increase the risk of cyclosporine toxicity.

Risk Factors: No specific risk factors known.

Related Drugs: The effect of allopurinol on *tacrolimus* is not established. Given the similarity in the metabolism of cyclosporine and tacrolimus, it is possible that allopurinol affects them similarly.

Management Options:
- *Circumvent/Minimize.* Adjustments of cyclosporine dosage may be needed.

- *Monitor* for altered cyclosporine concentrations and renal function if allopurinol is initiated, discontinued, or changed in dosage.

References:
1. Stevens SL et al. Cyclosporine toxicity associated with allopurinol. South Med J. 1992;85:1265.
2. Gorrie M et al. Allopurinol interaction with cyclosporin. Br Med J. 1994;308:113.

### Allopurinol (Zyloprim)

### Mercaptopurine (Purinethol)

Summary: Allopurinol increases the effect of mercaptopurine; mercaptopurine dose should be reduced and the patient monitored for toxicity.

Risk Factors: No specific risk factors known.

Related Drugs: **Azathioprine (Imuran)** interacts in a similar manner with allopurinol.

Management Options:

- *Circumvent/Minimize.* When allopurinol and mercaptopurine are given concomitantly, the mercaptopurine dose may need to be reduced to as little as 25% of the usual dose.
- *Monitor* for both excessive bone marrow suppression and adequate therapeutic response during cotherapy with these drugs.

References:

1. Calabro JJ et al. Case records of the Massachusetts General Hospital (Case 4-1972). N Engl J Med. 1972,286:205.
2. Coffey JJ et el. Effect of allopurinol on the pharmacokinetics of 6-mercaptopurine (NSC 755) in cancer patients. Cancer Res. 1972;32:1283.

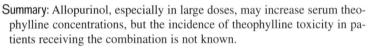

## Allopurinol (Zyloprim)

## Theophylline

Summary: Allopurinol, especially in large doses, may increase serum theophylline concentrations, but the incidence of theophylline toxicity in patients receiving the combination is not known.

Risk Factors:

- *Dosage Regimen.* Allopurinol doses ≥600 mg/day may inhibit the hepatic metabolism of theophylline.

Related Drugs: No information available.

Management Options:

- *Monitor* for evidence of altered theophylline effect if allopurinol therapy is initiated or discontinued, especially if large doses of allopurinol are used. Alteration of theophylline dose may be needed.

References:

1. Barry M et al. Allopurinol influences aminophenazone elimination. Clin Pharmacokinet. 1990;19:167.
2. Vozeh S et al. Influence of allopurinol on theophylline disposition in adults. Clin Pharmacol Ther. 1980;27:194.
3. Manfredi RL et al. Inhibition of theophylline metabolism by long-term allopurinol administration. Clin Pharmacol Ther. 1981;29:224.

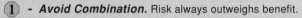

## Significance Classification

1 - *Avoid Combination.* Risk always outweighs benefit.

2 - *Usually Avoid Combination.* Use combination only under special circumstances.

3 - *Minimize Risk.* Take action as necessary to reduce risk.

### Allopurinol (Zyloprim)

### Vidarabine (Vira-A)

Summary: Allopurinol may increase vidarabine toxicity.

Risk Factors: No specific risk factors known.

Related Drugs: No information available.

Management Options:
- *Monitor.* Until additional information regarding this interaction is available, patients receiving allopurinol and vidarabine should be monitored carefully for signs of vidarabine toxicity.

References:
1. Friedman HM et al. Adenine arabinoside and allopurinol-possible adverse drug interaction. N Engl J Med. 1981;304:423.

### Allopurinol (Zyloprim)

### Warfarin (Coumadin)

Summary: Although the evidence is conflicting, allopurinol appears to enhance the hypoprothrombinemic response to oral anticoagulants in some patients; bleeding episodes have been reported in some cases.

Risk Factors: No specific risk factors known.

Related Drugs: Although data are limited, assume that all oral anticoagulants interact with allopurinol until proven otherwise.

Management Options:
- *Monitor.* Watch for an alteration in the hypoprothrombinemic response to oral anticoagulants when allopurinol is started, stopped, or changed in dosage; adjust oral anticoagulant dosage as needed.

References:
1. Jahnchen E et al. Interaction of allopurinol with phenprocoumon in man. Klin Wochenschr. 1977;55:759.
2. McInnes GT et al. Acute adverse reactions attributed to allopurinol in hospitalized patients. Ann Rheum Dis. 1981;40:245.
3. Barry M et al. Allopurinol influences aminophenazone elimination. Clin Pharmacokinet. 1990;19:167.

### Alprazolam (Xanax)

### Erythromycin

Summary: Erythromycin increases the plasma concentration and half-life of alprazolam. An increase in alprazolam effects may occur in some patients.

Risk Factors: No specific risk factors known.

Related Drugs: Erythromycin is known to increase the plasma concentrations of other benzodiazepines including *triazolam (Halcion)* and *midazolam (Versed)*. *Clarithromycin (Biaxin)* or *troleandomycin (TAO)* may produce similar reductions in the clearance of alprazolam.

Management Options:

*Consider Alternative.* Selection of a noninhibiting macrolide [e.g., azithromycin (Zithromax) or dirithromycin (Dynabac)] is likely to limit changes in alprazolam pharmacokinetics. Anxiolytics not metabolized by CYP3A4 such as lorazepam (Ativan) or temazepam (Restoril) could be substituted for alprazolam.

*Monitor.* Patients taking alprazolam chronically should be monitored for increased sedation during erythromycin administration.

References:

1. Yasui N et al. A kinetic and dynamic study of oral alprazolam with and without erythromycin in humans: in vivo evidence for the involvement of CYP3A4 in alprazolam metabolism. Clin Pharmacol Ther. 1996;59:514.

### Alprazolam (Xanax)
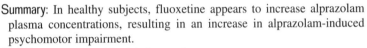
### Fluoxetine (Prozac)

Summary: In healthy subjects, fluoxetine appears to increase alprazolam plasma concentrations, resulting in an increase in alprazolam-induced psychomotor impairment.

Risk Factors: No specific risk factors known.

Related Drugs: The effect of selective serotonin reuptake inhibitors other than fluoxetine on alprazolam is not established, but *fluvoxamine (Luvox)* is known to inhibit CYP3A4, an isozyme important in the metabolism of alprazolam.

Management Options:

• *Circumvent/Minimize.* It would be prudent to use conservative doses of alprazolam in the presence of fluoxetine, until patient response is assessed. Advise patients receiving combined therapy to watch for excessive sedation.

• *Monitor* for altered alprazolam effect if fluoxetine is initiated, discontinued, or changed in dosage; adjust alprazolam dose as needed.

References:

1. Greenblatt DJ et al. Fluoxetine impairs clearance of alprazolam but not of clonazepam. Clin Pharmacol Ther. 1992;52:479.
2. Lasher TA et al. Pharmacokinetic pharmacodynamic evaluation of the combined administration of alprazolam and fluoxetine. Psychopharmacology. 1991;104:323.

### Altretamine (Hexalen)

### Imipramine (Tofranil)

Summary: Altretamine appears to increase the incidence of orthostatic hypotension caused by tricyclic antidepressants or monoamine oxidase inhibitors.

Risk Factors: No specific risk factors known.

Related Drugs: Theoretically, other tricyclic antidepressants or monoamine oxidase inhibitors might interact with altretamine.

Management Options:
- *Consider Alternative.* Antidepressants which are normally associated with a low incidence of orthostatic hypotension such as nortriptyline or selective serotonin reuptake inhibitors could be considered.
- *Circumvent/Minimize.* Patients receiving altretamine who require an antidepressant should be warned about orthostatic hypotension.
- *Monitor.* Monitor for orthostatic hypotension in patients receiving altretamine with either tricyclic antidepressants or monoamine oxidase inhibitors.

References:
1. Bruckner HW et al. Orthostatic hypotension as a complication of hexamethylmelamine antidepressant interaction. Cancer Treat Rep. 1983;67:516.

## Aminoglutethimide (Cytadren)

### Dexamethasone (Decadron)

Summary: Aminoglutethimide enhances the elimination of dexamethasone (and probably other corticosteroids) resulting in a marked reduction in corticosteroid response.

Risk Factors: No specific risk factors known.

Related Drugs: Theoretically, the metabolism of corticosteroids other than dexamethasone [e.g., **hydrocortisone (Cortef), cortisone, prednisone (Deltasone), prednisolone (Prelone), methylprednisolone (Medrol)**] also would be enhanced by aminoglutethimide, but it is not known whether they would be affected to the same degree as dexamethasone.

Management Options:
- *Monitor.* Dexamethasone dosage requirements are likely to increase considerably (e.g., up to twofold or more) in the presence of aminoglutethimide. Careful attention should be given to dexamethasone response when aminoglutethimide is initiated, discontinued, or changed in dosage.

References:
1. Kvinssland S et al. Aminoglutethimide as an inducer of microsomal enzymes. Part 1. Pharmacological aspects. Breast Cancer Res Treat. 1986;7(Suppl.):73.
2. Santen RJ et al. Successful medical adrenalectomy with aminoglutethimide. Role of altered drug metabolism. JAMA. 1974;230:1661.
3. Halpern J et al. A call for caution in the use of aminoglutethimide: negative interactions with dexamethasone and beta blocker treatment. J Med. 1984;15:59.

## Aminoglutethimide (Cytadren)

### Medroxyprogesterone (Provera)

Summary: Aminoglutethimide substantially lowers plasma medroxyprogesterone concentrations, but more study is needed to determine the degree to which this reduces the therapeutic response.

Risk Factors: No specific risk factors known.

**Related Drugs:** It is not known to what extent aminoglutethimide enhances the metabolism of progestins other than medroxyprogesterone, but consider the possibility.

**Management Options:**

- *Monitor* for altered medroxyprogesterone effect if aminoglutethimide is initiated, discontinued, or changed in dosage.

**References:**

1. Kvinssland S et al. Aminoglutethimide as an inducer of microsomal enzymes. Part 1. Pharmacological aspects. Breast Cancer Res Treat. 1986;7(Suppl.):73.
2. Van Deijk WA et al. Influence of aminoglutethimide on plasma levels of medroxyprogesterone acetate: its correlation with serum cortisol. Cancer Treat Rep. 1985; 69:85.

### Aminoglutethimide (Cytadren)

### Tamoxifen (Nolvadex)

**2**

**Summary:** Aminoglutethimide reduces tamoxifen concentrations and may reduce its clinical effect.

**Risk Factors:** No specific risk factors known.

**Related Drugs:** No information available.

**Management Options:**

- *Avoid Unless Benefit Outweighs Risk.* Aminoglutethimide generally should not be administered with tamoxifen since it lowers tamoxifen concentrations and does not enhance the response of breast cancer patients to tamoxifen therapy.
- *Monitor.* If combination is used, monitor tamoxifen response carefully.

**References:**

1. Lien EA et al. Decreased serum concentrations of tamoxifen and its metabolites induced by aminoglutethimide. Cancer Res. 1990;50:5851.

### Aminoglutethimide (Cytadren)

### Theophylline

**3**

**Summary:** Preliminary evidence from a limited number of patients indicates that aminoglutethimide reduces the serum concentration of theophylline.

**Risk Factors:** No specific risk factors known.

## Significance Classification

1. **- Avoid Combination.** Risk always outweighs benefit.

2. **- Usually Avoid Combination.** Use combination only under special circumstances.

3. **- Minimize Risk.** Take action as necessary to reduce risk.

Related Drugs: No information available.

Management Options:

- *Monitor.* Patients maintained on theophylline should have their theophylline concentrations monitored for several weeks following the initiation or discontinuation of aminoglutethimide. Adjustment of theophylline doses may be required for some patients to maintain their serum concentrations in the therapeutic range following the initiation or discontinuation of aminoglutethimide.

References:

1. Lonning PE et al. Mechanisms of action of aminoglutethimide as endocrine therapy of breast cancer. Drugs. 1988;35:685.
2. Lonning PE et al. Effect of aminoglutethimide on antipyrine, theophylline, and digitoxin disposition in breast cancer. Clin Pharmacol Ther. 1984;6:796.

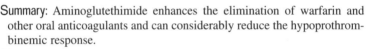

### Aminoglutethimide (Cytadren)

### Warfarin (Coumadin)

Summary: Aminoglutethimide enhances the elimination of warfarin and other oral anticoagulants and can considerably reduce the hypoprothrombinemic response.

Risk Factors:

- *Dosage Regimen.* The interaction appears to be dose related. In one study, plasma warfarin clearance was increased 41% by 250 mg/day of aminoglutethimide and 91% by 1000 mg/day of aminoglutethimide.[3]

Related Drugs: Although the reports involved warfarin and **acenocoumarol (Sintrom)**, it is likely that other oral anticoagulants interact similarly with aminoglutethimide.

Management Options:

- *Monitor.* In patients receiving warfarin or other oral anticoagulants, the hypoprothrombinemic response should be monitored carefully if aminoglutethimide is initiated, discontinued, or changed in dosage; oral anticoagulant dosage requirements are likely to change substantially. Warn patients accordingly.

References:

1. Kvinnsland S et al. Aminoglutethimide as an inducer of microsomal enzymes. Part 1. Pharmacological aspects. Breast Cancer Res Treat. 1986;7(Suppl.):73.
2. Lonning PE et al. Aminoglutethimide and warfarin. A new important drug interaction. Cancer Chemother Pharmacol. 1984;12:10.
3. Lonning PE et al. The influence of a graded dose schedule of aminoglutethimide on the disposition of the optical enantiomers of warfarin in patients with breast cancer. Cancer Chemother Pharmacol. 1986;17:177.

### Amiodarone (Cordarone)

### Cholestyramine (Questran)

Summary: Cholestyramine can decrease amiodarone plasma concentrations and antiarrhythmic efficacy.

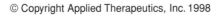

Risk Factors: No specific risk factors known.

Related Drugs: ***Colestipol (Colestid)*** also probably decreases amiodarone plasma concentrations.

Management Options:

- *Monitor.* Patients receiving cholestyramine and amiodarone should be observed for increased amiodarone dosage requirements. Discontinuation of cholestyramine may result in excessive accumulation of amiodarone and toxicity (arrhythmia, pneumonitis, thyroid abnormalities).

References:

1. Nitsch J et al. Enhanced elimination of amiodarone by cholestyramine. Dtsch Med Wochenschr. 1986;111:1241.

### Amiodarone (Cordarone)

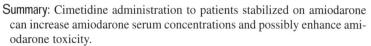

### Cimetidine (Tagamet)

Summary: Cimetidine administration to patients stabilized on amiodarone can increase amiodarone serum concentrations and possibly enhance amiodarone toxicity.

Risk Factors: No specific risk factors known.

Related Drugs: The effects of other $H_2$-receptor antagonists, such as ***ranitidine (Zantac)***, ***famotidine (Pepcid)***, and ***nizatidine (Axid)***, on amiodarone are unknown, but they probably would not affect amiodarone metabolism.

Management Options:

- *Monitor.* Amiodarone serum concentrations should be monitored in amiodarone-treated patients following the institution of cimetidine. Many weeks may be required for the maximum effects of this interaction to become evident. It also may take several weeks for amiodarone concentrations to return to normal after cimetidine is discontinued.

References:

1. Landau S et al. Cimetidine-amiodarone interaction. J Clin Pharmacol. 1988;38:909. Abstract.

### Amiodarone (Cordarone)

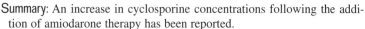

### Cyclosporine (Sandimmune)

Summary: An increase in cyclosporine concentrations following the addition of amiodarone therapy has been reported.

Risk Factors: No specific risk factors known.

Related Drugs: ***Tacrolimus (Prograf)*** also may be affected by amiodarone.

Management Options:

- *Monitor.* Watch for increased cyclosporine concentrations and evidence of toxicity (renal dysfunction) in patients started on amiodarone therapy.

References:
1. Nicolau DP et al. Amiodarone-cyclosporine interaction in heart transplant patient. J Heart Lung Transplant. 1992;11:564.
2. Chitwood KK et al. Cyclosporine-amiodarone interaction. Ann Pharmacother. 1993;27:569.
3. Mamprin F et al. Amiodarone-cyclosporine interaction in cardiac transplantation. Am Heart J. 1992;123:1725.

## Amiodarone (Cordarone)

### Digoxin (Lanoxin)

Summary: Amiodarone can cause digoxin to accumulate in the serum to concentrations that often are associated with toxicity.

Risk Factors: No specific risk factors known.

Related Drugs: The effect of amiodarone on *digitoxin (Crystodigin)* is not established but probably would be similar.

Management Options:

- *Circumvent/Minimize.* Digoxin doses probably will need to be reduced when amiodarone is added to therapy.

- *Monitor.* Patients should be monitored for changes in digoxin serum concentrations when amiodarone is initiated or discontinued during concurrent therapy. Several weeks may be required before new steady-state digoxin concentrations are achieved.

References:
1. Johnston A et al. The digoxin-amiodarone interaction. Br J Clin Pharmacol. 1987; 24:253P.
2. Ben-chetrit E et al. Case report: amiodarone-associated hypothyroidism—a possible cause of digoxin intoxication. Am J Med Sci. 1985;289:114.
3. Robinson K et al. The digoxin-amiodarone interaction. Cardiovasc Drugs Ther. 1989;3:25.

## Amiodarone (Cordarone)

### Diltiazem (Cardizem)

Summary: Amiodarone and diltiazem may result in cardiotoxicity with bradycardia and decreased cardiac output.

Risk Factors: No specific risk factors known.

Related Drugs: *Verapamil (Calan)* may produce similar effects when used with amiodarone. Dihydropyridine calcium channel blockers [e.g., *nifedipine (Procardia)*, *amlodipine (Norvasc)*, *felodipine (Plendil)*] would be unlikely to interact with amiodarone.

Management Options:

- *Monitor.* Until more information is available, patients receiving amiodarone should be monitored for signs of cardiac toxicity when diltiazem is administered concurrently.

References:
1. Lee TH et al. Sinus arrest and hypotension with combined amiodarone-diltiazem therapy. Am Heart J. 1985;109:163.

### Amiodarone (Cordarone)

### Flecainide (Tambocor)

Summary: When amiodarone is administered in conjunction with flecainide, the dose of flecainide required to maintain therapeutic plasma concentrations may be one-third less than that required when flecainide is administered alone.

Risk Factors: No specific risk factors known.

Related Drugs: Amiodarone may affect *encainide (Enkaid)* similarly.

Management Options:

- *Circumvent/Minimize.* Until more information is available, consider reducing the dose of flecainide by one-third to one-half when it is used in patients who already are being treated with amiodarone.

- *Monitor.* Patients should be observed for signs and symptoms consistent with altered flecainide serum concentrations when amiodarone is added to or discontinued from the regimens of patients taking flecainide. Because amiodarone has a long half-life, patients should be monitored for several weeks.

References:
1. Shea P et al. Flecainide and amiodarone interaction. J Am Coll Cardiol. 1986;7: 1127.
2. Funck-Brentano C et al. Variable disposition kinetics and electrocardiographic effects of flecainide during repeated dosing in humans: contribution of genetic factors, dose-dependent clearance, and interaction with amiodarone. Clin Pharmacol Ther. 1994;55:256.

### Amiodarone (Cordarone)

### Metoprolol (Lopressor)

Summary: The administration of metoprolol or propranolol (Inderal) to patients maintained on amiodarone may lead to bradycardia, cardiac arrest, or ventricular arrhythmia shortly after initiation of the beta blocker.

Risk Factors: No specific risk factors known.

Related Drugs: Two patients receiving amiodarone (1 for atrial flutter, 1 for ischemia) developed cardiac arrest or ventricular fibrillation within 2 hr

## Significance Classification

 - *Avoid Combination.* Risk always outweighs benefit.

 - *Usually Avoid Combination.* Use combination only under special circumstances.

 - *Minimize Risk.* Take action as necessary to reduce risk.

following 1 or 2 oral doses of propranolol.[2] If additive pharmacody-namic effects are partially responsible, all beta blockers [e.g., ***propranolol (Inderal)***] would be expected to interact in a similar manner. If reduction in beta blocker metabolism is responsible for this interaction, renally eliminated beta blockers [e.g., ***atenolol (Tenormin)***] would be expected to be less likely to interact.

Management Options:

- *Monitor.* Until additional information is available, patients main-tained on amiodarone should be observed carefully when beta blockers that undergo extensive hepatic metabolism are initiated. Although atenolol did not appear to interact with amiodarone in one case, there is insufficient evidence to recommend atenolol as an alternative.

References:

1. Leor J et al. Amiodarone and beta-adrenergic blockers: an interaction with meto-prolol but not with atenolol. Am Heart J. 1988;116:206.
2. Derrida JP et al. Amiodarone and propranolol, a dangerous association. Nouv Presse Med. 1979;8:1429.

## Amiodarone (Cordarone)

## Phenytoin (Dilantin)

Summary: The serum concentration of phenytoin can be increased consid-erably during concomitant amiodarone therapy and the serum concentra-tion of amiodarone can be reduced by concurrent phenytoin administra-tion.

Risk Factors: No specific risk factors known.

Related Drugs: ***Mephenytoin (Mesantoin)*** has been reported not to interact with amiodarone.

Management Options:

- *Monitor.* Patients being treated with phenytoin should have their phenytoin serum concentrations monitored carefully when amioda-rone is added to or removed from their drug regimen. This drug interaction may take several weeks to become fully apparent. In addition, patients taking amiodarone should be monitored for re-duced antiarrhythmic efficacy, and amiodarone serum concentra-tions should be monitored if phenytoin is added to their drug regi-men.

References:

1. Nolan PE Jr. et al. Pharmacokinetic interaction between intravenous phenytoin and amiodarone in healthy volunteers. Clin Pharmacol Ther. 1989;46:43.
2. Nolan PE et al. Evidence for an effect of phenytoin on the pharmacokinetics of ami-odarone. J Clin Pharmacol. 1990;30:1112.
3. Nolan PE et al. Steady-state interaction between amiodarone and phenytoin in nor-mal subjects. Am J Cardiol. 1990;65:1252.

## Amiodarone (Cordarone)

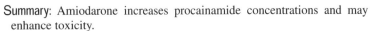

### Procainamide (Procan SR)

Summary: Amiodarone increases procainamide concentrations and may enhance toxicity.

Risk Factors: No specific risk factors known.

Related Drugs: No information available.

Management Options:
- *Circumvent/Minimize.* Procainamide dosages may need to be reduced by 25% to avoid toxicity.
- *Monitor.* Procainamide concentrations should be monitored and the patient observed for hypotension or arrhythmias when amiodarone is added to therapy.

References:
1. Windle J et al. Pharmacokinetic and electrophysiologic interaction of amiodarone and procainamide. Clin Pharmacol Ther. 1987;41:603.
2. Saal AK et al. Effect of amiodarone on serum quinidine and procainamide levels. Am J Cardiol. 1984;53:1264.

## Amiodarone (Cordarone)

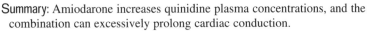

### Quinidine

Summary: Amiodarone increases quinidine plasma concentrations, and the combination can excessively prolong cardiac conduction.

Risk Factors: No specific risk factors known.

Related Drugs: No information available.

Management Options:
- *Monitor.* When amiodarone is added to quinidine therapy, monitor the cardiac status (e.g., QT interval prolongation) and plasma quinidine concentrations.

References:
1. Tartini R et al. Dangerous interaction between amiodarone and quinidine. Lancet. 1982;1:1327.
2. Saal AK et al. Effect of amiodarone on serum quinidine and procainamide levels. Am J Cardiol. 1984;53:1264.
3. Kerin NZ et al. The effectiveness and safety of the simultaneous administration of quinidine and amiodarone in the conversion of chronic atrial fibrillation. Am Heart J. 1993;125:1017.

## Amiodarone (Cordarone)

### Sotalol (Betapace)

Summary: A patient given amiodarone following chronic sotalol therapy developed hypotension and bradycardia, but a causal relationship for an interaction between the drugs was not established.

Risk Factors: No specific risk factors known.

Related Drugs: Beta blockers, including *metoprolol (Lopressor)* and *propranolol (Inderal)*, have been noted to produce bradycardia when administered with amiodarone.

Management Options:
- *Circumvent/Minimize.* It may be prudent to avoid the administration of amiodarone for several days to patients previously receiving drugs that depress myocardial conduction and contractility.
- *Monitor.* Until further information is available, patients receiving solatol (and perhaps other beta blockers) and amiodarone should be carefully monitored for hemodynamic depression.

References:
1. Warren R et al. Serious interaction of sotalol with amiodarone and flecainide. Med J Aust. 1990;152:227. Letter.

## Amiodarone (Cordarone)
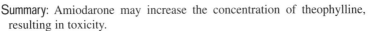

### Theophylline

Summary: Amiodarone may increase the concentration of theophylline, resulting in toxicity.

Risk Factors: No specific risk factors known.

Related Drugs: No information available.

Management Options:
- *Monitor.* Patients maintained on theophylline should be carefully observed for the development of theophylline toxicity (nausea, tachycardia, nervousness, tremor, seizures) following the addition of amiodarone. One or more weeks may be required for the onset and offset of this interaction due to the long half-life of amiodarone.

References:
1. Soto J et al. Possible theophylline-amiodarone interaction. DICP Ann Pharmacother. 1990;24:1115. Letter.

## Amiodarone (Cordarone)

### Warfarin (Coumadin)

Summary: Amiodarone enhances the hypoprothrombinemic response to warfarin.

Risk Factors: No specific risk factors known.

Related Drugs: *Acenocoumarol (Sintrom)* interacts similarly.

Management Options:
- *Circumvent/Minimize.* A decrease in the warfarin dose by one-third to one-half may be necessary to maintain the prothrombin time within the therapeutic range.
- *Monitor.* When amiodarone is administered to patients requiring oral anticoagulant therapy, the hypoprothrombinemic response should be monitored carefully. Because the onset and offset of this interaction

are delayed in some patients, close monitoring should continue for several weeks following initiation of amiodarone and for several months following discontinuation of amiodarone.

References:
1. O'Reilly RA et al. Interaction of amiodarone with racemic warfarin and its separated enantiomorphs in humans. Clin Pharmacol Ther. 1987;42:290.
2. Kerin NZ et al. The incidence, magnitude, and time course of the amiodarone-warfarin interaction. Arch Intern Med. 1988;148:1779.
3. Fodevila C et al. Amiodarone potentiates acenocoumarin. Thrombosis Res. 1989; 53:203.

## Amitriptyline (Elavil)

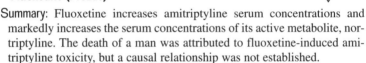

### Fluoxetine (Prozac)

Summary: Fluoxetine increases amitriptyline serum concentrations and markedly increases the serum concentrations of its active metabolite, nortriptyline. The death of a man was attributed to fluoxetine-induced amitriptyline toxicity, but a causal relationship was not established.

Risk Factors: No specific risk factors known.

Related Drugs: Since fluoxetine-induced inhibition of CYP2D6 is the likely mechanism, one would expect *paroxetine (Paxil)*, which is also a potent CYP2D6 inhibitor, to interact with amitriptyline in a similar manner. *Sertraline (Zoloft)* is only a weak CYP2D6 inhibitor and would theoretically be less likely to interact. *Fluvoxamine (Luvox)* has little or no effect on CYP2D6, but its ability to inhibit other cytochrome P450 isozymes might affect the metabolism of tricyclic antidepressants.

Management Options:
• *Monitor.* Although combinations of tricyclic antidepressants and selective serotonin reuptake inhibitors are frequently used with positive results, the patient's response to the tricyclic antidepressant must be carefully monitored if a selective serotonin reuptake inhibitor is initiated, discontinued, or changed in dosage.

References:
1. El-Yazigi A et al. Steady-state kinetics of fluoxetine and amitriptyline in patients treated with a combination of these drugs as compared with those treated with amitriptyline alone. J Clin Pharmacol. 1995;35:17.
2. Preskorn SH et al. Fatality associated with combined fluoxetine-amitriptyline therapy. JAMA. 1997;277:1682. Letter.

## Amitriptyline (Elavil)

### Guanfacine (Tenex)

Summary: Limited clinical information and theoretical considerations suggest that tricyclic antidepressants (TCAs) can inhibit the antihypertensive response to guanfacine.

Risk Factors: No specific risk factors known.

Related Drugs: Theoretically, any combination of a TCA [e.g., *imipramine (Tofranil)*] and a centrally-acting alpha agonist [*clonidine (Catapres)*, *guanabenz (Wytensin)*, guanfacine] would interact.

Management Options:

- *Consider Alternative.* If tricyclics are to be used, consider selecting an alternative antihypertensive agent. (But keep in mind that TCAs also may inhibit the effect of clonidine, guanabenz, guanethidine, bethanidine, and debrisoquin.)
- *Monitor.* Until more clinical evidence is available, monitor for reduced antihypertensive response when TCAs are added to guanfacine therapy. If guanfacine is withdrawn in the presence of TCAs, monitor for exaggerated rebound hypertension.

References:
1. Buckley M et al. Antagonism of antihypertensive effect of guanfacine by tricyclic antidepressants. Lancet. 1991;337:1173. Letter.

## Amitriptyline (Elavil)

## Isoproterenol (Isuprel)

Summary: Isolated case reports indicate that the combined use of isoproterenol and tricyclic antidepressants (TCAs) may predispose patients to cardiac arrhythmias, but the clinical importance of this interaction is not established.

Risk Factors:

- *Dosage Regimen.* It is possible that the risk is primarily in patients who take large doses of isoproterenol.

Related Drugs: Little is known regarding the effect of beta agonists other than isoproterenol [e.g., *albuterol (Proventil)*, *metaproterenol (Alupent)*, *terbutaline (Brethaire)*] in patients receiving TCAs. To the extent that these agents have less cardiac effects than isoproterenol, one would expect a reduced likelihood of cardiac interactions with TCAs.

Management Options:

- *Circumvent/Minimize.* Excessive use of isoproterenol or other beta-agonists should be avoided in any case, but it may be particularly important in patients receiving TCAs.

## Significance Classification

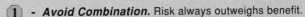 1 - *Avoid Combination.* Risk always outweighs benefit.

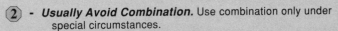 2 - *Usually Avoid Combination.* Use combination only under special circumstances.

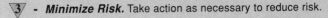 3 - *Minimize Risk.* Take action as necessary to reduce risk.

- *Monitor.* Although this interaction is not well documented, it would be prudent to monitor for cardiac arrhythmias if isoproterenol or other beta-agonists (especially in large doses) are used with TCAs.

References:
1. Kadar D. Amitriptyline and isoproterenol: fatal drug combinations. Can Med Assoc J. 1975;112:556. Letter.
2. Boakes AJ et al. Interactions between sympathomimetic amines and antidepressant agents in man. Br Med J. 1973;1:311.

## Amitriptyline (Elavil)

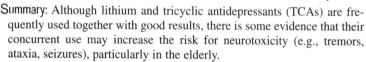

### Lithium (Eskalith)

Summary: Although lithium and tricyclic antidepressants (TCAs) are frequently used together with good results, there is some evidence that their concurrent use may increase the risk for neurotoxicity (e.g., tremors, ataxia, seizures), particularly in the elderly.

Risk Factors:
- *Age.* Elderly patients may be at higher risk.

Related Drugs: TCAs other than amitriptyline probably have a similar effect when combined with lithium.

Management Options:
- *Circumvent/Minimize.* Limited information suggests that using low doses of lithium may reduce the risk of neurotoxicity in geriatric patients without compromising its therapeutic effect.
- *Monitor.* Until further information is available, lithium and TCAs should be used cautiously in elderly patients. Monitor for evidence of neurotoxicity such as tremors, disorders of mentation, ataxia, and seizures.

References:
1. Camara EG. Lithium potentiation of antidepressant treatment in panic disorder. J Clin Psychopharmacol. 1990;10:225. Letter.
2. Lafferman J et al. Lithium augmentation for treatment-resistant depression in the elderly. J Geriatric Psychiatry Neurol. 1988;1:49.
3. Feder R. Lithium augmentation of clomipramine. J Clin Psychiatry. 1988;49:11.

## Amphotericin B (Fungizone)

### Cyclosporine (Sandimmune)

Summary: The administration of amphotericin B and cyclosporine probably increases the nephrotoxicity of both drugs.

Risk Factors: No specific risk factors known.

Related Drugs: No information available.

Management Options:
- *Circumvent/Minimize.* Alternative immunosuppression or antifungal therapy may be required to avoid or reverse renal toxicity.

- *Monitor.* Patients receiving both cyclosporine and amphotericin B should have their renal function monitored carefully.

References:
1. Kennedy MS et al. Acute renal toxicity with combined use of amphotericin B and cyclosporine after marrow transplantation. Transplantation. 1983;35:211.

## Amphotericin B (Fungizone)

### Gentamicin

Summary: The combination of aminoglycosides and amphotericin B may enhance the potential for nephrotoxicity.

Risk Factors:
- *Concurrent Diseases.* Renal dysfunction may increase the risk of nephrotoxicity.

Related Drugs: Other aminoglycosides may produce nephrotoxicity with amphotericin.

Management Options:
- *Consider Alternative.* The use of an alternative antibiotic or antifungal agent without nephrotoxicity would be prudent.
- *Monitor.* Patients on combined therapy with an aminoglycoside and amphotericin B should be monitored closely for deterioration of renal function.

References:
1. Churchill DN et al. Nephrotoxicity associated with combined gentamicin-amphotericin B therapy. Nephron. 1977;19:176.

## Amphotericin B (Fungizone)

### Succinylcholine (Anectine)

Summary: Prolonged muscle relaxation may accompany the use of amphotericin B and neuromuscular blocking agents.

Risk Factors: No specific risk factors known.

Related Drugs: Other drugs causing hypokalemia may cause a similar reaction with muscle relaxants like **atracurium (Tracrium)** and **vecuronium (Norcuron)**.

Management Options:
- *Monitor.* The potassium balance of patients on amphotericin B should be checked carefully before use of neuromuscular blocking agents.

References:
1. Miller RP et al. Amphotericin B toxicity. A follow-up report of 53 patients. Ann Intern Med. 1969;71:1089.
2. Cushard WG et al. Blastomycosis of bone. Treatment with intramedullary amphotericin B. J Bone Joint Surg. 1969;51A:704.

## Ampicillin

### Atenolol (Tenormin)

Summary: Ampicillin may reduce atenolol serum concentrations and a reduction of beta blocker effect is possible.

Risk Factors:
- *Dosage Regimen.* Ampicillin doses >1 gm appear to decrease the bioavailability of atenolol.

Related Drugs: No information available.

Management Options:
- *Monitor.* Until more data are available, watch for evidence of altered atenolol response when large doses of ampicillin are administered concomitantly.

References:
1. McLean AJ et al. Dose-dependence of atenolol-ampicillin interaction. Br J Clin Pharmacol. 1984;18:969.
2. Schafer-Korting M et al. Atenolol interaction with aspirin, allopurinol, and ampicillin. Clin Pharmacol Ther. 1983;33:283.

## Ampicillin

### Oral Contraceptives

Summary: Ampicillin probably impairs oral contraceptive efficacy occasionally.

Risk Factors: No specific risk factors known.

Related Drugs: The effect of other penicillins on oral contraceptives is not well established; however, reports of contraceptive failure have been noted with the concomitant use of a variety of antibiotics.

Management Options:
- *Circumvent/Minimize.* Since ampicillin often is given in relatively short courses, it may be best for patients to continue their oral contraceptive and use supplementary contraception during cycles in which ampicillin is used.

## Significance Classification

(1) - ***Avoid Combination.*** Risk always outweighs benefit.

(2) - ***Usually Avoid Combination.*** Use combination only under special circumstances.

(3) - ***Minimize Risk.*** Take action as necessary to reduce risk.

• *Monitor.* Patients should be told that spotting or breakthrough bleeding may be an indication that an interac-tion between ampicillin and an oral contraceptive is occurring.

References:

1. Friedman CI et al. The effect of ampicillin on oral contraceptive effectiveness. Obstet Gynecol. 1980;55:33.
2. DeSano EA et al. Possible interactions of antihistamines and antibiotics with oral contraceptive effectiveness. Fertil Steril. 1982;37:853.
3. Back DJ et al. The effects of ampicillin on oral contraceptive steroids in women. Br J Clin Pharmacol. 1982;14:43.

## Antacids

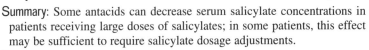

### Aspirin

Summary: Some antacids can decrease serum salicylate concentrations in patients receiving large doses of salicylates; in some patients, this effect may be sufficient to require salicylate dosage adjustments.

Risk Factors:

• *Dosage Regimen.* The lowering of serum salicylate concentrations by antacids is likely to occur only in patients receiving large doses of salicylate (e.g., several gm/day), since it is only with such doses that the renal excretion of unchanged salicylic acid is an important elimination pathway.

Related Drugs: Salicylates other than aspirin also would be affected by increases in urine pH.

Management Options:

• *Monitor.* In patients receiving large doses of salicylates (e.g., for arthritis), be alert for alteration in serum salicylate concentrations if antacids are initiated, discontinued, or changed in dosage. Adjustments in salicylate dosage may be required in some cases.

References:

1. Hansten PD et al. Effect of antacids and ascorbic acid on serum salicylate concentration. J Clin Pharmacol. 1980;24:326.
2. Shastri RA. Effect of antacids on salicylate kinetics. Int J Clin Pharmacol Ther Toxicol. 1985;23:480.
3. Kaniwa N et al. The bioavailabilies of aspirin from an aspirin aluminum and aspirin tablets and the effects of food and aluminum hydroxide gel. J Pharm Dyn. 1981;4:860.

## Antacids

### Cefpodoxime Proxetil (Vantin)

Summary: Antacids reduce the bioavailability and serum concentrations of cefpodoxime proxetil and could reduce the efficacy of the antibiotic.

Risk Factors: No specific risk factors known.

Related Drugs: Theoretically, any drug that substantially increases gastric pH also would reduce cefpodoxime absorption. This would include $H_2$-

receptor antagonists [e.g., *cimetidine (Tagamet)*, *famotidine (Pepcid)*, *nizatidine (Axid)*, *ranitidine (Zantac)*], proton pump inhibitors [e.g., *omeprazole (Prilosec)*, *lansoprazole (Prevacid)*] and other antacids.

Management Options:

- *Circumvent/Minimize.* Patients taking cefpodoxime should be advised to take the antibiotic between meals, preferably on an empty stomach. Antacids should not be administered for at least 2 hours before or after administration of cefpodoxime.

- *Monitor.* Be alert for evidence of reduced cefpodoxime response if antacids are used concurrently.

References:

1. Saathoff N et al. Pharmacokinetics of cefpodoxime proxetil and interactions with an antacid and an $H_2$-receptor antagonist. Antimicrob Agents Chemother. 1992;36:796.
2. Hughes GS et al. The effects of gastric pH and food on the pharmacokinetics of a new oral cephalosporin, cefpodoxime proxetil. Clin Pharmacol Ther. 1989;46:647.

## Antacids

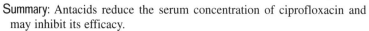

### Ciprofloxacin (Cipro)

Summary: Antacids reduce the serum concentration of ciprofloxacin and may inhibit its efficacy.

Risk Factors:

- *Diet/Food.* Binding interactions in the gastrointestinal tract tend to be greater in the fasting state than if there is food in the stomach.

- *Dosage Regimen.* The effects of antacids on quinolone absorption appear to be greater when large antacid doses are administered.

Related Drugs: The absorption of other quinolones is also reduced by antacids, but the absorption of *lomefloxacin (Maxaquin)* and *ofloxacin (Floxacin)* appears somewhat less affected by cations (e.g., antacids) than ciprofloxacin. Since *ranitidine (Zantac)* does not appear to affect ciprofloxacin absorption,[1,2] one would assume that other $H_2$-receptor antagonists [e.g., *cimetidine (Tagamet)*, *famotidine (Pepcid)*, *nizatidine (Axid)*] and proton pump inhibitors [e.g., *omeprazole (Prilosec)*, *lansoprazole (Prevacid)*] also would have no effect. *Sucralfate (Carafate)* dramatically reduces ciprofloxacin absorption.

Management Options:

- *Consider Alternative.* Since it may be difficult to separate the doses of magnesium-aluminum-hydroxide antacids and ciprofloxacin sufficiently to prevent their interaction, one could consider using $H_2$-receptor antagonists or proton pump inhibitors.

- *Circumvent/Minimize.* If antacids are used with oral ciprofloxacin, give the ciprofloxacin at least 2 hours before or 6 hours after the antacid.

- *Monitor* for reduced ciprofloxacin response if antacids are also taken.

References:
1. Nix DE et al. Effects of aluminum and magnesium antacids and ranitidine on the absorption of ciprofloxacin. Clin Pharmacol Ther. 1989;46:700.
2. Watson WA et al. Effects of timing of Maalox administration and ranitidine on ciprofloxacin (Cipro) absorption. Pharm Res. 1988:5(Suppl):S164. Abstract.
3. Brouwers JRBJ et al. Important reduction of ciprofloxacin absorption by sucralfate and magnesium citrate solution. Drug Invest. 1990;2:197.
4. Navarro AS et al. Comparative study of the influence of CA2+ on absorption parameters of ciprofloxacin and ofloxacin. J Antimicrob Chemother. 1994;34:119.

## Antacids

### Enoxacin (Penetrex)

Summary: Antacids reduce the serum concentration of enoxacin and may inhibit its efficacy.

Risk Factors:
- *Diet/Food.* Binding interactions in the gastrointestinal tract tend to be greater in the fasting state than if there is food in the stomach.
- *Dosage Regimen.* The effects of antacids on quinolone absorption appear to be greater when large antacid doses are administered.

Related Drugs: The absorption of other quinolones also is reduced by antacids. Given the effect of **ranitidine (Zantac)** on enoxacin absorption, other H$_2$-receptor antagonists [e.g., **cimetidine (Tagamet)**, **famotidine (Pepcid)**, **nizatidine (Axid)**] and proton pump inhibitors [e.g., **omeprazole (Prilosec)**, **lansoprazole (Prevacid)**] should be expected to reduce enoxacin absorption as well.

Management Options:
- *Circumvent/Minimize.* If antacids are used with oral enoxacin, give the enoxacin at least 2 hours before or 6 hours after the antacid.
- *Monitor* for reduced enoxacin response if antacids are also taken.

References:
1. Grasela TH et al. Inhibition of enoxacin absorption by antacids or ranitidine. Antimicrob Agents Chemother. 1989;33:615.
2. Lebsack M et al. Impact of gastric pH on ranitidine-enoxacin drug-drug interaction. J Clin Pharmacol. 1988;28:939. Abstract.

## Antacids

### Ephedrine

Summary: Large doses of sodium bicarbonate may increase serum concentrations of ephedrine.

Risk Factors: No specific risk factors known.

Related Drugs: Any drug that substantially alkalinizes the urine (e.g., carbonic anhydrase inhibitors) would be expected to inhibit ephedrine elimination. Some antacids other than **sodium bicarbonate** (e.g., **aluminum-**, **magnesium-**, and **calcium**-containing antacids) may slightly alkalinize the urine, but their effect on ephedrine excretion is probably not large. Sympathomimetic amines other than ephedrine have been shown to demonstrate pH dependent urinary excretion.

Management Options:

- *Monitor* for evidence of ephedrine toxicity (e.g., nervousness, insomnia, excitability) if the urine remains alkaline for more than a day or two. Monitor for altered ephedrine effect if sodium bicarbonate therapy is initiated, discontinued, or changed in dosage; adjust ephedrine dose as needed.

References:

1. Wilkinson GR et al. Absorption, metabolism and excretion of the ephedrines in man I. The influence of urinary pH and urine volume output. J Pharmacol Exp Ther. 1968;162:139.

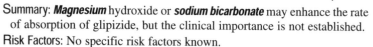

## Antacids

### Glipizide (Glucotrol)

Summary: ***Magnesium*** hydroxide or ***sodium bicarbonate*** may enhance the rate of absorption of glipizide, but the clinical importance is not established.

Risk Factors: No specific risk factors known.

Related Drugs: ***Aluminum*** hydroxide did not appear to interact. $H_2$-receptor antagonists [e.g., ***cimetidine (Tagamet), famotidine (Pepcid), nizatidine (Axid), ranitidine (Zantac)***] also have been reported to increase the hypoglycemic effect of glipizide. ***Glyburide (DiaBeta)*** absorption also appears to be increased by elevating gastric pH.

Management Options:

- *Circumvent/Minimize.* Until more information is available, it would be prudent to give glipizide 2 hours before or after antacids.
- *Monitor* for altered hypoglycemic effect of glipizide if antacids are initiated, discontinued, changed in dosage, or if the dosage interval between the antacid and glipizide is changed.

References:

1. Kivisto KT et al. Enhancement of absorption and effect of glipizide by magnesium hydroxide. Clin Pharmacol Ther. 1991;49:39.
2. Kivisto KT et al. Differential effects of sodium bicarbonate and aluminum hydroxide on the absorption and activity of glipizide. Eur J Clin Pharmacol. 1991;40:383.

## Antacids

### Glyburide (DiaBeta)

Summary: Antacid (***aluminum-magnesium*** hydroxides) increased glyburide serum concentrations, but the clinical importance of this effect is not established.

Risk Factors: No specific risk factors known.

Related Drugs: If the increased glyburide levels are due to increased gastric pH, all antacids would be expected to interact, as would $H_2$-receptor antagonists [e.g., ***cimetidine (Tagamet), famotidine (Pepcid), nizatidine (Axid)***] and proton pump inhibitors [e.g., **lansoprazole (Prevacid)**, **omeprazole (Prilosec)**]. Ranitidine does not alter glyburide pharmacokinetics.

Management Options:

- *Circumvent/Minimize.* Since the interaction is most likely due to increased gastric pH, one would expect that giving the glyburide at least 2 hours before or after the antacid should minimize the effect. If antacids are taken regularly, maintain a relatively constant interval between the antacid and glyburide so that any interaction will remain relatively constant.

- *Monitor* for altered hypoglycemic effect of glyburide if antacids are initiated, discontinued, changed in dosage, or if the dosing interval between the antacid and glyburide is changed.

References:

1. Zaccaro P et al. Influence of antacids on the bioavailability of glibenclamide. Drugs Exp Clin Res. 1989;15:165.

## Antacids

### Iron

**Summary:** Some antacids reduce the gastrointestinal absorption of iron; inhibition of the hematological response to iron has been reported.

**Risk Factors:** No specific risk factors known.

**Related Drugs:** Until more information is available, one should assume that all antacids (e.g., **magnesium** trisilicate, **sodium bicarbonate**, **calcium** carbonate, **Mylanta**, **aluminum** hydroxide antacids) can reduce iron absorption.

Management Options:

- *Circumvent/Minimize.* Antacids containing magnesium trisilicate, calcium carbonate, or sodium bicarbonate should be spaced as far apart as possible from oral iron preparations. Until further information is available, the same precaution should be observed with other antacids.

- *Monitor* for reduced iron response if antacids are also taken.

References:

1. Azarnoff DL et al. Drug interactions. Pharmacol Physicians. 1970;4(Feb):1.
2. Coste JF et al. *In vitro* interactions of oral hematinics and antacid suspensions. Curr Ther Res. 1977;22:205.
3. O'Neil-Cutting MA et al. The effect of antacids on the absorption of simultaneously ingested iron. JAMA. 1986;255:1468.

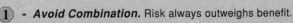
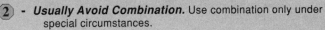

## Significance Classification

① - *Avoid Combination.* Risk always outweighs benefit.

② - *Usually Avoid Combination.* Use combination only under special circumstances.

③ - *Minimize Risk.* Take action as necessary to reduce risk.

## Antacids

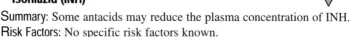

### Isoniazid (INH)

**Summary:** Some antacids may reduce the plasma concentration of INH.

**Risk Factors:** No specific risk factors known.

**Related Drugs:** Until more information is available, one should assume that all antacids (e.g., antacids containing *aluminum* and *magnesium*) can reduce INH absorption.

**Management Options:**
- *Circumvent/Minimize.* Give isoniazid 2 hours before or 6 hours after antacids.
- *Monitor* for reduced isoniazid response if antacids are also used.

**References:**
1. Hurwitz A et al. Effects of antacids on gastrointestinal absorption of isoniazid in rat and man. Am Rev Respir Dis. 1974;109:41.
2. Gallicano K et al. Effect of antacids in didanosine tablet on bioavailability of isoniazid. Antimicrob Agents Chemother. 1994;38:894.

## Antacids

### Ketoconazole (Nizoral)

**Summary:** Antacids may reduce ketoconazole concentrations.

**Risk Factors:** No specific risk factors known.

**Related Drugs:** Any agents that substantially increase gastric pH (e.g., $H_2$-receptor antagonists, proton pump inhibitors, *sodium bicarbonate*, and antacids containing *aluminum*, *magnesium*, or *calcium*) are likely to reduce the absorption of ketoconazole. *Itraconazole* absorption is similarly reduced by increased gastric pH, but *fluconazole (Diflucan)* is not.

**Management Options:**
- *Circumvent/Minimize.* Avoid antacids 2 hours before or after administration of ketoconazole.
- *Monitor* for reduced ketoconazole effect if antacids are also given.

**References:**
1. Van Der Meer JWM et al. The influence of gastric acidity on the bioavailability of ketoconazole. J Antimicrob Chemother. 1980;6:552.
2. Lelawongs P et al. Effect of food and gastric acidity on absorption of orally administered ketoconazole. Clin Pharm. 1988;7:228.
3. Carlson JA et al. Effect of pH on disintegration and dissolution of ketoconazole tablets. Am J Hosp Pharm. 1983;40:1334.

## Antacids

### Lomefloxacin (Maxaquin)

**Summary:** Antacids reduce the serum concentration of lomefloxacin and may inhibit its efficacy.

**Risk Factors:**
- *Diet/Food.* Binding interactions in the gastrointestinal tract tend to be greater in the fasting state than if there is food in the stomach.

• *Dosage Regimen.* The effects of antacids on quinolone absorption appear to be greater when large antacid doses are administered.

Related Drugs: The absorption of other quinolones also is reduced by antacids. Lomefloxacin absorption appears somewhat less affected by cations (e.g., antacids) than *ciprofloxacin (Cipro)* or *norfloxacin (Noroxin)*. $H_2$-receptor antagonists [e.g., *cimetidine (Tagamet), famotidine (Pepcid), nizatidine (Axid), ranitidine (Zantac)*] and proton pump inhibitors [e.g., *omeprazole (Prilosec), lansoprazole (Prevacid)*] are not known to affect lomefloxacin absorption.

Management Options:

• *Consider Alternative.* Since it may be difficult to separate the doses of antacid and lomefloxacin sufficiently to prevent their interaction, the use of $H_2$-receptor antagonists or proton pump inhibitors may be necessary for severe infections when patients require gastric acid reduction.

• *Circumvent/Minimize.* If antacids are used with oral lomefloxacin, give the lomefloxacin at least 2 hours before or 6 hours after the antacid.

• *Monitor* for reduced lomefloxacin response if antacids are also taken.

References:

1. Kunka RL et al. Effect of antacid on the pharmacokinetics of lomefloxacin. Pharm Res. 1988;10(Suppl.):S165. Abstract.

## Antacids

### Norfloxacin (Noroxin)

Summary: Antacids reduce the serum concentration of norfloxacin and probably inhibit its efficacy.

Risk Factors:

• *Diet/Food.* Binding interactions in the gastrointestinal tract tend to be greater in the fasting state than if there is food in the stomach.

• *Dosage Regimen.* The effects of antacids on quinolone absorption appear to be greater when large antacid doses are administered concurrently.

Related Drugs: The absorption of other quinolones also is reduced by antacids, but the absorption of *lomefloxacin (Maxaquin)* and *ofloxacin (Floxin)* appears somewhat less affected by cations (e.g., antacids) than norfloxacin. $H_2$-receptor antagonists [e.g., *cimetidine (Tagamet), famotidine (Pepcid), nizatidine (Axid), ranitidine (Zantac)*] and proton pump inhibitors [e.g., *omeprazole (Prilosec), lansoprazole (Prevacid)*] are not known to affect norfloxacin absorption.

Management Options:

• *Consider Alternative.* Since it may be difficult to separate the doses of antacid and norfloxacin sufficiently to prevent their interaction, the use of $H_2$-receptor antagonists or proton pump inhibitors may be necessary for severe infections when patients require gastric acid reduction.

- *Circumvent/Minimize.* If antacids are used with oral norfloxacin, give the norfloxacin at least 3 hours before or 6 hours after the antacid.

- *Monitor* for reduced norfloxacin response if antacids are also given.

References:

1. Nix DE et al. Inhibition of norfloxacin absorption by antacids. Antimicrob Agents Chemother. 1990;34:432.
2. Noyes M et al. Norfloxacin and absorption of magnesium-aluminum. Ann Intern Med. 1988;109:168. Letter.
3. Campbell NRC et al. Norfloxacin interaction with antacids and minerals. Br J Clin Pharmacol. 1992;33:115.

## Antacids

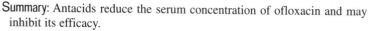

## Ofloxacin (Floxin)

Summary: Antacids reduce the serum concentration of ofloxacin and may inhibit its efficacy.

Risk Factors:

- *Diet/Food.* Binding interactions in the gastrointestinal tract tend to be greater in the fasting state than if there is food in the stomach.

- *Dosage Regimen.* Larger doses of antacids produce a greater reduction in ofloxacin absorption.

Related Drugs: The absorption of other quinolones also is reduced by antacids. Ofloxacin absorption appears somewhat less affected by cations (e.g., antacids) than *ciprofloxacin (Cipro)* or *norfloxacin (Noroxin)*. $H_2$-receptor antagonists [e.g., *cimetidine (Tagamet), famotidine (Pepcid), nizatidine (Axid), ranitidine (Zantac)*] and proton pump inhibitors [e.g., *omeprazole (Prilosec), lansoprazole (Prevacid)*] are not known to affect ofloxacin absorption.

Management Options:

- *Consider Alternative.* Calcium antacids, at least in small doses, appear to have little effect on the absorption of ofloxacin. One could also consider the use of $H_2$-receptor antagonists or proton pump inhibitors in place of antacids.

- *Circumvent/Minimize.* If antacids are used with oral ofloxacin, give the ofloxacin at least 2 hours before or 6 hours after the antacid.

- *Monitor* for reduced ofloxacin response if antacids are also given.

References:

1. Cabarga MM et al. Effects of two cations on gastrointestinal absorption of ofloxacin. Antimicrob Agents Chemother. 1991;35:2102.
2. Akerele JO et al. Influence of oral coadministered metallic drugs on ofloxacin pharmacokinetics. J Antimicrob Chemother. 1991;28:87.
3. Navarro AS et al. Comparative study of the influence of $Ca^{2+}$ on absorption parameters of ciprofloxacin and ofloxacin. J Antimicrob Chemother. 1994;34:119.

### Antacids

#### Penicillamine (Cuprimine)

Summary: Magnesium-aluminum hydroxides may reduce the bioavailability of penicillamine.

Risk Factors: No specific risk factors known.

Related Drugs: The effect of antacids other than magnesium-aluminum hydroxides on penicillamine absorption is not established.

Management Options:

- *Circumvent/Minimize.* Until more is known about this interaction, it would be prudent to give penicillamine 2 hours before or 6 hours after antacids.
- *Monitor* for reduced penicillamine response if antacids are also given.

References:

1. Osman MA et al. Reduction in oral penicillamine absorption by food, antacid, and ferrous sulfate. Clin Pharmacol Ther. 1983;33:465.

### Antacids

#### Pseudoephedrine (Sudafed)

Summary: Sodium bicarbonate in doses sufficient to alkalinize the urine may inhibit the elimination of pseudoephedrine markedly.

Risk Factors: No specific risk factors known.

Related Drugs: Any drug that significantly alkalinizes the urine (e.g., carbonic anhydrase inhibitors) would be expected to reduce the urinary excretion of pseudoephedrine. Nonsystemic antacids such as **magnesium-aluminum** hydroxides also may alkalinize the urine somewhat, but the extent to which this reduced pseudoephedrine elimination is not established. Sympathomimetic amines other than pseudoephedrine [e.g., **amphetamines**, **ephedrine**, **phenylpropanolamine (Propadrone)**] also have been shown to undergo pH dependent urinary excretion.

Management Options:

- *Consider Alternative.* If more than an occasional dose of sodium bicarbonate is used, consider using alternative antacid. (See Related Drugs.)

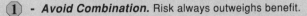

## Significance Classification

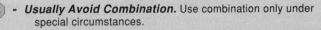

(1) - *Avoid Combination.* Risk always outweighs benefit.

(2) - *Usually Avoid Combination.* Use combination only under special circumstances.

3 - *Minimize Risk.* Take action as necessary to reduce risk.

- *Monitor* for enhanced pseudoephedrine effect (e.g., anxiety, tremor, palpitations, psychiatric changes) if large doses of sodium bicarbonate are taken concurrently.

References:
1. Brater DC et al. Renal excretion of pseudoephedrine. Clin Pharmacol Ther. 1980;28:690.
2. Kuntzman RG et al. The influence of urinary pH on the plasma half-life of pseudoephedrine in man and dog and a sensitive assay for its determination in human plasma. Clin Pharmacol Ther. 1971;12:62.

## Antacids

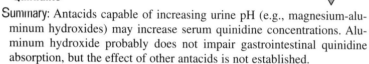

## Quinidine

Summary: Antacids capable of increasing urine pH (e.g., magnesium-aluminum hydroxides) may increase serum quinidine concentrations. Aluminum hydroxide probably does not impair gastrointestinal quinidine absorption, but the effect of other antacids is not established.

Risk Factors:
- *Diet/Food.* Diets that increase urine pH (e.g., large amounts of citrus juices) may add to the effect of antacids.

Related Drugs: $H_2$-receptor antagonists [e.g., *famotidine (Pepcid)*, *nizatidine (Axid)*, *ranitidine (Zantac)*] and proton pump inhibitors [e.g., *omeprazole (Prilosec)*, *lansoprazole (Prevacid)*] are not known to affect urine pH significantly, but *cimetidine (Tagamet)* inhibits the hepatic metabolism of quinidine and may increase its serum concentrations significantly.

Management Options:
- *Monitor* for altered quinidine effect if antacids are initiated, discontinued or changed in dosage. Current evidence does not suggest that it is necessary to space doses of quinidine from antacids.

References:
1. Remon JP et al. Interaction of antacids with antiarrhythmics. V. Effect of aluminum hydroxide and magnesium oxide on the bioavailability of quinidine, procainamide and propranolol in dogs. Arzneimittelforsch. 1983;33:117.
2. Romankiewicz JA et al. The noninterference of aluminum hydroxide gel with quinidine sulfate absorption: an approach to control quinidine-induced diarrhea. Am Heart J. 1978;96:518.
3. Mauro VF et al. Effect of aluminum hydroxide gel on quinidine gluconate absorption. DICP, Ann Pharmacother. 1990;24:252.

## Antacids

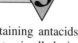

## Sodium Polystyrene Sulfonate Resin (Kayexalate)

Summary: Combined use of magnesium- or calcium-containing antacids with sodium polystyrene sulfonate resin may result in systemic alkalosis.

Risk Factors: No specific risk factors known.

Related Drugs: Theoretically, $H_2$-receptor antagonists [e.g., *cimetidine (Tagamet)*, *famotidine (Pepcid)*, *nizatidine (Axid)*, *ranitidine (Zantac)*] and proton pump inhibitors [e.g., *lansoprazole (Prevacid)*, *omeprazole (Prilosec)*] would not be expected to interact with sodium polystyrene sulfonate resin.

Management Options:

- *Consider Alternative.* Consider use of alternative to antacids (see Related Drugs).

- *Circumvent/Minimize.* Separating the time of administration of doses of antacid from the oral sodium polystyrene sulfonate resin would theoretically avoid the interaction; since it is not known how much of a separation would be necessary to avoid the interaction, separate doses by as much time as possible. Administering sodium polystyrene sulfonate resin rectally also would be expected to avoid this interaction.

- *Monitor.* If antacids and sodium polystyrene sulfonate resin are used concurrently, be alert for clinical or laboratory evidence of alkalosis.

References:

1. Schroeder ET. Alkalosis resulting from combined administration of a nonsystemic antacid and a cation-exchange resin. Gastroenterology. 1969;56:868.
2. Fernandez PC et al. Metabolic acidosis reversed by the combination of magnesium hydroxide and a cation-exchange resin. N Engl J Med. 1972;286:23.
3. Ziessman HA. Alkalosis and seizure due to a cation-exchange resin and magnesium hydroxide. South Med J. 1976;69:497.

## Antacids

### Tetracycline

Summary: Cotherapy with a tetracycline and an antacid containing divalent or trivalent cations (aluminum, calcium, magnesium) can reduce the serum concentration and efficacy of the tetracycline.

Risk Factors: No specific risk factors known.

Related Drugs: $H_2$-receptor antagonists [e.g., *cimetidine (Tagamet)*, *famotidine (Pepcid)*, *nizatidine (Axid)*, *ranitidine (Zantac)*] and proton pump inhibitors [e.g, *lansoprazole (Prevacid)*, *omeprazole (Prilosec)*] are not known to affect tetracycline. *Doxycycline (Vibramycin)* may interact similarly.[3]

Management Options:

- *Circumvent/Minimize.* Take oral tetracyclines 2 hr before or 6 hr after antacids. This may not completely avoid the interaction, but it should minimize it.

- *Monitor* for reduced tetracycline response if antacids are also used.

References:

1. Chin TF et al. Drug diffusion and bioavailability: tetracycline metallic chelation. Am J Hosp Pharm. 1975;32:625.
2. Neuvonen PJ. Interactions with the absorption of tetracyclines. Drugs. 1976;11:45.
3. Nix DE et al. Effect of oral aluminum containing antacids on the disposition of intravenous doxycycline. Pharm Res. 1988;5(Suppl.):S174. Abstract.

## Antacids

### Tocainide (Tonocard)

Summary: In a report involving healthy subjects, antacids that increase urine pH were found to increase tocainide serum concentrations. The degree to which this effect increases the potential for adverse reactions is unknown.

Risk Factors: No specific risk factors known.

Related Drugs: No information available.

Management Options:

• *Monitor.* Patients taking tocainide should be monitored more closely for excessive tocainide effect when antacids are concomitantly administered.

References:

1. Meneilly GP et al. The effect of antacid induced urinary alkalinization on the pharmacokinetics of tocainide. Pharmacotherapy. 1988;8:120. Abstract.

## Aspirin

### Captopril (Capoten)

Summary: Aspirin appears to inhibit both the antihypertensive effects of captopril and other angiotensin-converting enzyme (ACE) inhibitors and the favorable hemodynamic effects of ACE inhibitors in patients with congestive heart failure.

Risk Factors:

• *Dosage Regimen.* The inhibitory effect of aspirin on ACE inhibitors is probably dose related.

Related Drugs: The effect of aspirin is probably similar for all ACE inhibitors [e.g., **enalapril (Vasotec)**]. Other nonsteroidal anti-inflammatory drugs probably also inhibit ACE inhibitor effect, although it is possible that **sulindac (Clinoril)** interacts to a lesser degree. The effect of salicylates other than aspirin on ACE inhibitors is not established; theoretically, **nonacetylated salicylates** may be less likely to interact since they tend to have less inhibitory effect on prostaglandin synthesis.

Management Options:

• *Consider Alternative.* Acetaminophen is not known to affect ACE inhibitor response and may be a suitable alternative to aspirin as an analgesic or antipyretic.

## Significance Classification

① - *Avoid Combination.* Risk always outweighs benefit.

② - *Usually Avoid Combination.* Use combination only under special circumstances.

③ - *Minimize Risk.* Take action as necessary to reduce risk.

• *Monitor.* If more than occasional doses of aspirin are used in a patient on an ACE inhibitor, monitor for worsening of disease (hypertension and/or CHF). One should also be alert for evidence of reduced renal function.

References:
1. Smith SR et al. Effect of low-dose aspirin on thromboxane production and the antihypertensive effect of captopril. J Am Soc Nephrol. 1993;4:1133.
2. van Wijngaarden J et al. Effects of acetylsalicylic acid on peripheral hemodynamics in patients with chronic heart failure treated with angiotensin-converting enzyme inhibitors. J Cardiovasc Pharmacol. 1994;23:240.
3. Sioufi A et al. The absence of a pharmacokinetic interaction between aspirin and the angiotensin-converting enzyme inhibitor benazepril in healthy volunteers. Biopharm Drug Disposit. 1994;15:451.

## Aspirin
## Chlorpropamide (Diabinese)

Summary: Salicylate administration may enhance the hypoglycemic response to sulfonylureas, particularly chlorpropamide.

Risk Factors: No specific risk factors known.

Related Drugs: Similar cases of hypoglycemia have been reported with **tolbutamide (Orinase)**.[1] Aspirin also has been noted to reduce **glyburide (DiaBeta)** serum concentrations while enhancing its hypoglycemic effects.[2] **Insulin** is similarly affected by salicylates. More study in diabetic patients is needed to evaluate this interaction.

Management Options:
• *Monitor.* Be alert for evidence of altered response to oral hypoglycemics and insulin when salicylate therapy is started or stopped. Monitor blood glucose concentrations and watch for symptoms of hyper- or hypoglycemia.

References:
1. Cherner R et al. Prolonged tolbutamide-induced hypoglycemia. JAMA. 1963;185:883.
2. Kubacka RT et al. Effects of aspirin and ibuprofen on the pharmacokinetics and pharmacodynamics of in healthy subjects. Ann Pharmacother. 1996;30:20.
3. Richardson T et al. Enhancement by sodium salicylate of the blood glucose lowering effect of chlorpropamide—drug interaction or summation of similar effects? Br J Clin Pharmacol. 1986;22:43.

## Aspirin
## Diltiazem (Cardizem)

Summary: Diltiazem appears to enhance the antiplatelet activity of aspirin, but the clinical importance of this effect is not established.

Risk Factors: No specific risk factors known.

Related Drugs: **Verapamil (Calan)** may interact similarly; patients have developed bruising or petechiae following concomitant administration with aspirin.

Management Options:
- *Monitor.* Until further information is available, patients should be monitored for prolonged bleeding times when diltiazem or verapamil is coadministered with aspirin.

References:
1. Altman R et al. Diltiazem potentiates the inhibitory effect of aspirin on platelet aggregation. Clin Pharmacol Ther. 1988;44:320.
2. Ring ME et al. Antiplatelet effects of oral diltiazem, propranolol, and their combination. Br J Clin Pharmacol. 1987;24:615.
3. Yamauchi K et al. Effects of diltiazem hydrochloride on cardiovascular response, platelet aggregation and coagulating activity during exercise testing in systemic hypertension. Am J Card. 1986;57:609.

## Aspirin

## Ethanol (Ethyl Alcohol)

Summary: Ethanol appears to enhance aspirin-induced gastric mucosal damage and aspirin-induced prolongation of the bleeding time.

Risk Factors:
- *Diet/Food.* Theoretically, more concentrated alcohol (e.g., hard liquor) on an empty stomach would be more likely to enhance gastric mucosal damage from aspirin.

Related Drugs: Theoretically, salicylate preparations which are less likely to produce gastric mucosal injury [e.g., *effervescent buffered salicylates (Alka-Seltzer)*, *enteric coated aspirin (Ecotrin)*, *nonacetylated salicylates*] would be less likely to produce additive gastric mucosal damage when administered in the presence of alcohol. Also, salicylate-induced prolongation of the bleeding time can be avoided by using nonacetylated salicylates such as *choline salicylate (Arthropan)*, *salsalate (Disalcid)*, *choline magnesium salicylate*, and *sodium salicylate*; ethanol-induced potentiation of the salicylate-induced prolongation of the bleeding time by ethanol would not be a factor with these nonacetylated salicylates.

Management Options:
- *Consider Alternative.* Some forms of salicylate appear to be less likely to produce gastric mucosal injury than standard aspirin tablets. Such products include effervescent buffered products, enteric-coated products, and the nonacetylated salicylates. Theoretically, these preparations would be less likely to produce additive gastric mucosal damage with alcohol than standard aspirin tablets. (See Related Drugs for additional alternatives.)
- *Circumvent/Minimize.* Although concomitant use of ethanol and aspirin is not necessarily contraindicated, the possibility of enhanced GI bleeding should be considered. When possible, aspirin use within 8 to 10 hours of heavy alcohol use should be avoided.
- *Monitor.* Be alert for evidence of GI bleeding (e.g., melena, black stools, etc.).

References:
1. DeSchepper PJ et al. Gastrointestinal blood loss after diflunisal and after aspirin: effect of ethanol. Clin Pharmacol Ther. 1978;23:669.
2. Deykin D et al. Ethanol potentiation of aspirin-induced prolongation of the bleeding time. N Engl J Med. 1982;306:852.
3. Roine R et al. Aspirin increases blood alcohol concentrations in humans after ingestion of ethanol. JAMA. 1990;264:2406.

## Aspirin

### Griseofulvin (Grisactin)

Summary: Griseofulvin administration markedly reduced the plasma concentration of salicylate in a patient taking chronic aspirin therapy.

Risk Factors: No specific risk factors known.

Related Drugs: No information available.

Management Options:
- *Circumvent/Minimize.* Until the mechanism of this interaction is established, administration of an alternative antifungal agent should be considered in patients receiving aspirin.
- *Monitor.* Based on this initial case report, patients stabilized on aspirin therapy should be monitored for loss of efficacy following the concomitant administration of griseofulvin.

References:
1. Phillips KR et al. Griseofulvin significantly decreases serum salicylate concentrations. Pediatric Infect Disease J. 1993;12:350.

## Aspirin

### Methotrexate

Summary: Case reports, limited pharmacokinetic and epidemiological reports, and animal studies all indicate that salicylates may enhance methotrexate toxicity.

Risk Factors:
- *Dosage Regimen.* The risk of adverse effects from this interaction is primarily in patients receiving antineoplastic doses of methotrexate rather than the lower doses used to treat rheumatoid arthritis, psoriasis, and related diseases.

Related Drugs: All salicylates are likely to interact with methotrexate.

Management Options:
- *Avoid Unless Benefit Outweighs Risk.* Aspirin should generally be avoided in patients taking antineoplastic doses of methotrexate. The manufacturer of methotrexate also recommends that salicylates be avoided in patients receiving methotrexate. Patients receiving methotrexate should be reminded of the many nonprescription mixtures that contain salicylates.

• *Monitor.* If the combination is used, one should anticipate that a reduction in methotrexate dosage may be required. Serum methotrexate determinations would be helpful, and one should also monitor for excessive methotrexate effect (e.g., gastrointestinal toxicity, stomatitis, bone marrow suppression, hepatotoxicity, infection).

References:
1. Taylor JR et al. Effect of sodium salicylate and indomethacin on methotrexate-serum albumin binding. Arch Dermatol. 1977;113:588.
2. Aherne GW et al. Prolongation and enhancement of serum methotrexate concentrations by probenecid. Br Med J. 1978;1:1097.
3. Mandel MA. The synergistic effect of salicylates on methotrexate toxicity. Plast Reconstr Surg. 1976;57:733.

### Aspirin

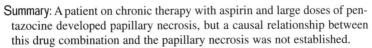

### Pentazocine (Talwin)

Summary: A patient on chronic therapy with aspirin and large doses of pentazocine developed papillary necrosis, but a causal relationship between this drug combination and the papillary necrosis was not established.

Risk Factors: No specific risk factors known.

Related Drugs: The effect of salicylates other than aspirin combined with pentazocine is not established.

Management Options:
• *Monitor.* Until more information is available, be alert for evidence of renal papillary necrosis (e.g., passing tissue via the urethra) in patients receiving large doses of pentazocine combined with aspirin.

References:
1. Muhalwas KK et al. Renal papillary necrosis caused by long-term ingestion of pentazocine and aspirin. JAMA. 1981;246:867.

### Aspirin

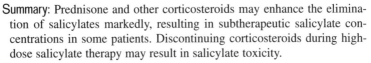

### Prednisone

Summary: Prednisone and other corticosteroids may enhance the elimination of salicylates markedly, resulting in subtherapeutic salicylate concentrations in some patients. Discontinuing corticosteroids during high-dose salicylate therapy may result in salicylate toxicity.

Risk Factors:
• *Dosage Regimen.* Patients taking large (antiarthritic) salicylate doses are at greater risk.

Related Drugs: Salicylates other than aspirin also can be expected to interact similarly with corticosteroids.

Management Options:
• *Monitor.* Corticosteroids and salicylates are frequently administered together, and their concomitant use is not contraindicated. However, salicylate dose requirements may be higher in the presence of corticosteroids, and patients should be watched for salicylate intoxi-

cation if the corticosteroid dose is reduced. The possibility that concomitant therapy may increase the incidence or severity of gastrointestinal ulceration also should be kept in mind.

References:

1. Koren G et al. Corticosteroids-salicylate interaction—a case of juvenile rheumatoid arthritis. Ther Drug Monit. 1987;9:177.
2. Edelman J et al. The effect of intra-articular steroids on plasma salicylate concentrations. Br J Clin Pharmacol. 1986;21:301.
3. Graham GG et al. Patterns of plasma concentrations and urinary excretion of salicylate in rheumatoid arthritis. Clin Pharmacol Ther. 1977;22:410.

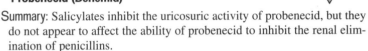

## Aspirin

### Probenecid (Benemid)

Summary: Salicylates inhibit the uricosuric activity of probenecid, but they do not appear to affect the ability of probenecid to inhibit the renal elimination of penicillins.

Risk Factors:

- *Dosage Regimen.* Doses of salicylate that do not produce serum salicylate concentrations >5 mg/dL do not appear to affect probenecid uricosuria significantly. Thus, occasional analgesic doses of salicylate may be insufficient to interact with probenecid.

Related Drugs: All salicylates probably interact with probenecid in a similar manner.

Management Options:

- *Circumvent/Minimize.* More than occasional small doses of salicylates should be avoided in patients receiving probenecid as a uricosuric agent. Available evidence suggests that patients receiving probenecid to prolong serum penicillin levels do not have to avoid salicylates.
- *Monitor* for reduced probenecid uricosuric effect if salicylates are given concurrently.

References:

1. Pascale LR et al. Inhibition of the uricosuric action of Benemid by salicylate. J Lab Clin Med. 1955;45:771.
2. Boger WP et al. Probenecid and salicylates: the question of interaction in terms of penicillin excretion. J Lab Clin Med. 1955;45:478.
3. Regal, RE. Aspirin and uricosurics: interaction revisited. Drug Intell Clin Pharm. 1987;21:219.

## Significance Classification

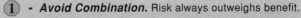

① - ***Avoid Combination.*** Risk always outweighs benefit.

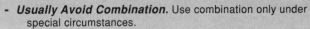

② - ***Usually Avoid Combination.*** Use combination only under special circumstances.

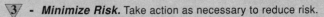

③ - ***Minimize Risk.*** Take action as necessary to reduce risk.

## Aspirin

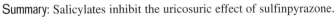

### Sulfinpyrazone (Anturane)

**Summary:** Salicylates inhibit the uricosuric effect of sulfinpyrazone.

**Risk Factors:** No specific risk factors known.

**Related Drugs:** All salicylates probably interact with sulfinpyrazone in a similar manner.

**Management Options:**
- *Circumvent/Minimize.* More than occasional small doses of salicylates should be avoided in patients receiving sulfinpyrazone.
- *Monitor* for reduced uricosuric effect of sulfinpyrazone if salicylates are given concurrently.

**References:**
1. Smith MJH et al. The Salicylates. A Critical Bibliographic Review. New York: Interscience Publishers; 1966:86–90.
2. Oyer JH et al. Suppression of salicylate-induced uricosuria by phenylbutazone. Am J Med Sci. 1966;251:1.
3. Yu TF et al. Mutual suppression of the uricosuric effects of sulfinpyrazone and salicylate: a study in interactions between drugs. J Clin Invest. 1963;42:1330.

## Aspirin

### Warfarin (Coumadin)

**Summary:** Aspirin (even in small doses) increases the risk of bleeding in anticoagulated patients by inhibiting platelet function and possibly by producing gastric erosions. Larger aspirin doses (e.g., >3 gm/day) may also enhance the hypoprothrombinemic response to warfarin. Nonetheless, the benefit of low-dose aspirin plus warfarin appears to outweigh the increased risk of bleeding in selected patients.

**Risk Factors:**
- *Dosage Regimen.* In most patients, more than 3 gm/day of aspirin is likely to have an intrinsic hypoprothrombinemic effect that would be additive with that of oral anticoagulants; the aspirin dosage required for this effect varies from patient to patient.

**Related Drugs: *Nonacetylated salicylates*** (e.g., choline salicylate, magnesium salicylate, salsalate, sodium salicylate) are probably safer with oral anticoagulants than aspirin, since such salicylates have minimal effects on platelet function and the gastric mucosa. Enteric-coated aspirin tends to produce less gastric mucosal damage,[1] but it would still be capable of increasing the hypoprothrombinemic response (if given in large doses) and inhibiting platelet function (in any dose).

**Management Options:**
- *Avoid Unless Benefit Outweighs Risk.* Aspirin should be combined with oral an anticoagulant only when used intentionally for additive anticoagulant effects. If the aspirin is being used as an analgesic or antipyretic, acetaminophen is probably safer to use with oral anticoagulants. If a salicylate is needed, nonacetylated salicylates are

probably safer (see Related Drugs). Patients should be warned that many nonprescription products contain aspirin and be advised to read the ingredients carefully.

- *Monitor.* If aspirin is used with oral anticoagulants, note that the increased bleeding risk is usually not accompanied by an increase in the hypoprothrombinemic response, especially when small doses of aspirin are used. Thus, particular attention should be directed to early detection of bleeding, especially from the GI tract.

References:
1. Hawthorne AB et al. Aspirin-induced gastric mucosal damage: prevention by enteric-coating and relation to prostaglandin synthesis. Br J Clin Pharmacol. 1991;32:77.
2. Turpie AGG et al. A comparison of aspirin with placebo in patients treated with warfarin after heart-valve replacement. New Engl J Med. 1993;329:524.
3. Hurlen M et al. Comparison of bleeding complications of warfarin and warfarin plus acetylsalicylic acid: a study in 3166 outpatients. J Int Med. 1994;236:299.

## Aspirin (Bayer)
## Zafirlukast (Accolate)

Summary: The manufacturer reports that aspirin can increase plasma concentrations of zafirlukast; adjustments in zafirlukast dose may be needed.

Risk Factors: No specific risk factors known.

Related Drugs: No information available.

Management Options:
- *Monitor* for altered zafirlukast effect if aspirin is initiated, discontinued, or changed in dosage. Adjust zafirlukast dose as needed.

References:
1. Zeneca Pharmaceuticals. Accolate manufacturer's product information. 1997.

## Astemizole (Hismanal)
## Erythromycin

Summary: Preliminary reports indicate that erythromycin and astemizole administration can cause QT interval prolongation and arrhythmia.

Risk Factors: No specific risk factors known.

Related Drugs: *Ketoconazole (Nizoral)* and *itraconazole (Sporanox)* interact similarly *in vitro*. *Troleandomycin (TAO)* and *clarithromycin (Biaxin)* also may inhibit astemizole metabolism. *Terfenadine (Seldane)* is also known to interact with erythromycin.

Management Options:
- *Avoid Combination.* It would be prudent to avoid giving the two drugs together. The use of sedating antihistamines or perhaps loratadine (Claritin) or cetirizine (Zyrtec) instead of astemizole would be preferred in patients taking erythromycin, ketoconazole, or itraconazole.

References:
1. Gelb LN, ed. FDA Medical Bull. 1993;23:2.

2. Goss JE et al. Torsades de pointes associated with astemizole (Hismanal) therapy. Arch Intern Med. 1993;153:2705.
3. Lavriisen K et al. The interaction of ketoconazole, itraconazole and erythromycin with the *in vitro* metabolism of antihistamines in human liver microsomes. Allergy. 1993;48(Suppl.):34.

## Astemizole (Hismanal)

## Fluvoxamine (Luvox)

Summary: Fluvoxamine appears to inhibit the enzyme that metabolizes astemizole, which theoretically could result in increased serum astemizole concentrations and cardiac arrhythmias; the combination should be avoided.

Risk Factors: No specific risk factors known.

Related Drugs: *Terfenadine (Seldane)* is also metabolized by CYP3A4 and can cause the same types of cardiac arrhythmias when combined with CYP3A4 inhibitors; thus, it may also interact adversely with fluvoxamine. *Loratadine (Claritin)* and *cetirizine (Zyrtec)* do not appear to produce cardiotoxicity when combined with CYP3A4 inhibitors.

Management Options:
- *Avoid Combination.* Although this interaction is based largely upon theoretical considerations, the combination of astemizole and fluvoxamine should be avoided.[2] The potential adverse effects of the interaction can be life threatening, and astemizole is generally used for symptomatic relief of allergic disorders. Theoretically, loratadine would be a safer nonsedating antihistamine in the presence of fluvoxamine.

References:
1. Fleishaker JC et al. A pharmacokinetic and pharmacodynamic evaluation of the combined administration of alprazolam and fluvoxamine. Eur J Clin Pharmacol. 1994;46:35.
2. Solvay Pharmaceuticals. Luvox prescribing information. 1996.

## Astemizole (Hismanal)

## Ketoconazole (Nizoral)

Summary: Ketoconazole administration can cause astemizole concentrations to increase and result in QT interval prolongation and arrhythmia.

Risk Factors: No specific risk factors known.

Related Drugs: Other antifungal agents [*miconazole (Monistat)*, *itraconazole (Sporanox)*, *fluconazole (Diflucan)*] are likely to increase astemizole concentrations. *Terfenadine (Seldane)* concentrations have been noted to increase when it is administered with antifungal agents. *Cetirizine (Zyrtec)* and *loratadine (Claritin)* appear to be less likely to produce side effects when administered with ketoconazole.

Management Options:
- *Avoid Combination.* It would be prudent to avoid giving the two drugs together. The use of sedating antihistamines or perhaps loratadine or cetirizine instead of astemizole would seem to be preferred in patients taking ketoconazole or other oral antifungal agents. If ketoconazole and astemizole are coadministered, monitor for cardiac arrhythmias.

References:
1. Gelb LN, ed. FDA Medical Bull. 1993;23:2.
2. Lavriisen K et al. The interaction of ketoconazole, itraconazole and erythromycin with the *in vitro* metabolism of antihistamines in human liver microsomes. Allergy. 1993;48(Suppl.):34.
3. Bishop R et al. Prolonged Q-T interval following astemizole overdose. Arch Emerg Med. 1989;6:63.

## Astemizole (Hismanal)

## Mibefradil (Posicor)

Summary: Mibefradil is likely to increase astemizole serum concentrations; cardiac arrhythmias may result. Pending further information on this interaction, the concomitant use of mibefradil and astemizole should be avoided.

Risk Factors: No specific risk factors known.

Related Drugs: Mibefradil administration causes an accumulation of **terfenadine (Seldane)** resulting in prolonged QTc intervals. Other calcium channel blockers [e.g., **amlodipine (Norvasc)**, **nifedipine (Procardia)**, **nicardipine (Cardene)**] would not be expected to change astemizole plasma concentrations. The metabolism of **fexofenadine (Allegra)**, **cetirizine (Zyrtec)**, and **loratadine (Claritin)** would be unlikely to be affected by concomitant mibefradil administration.

Management Options:
- *Use Alternative.* Due to the risk of a possibly serious arrhythmia, the combination of mibefradil and astemizole (or terfenadine) should be

## Significance Classification

① - *Avoid Combination.* Risk always outweighs benefit.

② - *Usually Avoid Combination.* Use combination only under special circumstances.

③ - *Minimize Risk.* Take action as necessary to reduce risk.

avoided. Noninteracting antihistamines are available and should be used in patients receiving mibefradil.

References:
1. Roche Laboratories, Inc. Mibefradil (Posicor) package insert. 1997.

### Atenolol (Tenormin)
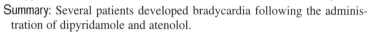
### Dipyridamole (Persantine)

Summary: Several patients developed bradycardia following the administration of dipyridamole and atenolol.

Risk Factors: No specific risk factors known.

Related Drugs: This interaction would be expected to occur with all beta blockers [e.g., *metoprolol (Lopressor)*]. A similar interaction would be expected with *adenosine (Adenocard)* and beta blockers.

Management Options:
- *Circumvent/Minimize.* Discontinuation of atenolol or other beta blockers before the administration of dipyridamole may be the most prudent approach.
- *Monitor.* Due to the potentially serious outcome of this interaction, patients taking beta-adrenergic blockers or other drugs known to have negative chronotropic or dromotropic effects should be observed carefully for signs of bradycardia following dipyridamole injections.

References:
1. Roach PJ et al. Asystole and bradycardia during dipyridamole stress testing in patients receiving beta blockers. Int J Cardiol. 1993;42:92.
2. Blumenthal MS et al. Cardiac arrest during dipyridamole imaging. Chest. 1988; 93:1103.
3. Picano E et al. Safety of intravenous high-dose dipyridamole echocardiography. Am J Cardiol. 1992;70:252.

### Atorvastatin (Lipitor)

### Erythromycin (E-Mycin)

Summary: Erythromycin increases the plasma concentration of atorvastatin; increased toxicity (hepatic dysfunction, myositis) may result.

Risk Factors: No specific risk factors known.

Related Drugs: *Clarithromycin (Biaxin)* and *troleandomycin (TAO)* may affect atorvastatin concentrations in a similar manner. *Dirithromycin (Dynabac)* and *azithromycin (Zithromycin)* would not be expected to alter atorvastatin metabolism, however, no data are available. Erythromycin is known to affect other HMG-CoA reductase inhibitors including *lovastatin (Mevacor)*. *Pravastatin (Pravachol)* does not appear to be affected by erythromycin.

The effect of erythromycin on other HMG-CoA reductase inhibitors is unknown, although *simvastatin (Zocor)* would likely be affected in a similar manner as lovastatin.

Management Options:
- *Consider Alternative.* Pravastatin may be a suitable alternative for patients taking erythromycin who require a HMG-CoA reductase inhibitor. Azithromycin or dirithromycin are macrolides that would be unlikely to interact with HMG-CoA reductase inhibitors.
- *Monitor.* Patients taking atorvastatin who receive erythromycin, clarithromycin, or TAO should be monitored for changes in hepatic function tests and the onset of muscle pains.

References:
1. Parke-Davis. Atorvastatin (Lipitor) package insert. 1997.

## Atracurium

## Gentamicin (Garamycin)

Summary: Aminoglycoside antibiotics like gentamicin potentiate the respiratory suppression produced by neuromuscular blockers.

Risk Factors:
- *Concurrent Diseases.* Patients with renal dysfunction are probably at greater risk.
- *Dosage Regimen.* Elevated aminoglycoside concentrations may lead to respiratory suppression.

Related Drugs: Other aminoglycosides [e.g., *tobramycin (Nebcin)*] also may produce enhanced neuromuscular blockade when administered in combination with neuromuscular blockers [e.g., *succinylcholine (Anectine)*, *vecuronium (Norcuron)*].

Management Options:
- *Avoid Unless Benefit Outweighs Risk.* Aminoglycoside antibiotics should be administered with extreme caution during surgery or in the immediate postoperative period.
- *Monitor.* Watch for respiratory depression; mechanical ventilation or treatment with anticholinesterase agents or calcium may be necessary.

References:
1. Kronenfeld MA et al. Recurrence of neuromuscular blockade after reversal of vecuronium in a patient receiving polymyxin/amikacin sternal irrigation. Anesthesiology. 1986;65:93.
2. Levanen J et al. Complete respiratory paralysis caused by a large dose of streptomycin and its treatment with calcium chloride. Ann Clin Res. 1975;7:47.
3. Lippman M et al. Neuromuscular blocking effects of tobramycin, gentamicin, and cefazolin. Anesth Analg. 1982;61:767.

## Azapropazone

## Methotrexate

**2**

Summary: A patient on chronic methotrexate developed evidence of methotrexate toxicity several days after starting azapropazone.

Risk Factors:

- *Dosage Regimen.* The risk of adverse effects from this interaction is primarily in patients receiving antineoplastic doses of methotrexate, rather than the lower doses used to treat rheumatoid arthritis, psoriasis, and related diseases.

- *Concurrent Diseases.* Particular caution is suggested in patients with pre-existing renal impairment [who may be more susceptible to nonsteroidal anti-inflammatory drug (NSAID)-induced renal failure].

Related Drugs: Several other NSAIDs also have been shown to increase methotrexate serum concentrations although the magnitude varies depending upon which NSAID is used at what dose.

Management Options:

- *Avoid Unless Benefit Outweighs Risk.* Until more information is available on this interaction, it would be prudent to avoid azapropazone (as well as other NSAIDs) in patients receiving antineoplastic doses of methotrexate. Although decreasing the methotrexate dosage would be expected to reduce the likelihood of toxicity, the magnitude of the required reduction in methotrexate dosage has not been established. Rarely, low-dose methotrexate may interact adversely with an NSAID, as with the patient described above.

- *Monitor.* Many patients receiving methotrexate for rheumatoid arthritis will require an NSAID for symptomatic treatment. These patients should be monitored closely for evidence of increased methotrexate toxicity.

References:

1. Furst DE et al. Effect of aspirin and sulindac on methotrexate clearance. J Pharm Sci. 1990;79:782.
2. Dupuis LL et al. Methotrexate-nonsteroidal antiinflammatory drug interaction in children with arthritis. J Rheumatol. 1990;17:1469.
3. Skeith KJ et al. Lack of significant interaction between low dose methotrexate and ibuprofen or flurbiprofen in patients with arthritis. J Rheumatol. 1990;17:1008.

## Significance Classification

1 - **Avoid Combination.** Risk always outweighs benefit.

2 - **Usually Avoid Combination.** Use combination only under special circumstances.

3 - **Minimize Risk.** Take action as necessary to reduce risk.

## Azapropazone

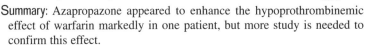

### Warfarin (Coumadin)

Summary: Azapropazone appeared to enhance the hypoprothrombinemic effect of warfarin markedly in one patient, but more study is needed to confirm this effect.

Risk Factors:
- *Concurrent Diseases.* Patients with peptic ulcer disease or a history of gastrointestinal bleeding are probably at greater risk.

Related Drugs: All NSAIDs inhibit platelet function, cause gastric erosions, and probably increase the risk of gastrointestinal bleeding. ***Phenylbutazone (Butazolidin)*** markedly increases warfarin response. Some NSAIDs, however, such as ***ibuprofen (Advil)***, ***naproxen (Naprosyn)***, and ***diclofenac (Voltaren)*** may be less likely to increase oral anticoagulant-induced hypoprothrombinemia than other NSAIDs.

Management Options:
- *Avoid Unless Benefit Outweighs Risk.* Since all NSAIDs probably increase the risk of gastrointestinal bleeding in patients on oral anticoagulants, use the combination only after careful consideration of the benefit versus risk. If a NSAID must be used with an oral anticoagulant it would be prudent to use NSAIDs that are unlikely to affect the hypoprothrombinemic response to oral anticoagulants. (See Related Drugs above.) If the NSAID is being used as an analgesic or antipyretic, acetaminophen is probably safer to use with oral anticoagulants. Nonacetylated salicylates (e.g., choline salicylate, magnesium salicylate, salsalate, sodium salicylate) are probably also safer with oral anticoagulants than NSAIDs, since such salicylates have minimal effects on platelet function and the gastric mucosa.
- *Monitor.* If any NSAID is used with an oral anticoagulant, one should monitor the prothrombin time carefully and watch for evidence of bleeding, especially from the gastrointestinal tract.

References:
1. McElnay JC et al. Interaction between azapropazone and warfarin. Br Med J. 1977;2:773. Letter.
2. Powell-Jackson PR. Interaction between azapropazone and warfarin. Br Med J. 1977;1:1193.
3. Shorr RI et al. Concurrent use of nonsteroidal anti-inflammatory drugs and oral anticoagulants places elderly persons at high risk for hemorrhagic peptic ulcer disease. Arch Intern Med. 1993;153:1665.

## Azathioprine (Imuran)

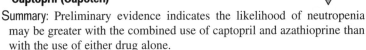

### Captopril (Capoten)

Summary: Preliminary evidence indicates the likelihood of neutropenia may be greater with the combined use of captopril and azathioprine than with the use of either drug alone.

Risk Factors: No specific risk factors known.

**Related Drugs:** Given that azathioprine is converted to mercaptopurine in the body, one would expect *mercaptopurine (6-MP)* to interact with angiotensin-converting enzyme (ACE) inhibitors in a similar manner. Little is known regarding the combined use of azathioprine or mercaptopurine with ACE inhibitors other than captopril.

**Management Options:**
- *Monitor.* Although evidence for an interaction between azathioprine and captopril is only preliminary, it would be prudent to monitor for laboratory and clinical evidence of bone marrow suppression in patients on both drugs.

**References:**
1. Edwards CRW et al. Successful reintroduction of captopril following neutropenia. Lancet. 1981;1:723.
2. Case DB et al. Successful low dose captopril rechallenge following drug-induced leukopenia. Lancet. 1981;1:1362.
3. Kirchertz EF et al. Successful low dose captopril rechallenge following drug-induced leukopenia. Lancet. 1981;1:1363.

## Azathioprine (Imuran)

### Warfarin (Coumadin)

**Summary:** Azathioprine appeared to inhibit the hypoprothrombinemic response to warfarin in one patient; more information is needed to establish the clinical importance.

**Risk Factors:** No specific risk factors known.

**Related Drugs:** *Mercaptopurine (6-MP)* also has been reported to inhibit the hypoprothrombinemic response to warfarin.

**Management Options:**
- *Monitor* for altered oral anticoagulant effect if azathioprine is initiated, discontinued, or changed in dosage. Adjust the anticoagulant dose as needed.

**References:**
1. Singleton JD et al. Warfarin and azathioprine: an important drug interaction. Am J Med. 1992;92:217.

## Benztropine (Cogentin)

### Haloperidol (Haldol)

**Summary:** Benztropine and other anticholinergics may inhibit the therapeutic response to neuroleptics; excess anticholinergic effects may occur.

**Risk Factors:** No specific risk factors known.

**Related Drugs:** Many combinations of antipsychotics and anticholinergics probably interact by one or more of the mechanisms described above. *Trihexyphenidyl (Artane)* apparently had a similar inhibitory effect on the therapeutic response to haloperidol in schizophrenic patients. However, there is also evidence that anticholinergics may reduce the GI absorption of *chlorpromazine (Thorazine)*. For example, trihexyphenidyl has been shown to reduce plasma chlorpromazine concentrations in schizophrenic patients,[1] and *orphenadrine (Norflex)* has been shown to reduce plasma concentrations and the pharmacologic response of chlorpromazine.[2]

Management Options:

- *Circumvent/Minimize.* Anticholinergics should not be used routinely in patients receiving neuroleptics. When the combination is needed, patients should take precautions to avoid heat stroke.
- *Monitor.* If the combination is used, be alert for evidence of reduced neuroleptic effects and for symptoms that may signal the onset of a dynamic ileus (e.g., constipation, abdominal pain, and distension).

References:

1. Rivera-Calimlim L et al. Effects of mode of management on plasma chlorpromazine in psychiatric patients. Clin Pharmacol Ther. 1973;14:978.
2. Loga S et al. Interactions of orphenadrine and phenobarbitone with chlorpromazine: plasma concentrations and effects in man. Br J Clin Pharmacol. 1975;2:197.
3. Schaffer CB et al. A case report of vomiting related to the interactions of antipsychotic and benzotropines. Am J Psychiatry. 1981;138:833

## Bepridil (Vascor)

## Digoxin (Lanoxin)

Summary: Bepridil increases digoxin serum concentrations; digoxin toxicity may result.

Risk Factors: No specific risk factors known.

Related Drugs: *Verapamil (Calan)*, *diltiazem (Cardizem)*, and *nitrendipine (Baypress)* appear to reduce digoxin elimination. *Digitoxin (Crystodigin)* is likely to be similarly affected.

Management Options:

- *Consider Alternative.* Nifedipine (Procardia),[1,2,3,4] isradipine (DynaCirc),[7] nicardipine (Cardene),[8] felodipine (Plendil),[5] and amlodipine (Norvasc)[6] do not appear to increase digoxin concentrations.
- *Circumvent/Minimize.* Digoxin dosages may need to be reduced when bepridil is added to a patient stabilized on digoxin.
- *Monitor.* Patients should be monitored for evidence of increased serum digitalis effects (e.g., bradycardia, heart block, gastrointestinal upset, mental changes) in the presence of bepridil therapy.

References:

1. Belz GG et al. Digoxin plasma concentrations and nifedipine. Lancet. 1981;1:844.
2. Kuhlmann J. Effects of nifedipine and diltiazem on plasma levels and renal excretion of beta-acetyldigoxin. Clin Pharmacol Ther. 1985;37:150.
3. Schwartz JB et al. Effect of nifedipine on serum digoxin concentration and renal digoxin clearance. Clin Pharmacol Ther. 1984;36:19.
4. Hutt HJ et al. Dose-dependence of the nifedipine/digoxin interaction? Arch Toxicol. 1986;Suppl. 9:209.
5. Kirch W et al. The felodipine/digoxin interaction. A placebo-controlled study in patients with heart failure. Br J Clin Pharmacol. 1988;26:644P. Abstract.
6. Schwartz JB. Effects of amlodipine on steady-state digoxin concentrations and renal digoxin clearance. J Cardiovasc Pharmacol. 1988;12:1.
7. Rodin SM et al. Comparative effects of verapamil and isradipine on steady-state digoxin kinetics. Clin Pharmacol Ther. 1988;43:668.

8. Debruyne D et al. Nicardipine does not significantly affect serum digoxin concentrations at the steady state of patients with congestive heart failure. Int J Clin Pharmacol. 1989;9:15.

## Bethanechol (Urecholine)

## Tacrine (Cognex)

Summary: Increased cholinergic effects may be seen when tacrine is combined with other cholinergic agents, like bethanechol.

Risk Factors: No specific risk factors known.

Related Drugs: Tacrine probably has additive effects with all cholinergic agents, including direct-acting cholinergics, as well as anticholinesterase agents, such as *ambenonium (Mytelase)*, *edrophonium (Tensilon)*, *neostigmine (Prostigmin)*, and *pyridostigmine (Mestinon)*.

Management Options:
- *Monitor* for excessive cholinergic response if tacrine is used with other cholinergic medications. Theoretically, it would be possible to reduce the dose of the cholinomimetic agent if tacrine is used concurrently without compromising the therapeutic response.

References:
1. Taylor P. Agents acting at the neuromuscular junction and autonomic ganglia. In: Hardman JG et al., eds. Goodman and Gilman's The Pharmacological Basis of Therapeutics. 9th ed. New York: Pergamon Press; 1996:177–197.

## Bismuth (Pepto-Bismol)

## Doxycycline (Vibramycin)

Summary: Bismuth can reduce the bioavailability of doxycycline significantly and could result in reduced antibacterial efficacy.

Risk Factors: No specific risk factors known.

Related Drugs: *Tetracycline* absorption is also affected by bismuth.

Management Options:
- *Use Alternative.* Patients taking tetracyclines for the treatment of infections should avoid bismuth. The use of doxycycline to prevent traveler's diarrhea should not include concomitant administration of bismuth.

References:
1. Albert KS et al. Decreased tetracycline bioavailability caused by a bismuth subsalicylate antidiarrheal mixture. J Pharmaceut Sci. 1979;68:586.
2. Ericsson CD et al. Influence of subsalicylate bismuth on absorption of doxycycline. JAMA. 1982;247:2266.

## Bismuth (Pepto-Bismol)

## Tetracycline

Summary: Bismuth can reduce the bioavailability of tetracycline significantly and could result in reduced antibacterial efficacy.

Risk Factors: No specific risk factors known.

Related Drugs: *Doxycycline (Vibramycin)* absorption is also affected by bismuth.

Management Options:
- *Use Alternative.* Patients taking tetracyclines for the treatment of infections should avoid bismuth. The use of doxycycline to prevent traveler's diarrhea should not include concomitant administration of bismuth.

References:
1. Albert KS et al. Decreased tetracycline bioavailability caused by a bismuth subsalicylate antidiarrheal mixture. J Pharmaceut Sci. 1979;68:586.

### Bromfenac (Duract)

### Lithium (Eskalith)

Summary: Since nonsteroidal anti-inflammatory drugs (NSAIDs) can increase lithium serum concentrations, bromfenac theoretically could also do so.

Risk Factors: No specific risk factors known.

Related Drugs: Other NSAIDs, except perhaps *sulindac (Clinoril)*, tend to increase lithium serum concentrations.

Management Options:
- *Monitor.* Be alert for evidence of lithium toxicity (nausea, vomiting, diarrhea, anorexia, coarse tremor, slurred speech, vertigo, confusion, lethargy; in severe cases, seizures, stupor, coma, and cardiovascular collapse). Adjust lithium dose as needed.

References:
1. Wyeth Laboratories. Duract manufacturer's product information. Philadelphia, PA: 1997.

### Bromfenac (Duract)

### Phenytoin (Dilantin)

Summary: Study in healthy subjects found a substantial reduction in bromfenac plasma concentrations in the presence of phenytoin, but the clinical importance of this effect is not established.

Risk Factors: No specific risk factors known.

## Significance Classification

 - *Avoid Combination.* Risk always outweighs benefit.

 - *Usually Avoid Combination.* Use combination only under special circumstances.

 - *Minimize Risk.* Take action as necessary to reduce risk.

**Related Drugs:** Other enzyme inducers (e.g., aminoglutethimide, barbiturates, carbamazepine, griseofulvin, phenytoin, primidone, rifabutin, rifampin, troglitazone) may also reduce bromfenac plasma concentrations.

**Management Options:**
- *Monitor* for reduced therapeutic effect of bromfenac if phenytoin is given concurrently. Adjust bromfenac dose as needed.

**References:**
1. Gumbhir K et al. Evaluation of pharmacokinetic interaction between bromfenac and phenytoin in healthy males. J Clin Pharmacol. 1997;37:160.
2. Wyeth Laboratories. Duract manufacturer's product information. Philadelphia, PA: 1997.

## Bromfenac (Duract)

## Warfarin (Coumadin)

**2**

**Summary:** Bromfenac does not appear to affect the hypoprothrombinemic response to warfarin, but cotherapy requires caution because of possible detrimental effects of bromfenac on the gastric mucosa and platelet function.

**Risk Factors:**
- *Concurrent Diseases.* Patients with peptic ulcer disease or a history of gastrointestinal (GI) bleeding are probably at greater risk for this interaction.
- *Dosage Regimen.* The risk of severe GI toxicity from bromfenac and other nonsteroidal anti-inflammatory drugs (NSAIDs) is directly related to the duration of NSAID therapy.

**Related Drugs:** All NSAIDs inhibit platelet function, cause gastric erosions, and increase the risk of GI bleeding. Thus, any combination of an oral anticoagulant with an NSAID would theoretically increase the risk of bleeding.

**Management Options:**
- *Avoid Unless Benefit Outweighs Risk.* Since all NSAIDs increase the risk of GI bleeding in patients on oral anticoagulants, use the combination only after careful consideration of the benefit versus risk. If the NSAID is being used as an analgesic or antipyretic, acetaminophen is probably safer to use with oral anticoagulants. Nonacetylated salicylates (e.g., choline salicylate, magnesium salicylate, salsalate, sodium salicylate) also are probably safer with oral anticoagulants than standard NSAIDs since they have minimal effects on platelet function and the gastric mucosa.
- *Monitor.* If any NSAID is used with an oral anticoagulant, one should monitor the prothrombin time carefully and watch for evidence of bleeding, especially from the gastrointestinal tract.

References:
1. Wyeth Laboratories. Duract manufacturer's product information. Philadelphia, PA: 1997.

## Bromocriptine (Parlodel)

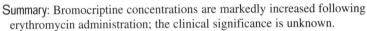

### Erythromycin

Summary: Bromocriptine concentrations are markedly increased following erythromycin administration; the clinical significance is unknown.

Risk Factors: No specific risk factors known.

Related Drugs: *Troleandomycin (TAO)* and *clarithromycin (Biaxin)* may also inhibit the metabolism of bromocriptine.

Management Options:
- *Monitor.* Patients maintained on bromocriptine should be observed for bromocriptine toxicity (hypotension, headache, nausea) during coadministration of erythromycin.

References:
1. Nelson MV et al. Pharmacokinetic evaluation of erythromycin and caffeine administered with bromocriptine in normal subjects. Clin Pharmacol Ther. 1990;47:694.

## Bromocriptine (Parlodel)

### Isometheptene (Midrin)

Summary: A patient on bromocriptine developed hypertension and ventricular tachycardia after taking isometheptene; the combination should be avoided until additional data are available.

Risk Factors: No specific risk factors known.

Related Drugs: Another sympathomimetic, *phenylpropanolamine*, has been associated with severe reactions when combined with bromocriptine.[1,2] Until this is resolved, one should assume that all sympathomimetics are capable of interacting adversely with bromocriptine.

Management Options:
- *Avoid Combination.* Even though a causal relationship for this interaction has not been established conclusively, it would be prudent to avoid isometheptene (and other sympathomimetics) in patients receiving bromocriptine.

References:
1. Kulig K et al. Bromocriptine-associated headache: possible life-threatening sympathomimetic interaction. Obstet Gynecol. 1991;78:941.
2. Chan JCN et al. Postpartum hypertension, bromocriptine and phenylpropanolamine. Drug Invest. 1994;8:254.
3. Gittelman DK. Bromocriptine associated with postpartum hypertension, seizures, and pituitary hemorrhage. Gen Hosp Psychiatry. 1991;13:278.

### Bromocriptine (Parlodel)

### Phenylpropanolamine

Summary: Isolated case reports suggest that phenylpropanolamine may increase the risk of hypertension and seizures in patients receiving bromocriptine; the combination should be avoided until additional data are available.

Risk Factors: No specific risk factors known.

Related Drugs: Another sympathomimetic, *isometheptene (Midrin)*, has been associated with hypertension and ventricular tachycardia when combined with bromocriptine.[2] Pending additional data, one should assume that all sympathomimetics are capable of interacting adversely with bromocriptine.

Management Options:
- *Avoid Combination.* Even though a causal relationship for this interaction has not been established conclusively, it would be prudent to avoid phenylpropanolamine (and other sympathomimetics) in patients receiving bromocriptine.

References:
1. Chan JCN et al. Postpartum hypertension, bromocriptine and phenylpropanolamine. Drug Invest. 1994;8:254.
2. Kulig K et al. Bromocriptine-associated headache: possible life-threatening sympathomimetic interaction. Obstet Gynecol. 1991;78:941.
3. Gittelman DK. Bromocriptine associated with postpartum hypertension, seizures, and pituitary hemorrhage. Gen Hosp Psychiatry. 1991; 13:278.

### Bromocriptine (Parlodel)

### Thioridazine (Mellaril)

Summary: Phenothiazines probably inhibit the ability of bromocriptine to lower serum prolactin concentrations in patients with pituitary adenomas. Theoretically, bromocriptine should inhibit the antipsychotic effects of phenothiazines, but clinical evidence suggests that this may be uncommon.

Risk Factors: No specific risk factors known.

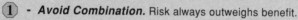

## Significance Classification

1. - *Avoid Combination.* Risk always outweighs benefit.
2. - *Usually Avoid Combination.* Use combination only under special circumstances.
3. - *Minimize Risk.* Take action as necessary to reduce risk.

Related Drugs: It is likely that a similar interference with bromocriptine response would be seen with other phenothiazines and related neuroleptics such as *haloperidol (Haldol)*, *chlorprothixene (Taractan)*, *pimozide (Orap)*, *thiothixene (Navane)*, *loxapine (Loxitane)*, and *molindone (Moban)*. Whether neuroleptics [e.g., *clozapine (Clozaril)*] that have less effect on serum prolactin concentrations would be less likely to interfere with the prolactin-lowering effect of bromocriptine is unknown.[2] A patient on *fluphenazine (Prolixin)* did not develop exacerbation of psychiatric symptoms while on bromocriptine for pituitary adenoma.[1]

Management Options:

- *Consider Alternative.* When possible, the combined use of bromocriptine and neuroleptics should be avoided.

- *Monitor.* When they are used concurrently, the patient should be monitored carefully for reduced effect of both drugs.

References:

1. Kellner C et al. Concurrent use of bromocriptine and fluphenazine. J Clin Psychiatry. 1985;46:455. Letter.
2. Ereshefsky L et al. Clozapine: an atypical antipsychotic agent. Clin Pharm. 1989;8:691.
3. Perovich RM et al. The behavioral toxicity of bromocriptine in patients with psychiatric illness. J Clin Psychopharmacol. 1989;9:417.

### Bumetanide (Bumex)

### Indomethacin (Indocin)

Summary: Indomethacin administration reduces the diuretic and antihypertensive efficacy of bumetanide.

Risk Factors: No specific risk factors known.

Related Drugs: Prostaglandin inhibitors other than indomethacin [e.g., other nonsteroidal anti-inflammatory drugs (NSAIDs)] may have a similar effect on bumetanide, but few data are available. *Aspirin*, however, may be less likely to interact with bumetanide. *Furosemide (Lasix)* is also affected by indomethacin.

Management Options:

- *Consider Alternative.* Aspirin may be less likely than NSAIDs to interfere with the response to bumetanide and, thus, may be a possible substitute for indomethacin. Because furosemide also is affected by indomethacin, it is not a viable alternative.

- *Monitor* for reduced diuretic and natriuretic response to bumetanide in the presence of indomethacin or other NSAIDs.

References:

1. Brater DC et al. Interaction studies with bumetanide and furosemide. J Clin Pharmacol. 1981;21:647.
2. Brater DC et al. Indomethacin and the response to butanimide. Clin Pharmacol Ther. 1980;27:421.
3. Kaufman J et al. Bumetanide-induced diuresis and natriuresis: effect of prostaglandin synthetase inhibition. J Clin Pharmacol. 1981;21:663.

### Bunazosin

### Enalapril (Vasotec)

Summary: Limited evidence suggests that patients receiving angiotensin-converting enzyme (ACE) inhibitors such as enalapril can have an exaggerated first dose hypotensive response to alpha blockers such as bunazosin.

Risk Factors: No specific risk factors known.

Related Drugs: Theoretically, one would expect this interaction to occur with any combination of an ACE inhibitor [e.g., *benazepril (Lotensin)*, *captopril (Capoten)*, *lisinopril (Prinivil)*] with alpha blockers such as *prazosin (Minipress)*, *terazosin (Hytrin)*, *doxazosin (Cardura)*, and *trimazosin*.

Management Options:

- *Circumvent/Minimize.* In patients receiving ACE inhibitors, initiation of therapy with bunazosin or other alpha blockers should be undertaken with caution and with conservative doses. Taking the initial doses of the alpha blocker at bedtime would be prudent.
- *Monitor.* Be alert for evidence of excessive hypotension.

References:
1. Baba T et al. Enhancement by an ACE inhibitor of first-dose hypotensive caused by an alpha blocker. N Engl J Med. 1990;322:1237.

### Buspirone (BuSpar)

### Erythromycin

Summary: Erythromycin administration results in a large increase in buspirone concentrations; increased buspirone side effects are likely to result.

Risk Factors: No specific risk factors known.

Related Drugs: Other macrolide antibiotics that inhibit CYP3A4 such as *clarithromycin (Biaxin)* and *troleandomycin (TAO)* are likely to produce similar effects on buspirone pharmacokinetics. Noninhibiting macrolides include *azithromycin (Zithromax)* and *dirithromycin (Dynabac)*. Other anxiolytics such as *midazolam (Versed)*, *alprazolam (Xanax)*, and *triazolam (Halcion)* are known to be inhibited by erythromycin. Anxiolytics not metabolized by CYP3A4 include *lorazepam (Ativan)* and *temazepam (Restoril)*.

Management Options:

- *Consider Alternative.* The use of a noninhibiting macrolide (see Related Drugs) should be considered for patients taking buspirone. Anxiolytics not metabolized by CYP3A4 could be substituted for buspirone.
- *Monitor.* Patients receiving buspirone should be monitored for increased sedation if erythromycin is administered.

References:
1. Kivisto KT et al. Plasma buspirone concentrations are greatly increased by erythromycin and itraconazole. Clin Pharmacol Ther. 1997;62:348.

## Buspirone (BuSpar)

## Fluoxetine (Prozac)

Summary: Isolated cases of reduced therapeutic response to buspirone or fluoxetine have been reported when the drugs were used together, and one patient on the combination developed a grand mal seizure. More study is needed to establish a causal relationship.

Risk Factors: No specific risk factors known.

Related Drugs: The effect of combining buspirone with other selective serotonin reuptake inhibitors is not established.

Management Options:
- *Monitor.* Until more information is available, monitor patients for altered response to either buspirone or fluoxetine when they are used together.

References:
1. Bodkin JA et al. Fluoxetine may antagonize the anxiolytic action of buspirone. J Clin Psychopharmacol. 1989;9:150. Letter.
2. Grady TA et al. Seizure associated with fluoxetine and adjuvant buspirone therapy. J Clin Psychopharmacol. 1992;12:70. Letter.
3. Tanquary J et al. Paradoxical reaction to buspirone augmentation of fluoxetine. J Clin Psychopharmacol. 1990;10:377. Letter.

## Buspirone (BuSpar)

## Itraconazole (Sporanox)

Summary: Itraconazole administration results in a large increase in buspirone concentrations; increased buspirone side effects are likely to result.

Risk Factors: No specific risk factors known.

Related Drugs: Other azole antifungals that inhibit CYP3A4 such as **ketoconazole (Nizoral)** are likely to produce similar effects on buspirone pharmacokinetics. Noninhibiting antifungals include **terbinafine (Lamisil)**. Other anxiolytics such as **midazolam (Versed)** and **triazolam (Halcion)** are known to be inhibited by itraconazole. Anxiolytics not metabolized by CYP3A4 include **lorazepam (Ativan)** and **temazepam (Restoril)**.

Management Options:
- *Consider Alternative.* The use of a noninhibiting antifungal (see Related Drugs) should be considered for patients taking buspirone. Anxiolytics not metabolized by CYP3A4 could be substituted for buspirone.

- *Monitor.* Patients receiving buspirone should be monitored for increased sedation if itraconazole is administered.

References:
1. Kivisto KT et al. Plasma buspirone concentrations are greatly increased by erythromycin and itraconazole. Clin Pharmacol Ther. 1997;62:348.

### Calcium

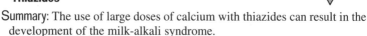

### Thiazides

Summary: The use of large doses of calcium with thiazides can result in the development of the milk-alkali syndrome.

Risk Factors:
- *Dosage Regimen.* Excessive doses of calcium appear to increase the risk of interaction.

Related Drugs: No information available.

Management Options:
- *Circumvent/Minimize.* Patients should be cautioned against excessive or prolonged self-administration of calcium, particularly if they are taking thiazides.
- *Monitor* for evidence of hypercalcemia in patients taking thiazides and calcium concurrently.

References:
1. Gora ML et al. Milk-alkali syndrome associated with use of chlorothiazide and calcium carbonate. Clin Pharm. 1989;8:227.
2. Hakim R et al. Severe hypercalcemia associated with hydrochlorothiazide and calcium carbonate therapy. Can Med Assoc J. 1979;8:591.

### Captopril (Capoten)

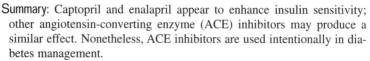

### Insulin

Summary: Captopril and enalapril appear to enhance insulin sensitivity; other angiotensin-converting enzyme (ACE) inhibitors may produce a similar effect. Nonetheless, ACE inhibitors are used intentionally in diabetes management.

Risk Factors: No specific risk factors known.

Related Drugs: Little is known regarding the effect of other ACE inhibitors on insulin sensitivity, but it may be similar to captopril and **enalapril (Vasotec)**.

Management Options:
- *Circumvent/Minimize.* Diabetic patients should be aware of an increased risk of hypoglycemia (symptoms include tachycardia, tremor, sweating) and potentially reduced antidiabetic drug requirements when ACE inhibitors are given concurrently.

## Significance Classification

1. - *Avoid Combination.* Risk always outweighs benefit.
2. - *Usually Avoid Combination.* Use combination only under special circumstances.
3. - *Minimize Risk.* Take action as necessary to reduce risk.

- *Monitor* for altered hypoglycemic effect if ACE inhibitor therapy is initiated, discontinued, or changed in dosage; adjust insulin dose as needed.

References:

1. Ferriere M et al. Captopril and insulin sensitivity. Ann Intern Med. 1985;102:134.
2. Arsuz-pacheco C et al. Hypoglycemia induced by angiotensin-converting enzyme inhibitors in patients with non-insulin-dependent diabetes receiving sulfonylurea therapy. Am J Med. 1990;89:811.
3. Herings RMC et al. Hypoglycaemia associated with use of inhibitors of angiotensin-converting enzyme. Lancet. 1995;345:1195.

## Carbamazepine (Tegretol)

### Clarithromycin (Biaxin)

Summary: Clarithromycin administration appears to increase carbamazepine concentrations; carbamazepine toxicity could result.

Risk Factors: No specific risk factors known.

Related Drugs: **Erythromycin** and **troleandomycin (TAO)** also are known to inhibit the metabolism of carbamazepine. **Azithromycin (Zithromax)** and **dirithromycin (Dynabac)** would be unlikely to decrease carbamazepine me-tabolism.

Management Options:

- *Consider Alternative.* Azithromycin does not appear to affect carbamazepine metabolism.
- *Monitor.* Until further information is available, patients maintained on carbamazepine should be carefully monitored for changing serum concentrations following the addition of clarithromycin.

References:

1. Albani F et al. Clarithromycin-carbamazepine interaction: a case report. Epilepsia. 1993;34:161.
2. Metz DC et al. *Helicobacter pylori* gastritis therapy with omeprazole and clarithromycin increases serum carbamazepine levels. Dig Dis Sci. 1995;40:912.6

## Carbamazepine (Tegretol)

### Clozapine (Clozaril)

Summary: Carbamazepine appears to considerably reduce clozapine plasma concentrations, but the clinical importance of this effect is not established.

Risk Factors: No specific risk factors known.

Related Drugs: Other enzyme-inducing anticonvulsants such as **phenytoin (Dilantin)**, **primidone (Mysoline)**, and barbiturates may have a similar effect.

Management Options:

- *Monitor.* Although more information is needed, one should monitor for altered clozapine response if carbamazepine therapy is initiated, discontinued, or changed in dosage.

References:

1. Jerling M et al. Fluvoxamine inhibition and carbamazepine induction of the metabolism of clozapine: evidence from a therapeutic drug monitoring service. Ther Drug Monit. 1994;16:368.
2. Tiihonen J et al. Carbamazepine induced changes in plasma levels of neuroleptics. Pharmacopsychiatry. 1995;28:26.

### Carbamazepine (Tegretol)

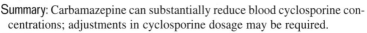

### Cyclosporine (Sandimmune)

Summary: Carbamazepine can substantially reduce blood cyclosporine concentrations; adjustments in cyclosporine dosage may be required.

Risk Factors: No specific risk factors known.

Related Drugs: Other enzyme-inducing anticonvulsants, such as *phenobarbital*, *phenytoin (Dilantin)*, and *primidone (Mysoline)*, also appear to reduce blood cyclosporine concentrations,[3] but in some cases *valproic acid (Depakene)* was successfully substituted for carbamazepine without evidence of interaction.[1,2] *Tacrolimus (Prograf)* probably is affected similarly by enzyme inducers.

Management Options:

- *Consider Alternative.* The interaction can be avoided (based upon limited clinical evidence) when valproic acid can be substituted for carbamazepine.

- *Monitor.* Be alert for evidence of altered cyclosporine effect if carbamazepine therapy is initiated or discontinued; monitor blood cyclosporine concentrations carefully.

References:

1. Schofield OMV et al. Cyclosporine A in psoriasis: interaction with carbamazepine. Br J Dermatol. 1990;122:425. Letter.
2. Hillebrand G et al. Valproate for epilepsy in renal transplant recipients receiving cyclosporine. Transplantation. 1987;43:915.
3. Yee GC et al. Pharmacokinetic drug interactions with cyclosporine (Part I). Clin Pharmacokinet. 1990;19:319.

### Carbamazepine (Tegretol)

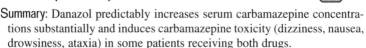

### Danazol (Danocrine)

Summary: Danazol predictably increases serum carbamazepine concentrations substantially and induces carbamazepine toxicity (dizziness, nausea, drowsiness, ataxia) in some patients receiving both drugs.

Risk Factors: No specific risk factors known.

Related Drugs: No information available.

Management Options:

- *Avoid Unless Benefit Outweighs Risk.* If possible, avoid danazol in patients receiving carbamazepine.

- *Monitor.* Patients on carbamazepine should be monitored for evidence of carbamazepine toxicity for several weeks after danazol is initiated. Carbamazepine dosage may need to be reduced. Stopping danazol therapy may result in decreasing carbamazepine serum concentrations and response, necessitating an increase in carbamazepine dosage.

References:
1. Kramer G et al. Carbamazepine-danazol drug interaction: its mechanism examined by a stable isotope technique. Ther Drug Monit. 1986;8:387.
2. Zielinski JJ et al. Clinically significant danazol-carbamazepine interaction. Ther Drug Monit. 1987;9:24.

## Carbamazepine (Tegretol)

### Diltiazem (Cardizem)

**2**

Summary: Diltiazem increases carbamazepine serum concentrations, and frequently results in carbamazepine toxicity.

Risk Factors: No specific risk factors known.

Related Drugs: Verapamil also can produce carbamazepine toxicity, but limited evidence suggests that nifedipine is less likely to do so. Felodipine undergoes extensive first-pass metabolism and is highly susceptible to enzyme induction; thus, it may be difficult to achieve therapeutic felodipine concentrations in the presence of carbamazepine. (Also see Carbamazepine/Verapamil and Carbamazepine/Felodipine monographs.)

Management Options:
- *Avoid Unless Benefit Outweighs Risk.* Given the high likelihood of carbamazepine toxicity with concurrent use and the possibility of reduced diltiazem effect, it would be best to avoid the combination if possible. (See Related Drugs section above for possible alternative calcium channel blockers.)
- *Monitor.* If the combination is used, monitor for carbamazepine toxicity (e.g., nausea, vomiting, dizziness, drowsiness, headache, diplopia, and confusion). Toxic symptoms are likely to occur within 2 to 3 days of starting diltiazem.

References:
1. Bahls F et al. Interactions between calcium channel blockers and the anticonvulsants carbamazepine and phenytoin. Neurol. 1991;41:740.
2. Gadde K et al. Diltiazem effect on carbamazepine levels in manic depression. J Clin Psych. 1990;10:378.
3. Ahmad S. Diltiazem-carbamazepine interaction. Am Heart J. 1990;120:1485.

## Carbamazepine (Tegretol)

### Doxycycline (Vibramycin)

**3**

Summary: Doxycycline serum concentrations may be reduced by carbamazepine.

Risk Factors: No specific risk factors known.

Related Drugs: The effect of carbamazepine on other tetracyclines has not been established, but an interaction does not seem likely since they are largely excreted renally.

Management Options:
- *Monitor.* When carbamazepine and doxycycline are used concomitantly, be alert for a decreased clinical response to doxycycline.

References:
1. Penttila O et al. Interaction between doxycycline and some antiepileptic drugs. Br Med J. 1974;2:470.

## Carbamazepine (Tegretol)

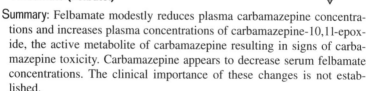

### Erythromycin

Summary: Erythromycin markedly increases serum carbamazepine concentrations; numerous cases of carbamazepine toxicity have been reported in patients receiving both drugs.

Risk Factors: No specific risk factors known.

Related Drugs: *Troleandomycin (TAO)* and *clarithromycin (Biaxin)* also may produce carbamazepine toxicity. *Azithromycin (Zithromax)* and *dirithromycin (Dynabac)* would not be likely to cause carbamazepine toxicity.

Management Options:
- *Consider Alternative.* If possible, erythromycin and troleandomycin should be avoided in patients receiving carbamazepine. Azithromycin does not appear to affect carbamazepine.
- *Monitor.* If erythromycin is used in patients receiving carbamazepine, they should be monitored for evidence of carbamazepine toxicity (dizziness, drowsiness, nausea, vomiting, ataxia, headache, nystagmus, blurred vision), and the dose of carbamazepine should be reduced if necessary. Carbamazepine dosage may need to be increased when the erythromycin is stopped.

References:
1. Jaster PJ et al. Erythromycin-carbamazepine interaction. Neurology. 1986;36:594.
2. McNab AJ et al. Heart block secondary to erythromycin-induced carbamazepine toxicity. Pediatrics. 1987;80:951.
3. Mitsch RA. Carbamazepine toxicity precipitated by intravenous erythromycin. Drug Intell Clin Pharm. 1989;23:878.

## Carbamazepine (Tegretol)

### Felbamate (Felbatol)

Summary: Felbamate modestly reduces plasma carbamazepine concentrations and increases plasma concentrations of carbamazepine-10,11-epoxide, the active metabolite of carbamazepine resulting in signs of carbamazepine toxicity. Carbamazepine appears to decrease serum felbamate concentrations. The clinical importance of these changes is not established.

Risk Factors: No specific risk factors known.

Related Drugs: No information available.

Management Options:
- *Monitor.* Serum concentrations of carbamazepine epoxide are not usually clinically available; therefore, patients need to be monitored for signs of carbamazepine toxicity that may occur concurrent with reductions in serum carbamazepine. Symptoms of carbamazepine toxicity include drowsiness, dizziness, nausea, vomiting, ataxia, headache, nystagmus, and blurred vision. It is not clear whether an alteration in felbamate dosage is needed when carbamazepine therapy is initiated or discontinued.

References:
1. Graves NM et al. Effects of felbamate on phenytoin and carbamazepine serum concentrations. Epilepsia. 1989;30:488.
2. Albani F et al. Effect of felbamate on plasma levels of carbamazepine and its metabolites. Epilepsia. 1991;32:130.
3. Wagner ML et al. Discontinuation of phenytoin and carbamazepine in patients receiving felbamate. Epilepsia. 1991;32:398.

### Carbamazepine (Tegretol)

### Felodipine (Plendil)

**2**

Summary: Felodipine bioavailability may be reduced dramatically in the presence of carbamazepine therapy.

Risk Factors: No specific risk factors known.

Related Drugs: Most calcium channel blockers have reduced bioavailability in the presence of enzyme inducers, but felodipine is probably one of the most markedly affected. Some calcium channel blockers (e.g., diltiazem and verapamil) can produce carbamazepine toxicity. (Also see Carbamazepine/Diltiazem and Carbamazepine/Verapamil monographs.)

Management Options:
- *Avoid Unless Benefit Outweighs Risk.* Since it may prove difficult to achieve therapeutic felodipine concentrations in the presence of carbamazepine, even if the felodipine dose is increased, it may be prudent to avoid concurrent use when possible. Keep in mind that the metabolism of most, if not all, calcium channel blockers is enhanced by enzyme inducers, and some calcium channel blockers (e.g., diltiazem, verapamil) regularly produce carbamazepine toxicity.

## Significance Classification

(1) - **Avoid Combination.** Risk always outweighs benefit.

(2) - **Usually Avoid Combination.** Use combination only under special circumstances.

(3) - **Minimize Risk.** Take action as necessary to reduce risk.

- *Monitor.* If felodipine or another calcium channel blocker is used with carbamazepine, monitor for reduced calcium channel blocker response.

References:
1. Capewell S et al. Gross reduction in felodipine bioavailability in patients taking anticonvulsants. Br J Clin Pharmacol. 1987;24:243P.

## Carbamazepine (Tegretol)

### Fluoxetine (Prozac)

Summary: Case reports describe carbamazepine toxicity, parkinsonism, and serotonin syndrome with concurrent use of fluoxetine, but data from pharmacokinetic studies are conflicting; one study found increased carbamazepine plasma concentrations, and another did not.

Risk Factors: No specific risk factors known.

Related Drugs: *Fluvoxamine (Floxyfral)* inhibits CYP3A4 and would be expected to inhibit carbamazepine metabolism. The effect of *paroxetine (Paxil)* and *sertraline (Zoloft)* on CYP3A4 is not established (but is being studied).

Management Options:
- *Monitor.* Until additional information is available to resolve this interaction, monitor for altered carbamazepine response if fluoxetine is initiated, discontinued, or changed in dosage. Also be alert for evidence of parkinsonism or a serotonin syndrome in patients receiving the combination.

References:
1. Grimsley SR et al. Increased carbamazepine plasma concentrations after fluoxetine coadministration. Clin Pharmacol Ther. 1991;50:10.
2. Spina E et al. Carbamazepine coadministration with fluoxetine or fluvoxamine. Ther Drug Monit. 1993;15:247.
3. Gidal BE et al. Evaluation of the effect of fluoxetine on the formation of carbamazepine epoxide. Ther Drug Monit. 1993;15:405.

## Carbamazepine (Tegretol)

### Fluvoxamine (Floxyfral)

Summary: Case reports suggest that fluvoxamine can increase plasma carbamazepine concentrations to toxic levels, while one study in epileptic patients found no effect of fluvoxamine on carbamazepine. More study is needed to resolve these conflicting results.

Risk Factors: No specific risk factors known.

Related Drugs: Isolated reports suggest that *fluoxetine (Prozac)* and *sertraline (Zoloft)* may increase carbamazepine serum concentrations, but a causal relationship was not established. Preliminary evidence suggests that *paroxetine (Paxil)* does not affect carbamazepine plasma concentrations, but more study is needed.

Management Options:
- *Monitor.* Until additional information is available to resolve this interaction, monitor for altered carbamazepine response if fluvoxamine is initiated, discontinued, or changed in dosage.

References:
1. Fritze J et al. Interaction between carbamazepine and fluvoxamine. Acta Psychiatr Scand. 1991;84:583.
2. Spina E et al. Carbamazepine coadministration with fluoxetine of fluvoxamine. Ther Drug Monit. 1993;15:247.

## Carbamazepine (Tegretol)

## Haloperidol (Haldol)

Summary: Carbamazepine appears to decrease serum haloperidol concentrations and inhibit the response to haloperidol in some patients.

Risk Factors: No specific risk factors known.

Related Drugs: The effect of carbamazepine on other butyrophenones is not established.

Management Options:
- *Monitor.* Be alert for evidence of reduced haloperidol effect if carbamazepine is given concurrently.

References:
1. Arana GW et al. Does carbamazepine-induced reduction of plasma haloperidol levels worsen psychotic symptoms? Am J Psychiatry. 1986;143:650.
2. Kidron R et al. Carbamazepine-induced reduction of blood levels of haloperidol in chronic schizophrenia. Biol Psychiatry. 1985;20:219.
3. Kahn EM et al. Change in haloperidol level due to carbamazepine: a complicating factor in combined medication for schizophrenia. J Clin Psychopharmacol. 1990; 10:54.

## Carbamazepine (Tegretol)

## Imipramine (Tofranil)

Summary: Preliminary evidence suggests that carbamazepine reduces serum concentrations of imipramine; other cyclic antidepressants probably are affected similarly.

Risk Factors: No specific risk factors known.

Related Drugs: Since cyclic antidepressants are metabolized primarily by the liver, one would expect most of them to be affected by carbamazepine. In one retrospective analysis, patients on concurrent carbamazepine therapy had significantly lower concentration/dose ratios of *amitriptyline (Elavil)* (n = 10) and *nortriptyline (Pamelor)* (n = 8) when compared to patients on monotherapy.[3] In addition, carbamazepine increased the oral clearance of single doses of *desipramine (Norpramin)* by 30% in 6 normal volunteers.[2] The effect of carbamazepine on other cyclic antidepressants is not known, but since most of them are extensively metabolized by the liver, they probably would also be affected by carbamazepine therapy.

Management Options:
- *Monitor.* Patients on chronic carbamazepine therapy may require larger than expected doses of cyclic and related antidepressants. Monitor patients for altered response to these antidepressants if carbamazepine therapy is started or stopped.

References:
1. De La Fuente JM. Carbamazepine-induced low plasma levels of tricyclic antidepressants. J Clin Psychopharmacol. 1991;12:67.
2. Spina E et al. The effect of carbamazepine on the 2-hydroxylation of desipramine. Psychopharmacology. 1995;117:413.
3. Jerling M et al. The use of therapeutic drug monitoring data to document kinetic drug interactions: an example with amitriptyline and nortriptyline. Ther Drug Monit. 1994;16:1.

### Carbamazepine (Tegretol)
### Isoniazid (INH)

Summary: Isoniazid appears to increase serum carbamazepine concentrations in most patients; symptoms of carbamazepine toxicity may occur. The interaction seems most likely to occur with INH doses of 200 mg/day or more, and carbamazepine toxicity may occur within the first day or two of INH therapy.

Risk Factors:
- *Dosage Regimen.* INH doses >200 mg/day can increase the risk of interaction.

Related Drugs: No information available.

Management Options:
- *Monitor.* Isoniazid is likely to reduce the dosage requirements for carbamazepine in a majority of patients. Watch for symptoms of carbamazepine toxicity (dizziness, drowsiness, nausea, vomiting, ataxia, headache, nystagmus, blurred vision), and monitor serum carbamazepine concentrations if possible. Monitor for evidence of reduced serum carbamazepine concentrations when INH is discontinued or reduced in dosage.

References:
1. Block SH. Carbamazepine-isoniazid interaction. Pediatrics. 1982;69:494.
2. Valsalan VC et al. Carbamazepine intoxication caused with isoniazid. Br Med J. 1982;285:261.
3. Wright JM et al. Isoniazid-induced carbamazepine toxicity and vice versa. N Engl J Med. 1982;307:1325.

### Carbamazepine (Tegretol)
### Isotretinoin (Accutane)

Summary: In one patient, isotretinoin decreased the area under the concentration-time curve (AUC) of both carbamazepine and carbamazepine epoxide, the active metabolite of carbamazepine. The clinical importance of this effect is unknown.

Risk Factors: No specific risk factors known.

Related Drugs: No information available.

Management Options:

- *Monitor.* Be alert for evidence of a reduced response to carbamazepine if isotretinoin is given concurrently. Until the clinical significance of this interaction is determined, monitor plasma concentrations of carbamazepine more frequently when the 2 drugs are given concurrently.

References:

1. Marsden JR. Effect of isotretinoin on carbamazepine pharmacokinetics. Br J Dermatol. 1988;119:403.

## Carbamazepine (Tegretol)

### Lamotrigine (Lamictal)

Summary: Lamotrigine may increase the carbamazepine epoxide to carbamazepine ratio and result in signs of carbamazepine toxicity. Carbamazepine reduces the concentrations of lamotrigine. The clinical importance of these changes in not established.

Risk Factors: No specific risk factors known.

Related Drugs: No information available.

Management Options:

- *Monitor.* Serum concentrations of carbamazepine epoxide usually are not clinically available; therefore, patients need to be monitored for signs of carbamazepine toxicity that may occur concurrent with reductions in serum carbamazepine. Symptoms of carbamazepine toxicity include drowsiness, dizziness, nausea, vomiting, ataxia, headache, nystagmus, and blurred vision. Doses of carbamazepine may need to be reduced. It is not clear whether an alteration in lamotrigine dosage is needed when carbamazepine therapy is initiated or discontinued.

References:

1. Warner T et al. Lamotrigine induced carbamazepine toxicity: an interaction with carbamazepine-10,11-epoxide. Epilepsy Res. 1992;11:147.
2. Graves N et al. Effect of lamotrigine on the carbamazepine epoxide concentrations. Epilepsia. 1991;32(Suppl. 3):13.
3. Pisani F et al. Single dose pharmacokinetics of carbamazepine-10,11-epoxide in patients on lamotrigine monotherapy. Epilepsy Res. 1994;19:245.

## Significance Classification

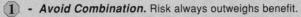

①  - *Avoid Combination.* Risk always outweighs benefit.

②  - *Usually Avoid Combination.* Use combination only under special circumstances.

③  - *Minimize Risk.* Take action as necessary to reduce risk.

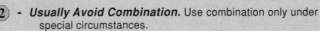

## Carbamazepine (Tegretol)

## Lithium (Eskalith)

**Summary:** Several cases of neurotoxicity (in the absence of toxic serum lithium concentrations) have been reported in patients receiving lithium and carbamazepine, but the combination also has been used to advantage in some manic patients. Lithium reverses carbamazepine-induced leukopenia but additive antithyroidal effects also can occur.

**Risk Factors:** No specific risk factors known.

**Related Drugs:** No information available.

**Management Options:**

- *Monitor.* Be alert for evidence of lithium toxicity when carbamazepine is given concurrently. It is not yet established whether plasma lithium concentrations are useful in monitoring this interaction since the carbamazepine might increase the effect of lithium without increasing plasma lithium concentrations.

**References:**

1. Chaudhry RP et al. Lithium and carbamazepine interaction: possible neurotoxicity. J Clin Psychiatry. 1983;44:30.
2. Laird KL et al. The use of carbamazepine and lithium in controlling a case of chronic rapid cycling. Pharmacotherapy. 1987;7:130.
3. Kramlinger KG et al. Addition of lithium carbonate to carbamazepine: hematological and thyroid effects. Am J Psychiatry. 1990;147:5.

## Carbamazepine (Tegretol)

## Mebendazole (Vermox)

**Summary:** Carbamazepine decreases plasma mebendazole concentrations. This may be most important when large oral doses of mebendazole are used for the treatment of *Echinococcus multilocularis* or *Echinococcus granulosus* (hydatid disease).

**Risk Factors:** No specific risk factors known.

**Related Drugs:** Theoretically, carbamazepine could affect *thiabendazole (Mintezol)* in a similar manner.

**Management Options:**

- *Consider Alternative.* No special precautions appear necessary during cotherapy with carbamazepine in patients receiving mebendazole to treat intestinal helminths. However, in patients receiving mebendazole for tissue-dwelling organisms, enzyme-inducing drugs should be avoided if possible. If carbamazepine is being used for seizures in such patients, valproic acid could be considered as an alternative to carbamazepine, since it does not appear to reduce plasma mebendazole concentrations.

- *Monitor.* If carbamazepine is used with mebendazole (for tissue-dwelling organisms) monitor for reduced mebendazole effect.

References:
1. Luder PJ et al. Treatment of hydatid disease with high oral doses of mebendazole. Long-term follow-up of plasma mebendazole levels and drug interactions. Eur J Clin Pharmacol. 1986;31:443.
2. Witassek F et al. Chemotherapy of larval echinococcus with mebendazole: microsomal liver function and cholestasis as determinants of plasma drug level. Eur J Clin Pharmacol. 1983;25:85.
3. Bekhti A et al. A correlation between serum mebendazole concentrations and the aminopyrine breath test. Implications in the treatment of hydatid disease. Br J Clin Pharmacol. 1986;21:223.

## Carbamazepine (Tegretol)

## Methadone (Dolophine)

Summary: Carbamazepine may decrease serum methadone concentrations, thereby increasing symptoms associated with narcotic withdrawal.

Risk Factors: No specific risk factors known.

Related Drugs: Other enzyme-inducing drugs [e.g., barbiturates, *phenytoin (Dilantin)*] may interact similarly.

Management Options:
• *Monitor.* Patients receiving enzyme inducers such as carbamazepine may require larger doses of methadone than patients who are not on enzyme inducers. Observe for symptoms of methadone withdrawal such as lacrimation, rhinorrhea, sweating, restlessness, insomnia, and piloerection.

References:
1. Bell J et al. The use of serum methadone levels in patients receiving methadone maintenance. Clin Pharmacol Ther. 1988;43:623.

## Carbamazepine (Tegretol)

## Metronidazole (Flagyl)

Summary: Metronidazole may increase carbamazepine plasma concentrations resulting in symptoms of toxicity (e.g., dizziness, nausea, diplopia).

Risk Factors: No specific risk factors known.

Related Drugs: No information available.

Management Options:
• *Monitor.* Until more definitive studies of this interaction are available, patients receiving carbamazepine should be monitored for altered response and plasma concentrations if metronidazole therapy is initiated or discontinued.

References:
1. Patterson BD. Possible interaction between metronidazole and carbamazepine. Ann Pharmacother. 1994;28:1303. Letter.

## Carbamazepine (Tegretol)

### Midazolam (Versed)

Summary: Carbamazepine markedly reduces the effect of oral midazolam, but parenteral midazolam is likely to be less affected.

Risk Factors:
- *Route of Administration.* Since the majority of the interaction is likely due to increased presystemic metabolism of oral midazolam by the gut wall and liver, parenteral midazolam is likely to be much less affected.

Related Drugs: *Triazolam (Halcion)* and *alprazolam (Xanax)* and to some extent *diazepam (Valium)* also are metabolized by CYP3A4 and would be expected to interact with enzyme inducers in a manner similar to midazolam.

Management Options:
- *Consider Alternative.* When midazolam is used orally as a sedative-hypnotic (as it is in several countries) patients receiving enzyme inducers such as carbamazepine are unlikely to respond unless very large doses of midazolam are used. Thus, it may be preferable to use alternative sedative-hypnotics in such patients.
- *Monitor.* Although parenteral midazolam is likely to be much less affected, monitor for inadequate midazolam effect and increase its dose if needed.

References:
1. Backman JT et al. Concentrations and effects of oral midazolam are greatly reduced in patients treated with carbamazepine or phenytoin. Epilepsia. 1996;37:253.

## Carbamazepine (Tegretol)

### Oral Contraceptives

Summary: Carbamazepine and other enzyme-inducing anticonvulsants, such as barbiturates, phenytoin, and primidone, can inhibit the effect of oral contraceptives, resulting in menstrual irregularities and unplanned pregnancies.

Risk Factors:
- *Dosage Regimen.* Oral contraceptives with lower doses of hormones can increase the risk of interaction.

Related Drugs: *Phenytoin (Dilantin)* interacts similarly. *Valproic acid* does not appear to affect the pharmacokinetics of oral contraceptives;[2] benzodiazepine anticonvulsants are unlikely to affect oral contraceptive efficacy.

Management Options:
- *Consider Alternative.* When pregnancy is to be avoided in women receiving carbamazepine or other enzyme-inducing anticonvulsants such as phenobarbital, phenytoin, and primidone, other means of contraception instead of, or in addition to, oral contraceptives should be considered. Although an oral contraceptive with a higher estrogen content would be preferable for some women who are

being treated with enzyme-inducing anticonvulsants, such a decision should be individualized based upon patient response (e.g., lack of breakthrough bleeding).

• *Monitor.* Spotting or breakthrough bleeding in patients taking oral contraceptives and enzyme-inducing anticonvulsants could indicate that the drugs are interacting, although lack of breakthrough bleeding does not ensure contraceptive protection.[3]

References:

1. Crawford P et al. The interaction of phenytoin and carbamazepine with combined oral contraceptive steroids. Br J Clin Pharmacol. 1990;30:892.
2. Crawford P et al. The lack of effect of sodium valproate on the pharmacokinetics of oral contraceptive steroids. Contraception. 1986;33:23.
3. Mattson RH et al. Use of oral contraceptives by women with epilepsy. JAMA. 1986;256:238.

## Carbamazepine (Tegretol)

### Phenytoin (Dilantin)

**Summary:** Combined use of phenytoin and carbamazepine may decrease the serum concentrations of both drugs. In some patients, however, phenytoin concentrations may increase or stay the same when carbamazepine is added.

**Risk Factors:** No specific risk factors known.

**Related Drugs:** No information available.

**Management Options:**

• *Monitor.* During coadministration of phenytoin and carbamazepine, serum concentrations of carbamazepine and phenytoin could decrease or phenytoin serum concentrations could increase. Plasma concentrations of both phenytoin and carbamazepine should be monitored during dosage changes. Patients also should be monitored clinically to determine if a change of dosage of either drug is required.

References:

1. Levy RH et al. Pharmacokinetics of carbamazepine in normal man. Clin Pharmacol Ther. 1977;17:657.
2. Zielinski JJ et al. Dual effects of carbamazepine-phenytoin interaction. Ther Drug Monit. 1987;9:21.
3. Brown TR et al. Carbamazepine increases phenytoin serum concentrations and reduces phenytoin clearance. Neurology. 1988;38:1146.

## Significance Classification

① - *Avoid Combination.* Risk always outweighs benefit.

② - *Usually Avoid Combination.* Use combination only under special circumstances.

③ - *Minimize Risk.* Take action as necessary to reduce risk.

### Carbamazepine (Tegretol)

### Propoxyphene (Darvocet-N)

Summary: Propoxyphene markedly increases plasma carbamazepine concentrations; carbamazepine toxicity is likely to occur in most patients receiving both drugs.

Risk Factors: No specific risk factors known.

Related Drugs: Other analgesics have not been shown to interact with carbamazepine.

Management Options:
- *Use Alternative.* Use analgesics other than propoxyphene in patients receiving carbamazepine.

References:
1. Hansen BS et al. Influence of dextropropoxyphene on steady state serum levels and protein binding of three antiepileptic drugs in man. Acta Neurol Scand. 1980; 61:357.
2. Kubacka RT et al. Carbamazepine-propoxyphene interaction. Clin Pharm. 1983; 2:104.
3. Yu YL et al. Interaction between carbamazepine and dextropropoxyphene. Postgrad Med J. 1986;62:231.

### Carbamazepine (Tegretol)

### Theophylline

Summary: Carbamazepine may reduce serum theophylline concentrations, thus increasing theophylline dosage requirements.

Risk Factors: No specific risk factors known.

Related Drugs: No information available.

Management Options:
- *Monitor.* Be alert for evidence of altered theophylline serum levels when carbamazepine is initiated, discontinued, or changed in dosage.

References:
1. Reed RC et al. Phenytoin-theophylline-quinidine interactions. N Engl J Med. 1983; 308:724.
2. Rosenberry KR et al. Reduced theophylline half-life induced by carbamazepine therapy. J Pediatr. 1983;102:472.

### Carbamazepine (Tegretol)

### Thyroid

Summary: Carbamazepine appears to increase the elimination of thyroid and may increase the requirements for thyroid in hypothyroid patients.

Risk Factors: No specific risk factors known.

Related Drugs: Other enzyme inducers [e.g., **phenytoin (Dilantin)**, **rifampin (Rifadin)**] also appear to interact similarly.

Management Options:
- *Monitor.* If carbamazepine therapy is initiated or discontinued in hypothyroid patients receiving thyroid replacement therapy, be alert for clinical and laboratory evidence of altered circulating thyroid concentrations. Adjust thyroid dosage as needed.

References:
1. Isley WL. Effect of rifampin therapy on thyroid function tests in a hypothyroid patient on replacement L-thyroxine. Ann Intern Med. 1987;107:517.
2. Connell JMC et al. Changes in circulating thyroid hormones during short-term hepatic enzyme induction with carbamazepine. Eur J Clin Pharmacol. 1984;26:453.
3. Cathro DM et al. Case report: Sub-normal serum thyroxine levels associated with carbamazepine and valproic acid treatment. Nebr Med J. 1985;70:235.

## Carbamazepine (Tegretol)
## Troleandomycin (TAO)

Summary: Troleandomycin may increase plasma carbamazepine concentrations; carbamazepine toxicity has occurred in some patients receiving both drugs.

Risk Factors: No specific risk factors known.

Related Drugs: **Erythromycin** and **clarithromycin (Biaxin)** appear to inhibit carbamazepine metabolism. **Azithromycin (Zithromax)** and **dirithromycin (Dynabac)** would be unlikely to interact with carbamazepine.

Management Options:
- *Consider Alternative.* Avoid concomitant use of troleandomycin and carbamazepine if possible. Azithromycin does not appear to alter carbamazepine metabolism.
- *Monitor.* When both drugs are used, monitor for evidence of carbamazepine toxicity (dizziness, drowsiness, nausea, vomiting, ataxia, headache, nystagmus, blurred vision), and measure plasma carbamazepine concentrations as needed. Monitor for evidence of reduced serum carbamazepine concentrations when troleandomycin is discontinued or reduced in dosage.

References:
1. Dravet C et al. Interaction between carbamazepine and triacetyloleandomycin. Lancet. 1977;2:810. Letter.
2. Mesdjian E et al. Carbamazepine intoxication due to triacetyloleandomycin administration in epileptic patients. Epilepsia. 1980;21:489.

## Carbamazepine (Tegretol)
## Valproic Acid (Depakene)

Summary: Valproic acid can increase, decrease, or have no effect on carbamazepine serum concentrations.[1] Plasma concentrations of carbamazepine-epoxide, the active metabolite, also can increase. Carbamazepine decreases plasma concentrations of valproic acid and larger doses of valproic acid are required to maintain therapeutic steady-state concentrations.[2,3]

Risk Factors: No specific risk factors known.

Related Drugs: No information available.

Management Options:

- *Monitor.* The unpredictability of the effect of valproic acid on total carbamazepine plasma concentrations and carbamazepine-epoxide (which is not routinely monitored) makes interpretation of carbamazepine plasma concentrations difficult when the 2 drugs are used concurrently. Carbamazepine-epoxide contributes significantly to the therapeutic and, possibly, the toxic effects of carbamazepine. Patients should be monitored for symptoms of carbamazepine toxicity and serum carbamazepine concentrations should be measured. Symptoms of carbamazepine toxicity include drowsiness, dizziness, nausea, vomiting, ataxia, headache, nystagmus, and blurred vision. Monitor for a decreased therapeutic response to carbamazepine when valproic acid is discontinued or reduced in dosage. An increase in valproic acid dose may be needed if carbamazepine is added. Monitor for evidence of valproic acid toxicity if carbamazepine is discontinued or reduced in dosage.

References:

1. Acid DJ et al. Sodium valproate in the treatment of intractable seizure disorders: a clinical and electroencephalographic study. Neurology. 1978;28:152.
2. Kondo T et al. The effects of phenytoin and carbamazepine on serum concentrations of mono-unsaturated metabolites of valproic acid. Br J Clin Pharmacol. 1990; 29:116–19.
3. Jann MW et al. Increased valproate serum concentrations upon carbamazepine cessation. Epilepsia. 1988;29:578.

## Carbamazepine (Tegretol)

### Verapamil (Calan)

Summary: Verapamil increases carbamazepine serum concentrations, and frequently results in carbamazepine toxicity.

Risk Factors: No specific risk factors known.

Related Drugs: Diltiazem also can produce carbamazepine toxicity, but limited evidence suggests that nifedipine is less likely to do so. Felodipine undergoes extensive first-pass metabolism and is highly susceptible to enzyme induction; thus, it may be difficult to achieve therapeutic felodipine concentrations in the presence of carbamazepine. (Also see Carbamazepine/Diltiazem and Carbamazepine/Felodipine monographs.)

Management Options:

- *Avoid Unless Benefit Outweighs Risk.* Given the high likelihood of carbamazepine toxicity with concurrent use and the possibility of reduced verapamil effect, it would be best to avoid the combination if possible. (See Related Drugs section above for possible alternative calcium channel blockers.)

- *Monitor.* If the combination is used, monitor for carbamazepine toxicity (e.g., nausea, vomiting, dizziness, drowsiness, headache, diplopia, and confusion). Toxic symptoms are likely to occur within 2 to 3 days of starting the verapamil.

References:
1. Macphee GJ et al. Verapamil potentiates carbamazepine neurotoxicity: a clinically important inhibitory interaction. Lancet. 1986;1:700.
2. Beattie B et al. Verapamil-induced carbamazepine neurotoxicity. Eur Neurol. 1988;28:104.
3. Bahls F et al. Interactions between calcium channel blockers and the anticonvulsants carbamazepine and phenytoin. Neurol. 1991;41:740.

## Carbamazepine (Tegretol)

### Warfarin (Coumadin)

Summary: Carbamazepine inhibits the hypoprothrombinemic response to oral anticoagulants; adjustments in anticoagulant dosage may be required during cotherapy.

Risk Factors: No specific risk factors known.

Related Drugs: Oral anticoagulants other than warfarin are likely to be similarly affected by carbamazepine.

Management Options:

- *Monitor.* Patients taking oral anticoagulants should be monitored for altered hypoprothrombinemic response to warfarin if carbamazepine therapy is initiated, discontinued, or changed in dosage; the anticoagulant dose should be adjusted as needed.

References:
1. Hansen JM et al. Carbamazepine-induced acceleration of diphenylhydantoin and warfarin metabolism in man. Clin Pharmacol Ther. 1971;12:539.
2. Kendall AG et al. Warfarin-carbamazepine interaction. Ann Intern Med. 1981; 94:280.
3. Massey EW. Effect of carbamazepine on coumadin metabolism. Ann Neurol. 1983;13:691.

## Significance Classification

(1) - *Avoid Combination.* Risk always outweighs benefit.

(2) - *Usually Avoid Combination.* Use combination only under special circumstances.

(3) - *Minimize Risk.* Take action as necessary to reduce risk.

## Carbenicillin (Geocillin)

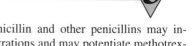

## Methotrexate (Mexate)

Summary: Administration of carbenicillin and other penicillins may increase methotrexate serum concentrations and may potentiate methotrexate toxicity.

Risk Factors: No specific risk factors known.

Related Drugs: Other penicillins administered in large doses could have similar effects on methotrexate. This effect also has been observed during *mezlocillin (Mezlin)* administration with methotrexate.[2]

Management Options:
- *Monitor.* Patients should be monitored for evidence of enhanced methotrexate effect and possible toxicity (e.g., mucositis, leukopenia) when large doses of carbenicillin or other penicillins are given concurrently.

References:
1. Gibson DL et al. Midyear Clinical Meeting Abstracts. American Society of Hospital Pharmacists. New Orleans;1981:305 Dec 6–10.
2. Dean R et al. Possible methotrexate-mezlocillin interaction. Am J Pediatr Hematol Oncol. 1992;141:88. Letter.
3. Mayall B et al. Neutropenia due to low-dose methotrexate therapy for psoriasis and rheumatoid arthritis may be fatal. Med J Aust. 1991;155:480.

## Carboplatin (Paraplatin)

## Gentamicin (Garamycin)

Summary: The combination of carboplatin and aminoglycoside antibiotics causes more hearing loss than would be expected with either agent alone.

Risk Factors: No specific risk factors known.

Related Drugs: It is likely that other aminoglycosides such as *amikacin (Amikin)*, *kanamycin (Kantrex)*, *netilmicin (Netromycin)*, *streptomycin*, and *tobramycin (Nebcin)* also may result in additive ototoxicity with carboplatin.

Management Options:
- *Consider Alternative.* Alternatives to aminoglycosides should be considered in patients receiving high doses of carboplatin.
- *Monitor.* If aminoglycosides are used be alert for evidence of ototoxicity.

References:
1. Lee EJ et al. Phase I and pharmacokinetic trial of carboplatin in refractory adult leukemia. J Natl Cancer Inst. 1988;80:131–35.

## Carmustine (BiCNU)

## Cimetidine (Tagamet)

Summary: Epidemiological evidence indicates that cimetidine increases the myelotoxicity of carmustine.

Risk Factors: No specific risk factors known.

Related Drugs: Little is known regarding the effect of cimetidine on the myelosuppressive effect of other cytotoxic drugs, but one should be alert for such effects. Isolated reports indicate that *chloramphenicol (Chloromycetin)*[1] and *phenytoin (Dilantin)*[2,3] may be more myelosuppressive in the presence of cimetidine. A similar interaction has been reported with *lomustine*, another nitrosourea.[4] Severe myelosuppression developed in a 55-year-old male receiving lomustine and cimetidine, and resolved rapidly upon discontinuation of cimetidine. Myelosuppression from subsequent doses of lomustine, after the cimetidine had been discontinued, was less severe. The effect of other $H_2$-receptor antagonists such as *famotidine (Pepcid), nizatidine (Axid)*, and *ranitidine (Zantac)* on carmustine is not established; theoretically they may be less likely to interact.

Management Options:
- *Monitor.* Until more is known regarding the incidence and magnitude of this potential interaction, one should monitor carefully for evidence of excessive bone marrow suppression when cimetidine is used concurrently with carmustine or other myelosuppressive drugs.
- *Consider Alternative.* Other $H_2$-receptor antagonists theoretically would be less likely to interact.

References:
1. Farber BF et al. Rapid development of aplastic anemia after intravenous chloramphenicol and cimetidine therapy. South Med J. 1981;74:1257.
2. Sazie E et al. Severe granulocytopenia with cimetidine and phenytoin. Ann Intern Med. 1980;93:151.
3. Al-Kawas FH et al. Cimetidine and agranulocytosis. Ann Intern Med. 1979;90:992.
4. Hess WA et al. Combination of lomustine and cimetidine in the treatment of a patient with malignant glioblastoma: a case report. Cancer Treat Rep. 1985;69:733. Letter.

## Cefamandole (Mandol)
## Ethanol (Ethyl Alcohol)

Summary: Cefamandole and some other cephalosporins may cause a disulfiram-like reaction when administered with ethanol.

Risk Factors: No specific risk factors known.

Related Drugs: *Cefoperazone (Cefobid), cefotetan (Cefotan)*, and *moxalactam (Moxam)* also produce disulfiram reactions following alcohol ingestion.

Management Options:
- *Circumvent/Minimize.* Patients should be counseled to avoid alcohol while taking the cephalosporins noted above and for 2 to 3 days after discontinuing the cephalosporin.
- *Monitor.* If ethanol is administered to a patient taking cefamandole or other cephalosporins, be alert for flushing, nausea, headache, or tachycardia.

References:
1. Elenbaas RM et al. On the disulfiram-like activity of moxalactam. Clin Pharmacol Ther. 1982;32:347.

2. Buening MK et al. Disulfiram-like reaction to beta-lactams. JAMA.1981;245:2027.

3. Kline SS et al. Cefotetan-induced disulfiram-type reactions and hypoprothrombinemia. Antimicrob Agents Chemother. 1987;31:1328.

---

### Cefpodoxime Proxetil (Vantin)

### Ranitidine (Zantac)

Summary: Serum concentrations of cefpodoxime proxetil are reduced by concomitant administration of agents that increase gastric pH; antibiotic efficacy may be reduced.

Risk Factors: No specific risk factors known.

Related Drugs: *Cefuroxime axetil (Ceftin)* concentrations are reduced by ranitidine. *Cefetamet pivoxil* and *cefixime (Suprax)* appear to be unaffected by concurrent ranitidine administration. Other $H_2$-receptor antagonists [e.g., *cimetidine (Tagamet), famotidine (Pepcid), nizatidine (Axid)*], antacids, and proton pump inhibitors [e.g., *omeprazole (Prilosec), lansoprazole (Prevacid)*] would be expected to have similar effects.

Management Options:

• *Consider Alternative.* Cefetamet pivoxil pharmacokinetics were not affected by Maalox or ranitidine administration;[1] similarly, cefixime pharmacokinetics were unaffected by antacids.[2] Pending determination of the clinical importance of the changes in serum concentrations, patients receiving cefpodoxime proxetil or cefuroxime axetil should avoid agents that increase gastric pH.

• *Monitor.* If the drugs are used together, watch for diminished antibiotic effect.

References:

1. Blouin RA et al. Influence of antacid and ranitidine on the pharmacokinetics of oral cefetamet pivoxil. Antimicrob Agents Chemother. 1990;34:1744.

2. Petitjean O et al. Study of a possible pharmacokinetic interaction between cefixime and two antacids. Presse Med. 1989;18:1596.

3. Saathoff N et al. Pharmacokinetics of cefpodoxime proxetil and interactions with an antacid and an $H_2$-receptor antagonist. Antimicrob Agents Chemother. 1992; 36:796.

---

### Cefuroxime (Ceftin)

### Ranitidine (Zantac)

Summary: Serum concentrations of cefpodoxime proxetil and cefuroxime axetil are reduced by concomitant administration of agents that increase gastric pH; antibiotic efficacy may be reduced.

Risk Factors: No specific risk factors known.

Related Drugs: *Cefpodoxime (Vantin)* concentrations are reduced following ranitidine administration. *Cefetamet pivoxil* and *cefixime (Suprax)* appear to be unaffected by concurrent ranitidine administration. Other $H_2$-receptor antagonists [e.g., *cimetidine (Tagamet), famotidine (Pepcid), nizatidine (Axid)*] antacids [e.g., *sodium bicarbonate, aluminum* hydroxide *(Amphojel)*], and proton pump inhibitors [e.g., *omeprazole (Prilosec), lansoprazole (Prevacid)*] would be expected to have similar effects.

Management Options:

- *Consider Alternative.* Cefetamet pivoxil pharmacokinetics were not affected by Maalox or ranitidine administration;[1] similarly, cefixime (Suprax) pharmacokinetics were unaffected by antacids.[2] Pending determination of the clinical importance of the changes in serum concentrations, patients receiving cefpodoxime proxetil or cefuroxime axetil should avoid agents that increase gastric pH.
- *Monitor.* If the drugs are used together, watch for diminished antibiotic effect.

References:

1. Blouin RA et al. Influence of antacid and ranitidine on the pharmacokinetics of oral cefetamet pivoxil. Antimicrob Agents Chemother. 1990;34:1744.
2. Petitjean O et al. Study of a possible pharmacokinetic interaction between cefixime and two antacids. Presse Med. 1989;18:1596.
3. Saathoff N et al. Pharmacokinetics of cefpodoxime proxetil and interactions with an antacid and an $H_2$-receptor antagonist. Antimicrob Agents Chemother. 1992; 36:796.

## Cephaloridine

## Furosemide (Lasix)

Summary: The combined use of furosemide and cephaloridine may result in enhanced nephrotoxicity, but only limited evidence indicates that furosemide plus cephalothin would have the same effect.

Risk Factors:

- *Concurrent Diseases.* Renal dysfunction can increase the risk of nephrotoxicity.

Related Drugs: *Cephalothin (Keflin)* interacts similarly. Additionally, *ethacrynic acid (Edecrin)* may affect cephaloridine similarly.

Management Options:

- *Consider Alternative.* If possible, select a cephalosporin other than cephalothin or cephaloridine for patients receiving furosemide.
- *Monitor* renal function in patients with pre-existing renal disease receiving furosemide and cephaloridine.

## Significance Classification

1. - *Avoid Combination.* Risk always outweighs benefit.
2. - *Usually Avoid Combination.* Use combination only under special circumstances.
3. - *Minimize Risk.* Take action as necessary to reduce risk.

References:
1. Simpson IJ. Nephrotoxicity and acute renal failure associated with cephalothin and cephaloridine. NZ Med J. 1971;74:312.
2. Gabriel R et al. Reversible encephalopathy and acute renal failure after cephaloridine. Br Med J. 1970;4:283.
3. Norrby R et al. Interaction between cephaloridine and furosemide in man. Scand J Infect Dis. 1976;8:209.

## Charcoal

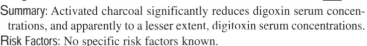

### Digoxin (Lanoxin)

Summary: Activated charcoal significantly reduces digoxin serum concentrations, and apparently to a lesser extent, digitoxin serum concentrations.

Risk Factors: No specific risk factors known.

Related Drugs: **Digitoxin (Crystodigin)** concentrations are also reduced by concomitant charcoal administration, but to an apparently lesser extent than digoxin.

Management Options:
- *Avoid Unless Benefit Outweighs Risk.* Activated charcoal should not be administered to patients taking digoxin since loss of the therapeutic effect of digoxin is likely. This combination might be of benefit in patients with digitalis glycoside intoxication.
- *Monitor.* Patients taking digoxin or digitoxin should be watched for reduced glycoside concentrations if charcoal is coadministered.

References:
1. Neuvonen PJ et al. Effects of resins and activated charcoal on the absorption of digoxin, carbamazepine and furosemide. Br J Clin Pharmacol. 1988;25:229.
2. Reissell P et al. Effect of administration of activated charcoal and fibre on absorption, excretion and steady blood levels of digoxin and digitoxin. Evidence for intestinal secretion of the glycosides. Acta Med Scand. 1982;(Suppl. 668):88.
3. Neuvonen PJ et al. Reduction of absorption of digoxin, phenytoin and aspirin by activated charcoal in man. Eur J Clin Pharmacol. 1978;13:213.

## Chloral Hydrate (Noctec)

### Ethanol (Ethyl Alcohol)

Summary: Ethanol and chloral hydrate have at least additive central nervous system (CNS)-depressant effects; combined use may be dangerous in patients performing tasks requiring alertness.

Risk Factors: No specific risk factors known.

Related Drugs: Alcohol would be expected to increase the CNS depression of all sedative-hypnotic drugs.

Management Options:
- *Circumvent/Minimize.* Patients taking chloral hydrate should be warned of the combined CNS depressant activity with ethanol. Patients with cardiovascular disease who are taking chloral hydrate should be quite careful about ingesting ethanol because the tachycardia and hypotension associated with the vasodilation reaction could adversely affect their disease.

• *Monitor.* If the combination is used, monitor for excessive CNS depression, as well as flushing, headache, and tachycardia.

References:
1. Gessner PK et al. A study of the interaction of the hypnotic effects and of the toxic effects of chloral hydrate and ethanol. J Pharmacol Exp Ther. 1970;174:247.
2. Sellers EM et al. Interaction of chloral hydrate and ethanol in man. I. Metabolism. Clin Pharmacol Ther. 1972;13:37.
3. Sellers EM et al. Interaction of chloral hydrate and ethanol in man. II. Hemodynamics and performance. Clin Pharmacol Ther. 1972;13:50.

### Chloral Hydrate (Noctec)
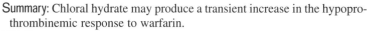
### Warfarin (Coumadin)

Summary: Chloral hydrate may produce a transient increase in the hypoprothrombinemic response to warfarin.

Risk Factors: No specific risk factors known.

Related Drugs: Alternative sedative/hypnotic drugs unlikely to interact with oral anticoagulants include *flurazepam (Dalmane)*, *chlordiazepoxide (Librium)*, *diazepam (Valium)*, or *diphenhydramine (Benadryl)*. Barbiturates would not be suitable alternatives, since they can enhance oral anticoagulant metabolism.

Management Options:
• *Consider Alternative.* Even though the interaction between chloral hydrate and warfarin usually does not cause adverse effects, it is preferable to use hypnotic drugs that do not appear to interact with anticoagulants, such as flurazepam or diazepam.
• *Monitor.* When chloral hydrate is given to a patient receiving an oral anticoagulant, the patient should be monitored for excessive hypoprothrombinemia during the first several days of chloral hydrate therapy. However, long-term coadministration of the 2 drugs probably does not increase the hazard of bleeding significantly.

References:
1. Udall JA. Warfarin-chloral hydrate interaction: pharmacological activity and clinical significance. Ann Intern Med. 1974;81:341.
2. Udall JA. Clinical implications of warfarin interactions with five sedatives. Am J Cardiol. 1975;35:67.
3. Galinsky RE et al. "Post hoc" and hypoprothrombinemia. Ann Intern Med. 1975;83:286.

### Chloramphenicol (Chloromycetin)
### Chlorpropamide (Diabinese)

Summary: Chloramphenicol may increase the hypoglycemic effects of chlorpropamide.

Risk Factors: No specific risk factors known.

Related Drugs: Chloramphenicol has been reported to increase the half-life of *tolbutamide (Orinase)*. The effect of chloramphenicol on other oral antidiabetics is unknown.

Management Options:
- *Monitor.* Patients receiving tolbutamide or chlorpropamide who receive chloramphenicol concurrently should be monitored for hypoglycemia.

References:
1. Petitpierre B et al. Behavior of chlorpropamide in renal insufficiency and under the effect of associated drug therapy. Int J Clin Pharmacol Ther Toxicol. 1972;6:120.
2. Christensen LK et al. Inhibition of drug metabolism by chloramphenicol. Lancet. 1969;2:1397.
3. Brunova E et al. Interaction of tolbutamide and chloramphenicol in diabetic patients. Int J Clin Pharmacol. 1977;15:7.

### Chloramphenicol (Chloromycetin)
### Dicumarol

Summary: Chloramphenicol may enhance the hypoprothrombinemic response to dicumarol and possibly other oral anticoagulants.

Risk Factors:
- *Diet/Food.* Dietary deficiency of vitamin $K^8$ can increase the risk of interaction.

Related Drugs: Although the effect of chloramphenicol on the metabolism of **warfarin (Coumadin)** and other oral anticoagulants has not been established, theoretical considerations suggest that it would be similar to the effect on dicumarol. Warfarin would be expected to interact similarly with chloramphenicol because chloramphenicol is known to inhibit CYP2C9, the enzyme primarily responsible for warfarin metabolism.

Management Options:
- *Use Alternative.* Concomitant use of chloramphenicol and dicumarol should be avoided. Warfarin may not be an acceptable alternative anticoagulant.

References:
1. Koch-Weser J et al. Drug interactions with coumarin anticoagulants (First of two parts). N Engl J Med. 1971;285:487.
2. Koch-Weser J et al. Drug interactions with coumarin anticoagulants (Second of two parts). N Engl J Med. 1971;285:547.
3. Ansell JE et al. The spectrum of vitamin K deficiency. JAMA. 1977;238:40.

## Significance Classification

(1) - **Avoid Combination.** Risk always outweighs benefit.

(2) - **Usually Avoid Combination.** Use combination only under special circumstances.

(3) - **Minimize Risk.** Take action as necessary to reduce risk.

## Chloramphenicol (Chloromycetin)

### Phenobarbital

**Summary:** Chloramphenicol can increase serum barbiturate concentrations, and barbiturates can reduce chloramphenicol concentrations.

**Risk Factors:** No specific risk factors known.

**Related Drugs:** Other barbiturates may be similarly affected by chloramphenicol and could reduce chloramphenicol concentrations as well.

**Management Options:**

- *Circumvent/Minimize.* Increased chloramphenicol dosage may be needed in some patients.

- *Monitor.* In patients receiving phenobarbital (and possibly other barbiturates), watch for evidence of reduced chloramphenicol effect. Also be alert for evidence of increased effect of phenobarbital (and possibly other barbiturates) when chloramphenicol is given concurrently.

**References:**

1. Koup JR et al. Interaction of chloramphenicol with phenytoin and phenobarbital. Case report. Clin Pharmacol Ther. 1978;24:571.
2. Bloxham RA et al. Chloramphenicol and phenobarbitone. A drug interaction. Arch Dis Child. 1979;54:76.

## Chloramphenicol (Chloromycetin)

### Phenytoin (Dilantin)

**Summary:** Chloramphenicol predictably increases serum phenytoin concentrations; symptoms of phenytoin toxicity have occurred. Phenytoin also may affect serum chloramphenicol concentrations, but results have been conflicting.

**Risk Factors:** No specific risk factors known.

**Related Drugs:** No information available.

**Management Options:**

- *Consider Alternative.* If possible, avoid chloramphenicol use in patients receiving phenytoin.

- *Monitor.* Patients who receive both phenytoin and chloramphenicol should be watched closely for signs of phenytoin toxicity (e.g., nystagmus, lethargy, ataxia, rash).

**References:**

1. Saltiel MS et al. Phenytoin-chloramphenicol interaction. Drug Intel Clin Pharm. 1980;14:221.
2. Powell DA et al. Interactions among chloramphenicol, phenytoin, and phenobarbital in a pediatric patient. J Pediatr. 1981;98:1001.
3. Krasinski K et al. Pharmacologic interactions among chloramphenicol, phenytoin and phenobarbital. Pediatr Infect Dis. 1982;1:232.

### Chloramphenicol (Chloromycetin)

### Rifampin (Rifadin)

Summary: Rifampin can reduce chloramphenicol concentrations, potentially reducing its antibacterial efficacy.

Risk Factors: No specific risk factors known.

Related Drugs: No information available.

Management Options:
- *Consider Alternative.* If possible, avoid rifampin use in patients receiving chloramphenicol.
- *Monitor.* Chloramphenicol concentrations should be monitored when rifampin is administered concomitantly.

References:
1. Prober CG. Effect of rifampin on chloramphenicol levels. N Engl J Med. 1985; 312:788.
2. Kelly HW et al. Interaction of chloramphenicol and rifampin. J Pediatr. 1988; 12:817.

### Chlordiazepoxide (Librium)

### Ketoconazole (Nizoral)

Summary: Ketoconazole increases chlordiazepoxide concentrations, but the degree to which chlordiazepoxide adverse effects are increased is not established.

Risk Factors: No specific risk factors known.

Related Drugs: Other antifungal agents [e.g., *itraconazole (Sporanox)*, *fluconazole (Diflucan)*] are likely to increase chlordiazepoxide concentrations. Ketoconazole also inhibits the metabolism of *alprazolam (Xanax)*, *midazolam (Versed)*, and *triazolam (Halcion)*.

Management Options:
- *Monitor.* Patients on chronic chlordiazepoxide who receive ketoconazole should be observed for increased sedation.

References:
1. Brown MW et al. Effect of ketoconazole on hepatic oxidative drug metabolism. Clin Pharmacol Ther. 1985;37:290.

### Chloroquine (Aralen)

### Chlorpromazine (Thorazine)

Summary: Chlorpromazine concentrations are increased by chloroquine and other antimalarial agents; the clinical significance of these changes is unknown.

Risk Factors: No specific risk factors known.

Related Drugs: Other phenothiazines may be similarly affected by chloroquine and other antimalarials. Other antimalarials [e.g., *amodiaquine*, *sulfadoxine-pyrimethamine (Fansidar)*] affect chlorpromazine similarly.

Management Options:
- *Monitor.* Patients maintained on chlorpromazine should be monitored for increased neuroleptic effects if antimalarial agents are prescribed.

References:
1. Makanjuola ROA et al. Effects of antimalarial agents on plasma levels of chlorpromazine and its metabolites in schizophrenic patients. Trop Geogr Med. 1988;40:31.

## Chloroquine (Aralen)
## Cyclosporine (Sandimmune)

Summary: Patients stabilized on cyclosporine may develop elevated cyclosporine concentrations following the addition of chloroquine. Signs and symptoms of cyclosporine toxicity may accompany the interaction.

Risk Factors: No specific risk factors known.

Related Drugs: *Tacrolimus (Prograf)* may be affected similarly by concurrently administered chloroquine.

Management Options:
- *Circumvent/Minimize.* Cyclosporine dosages may require reduction during concomitant chloroquine treatment.
- *Monitor.* Patients taking cyclosporine should be observed carefully for increased cyclosporine concentrations if chloroquine is administered concurrently.

References:
1. Finielz P et al. Interaction between cyclosporin and chloroquine. Nephron. 1993;65:333. Letter.
2. Nampoory MRN et al. Drug interaction of chloroquine with ciclosporin. Nephron. 1992;62:108. Letter.

## Chloroquine (Aralen)
## Methotrexate (Mexate)

Summary: Methotrexate concentrations are reduced by concomitant chloroquine administration; the clinical significance is unknown but some patients could experience reduced methotrexate efficacy.

Risk Factors: No specific risk factors known.

Related Drugs: *Hydroxychloroquine (Plaquenil)* may affect methotrexate in a similar manner.

Management Options:
- *Monitor.* Until more information is available, patients receiving methotrexate should be monitored for loss of efficacy during chloroquine coadministration.

References:
1. Seidman P et al. Chloroquine reduces the bioavailability of methotrexate in patients with rheumatoid arthritis. Arthritis Rheum. 1994;37:830.

### Chloroquine (Aralen)

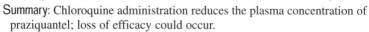

### Praziquantel (Biltricide)

Summary: Chloroquine administration reduces the plasma concentration of praziquantel; loss of efficacy could occur.

Risk Factors: No specific risk factors known.

Related Drugs: *Hydroxychloroquine (Plaquenil)* could affect praziquantel in a similar manner.

Management Options:
- *Monitor.* Until more information is available, patients taking praziquantel should be monitored for reduced plasma concentrations and possible loss of efficacy if they receive chloroquine concurrently.

References:
1. Masimirembwa CM et al. The effect of chloroquine on the pharmacokinetics and metabolism of praziquantel in rats and in humans. Biopharm Drug Dispos. 1994; 15:33.

### Chlorpromfazine (Thorazine)

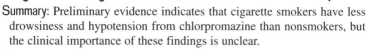

### Cigarette Smoking

Summary: Preliminary evidence indicates that cigarette smokers have less drowsiness and hypotension from chlorpromazine than nonsmokers, but the clinical importance of these findings is unclear.

Risk Factors: No specific risk factors known.

Related Drugs: Little is known regarding the effect of cigarette smoking on the response of other phenothiazines or neuroleptics. It is possible that some of them are similarly affected by cigarette smoking.

Management Options:
- *Monitor.* Be alert for evidence of increased neuroleptic dosage requirements in cigarette smokers and for reduced neuroleptic dosage requirements in patients who stop cigarette smoking.

References:
1. Swett C Jr et al. Hypotension due to chlorpromazine: relation to cigarette smoking, blood pressure and dosage. Arch Gen Psychiatry. 1977;34:661.
2. Panguck EJ et al. Cigarette smoking and chlorpromazine disposition and actions. Clin Pharmacol Ther. 1982;31:533.
3. Stimmel GL et al. Chlorpromazine plasma levels, adverse effects, and tobacco smoking: case report. J Clin Psychiatry. 1983;44:420.

## Significance Classification

**(1)** - *Avoid Combination.* Risk always outweighs benefit.

**(2)** - *Usually Avoid Combination.* Use combination only under special circumstances.

**(3)** - *Minimize Risk.* Take action as necessary to reduce risk.

## Chlorpromazine (Thorazine)

## Clonidine (Catapres)

Summary: Isolated cases of severe hypotensive episodes or delirium have been reported following the concurrent use of clonidine and chlorpromazine, but a causal relationship has not been established.

Risk Factors: No specific risk factors known.

Related Drugs: Other antipsychotics also may interact with clonidine. The combined use of clonidine and *fluphenazine (Prolixin)* was associated with delirium (confusion, disorientation, agitation) in a 33-year-old man,[3] but a causal relationship was not established. Additionally, the combined use of *haloperidol (Haldol)* and clonidine was associated with a case of hypotension.[1] Although little is known regarding the effect of centrally acting alpha-agonists other than clonidine such as *guanabenz (Wytensin)* and *guanfacine (Tenex)*, consider the possibility that they interact with neuroleptic drugs until clinical information is available.

Management Options:
- *Monitor.* Watch for additive hypotensive effects when clonidine and neuroleptics are used concurrently, especially when the neuroleptic is initiated in a patient with impaired cardiac function.

References:
1. Gruncillo RJ et al. Severe hypotension associated with concurrent clonidine and antipsychotic medication. Am J Psychiatry. 1985;142:274.
2. McEvoy GK, ed. AHFS Drug Information 89. Bethesda, MD: American Society of Hospital Pharmacists; 1995:1189.
3. Allen RM et al. Delirium associated with combined fluphenazine-clonidine therapy. J Clin Psychiatry. 1979;40:236.

## Chlorpromazine (Thorazine)

## Epinephrine (Adrenalin)

Summary: Chlorpromazine, and possibly some other phenothiazines, may reverse the pressor response of epinephrine.

Risk Factors: No specific risk factors known.

Related Drugs: Neuroleptics such as *thioridazine (Mellaril)* and *clozapine (Clozaril)* could theoretically interact with epinephrine similarly, but other neuroleptics with a low incidence of postural hypotension may have less effect on alpha-adrenergic receptors and may be less likely to affect epinephrine response [e.g., *fluphenazine (Prolixin)*, *trifluoperazine (Stelazine)*, *haloperidol (Haldol)*, *loxapine (Loxitane)*, *molindone (Moban)*, and *pimozide (Orap)*].

Management Options:
- *Consider Alternative.* It has been suggested that in neuroleptic-treated patients with hypotension, alpha-adrenergic agonists with little beta-adrenergic activity [e.g., phenylephrine (Neo-Synephrine), lev-

arterenol (Levophed)] would be more effective in increasing the blood pressure than epinephrine.[2,3]

- *Monitor* the blood pressure when epinephrine is given to hypotensive patients receiving neuroleptics, particularly chlorpromazine, thioridazine, or clozapine.

References:
1. Yagiela JA et al. Drug interaction and vasoconstrictors used in local anesthetic solutions. Oral Surg Oral Med Oral Pathol. 1985;59:565.
2. Gonzales ER. Catecholamine selection for vasopressor-dependent patients. Clin Pharm. 1988;7:493.
3. Alexander CS. Epinephrine not contraindicated in cardiac arrest attributed to phenothiazine. JAMA. 1976;236:405.

## Chlorpromazine (Thorazine)

## Guanethidine (Ismelin)

Summary: Phenothiazines may inhibit the antihypertensive response to guanethidine.

Risk Factors: No specific risk factors known.

Related Drugs: *Guanadrel (Hylorel)* is pharmacologically similar to guanethidine and also may be inhibited by phenothiazines.

Management Options:
- *Consider Alternative.* Consider using an antihypertensive agent other than guanethidine (or drugs related to guanethidine such as guanadrel). Keep in mind that the intrinsic hypotensive effect of phenothiazines might enhance the effect of antihypertensives other than guanethidine or guanadrel.
- *Monitor.* If the combination is used, monitor blood pressure for evidence of the interaction. If guanethidine antagonism is noted, consider increasing the guanethidine dose, or using an alternative antihypertensive agent.

References:
1. Ober KF et al. Drug interactions with guanethidine. Clin Pharmacol Ther. 1973;14:190.
2. Lahti RA et al. The tricyclic antidepressants: inhibition of norepinephrine uptake as related to potentiation of norepinephrine and clinical efficacy. Biochem Pharmacol. 1971;20:482.
3. Janowsky DS et al. Antagonism of guanethidine by chlorpromazine. Am J Psychiatry. 1973;130:808.

## Chlorpromazine (Thorazine)

## Levodopa (Larodopa)

Summary: Phenothiazines and related neuroleptic agents may inhibit the antiparkinsonian effect of levodopa.

Risk Factors: No specific risk factors known.

Related Drugs: Levodopa also probably is inhibited by butyrophenones [e.g., *haloperidol (Haldol)*] and other neuroleptics.

Management Options:
- *Avoid Unless Benefit Outweighs Risk.* If possible, avoid administration of phenothiazines and other neuroleptics to patients receiving levodopa.
- *Monitor* for reduced levodopa effect if phenothiazines are used.

References:
1. Mims RB et al. Inhibition of L-dopa-induced growth hormone stimulation by pyridoxine and chlorpromazine. J Clin Endocrinol Metab. 1975;40:256.
2. Yaryura-Tobias JA et al. Action of L-dopa in a drug-induced extrapyramidalism. Dis Nerv Syst. 1970;31:60.
3. Yahr MD et al. Drug therapy of parkinsonism. N Engl J Med. 1972;287:20.

## Chlorpromazine (Thorazine)

### Lithium (Eskalith)

Summary: Combined use of lithium and chlorpromazine may lower serum concentrations of both drugs. Rare cases of severe neurotoxicity have been reported in acute manic patients receiving lithium and phenothiazines, especially thioridazine.

Risk Factors:
- *Concurrent Diseases.* Patients with acute manic symptoms appear to be more likely to manifest neurotoxicity with the concurrent use of lithium and phenothiazines.

Related Drugs: Consider the possibility that lithium interacts with other phenothiazines [especially *thioridazine (Mellaril)*] as well. The combined use of *haloperidol (Haldol)* and lithium has been implicated in the production of severe neurotoxic symptoms.

Management Options:
- *Monitor* for neurotoxicity (e.g., delirium, seizures, encephalopathy) with the concurrent use of lithium and phenothiazines (especially thioridazine) in patients with acute manic symptoms. Chronic therapy with these combinations appears less likely to result in an adverse interaction. Although the clinical importance of the pharmacokinetic interactions of phenothiazine and lithium is not well established, be alert for evidence of reduced phenothiazine response in the presence of lithium therapy.

References:
1. Yassa R. A case of lithium-chlorpromazine interaction. J Clin Psychiatry. 1986;47:90.
2. Bailine SH et al. Neurotoxicity induced by combined lithium-thioridazine treatment. Biol Psychiatry. 1986;21:834.
3. Miller F et al. Lithium-neuroleptic neurotoxicity in the elderly bipolar patient. J Clin Psychopharmacol. 1986;6:176.

## Chlorpromazine (Thorazine)

### Meperidine (Demerol)

Summary: The combination of chlorpromazine and meperidine may result in hypotension and excessive central nervous system (CNS) depression.

Risk Factors: No specific risk factors known.

Related Drugs: Whether other combinations of neuroleptics and narcotic analgesics would produce similar effects is unknown, but, in general, one might expect enhanced respiratory depression and hypotension with such combinations.

Management Options:
- *Monitor.* Be alert for evidence of excessive CNS depression, hypotension, and respiratory depression when meperidine and chlorpromazine are used concurrently. Until more information is available, caution also is advised for other combinations of neuroleptics and narcotic analgesics.

References:
1. Stambaugh JE et al. Drug interaction: meperidine and chlorpromazine, a toxic combination. J Clin Pharmacol. 1981;21:140.
2. Swett C et al. Hypotension due to chlorpromazine. Arch Gen Psychiatry. 1977;34: 661.

## Chlorpromazine (Thorazine)

### Orphenadrine (Norflex)

Summary: The combination of orphenadrine and chlorpromazine may result in lower serum chlorpromazine concentrations and excessive anticholinergic effects. Also, a patient on chlorpromazine and orphenadrine developed hypoglycemia; the clinical importance of this effect is unclear.

Risk Factors: No specific risk factors known.

Related Drugs: The effect of orphenadrine combined with other phenothiazines is not established. There was no mention of adverse effects due to drug interaction in 6 patients who were receiving orphenadrine and *fluphenazine (Prolixin)*.[2]

Management Options:
- *Monitor.* In patients on concomitant neuroleptics and orphenadrine, be alert for evidence of excessive anticholinergic effects (especially ileus), reduced neuroleptic plasma concentrations, or hypoglycemia.

References:
1. Loga S et al. Interactions of orphenadrine and phenobarbitone with chlorpromazine: plasma concentrations and effects in man. Br J Clin Pharmacol. 1975;2:197.
2. Fleming P et al. Levodopa in drug-induced extrapyramidal disorders. Lancet. 1970;2:1186. Letter.
3. Buckle RM et al. Hypoglycaemic coma occurring during treatment with chlorpromazine and orphenadrine. Br Med J. 1967;4:599.

## Chlorpromazine (Thorazine)

### Phenobarbital

Summary: Barbiturates may reduce some chlorpromazine concentrations, but the degree to which the therapeutic response to chlorpromazine is reduced is not established.

Risk Factors: No specific risk factors known.

Related Drugs: The effect of barbiturates on other neuroleptics is not established, but be aware of a possible reduction in the antipsychotic effect. There is also some evidence that *thioridazine (Mellaril)* may reduce serum phenobarbital concentrations.[4] One patient undergoing withdrawal from barbiturates and methaqualone developed fatal hyperthermia after he was given *haloperidol (Haldol)*.[5] It was proposed that the tendency of sedative-hypnotic withdrawal to produce hyperpyrexia was markedly enhanced by the ability of the haloperidol to interfere with thermoregulation.

Management Options:
- *Monitor.* It does not seem necessary to avoid concomitant use of neuroleptics and barbiturates, but monitor patients for evidence of a reduced effect of either drug if the combination is used.

References:
1. Loga S et al. Interactions of orphenadrine and phenobarbitone with chlorpromazine: plasma concentrations and effects in a man. Br J Clin Pharmacol. 1975;2:197.
2. Gay PE et al. Interaction between phenobarbital and thioridazine. Neurology. 1983; 33:1631.
3. Greenblatt DJ et al. Fatal hyperthermia following haloperidol therapy of sedative-hypnotic withdrawal. J Clin Psychiatry. 1978;39:673.

## Chlorpromazine (Thorazine)

## Propranolol (Inderal)

Summary: Propranolol and some beta blockers and neuroleptics such as chlorpromazine can increase the plasma concentrations of each other, resulting in accentuated pharmacologic responses of both drugs.

Risk Factors: No specific risk factors known.

Related Drugs: *Thiothixene (Navane)* and *thioridazine (Mellaril)* concentrations increase in patients treated with propranolol, while propranolol appears to have little effect on *haloperidol (Haldol)* concentrations. While other pairs of beta blockers and neuroleptics may interact in a similar manner, the interaction may not occur with beta blockers excreted primarily by the kidneys, such as *atenolol (Tenormin)* and *nadolol (Corgard)*.

Management Options:
- *Consider Alternative.* The use of beta blockers (e.g., nadolol) that are renally eliminated may lessen the magnitude of this interaction.

## Significance Classification

 - *Avoid Combination.* Risk always outweighs benefit.

 - *Usually Avoid Combination.* Use combination only under special circumstances.

 - *Minimize Risk.* Take action as necessary to reduce risk.

- *Monitor.* Patients receiving neuroleptics and beta blockers should be monitored for enhanced effects of both drugs. The dosage of one or both drugs may require reduction.

References:
1. Greendyke RM et al. Plasma propranolol levels and their effect on plasma thioridazine and haloperidol concentrations. J Clin Psychopharmacol. 1987;7:178.
2. Silver JM et al. Elevation of thioridazine plasma levels by propranolol. Am J Psychiatry. 1986;143:1290.
3. Miller FA. Adverse effects of combined propranolol and chlorpromazine therapy. Am J Psychiatry. 1982;139:1198.

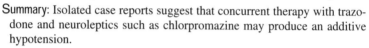

### Chlorpromazine (Thorazine)

### Trazodone (Desyrel)

Summary: Isolated case reports suggest that concurrent therapy with trazodone and neuroleptics such as chlorpromazine may produce an additive hypotension.

Risk Factors: No specific risk factors known.

Related Drugs: *Trifluoperazine (Stelazine)* appears to interact similarly.

Management Options:
- *Monitor* patients for hypotension if trazodone and neuroleptics are used concurrently.

References:
1. Asayesh K et al. Combination of trazodone and phenothiazines; a possible additive hypotensive effect. Can J Psychiatry. 1986;31:857.

### Chlorpropamide (Diabinese)

### Clofibrate (Atromid-S)

Summary: Clofibrate may enhance the effects of oral hypoglycemic drugs in some patients.

Risk Factors: No specific risk factors known.

Related Drugs: Other sulfonylureas may be similarly affected by clofibrate.

Management Options:
- *Monitor.* Patients treated with clofibrate and chlorpropamide or other sulfonylureas should be monitored more closely for hypoglycemia. This caution would apply especially when clofibrate is started or stopped in patients stabilized on a sulfonylurea.

References:
1. Ferrari C et al. Potentiation of hypoglycemic response to intravenous tolbutamide by clofibrate. N Engl J Med. 1976;294:613.
2. Daubresse JC et al. Clofibrate and diabetes control in patients treated with oral hypoglycaemic agents. Br J Clin Pharmacol. 1979;7:599.
3. Jain AK et al. Potentiation of hypoglycemic effect of sulfonylureas by halofenate. N Engl J Med. 1975;239:1283.

## Chlorpropamide (Diabinese)

### Erythromycin

**Summary:** A patient developed severe hepatic toxicity during the concomitant administration of erythromycin ethylsuccinate and chlorpropamide.

**Risk Factors:** No specific risk factors known.

**Related Drugs:** No information available.

**Management Options:**

- *Monitor.* Until more information is available on this potential interaction, patients taking chlorpropamide and erythromycin should be monitored for changes in hypoglycemic control and hepatotoxicity.

**References:**

1. Geubel AP et al. Prolonged cholestasis and disappearance of interlobular bile ducts following chlorpropamide and erythromycin ethylsuccinate: case of drug interaction? Liver. 1988;8:350.

## Chlorpropamide (Diabinese)

### Ethanol (Ethyl Alcohol)

**Summary:** Excessive ethanol intake may lead to altered glycemic control, most commonly hypoglycemia. An "Antabuse"-like reaction may occur in patients taking sulfonylureas.

**Risk Factors:** No specific risk factors known.

**Related Drugs:** Excessive ethanol may produce hypoglycemia in patients taking *insulin* or other oral hypoglycemic agents. Prolonged heavy intake of ethanol markedly decreases the half-life of *tolbutamide (Orinase)*, probably by inducing hepatic enzymes.[1,4,5] Ethanol ingestion may contribute to lactic acidosis in patients receiving *phenformin*.[2,3]

**Management Options:**

- *Avoid Combination.* Since an "Antabuse reaction" may occur following ethanol ingestion in patients receiving sulfonylureas, patients should be informed of this possibility when therapy is initiated. Ingestion of moderate-to-large amounts of ethanol should be avoided by patients on antidiabetic drugs because of the possible adverse effects of alcohol on diabetic control.

**References:**

1. Kater RMH et al. Increased rate tolbutamide metabolism in alcoholic patients. JAMA. 1969;207:363.
2. Johnson HK et al. Relationship of alcohol and hyperlactatemia in diabetic subjects treated with phenformin. Am J Med. 1968;45:98.
3. Kreisberg RA et al. Hyperlacticacidemia in man: ethanol-phenformin synergism. J Clin Endocrinol. 1972;34:29.
4. Carulli N et al. Alcohol-drugs interaction in man: alcohol and tolbutamide. Eur J Clin Invest. 1971;1:421.
5. Sotaniemi EA et al. Half-life of intravenous tolbutamide in the serum of patients in medical wards. Ann Clin Res. 1974;6:146.

## Cholestyramine (Questran)

### Diclofenac (Voltaren)

Summary: Single dose studies in healthy subjects suggest that cholestyramine substantially reduces the bioavailability of diclofenac; reduced diclofenac effect may occur.

Risk Factors: No specific risk factors known.

Related Drugs: Cholestyramine also reduces the serum concentrations of other nonsteroidal anti-inflammatory drugs such as ketoprofen, piroxicam, and tenoxicam. *Colestipol (Colestid)* also appears to inhibit the absorption of diclofenac, but to a somewhat lesser extent.

Management Options:
- *Consider Alternative.* Colestipol appears to reduce diclofenac absorption to a lesser extent than cholestyramine, but it still would be prudent to give the diclofenac 2 hours before or 6 hours after the colestipol.
- *Circumvent/Minimize.* Giving diclofenac 2 hours before or 6 hours after the cholestyramine would be expected to optimize the absorption of the diclofenac. Nonetheless, since diclofenac undergoes enterohepatic circulation, reduced diclofenac plasma concentrations may occur even if dosing of the drugs is separated.
- *Monitor* for reduced diclofenac effect, regardless of how far apart the doses are separated.

References:
1. Al-balla SR et al. The effects of cholestyramine and colestipol on the absorption of diclofenac in man. Int J Clin Pharmacol Ther. 1994;32;441.

## Cholestyramine (Questran)

### Digoxin (Lanoxin)

Summary: Cholestyramine appears to reduce the serum concentrations of digoxin and digitoxin, but the clinical impact in chronically treated patients has not been adequately assessed.

Risk Factors: No specific risk factors known.

Related Drugs: *Digitoxin (Crystodigin)* concentrations and pharmacologic activity were reduced after concomitant cholestyramine administration. *Colestipol (Colestid)* also has been noted to reduce digitalis glycoside concentrations.

## Significance Classification

 - *Avoid Combination.* Risk always outweighs benefit.

 - *Usually Avoid Combination.* Use combination only under special circumstances.

 - *Minimize Risk.* Take action as necessary to reduce risk.

Management Options:
- *Monitor.* Until more is known about this interaction, patients on digitalis glycosides should be watched for underdigitalization when cholestyramine is administered concurrently. Giving the digitalis product 2 or more hours before the cholestyramine may lessen the magnitude of the interaction.

References:
1. Brown DD et al. A steady-state evaluation of the effects of propantheline bromide and cholestyramine on the bioavailability of digoxin when administered as tablets or capsules. J Clin Pharmacol. 1985;25:360.
2. Pieroni RE et al. Use of cholestyramine resin in digitoxin toxicity. JAMA. 1981; 245:1939.
3. Neuvonen PJ et al. Effects of resins and activated charcoal on the absorption of digoxin, carbamazepine and furosemide. Br J Clin Pharmacol. 1988;25:229.

### Cholestyramine (Questran)

### Furosemide (Lasix)

Summary: Study in healthy subjects suggests that cholestyramine markedly reduces the bioavailability and diuretic response of furosemide.

Risk Factors: No specific risk factors known.

Related Drugs: *Colestipol (Colestid)* also substantially reduces the bioavailability of furosemide. The effect of cholestyramine and colestipol on other loop diuretics is not established.

Management Options:
- *Circumvent/Minimize.* Although the ability to circumvent the interaction by separating doses of furosemide from cholestyramine has not been systematically studied, giving furosemide 2 hours before or 6 hours after the cholestyramine would be expected to minimize the interaction.
- *Monitor* for altered furosemide response if cholestyramine therapy is initiated, discontinued, changed in dosage, or if the interval between doses of the 2 drugs is changed.

References:
1. Neuvonen PJ et al. Effects of resins and activated charcoal on the absorption of digoxin, carbamazepine and furosemide. Br J Clin Pharmacol. 1988;25:229.

### Cholestyramine (Questran)

### Hydrocortisone

Summary: Cholestyramine may lower plasma concentrations of oral hydrocortisone, possibly reducing its therapeutic effect.

Risk Factors: No specific risk factors known.

Related Drugs: The effect of cholestyramine on other corticosteroids is not established, but since corticosteroids are closely related structurally, it is possible that cholestyramine affects their absorption as well. *Colestipol*

*(Colestid)* probably interacts with corticosteroids in a manner similar to cholestyramine, but evidence is lacking.

Management Options:

- *Circumvent/Minimize.* Separate doses of oral hydrocortisone (and other corticosteroids) from cholestyramine as much as possible to minimize their mixing in the GI tract. Theoretically, giving the corticosteroid 2 hours before or 6 hours after the cholestyramine would optimize corticosteroid absorption. It also would be prudent to maintain a constant interval between the doses of corticosteroids and cholestyramine to minimize fluctuation of any interaction that does occur.

- *Monitor* patients for evidence of reduced corticosteroid response and increase the dose as needed when these drugs are used concurrently.

References:

1. Johansson C et al. Interaction by cholestyramine on the uptake of hydrocortisone in the GI tract. Acta Med Scand. 1978;204:509.

### Cholestyramine (Questran)

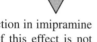

### Imipramine (Tofranil)

Summary: Cholestyramine may produce a modest reduction in imipramine plasma concentrations, but the clinical importance of this effect is not established.

Risk Factors: No specific risk factors known.

Related Drugs: Little is known about the effect of cholestyramine on antidepressants other than imipramine (e.g., *desipramine*), but consider the possibility of reduced antidepressant plasma concentrations if cholestyramine is taken concurrently. Theoretically, the binding resin *colestipol (Colestid)* also may interact with tricyclic antidepressants (TCAs).

Management Options:

- *Circumvent/Minimize.* Although the ability to circumvent the interaction by separating doses of imipramine before cholestyramine has not been systematically studied, giving imipramine 2 hours before or 6 hours after the cholestyramine would be expected to minimize the interaction.

- *Monitor* for altered TCA effect if cholestyramine is initiated, discontinued, or changed in dosage; adjust antidepressant dose as needed.

References:

1. Spina E et al. Decreased plasma concentrations of imipramine and desipramine following cholestyramine intake in depressed patients. Ther Drug Monit. 1994;16:432.

### Cholestyramine (Questran)

### Methotrexate (Mexate)

Summary: Preliminary evidence indicates that cholestyramine binds methotrexate in the gut and thus may reduce serum methotrexate concentrations. The degree to which this effect reduces the therapeutic response to methotrexate is not established.

Risk Factors: No specific risk factors known.

Related Drugs: The effect of *colestipol (Colestid)* on methotrexate is unknown, but it may be similar to that of cholestyramine.

Management Options:

- *Circumvent/Minimize.* Until clinical studies are performed, it would be prudent to separate oral doses of methotrexate from cholestyramine as much as possible.
- *Monitor.* Be alert for altered response to oral or parenteral methotrexate when cholestyramine is given concurrently.

References:

1. Erttmann R et al. Effect of oral cholestyramine on elimination of high-dose methotrexate. J Cancer Res Clin Oncol. 1985;110:48.
2. Ellman MH et al. Benefit of G-CSF for methotrexate-induced neutropenia in rheumatoid arthritis. Am J Med. 1992;92:337. Letter.
3. McAnena OJ et al. Alteration of methotrexate metabolism in rats by administration of an elemental liquid diet. Cancer. 1987;59:1091.

### Cholestyramine (Questran)

### Metronidazole (Flagyl)

Summary: Cholestyramine administration reduced the bioavailability of metronidazole in a single-dose study of healthy subjects.

Risk Factors: No specific risk factors known.

Related Drugs: *Colestipol (Colestid)* might affect metronidazole in a similar manner.

Management Options:

- *Circumvent/Minimize.* Patients should be advised to separate taking metronidazole from doses of cholestyramine as much as possible. Metronidazole should be taken at least 2 hours before the cholestyramine.
- *Monitor.* If metronidazole and bile acid binding resins are coadministered, watch for reduced metronidazole efficacy.

References:

1. Molokhia AM et al. Effect of concomitant oral administration of some adsorbing drugs on the bioavailability of metronidazole. Drug Dev Ind Pharm. 1987;13:1229.

### Cholestyramine (Questran)

### Piroxicam (Feldene)

Summary: Cholestyramine enhanced the elimination of piroxicam in one study, but the clinical importance of this effect is unknown.

Risk Factors: No specific risk factors known.

Related Drugs: The elimination of IV *tenoxicam*, a nonsteroidal anti-inflammatory drug (NSAID) related to piroxicam, also was enhanced by cholestyramine in this study.[1] Although little is known regarding the effect of cholestyramine on other NSAIDs, it would not be surprising to find that some of them also interact. The effect of another binding resin, **colestipol (Colestid)**, on the pharmacokinetics of piroxicam or other NSAIDs is not established, but some evidence suggests that colestipol binds drugs less avidly than cholestyramine.

Management Options:

- *Circumvent/Minimize.* Separate the doses of piroxicam and cholestyramine as much as possible.
- *Monitor* the patient for inadequate piroxicam response. If an inadequate piroxicam response appears to be related to the use of cholestyramine, consider the use of an alternative hypolipidemic agent and/or NSAID therapy.

References:

1. Meinertz T et al. Interruption of the enterohepatic circulation of phenprocoumon by cholestyramine. Clin Pharmacol Ther. 1977;21:731.
2. Jahnchen E et al. Enhanced elimination of warfarin during treatment with cholestyramine. Br J Clin Pharmacol. 1978;5:437.
3. Guentert TW et al. Accelerated elimination of tenoxicam and piroxicam by cholestyramine. Clin Pharmacol Ther. 1988;43:179. Abstract.

## Cholestyramine (Questran)

## Pravastatin (Pravachol)

Summary: Cholestyramine can inhibit the bioavailability of pravastatin, but this effect appears to be more than offset by the additive lipid-lowering effect of concurrent therapy.

Risk Factors: No specific risk factors known.

Related Drugs: **Colestipol (Colestid)** affects pravastatin similarly. Although little is known regarding the effect of bile acid binding resins on the absorption of other HMG-CoA reductase inhibitors such as **lovastatin (Mevacor)**, **simvastatin (Zocor)**, or **fluvastatin (Lescol)**, they may be similarly affected.

Management Options:

- *Circumvent/Minimize.* Cholestyramine or colestipol-induced reduction in pravastatin bioavailability probably is minimized by giving the cholestyramine or colestipol with meals and the pravastatin at bedtime. Other dosing schedules also may be suitable, but it would be best to avoid giving bile acid binding resins at the same time as pravastatin or other HMG-CoA reductase inhibitors.
- *Monitor* for reduced pravastatin effect if cholestyramine also is given.

References:

1. Pan HY et al. Pharmacokinetics and pharmacodynamics of pravastin alone and with cholestyramine in hypercholesterolemia. Clin Pharmacol Ther. 1990;48:201.
2. Pan HY. Clinical pharmacology of pravastatin, a selective inhibitor of HMG-CoA reductase. Eur J Clin Pharmacol. 1991;40:S15.

### Cholestyramine (Questran)

### Thyroid

Summary: Cholestyramine may reduce serum thyroid concentrations in patients receiving thyroid replacement therapy.

Risk Factors: No specific risk factors known.

Related Drugs: Until more information is available, assume that the absorption of all thyroid preparations can be reduced by cholestyramine administration. Although the effect of *colestipol (Colestid)* on thyroid absorption is not established, one should assume that it also interacts until proved otherwise.

Management Options:
- *Circumvent/Minimize.* The available evidence suggests that at least 4 to 5 hours should elapse between administration of cholestyramine and thyroid. Also, try to maintain a relatively constant interval between doses of the 2 drugs.
- *Monitor.* Even with the above precautions, monitor for altered thyroid response (e.g., serum thyroid-stimulating hormone concentrations) when cholestyramine is initiated, discontinued, changed in dosage, or when the interval between doses of the 2 drugs is changed for more than a few days.

References:
1. Northcutt RC et al. The influence of cholestyramine on thyroxine absorption. JAMA. 1969;208:1857.

### Cholestyramine (Questran)

### Valproic Acid (Depakene)

Summary: Cholestyramine inhibits the gastrointestinal (GI) absorption of valproic acid, but it is not known how often this would result in a clinically important reduction in valproic acid effect.

Risk Factors: No specific risk factors known.

Related Drugs: Theoretically, one would expect *colestipol (Colestid)* also to inhibit the absorption of valproic acid.

## Significance Classification

① - *Avoid Combination.* Risk always outweighs benefit.

② - *Usually Avoid Combination.* Use combination only under special circumstances.

③ - *Minimize Risk.* Take action as necessary to reduce risk.

Management Options:

- *Circumvent/Minimize.* Although the magnitude of the interaction appears small in most people, it would be prudent to take valproic acid at least 2 hours before or 6 hours after cholestyramine, and maintain a relatively constant interval between administration of the 2 drugs.
- *Monitor.* Even if the doses of the drugs are separated appropriately, it would be prudent to monitor for reduced effect, especially in the first few weeks of combined therapy.

References:

1. Malloy MJ et al. Effect of cholestyramine resin on single dose valproate pharmacokinetics. Int J Clin Pharmacol Ther. 1996;34:208.

### Cholestyramine (Questran)
### Warfarin (Coumadin)

Summary: Cholestyramine may inhibit the hypoprothrombinemic response to warfarin, phenprocoumon, and possibly other oral anticoagulants; colestipol (Colestid) might be less likely to interact.

Risk Factors: No specific risk factors known.

Related Drugs: **Phenprocoumon** interacts similarly. Some evidence suggests that **colestipol (Colestid)** is less likely than cholestyramine to interact with warfarin or phenprocoumon.[2,3]

Management Options:

- *Consider alternative* hypolipidemic therapy [but keep in mind that other agents also may interact with oral anticoagulants (e.g., clofibrate, gemfibrozil, and lovastatin)].
- *Circumvent/Minimize.* Giving the anticoagulant at least 2 hours before or 6 hours after the binding resin probably minimizes the impairment of oral anticoagulant absorption. However, any anticoagulant that undergoes enterohepatic circulation (e.g., warfarin, phenprocoumon) may be affected by cholestyramine therapy even if the doses are separated. The binding resin and the oral anticoagulant should consistently be given the same number of hours apart so that any interaction that does occur will be relatively consistent from day to day.
- *Monitor* for altered response to oral anticoagulants if a binding resin is initiated, discontinued, changed in dosage, or if the interval between the resin and the anticoagulant is changed.

References:

1. Jahnchen E et al. Enhanced elimination of warfarin during treatment with cholestyramine. Br J Clin Pharmacol. 1978;5:437.
2. Harvengt C et al. Effects of colestipol, a new bile acid sequestrant, on the absorption of phenprocoumon in man. Eur J Clin Pharmacol. 1973;6:19.
3. Upjohn Company. Colestid product information. Kalamazoo, MI: 1993.

### Cigarette Smoking

### Insulin

Summary: Cigarette smoking may increase glucose concentrations and decrease response to insulin administration.

Risk Factors: No specific risk factors known.

Related Drugs: No information available.

Management Options:
- *Monitor.* Patients should be informed that a change in smoking habits may change the response to insulin.

References:
1. Madsbad S et al. Influence of smoking on insulin requirement and metabolic status in diabetes mellitus. Diabetes Care. 1980;3:41.
2. Klemp P et al. Smoking reduces insulin absorption from subcutaneous tissue. Br Med J. 1982;284:237.

### Cigarette Smoking

### Oral Contraceptives

Summary: The risk of oral contraceptive-induced adverse cardiovascular events is increased by smoking.

Risk Factors:
- *Age.* Persons >35 years old are at greater risk.
- *Dosage Regimen.* Smoking greater than 15 cigarettes/day places women at greater risk.

Related Drugs: No information available.

Management Options:
- **Avoid combination.** Women taking oral contraceptives should be encouraged not to smoke; if they continue to smoke, they should consider using an alternative form of contraception.

References:
1. Goldbaum GM et al. The relative impact of smoking and oral contraceptive use on women in the United States. JAMA. 1987;258:1339.
2. Searle Laboratories. Ovulen Product Information. Chicago, IL: 1984.
3. Crawford FE et al. Oral contraceptive steroid plasma concentrations in smokers and nonsmokers. Br Med J. 1981;282:1829.

### Cigarette Smoking

### Quinine

Summary: Cigarette smokers have lower quinine serum concentrations than nonsmokers; clinical efficacy could be reduced.

Risk Factors: No specific risk factors known.

Related Drugs: No information available.

Management Options:
  • *Circumvent/Minimize.* Smokers requiring quinine therapy for malaria may need increased quinine doses to achieve a cure.
  • *Monitor.* Measurement of plasma quinine concentrations should be considered in smokers to ensure therapeutic plasma concentrations are attained.
References:
  1. Wanwimolruk S et al. Cigarette smoking enhances the elimination of quinine. Br J Clin Pharmacol. 1993;36:610.

### Cigarette Smoking

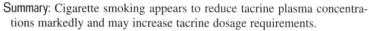

### Tacrine (Cognex)

Summary: Cigarette smoking appears to reduce tacrine plasma concentrations markedly and may increase tacrine dosage requirements.
Risk Factors: No specific risk factors known.
Related Drugs: No information available.
Management Options:
  • *Monitor* tacrine response, and keep in mind that smokers are likely to have higher tacrine dosage requirements than nonsmokers.
References:
  1. Parke-Davis. Cognex Product Information. Morris Plains, NJ: 1993.
  2. Watkins PB et al. Hepatotoxic effects of tacrine administration in patients with Alzheimer's disease. JAMA. 1994;271:992.
  3. Winker MA. Tacrine for Alzheimer's disease: which patient, what dose? JAMA. 1994;271:1023. Editorial.

### Cigarette Smoking

### Theophylline

Summary: Cigarette smoking increases the elimination of theophylline, thus increasing theophylline dosage requirements.
Risk Factors: No specific risk factors known.
Related Drugs: No information available.
Management Options:
  • *Monitor* theophylline response and serum concentrations. Keep in mind that smokers require considerably larger maintenance dosages of theophylline than nonsmokers in order to achieve adequate serum theophylline levels.
References:
  1. Jusko WJ et al. Enhanced biotransformation of theophylline in marijuana and tobacco smokers. Clin Pharmacol Ther. 1978;24:406.
  2. Pfeifer HJ et al. Clinical toxicity of theophylline in relations to cigarette smoking: a report from the Boston Collaborative Drug Surveillance. Chest. 1978;73:455.
  3. Powell JR et al. The influence of cigarette smoking and sex on theophylline disposition. Am Rev Resp Dis. 1977;116:17.

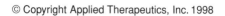

### Cimetidine (Tagamet)

### Cisapride (Propulsid)

Summary: Cimetidine substantially increased the bioavailability of cisapride in healthy subjects, but the clinical importance of the interaction is not established.

Risk Factors: No specific risk factors known.

Related Drugs: The effect of other $H_2$-receptor antagonists, such as **ranitidine (Zantac)**, **famotidine (Pepcid)**, and **nizatidine (Axid)**, on cisapride pharmacokinetics is not established; theoretically, they would be less likely to affect cisapride metabolism than cimetidine.

Management Options:
- *Consider Alternative.* Although there is little evidence to suggest that the combination is dangerous, given the potential severity of the adverse interaction, it would be prudent to use an alternative to cimetidine, such as ranitidine, famotidine, or nizatidine.
- *Monitor.* If the combination is used, monitor for evidence of ventricular arrhythmias (e.g., fainting, palpitations).

References:
1. Kirch W et al. Cisapride-cimetidine interaction: enhanced cisapride bioavailability and accelerated cimetidine absorption. Ther Drug Monit. 1989;11:411.
2. Galmiche P et al. Combined therapy with cisapride and cimetidine in severe reflux oesophagitis: a double blind controlled trial. Gut. 1988;29:675.

### Cimetidine (Tagamet)

### Citalopram

Summary: Cimetidine appears to moderately increase citalopram serum concentrations, but it is not known how often this would result in adverse outcomes.

Risk Factors: No specific risk factors known.

Related Drugs: **Famotidine (Pepcid)**, **nizatidine (Axid)**, and **ranitidine (Zantac)** theoretically are unlikely to interact with citalopram, but clinical studies are needed for confirmation. Theoretically, **omeprazole (Prilosec)** could interact with citalopram due to its ability to inhibit CYP2C19.

## Significance Classification

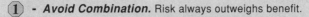 - *Avoid Combination.* Risk always outweighs benefit.

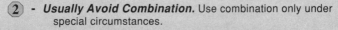 - *Usually Avoid Combination.* Use combination only under special circumstances.

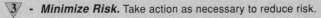 - *Minimize Risk.* Take action as necessary to reduce risk.

Management Options:
- *Consider Alternative.* Consider using an alternative $H_2$-receptor antagonist such as famotidine, nizatidine, or ranitidine.
- *Monitor.* If the combination is used, monitor for altered citalopram effect if cimetidine is initiated, discontinued, or changed in dosage; adjust citalopram dose as needed.

References:
1. Priskorn M et al. Pharmacokinetic interaction study of citalopram and cimetidine in healthy subjects. Eur J Clin Pharmacol. 1997;52:241. Letter.

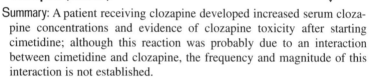

## Cimetidine (Tagamet)

### Clozapine (Clozaril)

Summary: A patient receiving clozapine developed increased serum clozapine concentrations and evidence of clozapine toxicity after starting cimetidine; although this reaction was probably due to an interaction between cimetidine and clozapine, the frequency and magnitude of this interaction is not established.

Risk Factors:
- *Dosage Regimen.* In most patients, clinically important inhibition of hepatic drug metabolism by cimetidine requires doses of 400 mg/day or more.

Related Drugs: It appears that **ranitidine (Zantac)** is preferable to cimetidine in patients receiving clozapine.[1] Theoretically, **famotidine (Pepcid)** and **nizatidine (Axid)** also would be unlikely to interact with clozapine.

Management Options:
- *Consider Alternative.* Until more information is available, it would be prudent to avoid the use of cimetidine in patients receiving clozapine. Theoretically, famotidine and nizatidine would be unlikely to interact and could be considered as alternatives.
- *Monitor.* If the combination is used, monitor for altered clozapine effect if cimetidine is initiated, discontinued, or changed in dosage. Adjust clozapine dosage as needed.

References:
1. Szymanski S et al. A case report of cimetidine-induced clozapine toxicity. J Clin Psychiatry. 1991;52:21.

## Cimetidine (Tagamet)

### Desipramine (Norpramin)

Summary: Limited clinical evidence suggests that cimetidine increases serum desipramine concentrations. Given the proven effect of cimetidine on tricyclic antidepressants closely related to desipramine, it seems likely that desipramine is affected similarly.

Risk Factors:
- *Dosage Regimen.* In most patients, clinically important inhibition of hepatic drug metabolism by cimetidine requires doses of 400 mg/day or more.

Related Drugs: Theoretically, **ranitidine (Zantac)**, **famotidine (Pepcid)**, and probably **nizatidine (Axid)** would be less likely to interact with desipramine. Other clinical studies suggest that cimetidine also inhibits the elimination of other tricyclic antidepressants such as imipramine and nortriptyline. Little clinical information is available on the effect of cimetidine on tricyclics such as **amitriptyline**, **amoxapine**, **protriptyline**, **trimipramine**, **maprotiline**, or **trazodone**. However, theoretical considerations would indicate that their elimination also might be reduced by cimetidine therapy.

Management Options:
- *Consider Alternative.* Consider using an alternative to cimetidine. Ranitidine, famotidine, and probably nizatidine are less likely to interact.
- *Monitor.* Until more information is available, be alert for altered desipramine effect if cimetidine therapy is initiated, discontinued, or changed in dosage.

References:
1. Miller DD et al. Cimetidine-imipramine interaction: a case report. Am J Psychiatry. 1983;140:351.

## Cimetidine (Tagamet)

## Diazepam (Valium)

**3**

Summary: Plasma levels of diazepam and several other benzodiazepines and/or their active metabolites can be increased by cimetidine, but the frequency of adverse effects associated with increased benzodiazepine concentration is unknown.

Risk Factors:
- *Age.* The elderly can be more susceptible to the sedative effects of benzodiazepines.
- *Dosage Regimen.* In most patients, clinically important inhibition of hepatic drug metabolism by cimetidine requires doses of 400 mg/day or more.

Related Drugs: Since **clorazepate (Tranxene)**, **halazepam (Paxipam)**, and **prazepam (Centrax)** are metabolized to active desmethyldiazepam, they probably also interact with cimetidine. **Clonazepam (Klonopin)** and **flurazepam (Dalmane)** undergo oxidative metabolism in the liver, and their elimination would be expected to be reduced by cimetidine. Cimetidine also reduces plasma clearance of **chlordiazepoxide (Librium)**, **desmethyldiazepam**, and probably also **alprazolam (Xanax)** and **triazolam (Halcion)**.[1-5] The pharmacokinetics of benzodiazepines that undergo glucuronide conjugation, such as *lorazepam (Ativan)*, *oxazepam (Serax)*, and *temazepam (Restoril)*, do not appear to be affected by cimetidine therapy.[5,6] *Ranitidine (Zantac)* appears to be less likely to interact with benzodiazepines than cimetidine; *famotidine (Pepcid)* and probably *nizatidine (Axid)* also appear unlikely to interact.

Management Options:

- *Consider Alternative.* Consider using an alternative to cimetidine. Ranitidine, famotidine, and probably nizatidine appear less likely to interact.

- *Monitor.* Patients receiving benzodiazepines that undergo oxidative metabolism should be watched for evidence of altered benzodiazepine response when cimetidine is initiated, discontinued, or changed in dosage.

References:

1. Desmond PV et al. Cimetidine impairs elimination of chlordiazepoxide (Librium) in man. Ann Intern Med. 1980;93:266.
2. Patwardhan RV et al. Lack of tolerance and rapid recovery of cimetidine-inhibited chlordiazepoxide (Librium) elimination. Gastroenterology. 1981;81:547.
3. Ruffalo RL et al. Cimetidine-benzodiazepine drug interaction. Am J Hosp Pharm. 1981;38:1365.
4. Greenblatt DJ et al. Old age, cimetidine, and disposition of alprazolam and triazolam. Clin Pharmacol Ther. 1983;33:253.
5. Klotz U et al. Influence of cimetidine on the pharmacokinetics of desmethyldiazepam and oxazepam. Eur J Clin Pharmacol. 1980;18:517.
6. Patwardhan RV et al. Cimetidine spares the glucuronidation of lorazepam and oxazepam. Gastroenterology. 1970;79:912.

## Cimetidine (Tagamet)

## Diltiazem (Cardizem)

**Summary:** Cimetidine can increase the serum concentration of diltiazem; excessive diltiazem effects may be seen.

**Risk Factors:** No specific risk factors known.

**Related Drugs:** Cimetidine also increases the concentrations of *nifedipine (Procardia)*, *nisoldipine (Sular)*, *nitrendipine (Baypress)*, and *verapamil (Calan)*. Other $H_2$-receptor antagonists, such as *ranitidine (Zantac)*, *famotidine (Pepcid)*, and *nizatidine (Axid)*, would be less likely to affect diltiazem concentrations.

Management Options:

- *Consider Alternative.* Ranitidine 150 mg BID does not appear to affect diltiazem concentrations.[1] Nizatidine and famotidine also would be unlikely to affect diltiazem pharmacokinetics.

- *Monitor.* Patients receiving diltiazem should be monitored carefully (e.g., bradycardia or hypotension) when cimetidine is added or deleted from their drug regimen.

References:

1. Winship LC et al. The effect of ranitidine and cimetidine on single-dose diltiazem pharmacokinetics. Pharmacotherapy. 1985;5:16.

### Cimetidine (Tagamet)

### Doxepin (Sinequan)

Summary: Cimetidine substantially increased serum concentrations of doxepin in healthy subjects, but it is not known how often this results in doxepin toxicity.

Risk Factors:
- *Dosage Regimen.* In most patients, clinically important inhibition of hepatic drug metabolism by cimetidine requires doses of 400 mg/day or more.

Related Drugs: Ranitidine does not appear to interact with doxepin. In 6 healthy men, **ranitidine (Zantac)** 150 mg BID had no effect on steady-state plasma doxepin concentrations.[1] Theoretically, **famotidine (Pepcid)** and **nizatidine (Axid)** also would be unlikely to affect doxepin metabolism. Other clinical studies suggest that cimetidine also inhibits the elimination of other tricyclic antidepressants (TCAs) such as **imipramine (Tofranil)**, **desipramine (Norpramin)**, and **nortriptyline (Pamelor)**. Little clinical information is available on the effect of cimetidine on TCAs such as **amitriptyline (Elavil)**, **amoxapine (Asendin)**, **protriptyline (Vivactil)**, **trimipramine (Surmontil)**, **maprotiline (Ludiomil)**, or **trazodone (Desyrel)**. However, theoretical considerations would indicate that their elimination also might be reduced by cimetidine therapy.

Management Options:
- *Consider Alternative.* Consider using an alternative to cimetidine, such as ranitidine, famotidine, or nizatidine.
- *Circumvent/Minimize.* In patients who are already receiving cimetidine and are about to begin a course of therapy with doxepin, consider using conservative doxepin doses until the patient's response to therapy can be evaluated.
- *Monitor.* In patients stabilized on doxepin who are then given cimetidine, be alert for evidence of doxepin toxicity (e.g., severe dry mouth, blurred vision, urinary retention, tachycardia, constipation, postural hypotension). If cimetidine is discontinued or its dose substantially reduced in a patient stabilized on both doxepin and cimetidine, the patient should be monitored for an inadequate response to the doxepin.

References:
1. Sutherland DL et al. The influence of cimetidine versus ranitidine on doxepin pharmacokinetics. Eur J Clin Pharmacol. 1987;32:159.
2. Smedley HM. Malignant breast change in man given two drugs associated with breast hyperplasia. Lancet. 1981;2:638.

### Cimetidine (Tagamet)

### Femoxetine

Summary: Preliminary study in healthy subjects suggests that cimetidine markedly increases femoxetine serum concentrations, but an increase in adverse effects was not observed.

Risk Factors: No specific risk factors known.
Related Drugs: The effect of $H_2$-receptor antagonists other than cimetidine on femoxetine pharmacokinetics is unknown; theoretically, *famotidine (Pepcid)*, *nizatidine (Axid)*, and *ranitidine (Zantac)* would not be expected to interact.
Management Options:
- *Consider Alternative.* Theoretically, other $H_2$-receptor antagonists such as ranitidine, famotidine or nizatidine would be less likely to interact with femoxetine; thus, their use may be preferred over cimetidine until more information is available on this interaction.
- *Monitor.* Patients receiving cimetidine may have lower dosage requirements for femoxetine. However, the results of this study suggest that femoxetine has little dose-dependent toxicity. Nonetheless, it would be prudent to monitor for alterations in therapeutic and toxic effects of femoxetine if cimetidine is initiated, discontinued, or changed in dosage.
References:
1. Schmidt J et al. Femoxetine and cimetidine: interaction in healthy volunteers. Eur J Clin Pharmacol. 1986;31:299.

### Cimetidine (Tagamet)
### Flecainide (Tambocor)

Summary: Cimetidine increases the plasma concentration of flecainide, but the clinical importance of this effect is not established.
Risk Factors:
- *Concurrent Diseases.* Patients with renal failure are more likely to experience this interaction.
Related Drugs: *Ranitidine (Zantac)*, *famotidine (Pepcid)*, and *nizatidine (Axid)* are less likely to interact with flecainide because they have little or no effect on hepatic metabolism.
Management Options:
- *Monitor.* Patients stabilized on flecainide (particularly those with renal disease) should be monitored for increased flecainide effect if cimetidine is added to their therapy.

## Significance Classification

1 - *Avoid Combination.* Risk always outweighs benefit.
2 - *Usually Avoid Combination.* Use combination only under special circumstances.
3 - *Minimize Risk.* Take action as necessary to reduce risk.

References:
1. Tjamdra-Maga TB et al. Altered pharmacokinetics of oral flecainide by cimetidine. Br J Clin Pharmacol. 1986;22:108.

## Cimetidine (Tagamet)

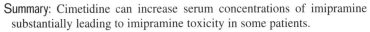

### Imipramine (Tofranil)

Summary: Cimetidine can increase serum concentrations of imipramine substantially leading to imipramine toxicity in some patients.

Risk Factors:

- *Dosage Regimen.* In most patients, clinically important inhibition of hepatic drug metabolism by cimetidine requires doses of 400 mg/day or more.

Related Drugs: *Ranitidine (Zantac)* does not appear to affect imipramine metabolism or pharmacokinetics.[2,3] Theoretically, it is unlikely that *famotidine (Pepcid)* and *nizatidine (Axid)* will interact with imipramine since these $H_2$-receptor antagonists have little effect on drug metabolism. Cimetidine also may increase serum concentrations of *desipramine (Norpramin)*, *doxepin (Sinequan)*, and *nortriptyline (Pamelor)*.

Management Options:

- *Consider Alternative.* Consider using an alternative to cimetidine (e.g., ranitidine, famotidine, nizatidine).
- *Circumvent/Minimize.* In patients who are already receiving cimetidine and are about to begin a course of therapy with imipramine, consider using conservative imipramine doses until the patient's response to therapy can be evaluated.
- *Monitor.* In patients stabilized on imipramine who are then given cimetidine, be alert for evidence of imipramine toxicity (e.g., severe dry mouth, blurred vision, urinary retention, tachycardia, constipation, and postural hypotension). If cimetidine is discontinued or its dose substantially reduced in a patient stabilized on both imipramine and cimetidine, the patient should be monitored for an inadequate response to the cyclic antidepressant.

References:
1. Shapiro PA. Cimetidine-imipramine interaction: case report and comments. Am J Psychiatry. 1984;141:152.
2. Wells BG et al. The effect of ranitidine and cimetidine on imipramine disposition. Eur J Clin Pharmacol. 1986;31:285.
3. Spine E et al. Differential effects of cimetidine and ranitidine on imipramine demethylation and desmethylimipramine hydroxylation by human liver microsomes. Eur J Clin Pharmacol. 1986;30:239.

## Cimetidine (Tagamet)

### Ketoconazole (Nizoral)

Summary: Cimetidine administration reduces ketoconazole concentrations.

Risk Factors: No specific risk factors known.

Related Drugs: Other oral imidazole antifungal [e.g., *fluconazole (Diflucan)*] agents may be affected similarly by cimetidine administration. Other $H_2$-receptor antagonists [e.g., *ranitidine (Zantac), famotidine (Pepcid), nizatidine (Axid)*] and proton pump inhibitors would be expected to reduce ketoconazole absorption.

Management Options:

- *Circumvent/Minimize.* Several recommendations have been made to avoid this interaction in patients with elevated gastric pH. The product information for ketoconazole suggests that each ketoconazole tablet should be dissolved in 4 mL of an aqueous solution of 0.2 N hydrochloric acid with the resulting mixture ingested with a straw (to avoid contact with teeth) and followed by a glass of water.[2] Others suggest that an easier and equally effective method is to give 2 capsules of glutamic acid hydrochloride (Acidulin) 15 minutes before the ketoconazole.[2]

- *Monitor.* Until more is known about this interaction, be alert for evidence of reduced ketoconazole effect when cimetidine or other agents that increase gastric pH are coadministered.

References:

1. Lelawongs P et al. Effect of food and gastric acidity on absorption of orally administered ketoconazole. Clin Pharm. 1988;7:228.
2. Nizoral. Physicians' Desk Reference. 47th ed. Oradell: Medical Economics Data; 1993:1172.
3. Blum RA et al. Effect of increased gastric pH on the relative bioavailability of fluconazole and ketoconazole. Pharm Res. 1990;7:S52. Abstract.

## Cimetidine (Tagamet)

## Lidocaine (Xylocaine)

Summary: Cimetidine modestly increases lidocaine serum concentrations, but it is not known how often this would cause lidocaine toxicity.

Risk Factors: No specific risk factors known.

Related Drugs: *Ranitidine (Zantac)* may be a good alternative to cimetidine because it has minimal effect on lidocaine disposition.[2] For similar reasons, it is unlikely that *famotidine (Pepcid)* and *nizatidine (Axid)* would interact with lidocaine.

Management Options:

- *Consider Alternative.* Ranitidine, famotidine, or nizatidine would be less likely to interact with lidocaine.

- *Monitor.* When cimetidine and lidocaine are given concurrently, patients should be monitored for lidocaine toxicity.

References:

1. Jackson JE et al. Effects of histamine-2 receptor blockade on lidocaine kinetics. Clin Pharmacol Ther. 1985;37:544.
2. Jackson JE et al. The effects of $H_2$-blockers on lidocaine disposition. Clin Pharmacol Ther. 1983;33:255.
3. Powell JR et al. Effect of duration of lidocaine infusion and route of cimetidine administration on lidocaine pharmacokinetics. Clin Pharm. 1986;5:993.

## Cimetidine (Tagamet)

### Melphalan (Alkeran)

Summary: Cimetidine administration appears to reduce the serum concentrations of melphalan, but the clinical importance of this effect is not established.

Risk Factors: No specific risk factors known.

Related Drugs: Other inhibitors of gastric acid secretion also may reduce the serum concentrations of melphalan, but little clinical information is available.

Management Options:
- *Monitor.* Until further information is available, patients treated with melphalan and cimetidine should be monitored for reduced melphalan activity.

References:
1. Sviland L et al. Interaction of cimetidine with oral melphalan. Cancer Chemother Pharmacol. 1987;20:173

## Cimetidine (Tagamet)

### Meperidine (Demerol)

Summary: Cimetidine may increase the effect of meperidine and possibly other narcotic analgesics; morphine may be less likely to interact than other narcotics.

Risk Factors: No specific risk factors known.

Related Drugs: *In vitro* studies also indicate that cimetidine may inhibit the hepatic microsomal metabolism of meperidine and fentanyl.[1,2] **Morphine** disposition was not affected by cimetidine pretreatment in 7 healthy men,[3] probably because morphine undergoes glucuronidation, a metabolic process little affected by cimetidine. Cimetidine may inhibit some of the cardiovascular effects of histamine, which is released in response to administration of narcotic analgesics. Pharmacodynamic interactions between cimetidine and narcotic analgesics are also possible but not well studied. **Ranitidine (Zantac)** is probably less likely to interact than cimetidine and thus may be preferable in patients receiving meperidine. Theoretically, **famotidine (Pepcid)** and **nizatidine (Axid)** also would be less likely to interact than cimetidine.

Management Options:
- *Consider Alternative.* Ranitidine may be preferable in patients receiving meperidine, as it is less likely to interact.
- *Monitor.* Until these interactions are better described, be alert for evidence of enhanced respiratory and CNS depression during combined therapy with cimetidine and narcotic analgesics.

References:
1. Knodell RG et al. Drug metabolism by rat and human hepatic microsomes in response to interaction with $H_2$-receptor antagonists. Gastroenterology. 1982;82:84.

2. Lee HR et al. Effect of histamine $H_2$-receptors on fentanyl metabolism. Pharmacologist. 1982;24:145.
3. Mojaverian P et al. Cimetidine does not alter morphine disposition in man. Br J Clin Pharmacol. 1982;14:309.

### Cimetidine (Tagamet)

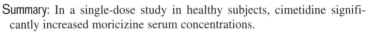

### Moricizine (Ethmozine)

Summary: In a single-dose study in healthy subjects, cimetidine significantly increased moricizine serum concentrations.

Risk Factors: No specific risk factors known.

Related Drugs: Theoretically, other $H_2$-receptor antagonists such as *ranitidine (Zantac)*, *famotidine (Pepcid)*, and *nizatidine (Axid)*, would be less likely to interact with moricizine.

Management Options:
- *Monitor.* Patients taking moricizine should be monitored for increased moricizine concentrations and increased cardiovascular effects if cimetidine is added.

References:
1. Biollaz J et al. Cimetidine inhibition of moricizine metabolism. Clin Pharmacol Ther. 1985;37:665.

### Cimetidine (Tagamet)

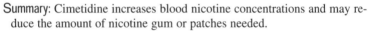

### Nicotine (Nicorette)

Summary: Cimetidine increases blood nicotine concentrations and may reduce the amount of nicotine gum or patches needed.

Risk Factors: No specific risk factors known.

Related Drugs: Ranitidine may reduce nicotine clearance as mentioned above. The effect of *famotidine (Pepcid)* and *nizatidine (Axid)* on nicotine elimination is unknown, but one would expect them to interact minimally as does *ranitidine (Zantac)*.

Management Options:
- *Circumvent/Minimize.* Patients on cimetidine therapy may not need to use as much nicotine gum or nicotine patches as those not on cimetidine. For smokers, it is possible that cimetidine therapy would

## Significance Classification

(1) - ***Avoid Combination.*** Risk always outweighs benefit.

(2) - ***Usually Avoid Combination.*** Use combination only under special circumstances.

(3) - ***Minimize Risk.*** Take action as necessary to reduce risk.

allow a reduction in the number of cigarettes smoked while maintaining the same blood nicotine concentrations.

• *Monitor:* Be alert for evidence of excessive nicotine response.

References:
1. Bendayan R et al. Effect of cimetidine and ranitidine on the hepatic and renal elimination of nicotine in humans. Eur J Clin Pharmacol. 1990;38:165.

## Cimetidine (Tagamet)

## Nifedipine (Procardia)

Summary: Cimetidine can increase the serum concentration of nifedipine; excessive nifedipine effects can occur.

Risk Factors: No specific risk factors known.

Related Drugs: *Ranitidine (Zantac)* appears to have a smaller effect on nifedipine serum concentrations but may increase nifedipine AUC by 13% to 48%.[1-7] If confirmed, other $H_2$-receptor antagonists [e.g., *famotidine (Pepcid)* and *nizatidine (Axid)*], *omeprazole (Prilosec)*, and *lansoprazole (Prevacid)* would be expected to have a similar effect. Increased nifedipine effects (headache, hypotension) could occur. Cimetidine also increases the concentrations of *diltiazem (Cardizem)*, *nisoldipine (Sular)*, *nitrendipine (Baypress)*, and *verapamil (Calan)*.

Management Options:
• *Monitor:* Patients receiving nifedipine should be carefully monitored when cimetidine or other drugs that alter gastric pH are added or deleted from their drug regimen.

References:
1. Kirch W et al. Einflub von cimetidine und ranitidin auf pharmakokinetic und antihypertensive effekt von nifedipin. Dtsch Med Wochenschr. 1983;108:1757.
2. Renwick AG et al. Factors affecting the pharmacokinetics of nifedipine. Eur J Clin Pharmacol. 1987;32:351.
3. Smith SR et al. Ranitidine and cimetidine; drug interactions with single and steady-state nifedipine administration. Br J Clin Pharmacol. 1987;23:311.
4. Adams LJ et al. Effect of ranitidine on bioavailability of nifedipine. Gastroenterology. 1986;90:1320. Abstract.
5. Kirch W et al. Ranitidine increases bioavailability of nifedipine. Clin Pharmacol Ther. 1985;37:204. Abstract.
6. Schwartz JB et al. Effect of cimetidine or ranitidine administration of nifedipine pharmacokinetics and pharmacodynamics. Clin Pharmacol Ther. 1988;43:673.
7. Khan A et al. The pharmacokinetics and pharmacodynamics of nifedipine at steady state during concomitant administration of cimetidine or high dose ranitidine. Br J Clin Pharmacol. 1991;32:519.

## Cimetidine (Tagamet)

## Nimodipine (Nimotop)

Summary: Cimetidine can increase the serum concentration of nimodipine; the clinical significance of this interaction is unknown.

Risk Factors: No specific risk factors known.

Related Drugs: Cimetidine also increases the concentrations of *diltiazem (Cardizem), nisoldipine (Sular), nifedipine (Procardia)*, and *verapamil (Calan)*. *Ranitidine (Zantac)* 300 mg/day for five days produced no change in the pharmacokinetics of nimodipine.[1] Other drugs that increase gastric pH [e.g., *omeprazole (Prilosec)*] may affect nimodipine similarly.

Management Options:
- *Monitor.* Patients receiving nimodipine should be monitored for excessive effects (headache, hypotension) when cimetidine is added or deleted from their drug regimen.

References:
1. Muck W et al. Influence of the H2-receptor antagonists cimetidine and ranitidine on the pharmacokinetics of nimodipine in healthy volunteers. Eur J Clin Pharmacol. 1992;42:325.

## Cimetidine (Tagamet) ⟨3⟩
### Nisoldipine (Sular)

Summary: Cimetidine can increase the serum concentration of nisoldipine; excessive nisoldipine effects may be seen.

Risk Factors:
- *Route of Administration.* Oral administration of nisoldipine increases the likelihood of this interaction.

Related Drugs: Cimetidine also increases the concentrations of *diltiazem (Cardizem), nifedipine (Procardia), nitrendipine (Baypress)*, and *verapamil (Calan)*. Other drugs that increase gastric pH [e.g., *famotidine (Pepcid), nizatidine (Axid), ranitidine (Zantac), omeprazole (Prilosec)*] may affect nisoldipine in a similar manner.

Management Options:
- *Monitor.* Patients receiving nisoldipine should be carefully monitored for altered hypotensive effects when cimetidine or other drugs that alter gastric pH are added or deleted from their drug regimen.

References:
1. van Harten J et al. Pharmacokinetics and hemodynamic effects of nisoldipine and its interaction with cimetidine. Clin Pharmacol Ther. 1988;43:332.

## Cimetidine (Tagamet) ⟨3⟩
### Nitrendipine (Baypress)

Summary: Cimetidine can increase the serum concentration of nitrendipine; excessive nitrendipine effects may be seen.

Risk Factors: No specific risk factors known.

Related Drugs: Cimetidine also increases the concentrations of *diltiazem (Cardizem), nisoldipine (Sular), nifedipine (Procardia)*, and *verapamil (Calan)*. *Ranitidine (Zantac)* 300 mg/day for 1 week increased the AUC of nitrendipine 50% without changing its hemodynamic effects.[1] Other drugs that increase gastric pH [e.g., *famotidine (Pepcid), nizatidine (Axid), omeprazole (Prilosec)*] may affect nitrendipine in a similar manner.

Management Options:
- *Monitor.* Patients receiving nitrendipine should be monitored carefully for altered hypotensive effects when cimetidine or other drugs that increase gastric pH are added or deleted from their drug regimen.

References:
1. Halabi A et al. Influence of ranitidine on kinetics of nitrendipine and on noninvasive hemodynamic parameters. Ther Drug Monit. 1990;12: 303. Letter.
2. Soons PA et al. Grapefruit juice and cimetidine inhibit stereoselective metabolism of nitrendipine in humans. Clin Pharmacol Ther. 1991;50:394.

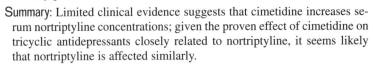

## Cimetidine (Tagamet)

## Nortriptyline (Pamelor)

Summary: Limited clinical evidence suggests that cimetidine increases serum nortriptyline concentrations; given the proven effect of cimetidine on tricyclic antidepressants closely related to nortriptyline, it seems likely that nortriptyline is affected similarly.

Risk Factors:
- *Dosage Regimen.* In most patients, clinically important inhibition of hepatic drug metabolism by cimetidine requires doses of 400 mg/day or more.

Related Drugs: The evidence suggests that *ranitidine (Zantac)* is unlikely to interact with cyclic antidepressants. Theoretically, it is unlikely that *famotidine (Pepcid)* and *nizatidine (Axid)* will interact with cyclic antidepressants since these H₂-receptor antagonists have little effect on drug metabolism. Cimetidine also may increase serum concentrations of *desipramine (Norpramin), doxepin (Sinequan), imipramine (Tofranil)*, and *protriptyline (Vivactil)*.

Management Options:
- *Consider Alternative.* Consider using an alternative to cimetidine (e.g., ranitidine, nizatidine, famotidine).
- *Circumvent/Minimize.* In patients who are already receiving cimetidine and are about to begin a course of therapy with nortriptyline, consider using conservative nortriptyline doses until the patient's response to therapy can be evaluated.
- *Monitor.* In patients stabilized on nortriptyline who are then given cimetidine, be alert for evidence of nortriptyline toxicity (e.g., severe dry mouth, blurred vision, urinary retention, tachycardia, constipation, and postural hypotension). If cimetidine is discontinued or its dose substantially reduced in a patient stabilized on both nortriptyline and cimetidine, the patient should be monitored for an inadequate nortriptyline response.

References:
1. Miller DD et al. Cimetidine's effect on steady-state serum nortriptyline concentrations. Drug Intell Clin Pharm. 1983;17:904.
2. Henauer SA et al. Cimetidine interaction with imipramine and nortriptyline. Clin Pharmacol Ther. 1984;35:183.

### Cimetidine (Tagamet)

### Paroxetine (Paxil)

Summary: Preliminary evidence suggests that cimetidine substantially increases paroxetine serum concentrations, but the clinical importance of the interaction is not established.

Risk Factors: No specific risk factors known.

Related Drugs: The effect of *ranitidine (Zantac)*, *famotidine (Pepcid)*, and *nizatidine (Axid)* on paroxetine pharmacokinetics is unknown; theoretically they would not be expected to interact.

Management Options:

• *Consider Alternative.* Theoretically, other $H_2$-receptor antagonists, such as ranitidine, famotidine, and nizatidine, would be less likely to interact with paroxetine; thus their use may be preferred over cimetidine until more information is available on this interaction.

• *Monitor* for alterations in therapeutic and toxic effects of paroxetine if cimetidine is initiated, discontinued, or changed in dosage. Patients receiving cimetidine may require lower doses of paroxetine. However, determining whether to adjust the dose of paroxetine and by how much may not be easy, since the degree to which paroxetine produces dose-dependent adverse effects is not well established.

References:

1. Greb WH et al. The effect of liver enzyme inhibition by cimetidine and enzyme induction by phenobarbitone on the pharmacokinetics of paroxetine. Acta Psychiatr Scand. 1989;80(Suppl. 350):95.

2. Bannister SJ et al. Evaluation of the potential for interactions of paroxetine with diazepam, cimetidine, warfarin, and digoxin. Acta Psychiatr Scand. 1989;80(Suppl. 350):102.

### Cimetidine (Tagamet)

### Phenytoin (Dilantin)

Summary: Cimetidine increases serum phenytoin concentrations; phenytoin intoxication occurs in some patients. Ranitidine may increase serum phenytoin concentrations in some patients, but the data are limited.

## Significance Classification

① - *Avoid Combination.* Risk always outweighs benefit.

② - *Usually Avoid Combination.* Use combination only under special circumstances.

③ - *Minimize Risk.* Take action as necessary to reduce risk.

Risk Factors:
- *Dosage Regimen.* Cimetidine doses of 400 mg/day may increase serum phenytoin slightly, but larger cimetidine doses can produce greater increases.

Related Drugs: **Ranitidine (Zantac)**, **famotidine (Pepcid)**, and **nizatidine (Axid)** do not appear to affect phenytoin metabolism.[1,2] Case reports have suggested that ranitidine may increase serum phenytoin concentrations, but the cases were complicated by other confounding variables.[3-5]

Management Options:
- *Consider Alternative.* Ranitidine, famotidine, and nizatidine would be preferable to cimetidine in most patients receiving phenytoin.
- *Monitor.* Be alert for evidence of phenytoin toxicity (e.g., nystagmus, ataxia, confusion) when cimetidine is given concurrently. In a patient well stabilized on both drugs, discontinuation of cimetidine may result in inadequate serum phenytoin concentrations.

References:
1. Watts RW et al. Lack of interaction between ranitidine and phenytoin. Br J Clin Pharmacol. 1983;15:499.
2. Sambol NC et al. Influence of famotidine (Fam) and cimetidine (Cim) on the disposition of phenytoin (Phe) and indocyanine green (ICG). Clin Pharmacol Ther. 1986;39:225. Abstract.
3. Bramhall D et al. Possible interaction of ranitidine with phenytoin. Drug Intell Clin Pharm. 1988;22:979.
4. Tse CST et al. Phenytoin concentration elevation subsequent to ranitidine administration. Ann Pharmacother. 1993;27:1448.
5. Tse CST et al. Phenytoin and ranitidine interaction. Ann Intern Med. 1994;120:892.

## Cimetidine (Tagamet)

## Praziquantel (Biltricide)

Summary: Cimetidine increases praziquantel concentrations; the changes clinical significance of these is unknown, but toxicity is possible.

Risk Factors: No specific risk factors known.

Related Drugs: Other $H_2$-receptor antagonists, such as **ranitidine (Zantac)**, **famotidine (Pepcid)**, and **nizatidine (Axid)**, would be unlikely to affect the metabolism of praziquantel.

Management Options:
- *Consider Alternative.* In patients not receiving anticonvulsants, an alternative $H_2$-receptor antagonist (e.g., ranitidine, famotidine, nizatidine) probably would avoid the interaction.
- *Monitor.* Patients who receive cimetidine and praziquantel should be monitored for increased praziquantel plasma concentrations and potential toxicity (headache, nausea, dizziness).

References:
1. Dachman WD et al. Cimetidine-induced rise in praziquantel levels in a patient with neurocysticercosis being treated with anticonvulsants. J Infect Dis. 1994;169:689.
2. Metwally A et al. Effect of cimetidine, bicarbonate and glucose on the bioavailability of different formulations of praziquantel. Arzneimittelforschung. 1995;45:460.

### Cimetidine (Tagamet)

### Procainamide (Procan SR)

Summary: Cimetidine may increase procainamide serum concentrations significantly; procainamide toxicity from this interaction has been reported.

Risk Factors:
- *Concurrent Diseases.* Patients with renal dysfunction are at particular risk.

Related Drugs: *Ranitidine (Zantac)* produces a small increase in procainamide concentrations; *famotidine (Pepcid)* appears to have no effect. Theoretically, *nizatidine (Axid)* is unlikely to interact. Although no data exist, proton pump inhibitors [e.g., *omeprazole (Prilosec)*] would be unlikely to alter procainamide clearance.

Management Options:
- *Consider Alternative.* Famotidine or nizatidine use would likely avoid the interaction.
- *Monitor.* Be alert for evidence of enhanced procainamide and NAPA response (wide QRS, QT interval) in the presence of cimetidine therapy. A reduction in procainamide dose may be necessary.

References:
1. Somogyi A et al. Cimetidine-procainamide pharmacokinetic interaction in man: evidence of competition for tubular secretion of basic drugs. Eur J Clin Pharmacol. 1983;25:339.
2. Lai MY et al. Dose dependent effect of cimetidine on procainamide disposition in man. Int J Clin Pharmacol Ther Toxicol. 1988;26:118.
3. Bauer LA et al. Procainamide-cimetidine drug interaction in elderly male patients. J Am Geriatr Soc. 1990;38:467.

### Cimetidine (Tagamet)

### Propafenone (Rythmol)

Summary: Cimetidine significantly increased propafenone concentration in 8 of 12 subjects stabilized on propafenone.

Risk Factors: No specific risk factors known.

Related Drugs: The effects of other $H_2$-receptor antagonists on propafenone are unknown; *ranitidine (Zantac)*, *nizatidine (Axid)*, and *famotidine (Pepcid)* would be expected to have little effect on propafenone.

Management Options:
- *Monitor.* Until further information is available, patients maintained on propafenone should be observed carefully for increased propafenone response if cimetidine is added or for a reduced response if cimetidine is removed from their drug regimen.

References:
1. Pritchett ELC et al. Pharmacokinetic and pharmacodynamic interactions of propafenone and cimetidine. J Clin Pharmacol. 1988;28:619.

## Cimetidine (Tagamet)

## Propranolol (Inderal)

Summary: Propranolol and other plasma concentrations of beta blockers that undergo significant hepatic metabolism (e.g., metoprolol, labetalol) may be increased by cimetidine therapy.

Risk Factors: No specific risk factors known.

Related Drugs: *Metoprolol (Lopressor)* pharmacokinetics (100 mg single dose) were not affected by cimetidine in one study,[5] but cimetidine substantially increased plasma concentrations of metoprolol 100 mg BID for 7 days in other studies.[3,4,8] The bioavailability of *labetalol (Normodyne)* was increased by 55% to 80% without significant change in systemic clearance after the administration of cimetidine 1.6 gm/day for 3 days,[6,7] while the bioavailability of *dilevalol* increased 11% and the area under the concentration-time curve (AUC) increased 20% following cimetidine 1.2 gm/day.[3] The renal clearance of *pindolol (Visken)* was reduced about 30% and its AUC increased about 45% with cimetidine 400 mg BID coadministration.[9] *Atenolol (Tenormin)*,[3,4,5] *penbutolol (Levatol)*,[2,3] and *nadolol (Corgard)*[1] appear to be affected minimally by cimetidine therapy. *Ranitidine (Zantac)* does not affect propranolol concentrations. *Famotidine (Pepcid)* and *nizatidine (Axid)* would be unlikely to affect propranolol concentrations.

Management Options:

- *Consider Alternative.* Atenolol or nadolol could be administered instead of hepatically metabolized beta blockers. Ranitidine, famotidine, nizatidine, antacids, or sucralfate (Carafate) also may be suitable alternatives to cimetidine, although beta blocker doses probably should be separated from antacids or sucralfate to minimize the possibility of impaired absorption of the beta blocker.

- *Monitor.* Be alert for evidence of altered response to propranolol, labetalol, and possibly other beta blockers when cimetidine therapy is initiated or discontinued.

References:

1. Duchin KL et al. Comparison of kinetic interaction of nadolol and propranolol with cimetidine. Am Heart J. 1984;108(Part 2):1084.
2. Spahn H et al. Penbutolol pharmacokinetics: the influence of concomitant administration of cimetidine. Eur J Clin Pharmacol. 1986;29:555.
3. Mutschler E et al. The interaction between $H_2$-receptor antagonists and beta-adrenoceptor blockers. Br J Clin Pharmacol. 1984;17:51S.
4. Kirch W et al. Interaction of metoprolol, propranolol and atenolol with concurrent administration of cimetidine. Klin Wochenschr. 1982;60:1401.
5. Houtzagers JJR et al. The effect of pretreatment with cimetidine on the bioavailability and disposition of atenolol and metoprolol. Br J Clin Pharmacol. 1982; 14:67.
6. Daneshmend TK et al. Cimetidine and bioavailability of labetalol. Lancet. 1981; 1:565.
7. Daneshmend TK et al. The effects of enzyme induction and enzyme inhibition of labetalol pharmacokinetics. Br J Clin Pharmacol. 1984;18:393.

8. Toon S et al. The racemic metoprolol H2-antagonist interaction. Clin Pharmacol Ther. 1988;43:283.
9. Somogyi AA et al. Stereoselective inhibition of pindolol renal clearance by cimetidine in humans. Clin Pharmacol Ther. 1992;51:379.

## Cimetidine (Tagamet)

### Quinidine

**Summary:** Cimetidine coadministration elevates quinidine serum concentrations; watch for evidence of quinidine toxicity.

**Risk Factors:** No specific risk factors known.

**Related Drugs:** While *ranitidine (Zantac)* would not be expected to alter quinidine metabolism, a case of ventricular bigeminy during quinidine and ranitidine coadministration has been reported.[3]

**Management Options:**

- *Consider Alternative.* Other $H_2$-receptor antagonists, such as ranitidine, famotidine (Pepcid), and nizatidine (Axid), are probably less likely to interact with quinidine than cimetidine.
- *Monitor.* Be alert for evidence of altered quinidine response when cimetidine is started or stopped. Serum quinidine determinations would be useful if the interaction is suspected.

**References:**

1. MacKichan JJ et al. Effect of cimetidine on quinidine bioavailability. Biopharm Drug Dispos. 1989;10:121.
2. Hardy BG et al. Lack of effect of cimetidine on the metabolism of quinidine: effect on renal clearance. Int J Clin Pharmacol Ther Toxicol. 1988;26:388.
3. Iliopoulou A et al. Quinidine-ranitidine adverse reaction. Eur Heart J. 1986;7:360. Letter.

## Cimetidine (Tagamet)

### Tacrine (Cognex)

**Summary:** Cimetidine substantially increases tacrine plasma concentrations, but the degree to which it increases tacrine adverse effects is not established.

**Risk Factors:**

- *Dosage Regimen.* In most patients, clinically important inhibition of hepatic drug metabolism by cimetidine requires doses of 400 mg/day or more.

**Related Drugs:** The effect of *ranitidine (Zantac)*, *famotidine (Pepcid)*, and *nizatidine (Axid)* on tacrine metabolism is not established, but an interaction would not be expected.

**Management Options:**

- *Consider Alternative.* Until the clinical importance of the cimetidine-tacrine interaction is established, consider using alternative $H_2$-receptor antagonists such as ranitidine, famotidine, or nizatidine.
- *Monitor.* If cimetidine and tacrine are used concurrently, monitor for excessive cholinergic response (e.g., nausea, vomiting, anorexia, diarrhea, abdominal pain) and adjust tacrine dosage as needed.

References:
1. Parke-Davis. Cognex Product Information. Morris Plains, NJ; 1993.
2. Madden S et al. An investigation into the formation of stable, protein-reactive and cytotoxic metabolites from tacrine in vitro. Studies with human and rat liver microsomes. Biochem Pharmacol. 1993;46:13.
3. Spaldin V et al. The effect of enzyme inhibition on the metabolism and activation of tacrine by human liver microsomes. Br J Clin Pharmacol. 1994;38:15.

## Cimetidine (Tagamet)

### Theophylline

Summary: Cimetidine increases serum theophylline concentrations, resulting in symptoms of theophylline toxicity in some patients.

Risk Factors:
- *Dosage Regimen.* The magnitude of this interaction increases as the dose of cimetidine increases.
- *Habits.* Cimetidine may have a greater effect in smokers and other patients with high basal theophylline clearance.

Related Drugs: $H_2$-receptor antagonists other than cimetidine, such as *famotidine (Pepcid)*, *nizatidine (Axid)*, and *ranitidine (Zantac)*, are unlikely to affect theophylline pharmacokinetics.

Management Options:
- *Consider Alternative.* Ranitidine does not appear to affect theophylline disposition and thus would be preferable to cimetidine in patients receiving theophylline. Famotidine and nizatidine are also unlikely to interact with theophylline.[3]
- *Monitor.* If cimetidine is used with theophylline, monitor for altered theophylline response if cimetidine therapy is initiated, discontinued, or changed in dosage; the dose of theophylline may need to be adjusted. In a patient already receiving cimetidine, initial doses of theophylline should be conservative until the dosage requirement is determined. Serum theophylline determinations would be useful in following this interaction.

References:
1. Grygiel JJ et al. Differential effects of cimetidine on theophylline metabolic pathways. Eur J Clin Pharmacol. 1984;265:335.
2. Boehning W et al. Effect of cimetidine and ranitidine on plasma theophylline in patients with chronic obstructive airways disease treated with theophylline and corticosteroids. Eur J Clin Pharmacol. 1990;38:43.
3. Lin JH et al. Comparative effect of famotidine and cimetidine on the pharmacokinetics of theophylline in normal volunteers. Br J Clin Pharmacol. 1987;24:669.

## Cimetidine (Tagamet)

### Tolbutamide (Orinase)

Summary: Tolbutamide, glipizide, and glyburide serum concentrations may be increased by cimetidine. Cimetidine may have independent effects on serum glucose.

Risk Factors: No specific risk factors known.

Related Drugs: ***Ranitidine (Zantac)*** does not alter tolbutamide pharmacokinetics. The effect of ***famotidine (Pepcid)*** and ***nizatidine (Axid)*** on sulfonylureas is unknown, but they may interact if increased gastric pH is involved in the observed changes with cimetidine and ranitidine. ***Glipizide (Glucotrol)*** and ***glyburide (Micronase)*** interact similarly with cimetidine. ***Sucralfate (Carafate)*** produced a significant but small (8%) reduction in the chlorpropamide AUC in healthy subjects.[2]

Management Options:

- *Consider Alternative.* Sucralfate may be a good alternative therapy for the treatment of ulcer disease in diabetics because it appears unlikely to alter glycemic control to a clinically significant degree.
- *Monitor.* Diabetics stabilized on any hypoglycemic therapy in whom $H_2$-receptor antagonist therapy is initiated or discontinued should be observed for altered glycemic responses.

References:

1. Feely J et al. Potentiation of the hypoglycemic response to glipizide in diabetic patients by histamine $H_2$-receptor antagonists. Br J Clin Pharmacol. 1993;35:321.
2. Letendre PW et al. Effect of sucralfate on the absorption and pharmacokinetics of chlorpropamide. J Clin Pharmacol. 1986;26:622.
3. Toon S et al. Effects of cimetidine, ranitidine and omeprazole on tolbutamide pharmacokinetics. J Pharm Pharmacol. 1995;47:85.

## Cimetidine (Tagamet)
## Verapamil (Calan)

Summary: Cimetidine can increase the serum concentration of verapamil; excessive verapamil effects may be seen.

Risk Factors: No specific risk factors known.

Related Drugs: Cimetidine also increases the concentrations of ***diltiazem (Cardizem), nisoldipine (Sular), nifedipine (Procardia)***, and ***nitrendipine (Baypress). Ranitidine (Zantac), famotidine (Pepcid)***, and ***nizatidine (Axid)*** would not be expected to alter verapamil metabolism.

Management Options:

- *Consider Alternative.* Although data is limited, other $H_2$-receptor antagonists [e.g., ranitidine (Zantac), famotidine (Pepcid), nizatidine (Axid)] would be unlikely to inhibit the metabolism of verapamil.

## Significance Classification

1. - *Avoid Combination.* Risk always outweighs benefit.
2. - *Usually Avoid Combination.* Use combination only under special circumstances.
3. - *Minimize Risk.* Take action as necessary to reduce risk.

• *Monitor.* Patients receiving verapamil should be monitored carefully for signs of toxicity (hypotension, bradycardia, heart block) when cimetidine is added to their drug regimen.

References:

1. Abernethy DR et al. Lack of interaction between verapamil and cimetidine. Clin Pharmacol Ther. 1985;38:342.
2. Loi C-M et al. Effect of cimetidine on verapamil disposition. Clin Pharmacol Ther. 1985;37:654.
3. Mikus G et al. Interaction of verapamil and cimetidine: stereochemical aspects of drug metabolism, drug disposition and drug action. J Pharmacol Exper Ther. 1990;253:1042.

## Cimetidine (Tagamet)

## Warfarin (Coumadin)

**2**

Summary: Cimetidine may increase the hypoprothrombinemic response to oral anticoagulants; the effect is usually modest, but bleeding has occurred in some patients receiving both drugs.

Risk Factors:

• *Dosage Regimen.* The interaction between cimetidine and warfarin is dose related. For example, cimetidine doses of 800 mg nightly tend to affect warfarin less than larger doses given two or more times daily, and 400 mg/day of cimetidine may be insufficient to produce clinically significant effects on warfarin in some patients.

Related Drugs: ***Ranitidine (Zantac), famotidine (Pepcid)***, and probably ***nizatidine (Axid)*** are unlikely to affect the hypoprothrombinemic response to warfarin.[2,3] ***Phenprocoumon*** does not appear to be affected by cimetidine.[1] ***Omeprazole (Prilosec)***, at least in doses of 20 mg/day, appears to produce a small increase in the hypoprothrombinemic response of warfarin. Cimetidine also inhibits the metabolism of ***acenocoumarol***[4] and possibly other oral anticoagulants with the exception of phenprocoumon (which undergoes glucuronide conjugation). Cimetidine does not appear to affect glucuronidation of drugs in the liver.

Management Options:

• *Use Alternative.* Use ranitidine, famotidine, or nizatidine instead of cimetidine in patients receiving oral anticoagulants. If cimetidine is used, monitor for altered oral anticoagulant effect if cimetidine is initiated, discontinued, or changed in dosage. Adjust the anticoagulant dose as needed.

References:

1. Harenberg J et al. Lack of effect of cimetidine on action of phenprocoumon. Eur J Clin Pharmacol. 1982;23:365.
2. Serlin MJ et al. Lack of effect of ranitidine on warfarin action. Br J Clin Pharmacol. 1981;12:791.
3. O'Reilly RA. Comparative interaction of cimetidine and ranitidine with racemic warfarin in man. Fed Proc. 1983;42:1175.
4. Kroon C et al. Interaction between single dose acenocoumarol and cimetidine or pentobarbitone: validation of a single dose model to predict interactions in steady state. Br J Clin Pharmacol. 1990;29:643P.

## Ciprofloxacin (Cipro)

## Diazepam (Valium)

Summary: The plasma concentrations of diazepam are increased by ciprofloxacin; the clinical significance of this interaction is unknown.

Risk Factors: No specific risk factors known.

Related Drugs: Other quinolones also may inhibit the metabolism of diazepam or compete with it at the GABA receptor. Other benzodiazepines may be inhibited by ciprofloxacin.

Management Options:
- *Monitor.* Patients stabilized on diazepam may experience increased plasma concentrations if ciprofloxacin is administered. Patients should be observed for any increased or prolonged diazepam effects (sedation, ataxia).

References:
1. Kamali F et al. The influence of steady-state ciprofloxacin on the pharmacokinetics and pharmacodynamics of a single dose of diazepam in healthy volunteers. Eur J Clin Pharmacol. 1993;44:365.

## Ciprofloxacin (Cipro)

## Didanosine (Videx)

Summary: The buffers contained in didanosine markedly reduce the plasma concentrations of ciprofloxacin and will likely reduce the efficacy of ciprofloxacin.

Risk Factors: No specific risk factors known.

Related Drugs: Other orally administered **quinolones** also would be expected to interact with didanosine. Drugs containing **magnesium** or **aluminum** will likely interact with ciprofloxacin in a similar manner.

Management Options:
- *Circumvent/Minimize.* To avoid this interaction, ciprofloxacin should be taken at least 2 hours before didanosine. Ciprofloxacin administration up to 6 hours after the didanosine will probably not avoid the interaction due to the persistence of aluminum and magnesium in the gut.[2]

- *Monitor.* Patient response to ciprofloxacin should be monitored if this combination is administered.

References:
1. Sahai J et al. Cations in the didanosine tablet reduce ciprofloxacin bioavailability. Clin Pharmacol Ther. 1993;53:292.
2. Nix DE et al. Effects of aluminum and magnesium antacids and ranitidine on the absorption of ciprofloxacin. Clin Pharmacol Ther. 1989;46:700.

## Ciprofloxacin (Cipro)

### Food

Summary: The administration of ciprofloxacin with milk or yogurt reduces ciprofloxacin concentrations; the clinical significance is unknown but could result in therapeutic failure in some patients.

Risk Factors: No specific risk factors known.

Related Drugs: *Lomefloxacin (Maxaquin)* and *temafloxacin* pharmacokinetics were not affected significantly by administration with meals.[1-3] Additionally, *ofloxacin (Floxin)* appears to be similarly unaffected. Some of the other quinolones may be similarly affected.

Management Options:

- *Consider Alternative.* Lomefloxacin, ofloxacin, or temafloxacin could be considered for use instead of ciprofloxacin.

- *Circumvent/Minimize.* Patients should be counseled to avoid taking ciprofloxacin with milk or yogurt.

- *Monitor.* Watch for decreased quinolone efficacy if administered with milk or high calcium foods. Quinolone administration with foods not high in calcium appears to be acceptable.

References:

1. Hooper WD et al. Effect of food on absorption of lomefloxacin. Antimicrob Agents Chemother. 1990;34:1797.
2. Granneman GR et al. The effect of food on the bioavailability of temafloxacin. Clin Pharmacokinet. 1992;22(Suppl. 1):48.
3. Lehto P et al. Different effects of products containing metal ions on the absorption of lomefloxacin. Clin Pharmacol Ther. 1994;56:477.

## Ciprofloxacin (Cipro)

### Foscarnet (Foscavir)

Summary: The combination of ciprofloxacin and foscarnet has resulted in tonic-clonic seizure activity in 2 patients; the potential significance of this purported interaction requires additional study.

Risk Factors: No specific risk factors known.

Related Drugs: Other quinolones potentially could produce a similar interaction with foscarnet.

Management Options:

- *Monitor.* Until further evidence of this purported interaction is available, patients receiving foscarnet and ciprofloxacin should be monitored for seizure activity.

References:

1. Fan-Havard P et al. Concurrent use of foscarnet and ciprofloxacin may increase the propensity for seizures. Ann Pharmacother. 1994;28:869.

## Ciprofloxacin (Cipro)

### Iron

**Summary:** The administration of iron salts with ciprofloxacin lowers the antibiotic serum concentration and may lead to therapeutic failure.

**Risk Factors:** No specific risk factors known.

**Related Drugs:** Other quinolones, including *norfloxacin (Noroxin)*, have been reported to be affected similarly by iron.[2,3] *Ofloxacin (Floxin)* absorption may be less affected by iron.[1,3]

**Management Options:**

- *Consider Alternative.* Patients taking ciprofloxacin (and probably other quinolones) should not take oral iron salts concurrently since serum ciprofloxacin concentrations may be subtherapeutic. Ofloxacin absorption may be less affected by iron.[1,3]
- *Circumvent/Minimize.* IV iron or IV ciprofloxacin doses could be considered to avoid the interaction. If ciprofloxacin is administered orally, give it at least 2 hours before any oral iron product.
- *Monitor.* If the drugs are used together, watch for lessened antibiotic effect.

**References:**

1. Akerele JO et al. Influence of oral co-administered metallic drugs on ofloxacin pharmacokinetics. J Antimicrob Chemother. 1991;28:87.
2. Campbell NCR et al. Norfloxacin interactions with antacids and minerals. Br J Clin Pharmacol. 1992;33:115.
3. Lehto P et al. The effect of ferrous sulphate on the absorption of norfloxacin, ciprofloxacin and ofloxacin. Br J Clin Pharmacol. 1994;37:82.

## Ciprofloxacin (Cipro)

### Metoprolol (Lopressor)

**Summary:** Ciprofloxacin increases the concentration of metoprolol enantiomers; the greatest effect is on the enantiomer with the least beta-blocking activity.

**Risk Factors:** No specific risk factors known.

**Related Drugs:** Quinolones reported to inhibit drug metabolism include ciprofloxacin, *enoxacin (Penetrex)*, *norfloxacin (Noroxin)*, *pipemidic acid*, and

---

## Significance Classification

(1) - ***Avoid Combination.*** Risk always outweighs benefit.

(2) - ***Usually Avoid Combination.*** Use combination only under special circumstances.

(3) - ***Minimize Risk.*** Take action as necessary to reduce risk.

---

*pefloxacin*. These quinolones also may inhibit metoprolol metabolism. Other beta blockers [e.g., *propranolol (Inderal)*] may be affected similarly by ciprofloxacin administration.

Management Options:
- *Monitor.* Since patients stabilized on oral metoprolol might experience increased beta blockade during concomitant ciprofloxacin administration, they should be monitored for bradycardia, heart failure, or prolonged atrioventricular conduction.

References:
1. Waite NM et al. Disposition of the (+) and (-) isomers of metoprolol following ciprofloxacin treatment. Pharmacotherapy. 1990;10:236. Abstract.

## Ciprofloxacin (Cipro)
## Pentoxifylline (Trental)

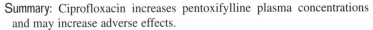

Summary: Ciprofloxacin increases pentoxifylline plasma concentrations and may increase adverse effects.

Risk Factors: No specific risk factors known.

Related Drugs: Other quinolones that inhibit metabolism [e.g., *enoxacin (Penetrex)*, *norfloxacin (Noroxin)*, *pipemidic acid*, *pefloxacin*] would be expected to produce a similar reaction.

Management Options:
- *Monitor.* Patients taking pentoxifylline should be monitored for increased pentoxifylline effects and side effects (flushing, nausea, headache) if ciprofloxacin is administered.

References:
1. Cleary JD et al. Ciprofloxacin (CIPRO) and pentoxifylline (PTF): a clinically significant drug interaction. Pharmacotherapy. 1992;12:259. Abstract.

## Ciprofloxacin (Cipro)
## Phenytoin (Dilantin)

Summary: Preliminary evidence suggests that ciprofloxacin administration may elevate plasma phenytoin concentrations modestly.

Risk Factors: No specific risk factors known.

Related Drugs: Other quinolones that inhibit metabolism [e.g., *enoxacin (Penetrex)*, *norfloxacin (Noroxin)*, *pipemidic acid*, *pefloxacin*] would be expected to produce a similar reaction.

Management Options:
- *Monitor.* Until further data are available, monitor patients for phenytoin toxicity (e.g., nystagmus, ataxia, confusion, dizziness, slurred speech, involuntary muscular movements) when ciprofloxacin is started. Serum phenytoin determinations may also be useful. When

ciprofloxacin therapy is stopped in the presence of phenytoin therapy, monitor the patient for a reduced phenytoin effect.

References:
1. Schroeder D et al. Effect of ciprofloxacin on serum phenytoin concentrations in epileptic patients. Pharmacotherapy. 1991;11:276. Abstract.
2. Hull RL. Possible phenytoin-ciprofloxacin interaction. Ann Pharmacother. 1993; 27:1283. Letter.
3. Job ML et al. Effect of ciprofloxacin on the pharmacokinetics of multiple-dose phenytoin serum concentrations. Ther Drug Monit. 1994;16:427.

### Ciprofloxacin (Cipro)

### Sucralfate (Carafate)

Summary: The administration of sucralfate markedly reduced ciprofloxacin serum concentrations; loss of antibiotic effect may occur.

Risk Factors: No specific risk factors known.

Related Drugs: Sucralfate inhibits the absorption of *fleroxacin*, *norfloxacin (Noroxin)*, and *ofloxacin (Floxin)*. Antacids containing *aluminum* also inhibit ciprofloxacin absorption.

Management Options:
- *Consider Alternative.* If dosage separation is not possible, an alternative to sucralfate (e.g., $H_2$-receptor antagonist, omeprazole, but *not* an antacid) should be considered.
- *Circumvent/Minimize.* The coadministration of ciprofloxacin and sucralfate should be avoided if possible. Ciprofloxacin should be administered several hours before sucralfate or 6 hours after.[3]
- *Monitor.* If sucralfate and a quinolone are coadministered, monitor the patient for reduced antibiotic efficacy.

References:
1. Brouwers JRBJ et al. Important reduction of ciprofloxacin absorption by sucralfate and magnesium citrate solution. Drug Invest. 1990; 2:197.
2. Garrelts JC et al. Sucralfate significantly reduces ciprofloxacin concentrations in serum. Antimicrob Agents Chemother. 1990;34:931.
3. Van Slooten AD et al. Combined use of ciprofloxacin and sucralfate. DICP, Ann Pharmacother. 1991;25:578.

### Ciprofloxacin (Cipro)

### Theophylline

Summary: Ciprofloxacin increases the serum concentration of theophylline and can induce theophylline toxicity.

Risk Factors:
- *Dosage Regimen.* High doses of ciprofloxacin place one at greater risk.

Related Drugs: Quinolones reported to inhibit the metabolism of drugs include *enoxacin (Penetrex)*, *norfloxacin (Noroxin)*, *pipemidic acid*, and *pefloxacin*.

Management Options:

- *Consider Alternative.* Quinolones reported to produce no or minor changes in theophylline kinetics include fleroxacin, flosequinan, lomefloxacin (Maxaquin), ofloxacin (Floxin), rufloxacin, sparfloxacin, and temafloxacin.

- *Monitor.* Patients maintained on theophylline should be monitored for increased serum theophylline concentrations and signs of toxicity (palpitations, tachycardia, nausea, tremor) during concomitant administration of ciprofloxacin.

References:

1. Karki SD et al. Seizure with ciprofloxacin and theophylline combined therapy. DICP, Ann Pharmacother. 1990;24:595.
2. Loi CM et al. Individual and combined effects of cimetidine and ciprofloxacin on theophylline metabolism in male nonsmokers. Br J Clin Pharmacol. 1993;36:195.
3. Batty KT et al. The effect of ciprofloxacin on theophylline pharmacokinetics in healthy subjects. Br J Clin Pharmacol. 1995;39:305.

## Ciprofloxacin (Cipro)

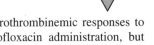

### Warfarin (Coumadin)

Summary: Several cases of enhanced hypoprothrombinemic responses to warfarin have been associated with ciprofloxacin administration, but prospective trials have not supported this observation.

Risk Factors:

- *Concurrent Diseases.* Fever may enhance the catabolism of clotting factors thus enhancing the oral anticoagulant effect.

Related Drugs: **Norfloxacin (Noroxin)** and **ofloxacin (Floxin)** have been noted to increase INRs in a few case reports.

Management Options:

- *Consider Alternative.* Using an antibiotic other than ciprofloxacin to avoid the potential interaction should be considered.

- *Monitor.* In patients receiving oral anticoagulants, monitor for altered hypoprothrombinemic response when ciprofloxacin is initiated or discontinued and adjust the anticoagulant dose as needed.

References:

1. Renzi R et al. Ciprofloxacin interaction with sodium warfarin: a potentially dangerous side effect. Am J Emerg Med. 1991;9:551.
2. Johnson KC et al. Drug interaction. J Fam Pract. 1991;33:338.
3. Rindone JP et al. Hypoprothrombinemic effect of warfarin not influenced by ciprofloxacin. Clin Pharm. 1991;10:136.

## Ciprofloxacin (Cipro)

### Zinc

Summary: The administration of multivitamins with zinc may reduce the serum concentration of ciprofloxacin; however the clinical significance appears to be minimal.

Risk Factors: No specific risk factors known.

Related Drugs: The absorption of other quinolones [e.g., **norfloxacin (Noroxin)**, **enoxacin (Penetrex)**] is likely to be reduced by zinc.

Management Options:

- *Circumvent/Minimize.* Patients taking ciprofloxacin, and probably other quinolone antibiotics, should avoid the concomitant administration of oral multivitamins containing zinc. If the drugs are used together, administer the ciprofloxacin at least 2 hours before the zinc.
- *Monitor.* Watch for antibiotic failure when zinc and a quinolone are coadministered.

References:

1. Polk RE et al. Effect of ferrous sulfate and multivitamins with zinc on absorption of ciprofloxacin in normal volunteers. Antimicrob Agents Chemother. 1989;33: 1841.

## Cisapride (Propulsid)

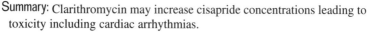

## Clarithromycin (Biaxin)

Summary: Clarithromycin may increase cisapride concentrations leading to toxicity including cardiac arrhythmias.

Risk Factors:

- *Concurrent Diseases.* Pre-existing cardiovascular disease and/or an electrolyte imbalance may increase the risk of the interaction.

Related Drugs: **Ketoconazole (Nizoral)** can increase cisapride concentrations. **Troleandomycin** and **erythromycin** also may inhibit cisapride metabolism. **Azithromycin (Zithromax)** and **dirithromycin (Dynabac)** would not be expected to inhibit cisapride metabolism.

Management Options:

- *Avoid Unless Benefit Outweighs Risk.* Patients who are receiving cisapride and require clarithromycin should have their cisapride temporarily discontinued. Metoclopramide (Reglan) or an $H_2$-receptor antagonist could be considered as a substitute for cisapride.
- *Monitor.* If cisapride is used with clarithromycin, monitor patient for arrhythmias and prolonged QT intervals.

References:

1. Janssen Pharmaceutica. Propulsid prescribing information. 1995.

## Cisapride (Propulsid)

## Erythromycin

Summary: Erythromycin may increase cisapride concentrations leading to toxicity including cardiac arrhythmias.

Risk Factors:

- *Concurrent Diseases.* Pre-existing cardiovascular disease and/or electrolyte imbalance may increase the risk of the interaction.

Related Drugs: ***Ketoconazole (Nizoral)*** can increase cisapride concentrations. ***Troleandomycin*** and ***clarithromycin (Biaxin)*** also may inhibit cisapride metabolism.

Management Options:

- *Avoid Unless Benefit Outweighs Risk.* Patients who are receiving cisapride and require erythromycin should have their cisapride temporarily discontinued. Metoclopramide (Reglan) or an $H_2$-receptor antagonist could be considered as a substitute for cisapride.
- *Monitor.* If cisapride is used with erythromycin, monitor patient for arrhythmias and prolonged QT intervals.

References:
1. Janssen Pharmaceutica. Propulsid prescribing information. Physicians' Desk Reference. 49th Edition. Montvale, NJ; 1995:1191–93.

### Cisapride (Propulsid)
### Itraconazole (Sporanox)

Summary: Itraconazole may increase cisapride concentrations and lead to toxicity including arrhythmias.

Risk Factors:

- *Concurrent Diseases.* Pre-existing cardiovascular disease and/or electrolyte imbalance may increase the risk of the interaction.

Related Drugs: *In vitro* studies have shown ***ketoconazole (Nizoral)*** and ***miconazole (Monistat)*** could interact with cisapride in a similar manner. ***Fluconazole (Diflucan)*** appears to produce less *in vitro* inhibition, but caution is warranted if this agent is administered (especially at high doses) with cisapride, particularly in patients with other risk factors for arrhythmias (hypokalemia, cardiovascular disease, antiarrhythmic drug therapy). Itraconazole would not be expected to alter the elimination of ***metoclopramide (Reglan)***.

Management Options:

- *Avoid Unless Benefit Outweighs Risk.* Patients who are receiving cisapride and require itraconazole should have their cisapride temporarily discontinued. The use of $H_2$-receptor antagonists or proton pump inhibitors is not recommended because they reduce the absorption of oral antifungal agents. Metoclopramide therapy could be considered as a substitute for cisapride.

## Significance Classification

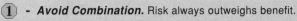

1. - ***Avoid Combination.*** Risk always outweighs benefit.

2. - ***Usually Avoid Combination.*** Use combination only under special circumstances.

3. - ***Minimize Risk.*** Take action as necessary to reduce risk.

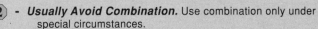

- *Monitor.* Pending further information on this interaction, the manufacturer recommends avoiding the concomitant use of itraconazole and cisapride. If they are coadministered, monitor patients carefully for arrhythmias and prolonged QT intervals.

References:
1. Janssen Pharmaceutica. Propulsid prescribing information. Physicians' Desk Reference. 49th Edition. Montvale, NJ; 1995:1191–93.

### Cisapride (Propulsid)

### Ketoconazole (Nizoral)

Summary: Ketoconazole increases cisapride concentrations and may lead to toxicity, including arrhythmias.

Risk Factors:
- *Concurrent Diseases.* Pre-existing cardiovascular disease and/or electrolyte imbalance may increase the risk of the interaction.

Related Drugs: Other antifungal inhibitors of CYP3A4 [e.g., *itraconazole (Sporanox), fluconazole (Diflucan), miconazole (Monistat)*] are likely to increase cisapride concentrations. Ketoconazole would not be expected to alter the elimination of *metoclopramide (Reglan)*.

Management Options:
- *Avoid Unless Benefit Outweighs Risk.* Until further information on this interaction is available, the manufacturer recommends avoiding the concomitant use of ketoconazole and cisapride. The use of $H_2$-receptor antagonists or proton pump inhibitors (omeprazole, lansoprazole) is not recommended because they may reduce the absorption of some oral antifungal agents. Metoclopramide therapy could be considered as a substitute for cisapride.

- *Monitor.* Patients who are receiving cisapride, particularly in patients with other risk factors for arrhythmias, and require ketoconazole should be monitored for arrhythmias and prolonged QT intervals.

References:
1. Janssen Pharmaceutica. Propulsid prescribing information. Physicians' Desk Reference. 49th Edition. Montvale, NJ; 1995:1191–93.

### Cisapride (Propulsid)

### Mibefradil (Posicor)

Summary: Mibefradil is likely to increase cisapride serum concentrations, potentially resulting in adverse effects including cardiac arrhythmias. Pending further information on this interaction, the concomitant use of mibefradil and cisapride should be avoided.

Risk Factors: No specific risk factors known.

Related Drugs: Other calcium channel blockers [e.g., *amlodipine (Norvasc), nifedipine (Procardia), nicardipine (Cardene)*] would not be expected to change cisapride plasma concentrations. The metabolism of *metoclo-*

*pramide (Reglan)* would be unlikely to be affected by concomitant mibefradil administration. Mibefradil is known to inhibit the metabolism of other CYP3A4 substrates [e.g., *terfenadine (Seldane)*].

Management Options:

- *Use Alternative.* Due to the risk of a possibly serious arrhythmia, the combination of mibefradil and cisapride should be avoided. Noninteracting alternatives are available and should be considered in patients requiring a prokinetic agent and a calcium channel blocker.

References:

1. Roche Laboratories, Inc. Mibefradil (Posicor) package insert. 1997.

## Cisapride (Propulsid)

## Miconazole (Monistat)

Summary: IV miconazole may increase cisapride concentrations and lead to toxicity including arrhythmias.

Risk Factors:

- *Concurrent Diseases.* Pre-existing cardiovascular disease and/or electrolyte imbalance may increase the risk of interaction.

Related Drugs: Other antifungal agents that inhibit CYP3A4 [e.g., *ketoconazole (Nizoral)*, *itraconazole (Sporanox)*, *fluconazole (Diflucan)*] are likely to increase cisapride concentrations. Miconazole would not be expected to alter the elimination of metoclopramide (Reglan).

Management Options:

- *Avoid Unless Benefit Outweighs Risk.* Until further information is available, the manufacturer recommends avoiding the concomitant use of miconazole and cisapride. Patients who are receiving cisapride and require miconazole should have their cisapride temporarily discontinued. Metoclopramide therapy could be considered as a substitute for cisapride.

- *Monitor.* If a patient requires both cisapride and miconazole, monitor for cardiac arrhythmias and prolonged QT intervals.

References:

1. Janssen Pharmaceutica. Propulsid prescribing information. Physicians' Desk Reference. 49th Edition. Montvale, NJ; 1995:1191–1193.

## Cisapride (Propulsid)

## Troleandomycin (TAO)

Summary: Troleandomycin may increase cisapride concentrations and lead to toxicity including arrhythmias.

Risk Factors:

- *Concurrent Diseases.* Pre-existing cardiovascular disease and/or electrolyte imbalance may increase the risk of the interaction.

Related Drugs: *Erythromycin* and *clarithromycin (Biaxin)* also may inhibit cisapride metabolism.

Management Options:
- Avoid Unless Benefit Outweighs Risk. Patients who are receiving cisapride and require troleandomycin should have their cisapride temporarily discontinued. Metoclopramide (Reglan) or an H2-receptor antagonist could be considered as a substitute for cisapride. Azithromycin (Zithromax) could be substituted for TAO.
- *Monitor.* If cisapride is used with troleandomycin, monitor patients for arrhythmias and prolonged QT intervals.

References:
1. Janssen Pharmaceutica. Propulsid prescribing information. Physicians' Desk Reference. 49th Edition. Montvale, NJ; 1995:1191–93.

### Cisplatin (Platinol)

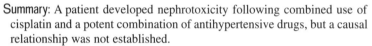

### Diazoxide (Hyperstat)

Summary: A patient developed nephrotoxicity following combined use of cisplatin and a potent combination of antihypertensive drugs, but a causal relationship was not established.

Risk Factors: No specific risk factors known.

Related Drugs: Theoretically, any potent hypotensive drug regimen could increase cisplatin or *carboplatin* nephrotoxicity.

Management Options:
- *Monitor* renal function if potent antihypertensive drugs are used with cisplatin.

References:
1. Markman M et al. Nephrotoxicity with cisplatin and antihypertensive medications. Ann Intern Med. 1982;96:257.

### Cisplatin (Platinol)

### Ethacrynic Acid (Edecrin)

Summary: Severe ototoxicity has been noted in animals given cisplatin and ethacrynic acid.

Risk Factors: No specific risk factors known.

Related Drugs: *Furosemide (Lasix)* and *bumetanide (Bumex)* appear to be less ototoxic than ethacrynic acid and might be less likely to cause ototoxicity when combined with cisplatin.

Management Options:
- *Avoid Unless Benefit Outweighs Risk.* Avoid concurrent use of ethacrynic acid and cisplatin if possible.
- *Monitor.* If any loop diuretic is used with cisplatin, the patient should be monitored carefully for ototoxicity.

References:
1. Komune S et al. Potentiating effects of cisplatin and ethacrynic acid in ototoxicity. Arch Otolaryngol. 1981;107:594.

### Cisplatin (Platinol)

### Gentamicin

Summary: Cisplatin may enhance the nephrotoxicity of aminoglycosides like gentamicin, but the clinical importance is not established.

Risk Factors:
- *Concurrent Diseases.* Renal dysfunction places one at particular risk for the interaction.

Related Drugs: Other aminoglycosides may increase the risk of nephrotoxicity with cisplatin. **Carboplatin** may interact in a similar manner with aminoglycosides.

Management Options:
- *Consider Alternative.* Select an antibiotic other than an aminoglycoside.
- *Monitor.* Patients receiving the combination should be observed for renal dysfunction or hypomagnesemia.

References:
1. Dentino M et al. Long term effect of cis-diaminedichloride platinum (CDDP) on renal functions and structure in man. Cancer. 1978;41:1274.

### Cisplatin (Platinol)

### Phenytoin (Dilantin)

Summary: Phenytoin levels may be decreased by antineoplastic drugs like cisplatin, which may result in increased seizure activity or increased phenytoin dosage requirement.

Risk Factors: No specific risk factors known.

Related Drugs: A 46-year-old male receiving chronic phenytoin experienced increased seizure activity associated with subtherapeutic phenytoin levels following chemotherapy with methotrexate, vinblastine, and carmustine.[2] In another case, a pharmacokinetic study of intravenous phenytoin was performed in a 10-year-old boy with acute lymphocytic leukemia being treated with prednisone, vincristine, methotrexate, leucovorin, and mercaptopurine. The clearance of phenytoin was more than doubled on the seventh day after starting chemotherapy. Plasma protein binding of phenytoin was unchanged.[3]

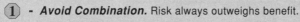

## Significance Classification

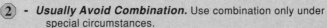

(1) - *Avoid Combination.* Risk always outweighs benefit.

(2) - *Usually Avoid Combination.* Use combination only under special circumstances.

(3) - *Minimize Risk.* Take action as necessary to reduce risk.

Management Options:
- *Circumvent/Minimize.* Case reports suggest that phenytoin levels will begin to return to normal 2–3 weeks following chemotherapy. If a patient had required a dosage increase to maintain a therapeutic level following chemotherapy, it would be important to anticipate this and reduce the dosage accordingly to prevent phenytoin toxicity from developing.
- *Monitor.* Patients should have phenytoin levels monitored 2–3 days after a dose of chemotherapy. If the phenytoin concentration has decreased significantly, the phenytoin dosage should be adjusted accordingly, and phenytoin concentrations should be monitored weekly.

References:
1. Grossman SA et al. Decreased phenytoin levels in patients receiving chemotherapy. Am J Med. 1989;87:505.
2. Bollini P et al. Decreased phenytoin level during antineoplastic therapy: a case report. Epilepsia. 1983;24:75.
3. Jarosinski PF et al. Altered phenytoin clearance during intensive chemotherapy for acute lymphoblastic leukemia. J Pediatr. 1988;112:996.

**Citalopram**

**Moclobemide**

Summary: Combined overdose of citalopram and moclobemide has resulted in fatal serotonin syndrome, but the danger of combining therapeutic doses of the two drugs is not known.

Risk Factors:
- *Dosage Regimen.* The observed reactions occurred in overdose situations.

Related Drugs: In a preliminary report on the use of therapeutic moclobemide doses with another SSRI, *fluoxetine (Prozac)*, no unexpected side effect occurred.[3] Little is known regarding the effect of moclobemide combined with selective serotonin reuptake inhibitors other than citalopram or fluoxetine.

Management Options:
- *Avoid Unless Benefit Outweighs Risk.* Although it is possible that the danger of concomitant use of citalopram and moclobemide is restricted to overdoses, the lack of safety data at therapeutic doses dictates extreme caution in using this combination.
- *Monitor.* If the combination is used, careful monitoring and conservative dosing would be prudent.

References:
1. Beasley CM et al. Possible monoamine oxidase inhibitor-serotonin reuptake inhibitor interaction: fluoxetine clinical data and preclinical findings. J Clin Psychopharmacol. 1993;13:312.
2. Graber MA et al. Sertraline-phenelzine drug interaction: a serotonin syndrome reaction. Ann Pharmacother. 1994;28:732.
3. Dingemanse J et al. Pharmacodynamic and pharmacokinetic interactions between fluoxetine and moclobemide. Clin Pharmacol Ther. 1993;53:178. Abstract.

## Clarithromycin (Biaxin)

### Cyclosporine (Sandimmune)

Summary: Cyclosporine concentrations are likely to be increased by concomitant clarithromycin administration; toxic cyclosporine concentrations and renal toxicity may result.

Risk Factors:
- *Concomitant Diseases.* Renal dysfunction can increase the risk of interaction.[1]

Related Drugs: **Erythromycin,**[2] and to a lesser extent, **josamycin**[3] and **roxithromycin**[4] also have been noted to increase cyclosporine concentrations; **azithromycin (Zithromax)** and **dirithromycin (Dynabac)** would be unlikely to inhibit cyclosporine metabolism. **Tacrolimus (Prograf)** is similarly affected by macrolide administration.

Management Options:
- *Monitor.* Patients stabilized on cyclosporine should have their cyclosporine concentrations carefully monitored and doses adjusted as required during clarithromycin administration.

References:
1. Neu HC. The development of macrolides: clarithromycin in perspective. J Antimicrob Chemother. 1991;27(Suppl. A):1.
2. Harnett JD et al. Erythromycin-cyclosporine interaction in renal transplant recipients. Transplantation. 1987;43:316.
3. Kreft-Jais C et al. Effect of josamycin on plasma cyclosporine levels. Eur J Clin Pharmacol. 1987;32:327.
4. Billaud EM et al. Interaction between roxithromycin and cyclosporin in heart transplant patients. Clin Pharmacol Ther. 1990;19:499.

## Clarithromycin (Biaxin)

### Ergotamine (Ergostat)

Summary: The coadministration of clarithromycin and ergotamine may result in ergotism including hypertension and ischemia.

Risk Factors: No specific risk factors known.

Related Drugs: **Erythromycin** also has been reported to cause ergotamine toxicity.[2] While no data is available, **azithromycin (Zithromax)** or **dirithromycin (Dynabac)** would be unlikely to inhibit the metabolism of ergotamine.

Management Options:
- *Use Alternative.* The use of macrolides such as azithromycin or dirithromycin that do not inhibit drug metabolism would be preferable in patients with migraine headaches who require ergotamine for acute migraine attacks.

References:
1. Horowitz RS et al. Clinical ergotism with lingual ischemia induced by clarithromycin-ergotamine interaction. Arch Intern Med. 1996;156:456.
2. Ghali R et al. Erythromycin-associated ergotamine intoxication: arteriographic and electrophysiologic analysis of a rare cause of severe ischemia of the lower extremities and associated ischemic neuropathy. Ann Vasc Surg. 1993;7:291.

### Clarithromycin (Biaxin)

### Indinavir (Crixivan)

Summary: Clarithromycin can increase indinavir serum concentrations possibly resulting in toxicity. Indinavir increased clarithromycin concentrations; the clinical significance of these changes is unknown.

Risk Factors: No specific risk factors known.

Related Drugs: Clarithromycin produces a small increase in **ritonavir (Norvir)** serum concentrations that are unlikely to produce toxicity. Ritonavir significantly increased clarithromycin concentrations. Other macrolides [e.g., **erythromycin, troleandomycin (TAO)**] are likely to affect indinavir in a similar manner. **Dirithromycin (Dynabac)** and **azithromycin (Zithromax)** would not be likely to inhibit indinavir metabolism.

Management Options:
- *Circumvent/Minimize.* The dose of indinavir may require reduction during administration of clarithromycin or certain other macrolides.
- *Monitor.* Patients should be monitored for possible indinavir toxicity (e.g., nausea, vomiting, and headache).

References:
1. Merck and Co., Inc. Crixivan prescribing information. 1996.

### Clarithromycin (Biaxin)

### Itraconazole (Sporanox)

Summary: Itraconazole concentrations are nearly doubled during concomitant clarithromycin administration; an increase in itraconazole side effects is possible.

Risk Factors:
- *Route of Administration.* Oral administration of clarithromycin is likely to produce a greater effect on itraconazole concentrations than intravenous dosing.

Related Drugs: It is possible that other macrolide antibiotics (e.g., **erythromycin**) could alter itraconazole pharmacokinetics in a similar manner. Macrolide antibiotics that have little effect on CYP3A4 activity include **azithromycin (Zithromax)** or **dirithromycin (Dynabac)**.

Management Options:
- *Consider Alternative.* Macrolide antibiotics that have little effect on CYP3A4 activity (see Related Drugs) should be considered for patients taking itraconazole.
- *Monitor.* Patients receiving both drugs should be observed for increased itraconazole side effects (e.g., nausea, vomiting, headache) during the coadministration of clarithromycin.

References:
1. Hardin TC et al. Evaluation of the pharmacokinetic interaction between itraconazole and clarithromycin following chronic oral dosing in HIV-infected patients. Pharmacotherapy. 1997;17:52. Abstract.

## Clarithromycin (Biaxin)

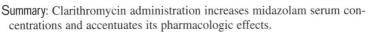

## Midazolam (Versed)

Summary: Clarithromycin administration increases midazolam serum concentrations and accentuates its pharmacologic effects.

Risk Factors:
- *Route of Administration.* The oral administration of midazolam would increase the risk of this interaction.

Related Drugs: *Erythromycin* and *roxithromycin* have been reported to inhibit the metabolism of midazolam. *Azithromycin (Zithromax)* does not appear to significantly affect midazolam metabolism and *dirithromycin (Dynabac)* would not be expected to inhibit midazolam metabolism. Clarithromycin is likely to reduce the metabolism of other benzodiazepines such as *diazepam (Valium)* which are metabolized by CPY3A4; however, *temazepam (Restoril)* which is metabolized by conjugation would not be expected to interact. Other benzodiazepines [e.g., *lorazepam (Ativan), oxazepam (Prilosec)* that are eliminated by CYP3A4 would be unlikely to be affected by clarithromycin.

Management Options:
- *Use Alternative.* The risk of prolonged sedation during the concomitant use of midazolam and clarithromycin suggests avoiding the combination. Azithromycin (Zithromax) does not appear to significantly affect midazolam metabolism. Temazepam is metabolized by conjugation and would not be expected to be affected by clarithromycin.

References:
1. Yeates RA et al. Interaction between midazolam and clarithromycin: comparison with azithromycin. Int J Clin Pharmacol Ther. 1996;34:400.

## Clarithromycin (Biaxin)

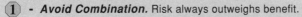

## Tacrolimus (Prograf)

Summary: Tacrolimus concentrations may increase during clarithromycin administration; nephrotoxicity could result.

Risk Factors: No specific risk factors known.

Related Drugs: *Erythromycin* also has been reported to increase tacrolimus concentrations.[2] *Troleandomycin (TAO)* would be expected to affect tacro-

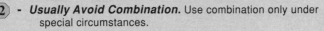

## Significance Classification

1 - *Avoid Combination.* Risk always outweighs benefit.

2 - *Usually Avoid Combination.* Use combination only under special circumstances.

3 - *Minimize Risk.* Take action as necessary to reduce risk.

limus in a similar manner. *Azithromycin (Zithromax)* and **dirithromycin (Dynabac)** would be unlikely to increase tacrolimus concentrations. Clarithromycin would be expected to affect **cyclosporine (Sandimmune)** in a similar manner.

Management Options:

- *Monitor.* Until more information is available, patients receiving tacrolimus should be monitored carefully for decreasing renal function and increasing tacrolimus serum concentrations following the addition of clarithromycin.

References:

1. Wolter K et al. Interaction between FK 506 and clarithromycin in a renal transplant patient. Eur J Clin Pharmacol. 1994;47:207. Letter.
2. Shaeffer MS et al. Interaction between FK506 and erythromycin. Ann Pharmacother. 1994;28:280. Letter.

## Clarithromycin (Biaxin)

## Terfenadine (Seldane)

Summary: Clarithromycin appears to increase terfenadine and terfenadine carboxylate plasma concentrations. Cardiac arrhythmias could result from elevated terfenadine concentrations.

Risk Factors: No specific risk factors known.

Related Drugs: **Erythromycin** and **troleandomycin** have been reported to inhibit the metabolism of terfenadine. *Azithromycin (Zithromax)* and **dirithromycin (Dynabac)** would be unlikely to increase terfenadine concentrations. **Astemizole (Hismanol)** is likely to be similarly affected by clarithromycin.

Management Options:

- *Use Alternative.* Astemizole may not be a safe alternative to terfenadine since it has been associated with arrhythmias when administered with drugs that inhibit its metabolism. The use of sedating antihistamines, loratadine (Claritin), fexofenadine, or cetirizine (Zyrtec) may be preferable in patients who require antihistamine therapy during clarithromycin treatment. Azithromycin may be substituted for clarithromycin in some cases. Patients taking both clarithromycin and terfenadine should be monitored for changes in cardiac conduction.

References:

1. Honig P et al. Comparison of the effect of the macrolide antibiotics erythromycin, clarithromycin and azithromycin on terfenadine steady-state pharmacokinetics and electrocardiographic parameters. Drug Invest. 1994;7:148.

## Clobazam (Frisium)

## Phenytoin (Dilantin)

Summary: Case reports suggest that clobazam addition to phenytoin can lead to clinically obvious phenytoin toxicity in patients who have been taking maximum tolerated phenytoin doses.

Risk Factors: No specific risk factors known.
Related Drugs: No information available.
Management Options:
- *Monitor.* Be alert for signs of increased phenytoin concentrations when clobazam is initiated, especially in patients maintained at high therapeutic phenytoin concentrations.

References:
1. Zifkin et al. Phenytoin toxicity due to interaction with clobazam. Neurology. 1991;41:313.

## Clofibrate (Atromid)

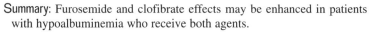

## Furosemide (Lasix)

Summary: Furosemide and clofibrate effects may be enhanced in patients with hypoalbuminemia who receive both agents.
Risk Factors:
- *Concurrent Diseases.* Risk appears higher in nephrotic syndrome or other disorders resulting in hypoalbuminemia.

Related Drugs: It is not known whether other fibric acids such as **gemfibrozil (Lopid)** would interact with furosemide, nor is it known whether loop diuretics other than furosemide would interact with clofibrate.
Management Options:
- *Consider Alternative.* In patients with hypoalbuminemia who are receiving furosemide, consider using hypolipidemic agents other than clofibrate.
- *Circumvent/Minimize.* If furosemide and clofibrate are used concurrently in patients with hypoalbuminemia, consider using conservative doses of 1 or both drugs until patient response is determined.
- *Monitor.* If furosemide and clofibrate are used concurrently in patients with hypoalbuminemia, monitor for evidence of myopathy (muscle pain and/or weakness) and for excessive diuretic effect.

References:
1. Bridgman JF et al. Complications during clofibrate treatment of nephrotic-syndrome hyperlipoproteinemia. Lancet. 1972;2:506.
2. Prandota J et al. Furosemide binding to human albumin and plasma of nephrotic children. Clin Pharmacol Ther. 1975;17:159.

## Clofibrate (Atromid)

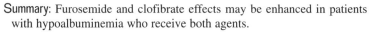

## Rifampin (Rifadin)

Summary: Clofibrate serum concentrations can be reduced by rifampin.
Risk Factors: No specific risk factors known.
Related Drugs: No information available.
Management Options:
- *Circumvent/Minimize.* An increased dose of clofibrate may be necessary during rifampin coadministration.

- *Monitor.* When rifampin therapy is prolonged in patients on clofibrate, monitor serum lipid levels to detect inhibition of clofibrate effect.

References:
1. Houin G et al. Clofibrate and enzymatic induction in man. Int J Clin Pharmacol. 1978;16:150.

## Clofibrate (Atromid)

### Warfarin (Coumadin)

Summary: Clofibrate increases the hypoprothrombinemic effect of warfarin and probably other oral anticoagulants; serious bleeding episodes have occurred in some patients receiving warfarin and clofibrate.

Risk Factors: No specific risk factors known.

Related Drugs: *Gemfibrozil (Lopid)*, *lovastatin (Mevacor)*, and *simvastatin (Zocor)* also may increase the effect of oral anticoagulants while *cholestyramine (Questran)* and *colestipol (Colestid)* may reduce their effect.

Management Options:
- *Avoid Unless Benefit Outweighs Risk.* Concomitant therapy with clofibrate and oral anticoagulants should be avoided if possible. If oral anticoagulant therapy is begun in a patient receiving clofibrate, anticoagulant doses probably should be conservative until the maintenance dose is established.
- *Monitor* for altered oral anticoagulant effect if clofibrate is initiated, discontinued, or changed in dosage.

References:
1. Williams JRB et al. Effect of concomitantly administered drugs on the control of long term anticoagulant therapy. Q J Med. 1976;45:63.
2. Bjornsson TD et al. Clofibrate displaces warfarin from plasma proteins in man: an example of a pure displacement interaction. J Pharmacol Exp Ther. 1979;210:316.
3. Bjornsson TD et al. Interaction of clofibrate with warfarin: effect of clofibrate on the disposition of the optical enantiomorphs of warfarin. J Pharmacokinet Biopharm. 1977;5:495.

## Clomipramine (Anafranil)

### Fluvoxamine (Luvox)

Summary: Fluvoxamine substantially increased clomipramine serum concentrations in 1 patient, probably by inhibition of clomipramine metabolism; adjustments in clomipramine dosage may be needed.

Risk Factors: No specific risk factors known.

Related Drugs: Other combinations of tricyclic antidepressants and selective serotonin reuptake inhibitors also may interact (see Desipramine-Fluoxetine monograph and Index).

Management Options:
- *Monitor* for evidence of excessive clomipramine effect if fluvoxamine is given concurrently; adjust the clomipramine dosage as needed.

References:
   1. Oesterheld J et al. Grapefruit juice and clomipramine: shifting metabolic ratios. J Clin Psychopharmacol. 1997;17:62. Letter.

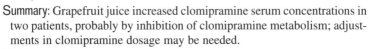

### Clomipramine (Anafranil)

### Grapefruit Juice

Summary: Grapefruit juice increased clomipramine serum concentrations in two patients, probably by inhibition of clomipramine metabolism; adjustments in clomipramine dosage may be needed.

Risk Factors: No specific risk factors known.

Related Drugs: The effect of grapefruit juice on other tricyclic antidepressants is not established.

Management Options:
   • *Monitor* for evidence of excessive clomipramine effect if it is taken with grapefruit juice; adjust the clomipramine dosage as needed.

References:
   1. Oesterheld J et al. Grapefruit juice and clomipramine: shifting metabolic ratios. J Clin Psychopharmacol. 1997;17:62. Letter.

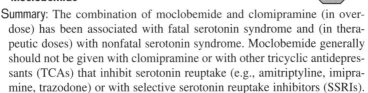

### Clomipramine (Anafranil)

### Moclobemide

Summary: The combination of moclobemide and clomipramine (in overdose) has been associated with fatal serotonin syndrome and (in therapeutic doses) with nonfatal serotonin syndrome. Moclobemide generally should not be given with clomipramine or with other tricyclic antidepressants (TCAs) that inhibit serotonin reuptake (e.g., amitriptyline, imipramine, trazodone) or with selective serotonin reuptake inhibitors (SSRIs).

Risk Factors: No specific risk factors known.

Related Drugs: Other antidepressants that inhibit serotonin reuptake such as SSRIs, *amitriptyline (Elavil)*, *imipramine (Tofranil)*, and *trazodone (Desyrel)* also would be expected to interact adversely with moclobemide.

Management Options:
   • *Avoid Unless Benefit Outweighs Risk.* Combined use of moclobemide and clomipramine should be avoided. Other TCAs that can inhibit serotonin uptake (e.g., amitriptyline, imipramine, trazodone)

## Significance Classification

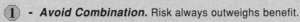 - *Avoid Combination.* Risk always outweighs benefit.

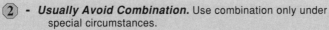 - *Usually Avoid Combination.* Use combination only under special circumstances.

③ - *Minimize Risk.* Take action as necessary to reduce risk.

probably also should be avoided in patients taking moclobemide unless additional data prove that they are safe. SSRIs probably also should be avoided with moclobemide, although some combinations may be safe. If a patient develops serotonin syndrome from one of these interactions, intensive supportive therapy is needed to treat convulsions, hyperthermia, and cardiorespiratory problems. Some also have recommended the use of methysergide (a serotonin antagonist) and dantrolene (for muscle rigidity and hyperpyrexia).[1]

- *Monitor.* If the combination is used, be alert for evidence of serotonin syndrome which can result in neurologic findings (e.g., dizziness, tremor, myoclonus, rigidity, seizures, incoordination, and coma), psychiatric symptoms (e.g., agitation, confusion, hypomania), and disorders of temperature regulation (e.g., fever, sweating, shivering); severe cases can be fatal.

References:
1. Neuvonen PJ et al. Five fatal cases of serotonin syndrome after moclobemide-citalopram or moclobemide-clomipramine overdoses. Lancet. 1993;342:1419. Letter.
2. Spigset O et al. Serotonin syndrome caused by a moclobemide-clomipramine interaction. Br Med J. 1993;306:248.

## Clomipramine (Anafranil)
### Phenelzine (Nardil)

**Summary:** Clomipramine and imipramine should be avoided in patients receiving phenelzine or other nonselective monoamine oxidase inhibitors (MAOIs).

**Risk Factors:** No specific risk factors known.

**Related Drugs:** Other antidepressants that inhibit serotonin reuptake such as *amitriptyline (Elavil)*, *imipramine (Tofranil)*, and *trazodone (Desyrel)* also would be expected to interact adversely with nonselective MAOIs, including *tranylcypromine (Parnate)*, and *isocarboxazid*. Other TCAs also may interact with MAOIs, but some TCAs and nonselective MAOIs can be given together safely if the following precautions are observed: 1) avoid large doses, 2) give the drugs orally, 3) avoid clomipramine and imipramine, and 4) monitor the patient closely.[1-11]

**Management Options:**
- *Avoid Combination.* Combined use of clomipramine or imipramine with nonselective MAOIs should be avoided.

References:
1. Kline NS. Experimental use of monoamine oxidase inhibitors with tricyclic antidepressants (Questions and Answers). JAMA. 1974;227:807.
2. De La Fuente RJ et al. Mania induced by tricyclic-MAOI combination therapy in bipolar treatment-resistant disorder: case reports. J Clin Psychiatry. 1986;47:40.

3. Beaumont G. Drug interactions with clomipramine (Anafranil). J Int Med Res. 1973;1:480.
4. White K et al. The combined use of MAOIs and tricyclics. J Clin Psychiatry. 1984;45:67.
5. Winston F. Combined antidepressant therapy. Br J Psychiatry. 1971;118:301.
6. Schuckit U et al. Tricyclic antidepressants and monoamine oxidase inhibitors. Combination therapy in the treatment of depression. Arch Gen Psychiatry. 1971;24: 509.
7. Spiker DG et al. Combining tricyclic and monoamine oxidase inhibitor antidepressants. Arch Gen Psychiatry. 1976;33:828.
8. Ananth J et al. A review of combined tricyclic and MAOI therapy. Compr Psychiatry. 1977;18:221.
9. White K. Tricyclic overdose in a patient given combined tricyclic-MAOI treatment. Am J Psychiatry. 1978;135:1411.
10. Young JPR et al. Controlled trial of trimipramine, monoamine oxidase inhibitors, and combined treatment in depressed outpatients. Br Med J. 1979;2:1315.
11. White K. Combined tricyclic and monoamine-oxidase inhibitor antidepressant treatment. West J Med. 1983;138:406.

## Clonazepam (Klonopin)

## Valproic Acid (Depakene)

Summary: Absence seizures have been reported in patients receiving valproic acid and clonazepam, but a causal relationship has not been established.

Risk Factors: No specific risk factors known.

Related Drugs: No information available.

Management Options:

- *Monitor.* If absence seizures increase with combined clonazepam and valproic acid, an alternative anticonvulsant regimen should be considered.

References:

1. Jeavons PM et al. Treatment of generalized epilepsies of childhood and adolescence with sodium valproate ("epilim"). Dev Med Child Neurol. 1977;19:9.
2. Browne TR. Interaction between clonazepam and sodium valproate. N Engl J Med. 1979;300:678.

## Clonidine (Catapres)

## Cyclosporine (Sandimmune)

Summary: Limited clinical evidence suggests that clonidine increases cyclosporine blood concentrations; more study is needed to establish the incidence and magnitude of this interaction.

Risk Factors: No specific risk factors known.

Related Drugs: The effect of clonidine on *tacrolimus (Prograf)* is not established, but the drug interactions of cyclosporine and tacrolimus tend to be similar.

Management Options:
- *Monitor* for altered cyclosporine blood concentrations if clonidine is initiated, discontinued, or changed in dosage; adjust cyclosporine dose as needed.

References:
1. Gilbert RD et al. Interaction between clonidine and cyclosporine A. Nephron. 1995;71:105. Letter.
2. Luke J et al. Prevention of cyclosporine-induced nephrotoxicity with transdermal clonidine. Clin Pharmacol. 1990;9:49.

### Clonidine (Catapres)

### Desipramine (Norpramin)

Summary: Tricyclic antidepressants (TCAs) such as desipramine can inhibit the antihypertensive response to clonidone; preliminary evidence indicates that TCAs also may enhance the hypertensive response to abrupt clonidine withdrawal.

Risk Factors:
- *Dosage Regimen.* Abrupt withdrawal of clonidine in the presence of a TCA may lead to an exaggerated hypertensive response.

Related Drugs: Little is known regarding the effect of other TCAs [e.g., *imipramine (Tofranil)*, *amitriptyline (Elavil)*] on clonidine response; assume that they interact until proven otherwise. *Trazodone (Desyrel)* reportedly inhibits the hypotensive response to clonidine, but more evidence is needed.[1] Theoretically, *maprotiline (Ludiomil)* would be less likely to interact with clonidine than other TCAs, but clinical studies are lacking. The tetracyclic drug *mianserin* has minimal effects on clonidine response in both healthy subjects and patients with essential hypertension.[2-4] Clonidine-like drugs such as *guanabenz (Wytensin)* and *guanfacine (Tenex)* theoretically also would interact with TCAs.

Management Options:
- *Avoid Unless Benefit Outweighs Risk.* If possible, concomitant use of clonidine and tricyclic antidepressants should be avoided. Since TCAs also appear to interact with guanethidine (Ismelin), bethanidine, and debrisoquin, these drugs would not be suitable alterna-

## Significance Classification

1 - *Avoid Combination.* Risk always outweighs benefit.

2 - *Usually Avoid Combination.* Use combination only under special circumstances.

3 - *Minimize Risk.* Take action as necessary to reduce risk.

tives. Methyldopa (Aldomet) apparently can be used safely with TCAs, but methyldopa has other disadvantages. In any case, blood pressure should be monitored if TCAs are initiated, discontinued, or changed in dosage in a patient on antihypertensive drugs.

- *Monitor.* If TCAs and clonidine are used concurrently, monitor blood pressure carefully when the TCA is started and also if the clonidine is withdrawn. Gradual tapering of the clonidine dosage may be helpful in reducing the likelihood of severe rebound hypertension.

References:

1. Barnes JS et al. Lack of interaction between tricyclic antidepressants and clonidine at the alpha-2-adrenoceptor on human platelets. Clin Pharmacol Ther. 1982;32:744.
2. Elliott HL et al. Pharmacodynamics studies on mianserin and its interaction with clonidine. Eur J Clin Pharmacol. 1981;21:97.
3. Elliot HL et al. Absence of an effect of mianserin on the actions of clonidine or methyldopa in hypertensive patients. Eur J Clin Pharmacol. 1983;24:15.
4. Elliot HL et al. Assessment of the interaction between mianserin and centrally-acting antihypertensive drugs. Br J Clin Pharmacol. 1983;15:323S.

## Clonidine (Catapres)
### Insulin

**Summary:** Clonidine may diminish the symptoms of hypoglycemia.

**Risk Factors:** No specific risk factors known.

**Related Drugs:** *Guanfacine (Tenex)* and *guanabenz (Wytensin)* theoretically would produce a similar effect during hypoglycemic episodes.

**Management Options:**

- *Monitor.* Patients receiving antidiabetic drugs and clonidine should be aware that clonidine may suppress the signs and symptoms of hypoglycemia.

References:

1. Hedeland H et al. The effect of insulin-induced hypoglycaemia on plasma renin activity and urinary catecholamines before and following clonidine (Catapres) in man. Acta Endocrinol. 1972;71:321.
2. Guthrie GP et al. Effect of transdermal clonidine on the endocrine responses to insulin-induced hypoglycemia in essential hypertension. Clin Pharmacol Ther. 1989;45:417.

## Clonidine (Catapres)
### Nitroprusside (Nipride)

**Summary:** Cases of severe hypotensive reactions with the combined use of clonidine and nitroprusside have been reported.

**Risk Factors:** No specific risk factors known.

**Related Drugs:** Although little is known regarding the effect of centrally acting alpha-agonists other than clonidine, such as *guanabenz (Wytensin)* and *guanfacine (Tenex)*, consider the possibility that they interact with nitroprusside until clinical information is available.

Management Options:

- *Monitor* for excessive hypotensive effects when clonidine is used in patients who are receiving nitroprusside or who have very recently received it.

References:

1. Cohen IM et al. Danger in nitroprusside therapy. Ann Intern Med. 1976;85:205. Letter.

## Clonidine (Catapres)

## Propranolol (Inderal)

Summary: Hypertension occurring upon withdrawal of clonidine may be exacerbated by noncardioselective [e.g., propranolol, nadolol (Corgard)] beta blocker therapy.

Risk Factors:

- *Order of Administration.* Withdrawal of clonidine during noncardioselective beta blocker therapy.

Related Drugs: Centrally acting alpha-agonists other than clonidine, such as *guanabenz (Wystensin)* and *guanfacine (Tenex)*, also can produce rebound hypertension when discontinued; thus, one should assume that beta-adrenergic blockers can enhance this hypertensive reaction until proven otherwise. *Sotalol (Betapace)* appears to affect clonidine similarly.

Management Options:

- *Consider Alternative.* The use of labetalol (Normodyne) (which has both alpha- and beta-blocking activity) may prove useful in preventing rebound hypertension following clonidine withdrawal.[3] Cardioselective beta block-ers [e.g., atenolol (Tenormin), metoprolol (Lopressor)] would be less likely to produce rebound hypertension.

- *Circumvent/Minimize.* In patients receiving both nonselective beta-adrenergic blockers and clonidine, the beta blocker could be withdrawn before the clonidine to reduce the danger of rebound hypertension.

- *Monitor.* If clonidine is withdrawn while the patient remains on a beta-adrenergic blocker, the patient should be monitored very carefully for a hypertensive response.

References:

1. Warren SE et al. Clonidine and propranolol paradoxical hypertension. Arch Intern Med. 1979;139:253.
2. Lilja M et al. Interaction of clonidine and beta blockers. Acta Med Scand. 1980;207:173.
3. Rosenthal T et al. Use of labetalol in hypertensive patients during discontinuation of clonidine therapy. Eur J Clin Pharmacol. 1981;20:237.

## Clotrimazole (Mycelex)

## Tacrolimus (Prograf)

Summary: Clotrimazole troche administration appears to result in increased tacrolimus concentrations and possibly enhanced nephrotoxicity; more study is needed to clarify this interaction.

Risk Factors: No specific risk factors known.

Related Drugs: **Fluconazole (Diflucan)** (and perhaps other antifungal agents) administration increases tacrolimus concentration. **Cyclosporine (Sandimmune)** may be similar affected by clotrimazole.

Management Options:
- *Monitor.* Until more information is available, patients taking tacrolimus should be monitored carefully for increased serum concentrations of tacrolimus and creatinine during concomitant administration of clotrimazole.

References:
1. Mieles L et al. Interaction between FK506 and clotrimazole in a liver transplant recipient. Transplantation. 1991;52:1086.

## Clozapine (Clozaril)

## Diazepam (Valium)

Summary: Isolated cases of cardiorespiratory collapse have been reported in patients receiving diazepam and clozapine, but a causal relationship has not been established.

Risk Factors: No specific risk factors known.

Related Drugs: **Lorazepam (Ativan)** also has been associated with similar reactions when combined with clozapine, but a causal relationship has not been established.

Management Options:
- *Monitor.* Although a causal relationship has not been established for this interaction, the severity of the reaction dictates that patients receiving clozapine and diazepam be monitored closely for evidence of respiratory depression and hypotension, especially during the first few weeks of therapy and after an increase in the dose of either drug. Until more information is available, the same precautions also should pertain to the use of clozapine concurrently with benzodiazepines other than diazepam.

References:
1. Sassim N et al. Adverse drug reactions with clozapine and simultaneous application of benzodiazepines. Pharmacopsychiatry. 1988;21:306.
2. Finkel M et al. Clozapine—a novel antipsychotic agent. N Engl J Med. 1991; 325:518. Letter.
3. Frankenburg F et al. Clozapine—a novel antipsychotic agent. N Engl J Med. 1991,325:518. Letter.

## Clozapine (Clozaril)

### Erythromycin

**Summary:** A patient receiving clozapine developed elevated plasma concentrations and a seizure following the addition of erythromycin therapy.

**Risk Factors:** No specific risk factors known.

**Related Drugs:** *Troleandomycin (TAO)* or *clarithromycin (Biaxin)* also may inhibit the metabolism of clozapine. *Azithromycin (Zithromax)* and *dirithromycin (Dynabac)* would be unlikely to inhibit the metabolism of clozapine.

**Management Options:**
- *Use Alternative.* Noninteracting antibiotics (e.g., azithromycin, dirithromycin) are preferable in patients receiving clozapine.

**References:**
1. Funderburg LG et al. Seizure following the addition of erythromycin to clozapine treatment. Am J Psychiatry. 1994;151:12. Letter.

## Clozapine (Clozaril)

### Fluvoxamine (Floxyfral)

**Summary:** Fluvoxamine can markedly increase clozapine plasma concentrations; dosage adjustments are likely to be needed.

**Risk Factors:** No specific risk factors known.

**Related Drugs:** The effect of selective serotonin reuptake inhibitors (SSRIs) other than fluvoxamine on clozapine is not established, but *fluoxetine (Prozac)*, *paroxetine (Paxil)*, and *sertraline (Zoloft)* appear to have little effect on cytochrome P4501A2.

**Management Options:**
- *Use Alternative.* Given the large magnitude of the increases in clozapine plasma concentrations due to fluvoxamine, an SSRI other than fluvoxamine generally would be preferable. If fluvoxamine is used, adjustments in clozapine dosage are likely to be needed. Monitor for altered clozapine response if fluvoxamine therapy is initiated, discontinued, or changed in dosage.

## Significance Classification

1. - *Avoid Combination.* Risk always outweighs benefit.

2. - *Usually Avoid Combination.* Use combination only under special circumstances.

3. - *Minimize Risk.* Take action as necessary to reduce risk.

References:
1. Heimke C et al. Elevated levels of clozapine in serum after addition of fluvoxamine. J Clin Psychopharmacol. 1994;14:279. Letter.
2. Jerling M et al. Fluvoxamine inhibition and carbamazepine induction of the metabolism of clozapine: evidence from a therapeutic drug monitoring service. Ther Drug Monit. 1994;16:368.

## Clozapine (Clozaril)

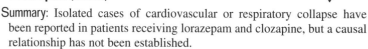

## Lorazepam (Ativan)

Summary: Isolated cases of cardiovascular or respiratory collapse have been reported in patients receiving lorazepam and clozapine, but a causal relationship has not been established.

Risk Factors: No specific risk factors known.

Related Drugs: *Diazepam* also has been associated with similar reactions when combined with clozapine, but a causal relationship has not been established.

Management Options:
- *Monitor.* Although a causal relationship has not been established for this interaction, the severity of the reaction dictates that patients receiving clozapine and lorazepam be monitored closely for evidence of respiratory depression and hypotension, especially during the first few weeks of therapy and after an increase in the dose of either drug. Until more information is available, the same precautions also should pertain to the use of clozapine concurrently with benzodiazepines other than lorazepam.

References:
1. Friedman LJ et al. Clozapine—a novel antipsychotic agent. N Engl J Med. 1991;325:518. Letter.
2. Sassim N et al. Adverse drug reactions with clozapine and simultaneous application of benzodiazepines. Pharmacopsychiatry. 1988;21:306.
3. Klimke A et al. Sudden death after intravenous application of lorazepam in a patient treated with clozapine. Am J Psychiatry. 1994;151:780. Letter.

## Clozapine (Clozaril)

## Valproic Acid (Depakene)

Summary: Several patients stabilized on clozapine developed substantial reductions in clozapine total serum concentrations after valproic acid was started, but clozapine therapeutic response was not affected.

Risk Factors: No specific risk factors known.

Related Drugs: No information available.

Management Options:
- *Monitor.* Until more data are available, one should monitor for altered clozapine response if valproic acid therapy is initiated, discontinued, or changed in dosage. When interpreting clozapine serum

concentrations, keep in mind that if displacement of clozapine from plasma protein binding is involved, subtherapeutic total clozapine levels may not indicate subtherapeutic unbound levels.

References:
1. Finley P et al. Potential impact of valproic acid therapy on clozapine disposition. Biol Psychiatry. 1994;36:487.

## Cocaine

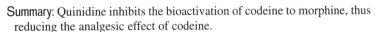

## Propranolol (Inderal)

Summary: Propranolol increases the angina-inducing potential of cocaine; other beta-adrenergic blockers would be expected to have similar effects.

Risk Factors: No specific risk factors known.

Related Drugs: Other beta blockers are likely to produce a similar reaction.

Management Options:
- *Consider Alternative.* The use of cocaine for local anesthesia also might pose an increased risk to patients taking beta blockers. Other local anesthetics should be considered for use.
- *Monitor.* Patients, particularly those with coronary artery disease, taking beta-adrenergic blockers should be cautioned regarding the potential for angina during cocaine use.

References:
1. Lange RA et al. Potentiation of cocaine-induced coronary vasoconstriction by beta-adrenergic blockade. Ann Intern Med. 1990;112:897.

## Codeine

## Quinidine

Summary: Quinidine inhibits the bioactivation of codeine to morphine, thus reducing the analgesic effect of codeine.

Risk Factors:
- *Pharmacogenetics.* Only patients with the extensive metabolizer CYP2D6 phenotype (EMs) would be expected to experience this interaction. Poor metabolizers (PMs) do not have the gene for production of CYP2D6, so there would be no CYP2D6 for the quinidine to inhibit. About 8% of whites are deficient in CYP2D6, but the deficiency is rare in Asians, usually ≤2%.[1,2]

Related Drugs: The analgesic effect of *dihydrocodeine (Synalgos-DC)* and *hydrocodone (Vicodin)* also may be dependent on conversion to morphine-like active metabolites, and early evidence suggests that quinidine can reduce their analgesic efficacy.[1–3] *Tramadol (Ultram)* appears to be partially dependent upon CYP2D6 for analgesic activity, but theoretically would be less affected than codeine by quinidine therapy.[4] Early pharmacodynamic evidence suggests that *oxycodone (Percodan)* does not require conversion by CYP2D6 to an active metabolite.[5,6] Theoretically, oxycodone would not be affected by quinidine, but more study is needed.

Management Options:
- *Consider Alternative.* Consider use of an analgesics other than codeine, dihydrocodeine, hydrocodone, or tramadol. (See Related Drugs.)
- *Monitor.* If codeine and quinidine are used together, monitor for reduced analgesic effect.

References:
1. Fromm MF et al. Dihydrocodeine: a new opioid substrate for the polymorphic CYP2D6 in humans. Clin Pharmacol Ther. 1995;58:374.
2. Hufschmid E et al. Exploration of the metabolism of dihydrocodeine via determination of its metabolites in human urine using micellar electrokinetic capillary chromatography. J Chromatogr B Biomed Appl. 1995;668:159.
3. Otton SV et al. CYP2D6 phenotype determines the metabolic conversion of hydrocodone to hydromorphone. Clin Pharmacol Ther. 1993;54:463.
4. Poulsen L et al. The hypoalgesic effect of tramadol in relation to CYP2D6. Clin Pharmacol Ther. 1996;60:636.
5. Poyhia R et al. A review of oxycodone's clinical pharmacokinetics and pharmacodynamics. J Pain Symptom Manage. 1993;8:63.
6. Kaiko RF et al. Pharmacokinetic-pharmacodynamic relationships of controlled-release oxycodone. Clin Pharmacol Ther. 1996;59:52.

## Colchicine

### Cyclosporine (Sandimmune)

Summary: Cyclosporine blood concentrations increased and nephrotoxicity developed after administration of colchicine in renal transplant patients.

Risk Factors: No specific risk factors known.

Related Drugs: *Tacrolimus (Prograf)* and cyclosporine tend to have similar interactions, but it is not known if tacrolimus interacts with colchicine.

Management Options:
- *Monitor* for altered cyclosporine blood concentrations and renal function if colchicine is initiated, discontinued or changed in dosage. *Note*: Cyclosporine commonly induces hyperuricemia by decreasing urate clearance.[1] Colchicine must be used with caution in patients with decreased renal function because they are at increased risk for neuromuscular toxicity and bone marrow dysplasia.[2]

References:
1. Lin HY et al. Cyclosporine-induced hyperuricemia and gout. N Engl J Med. 1989; 321:287.
2. Kuncl RE et al. Colchicine myopathy and neuropathy. N Engl J Med. 1987; 316:1562.
3. Yussim A et al. Gastrointestinal, hepatorenal, and neuromuscular toxicity caused by cyclosporine-colchicine interaction in renal transplantation. Transplant Proc. 1994; 26:2825.

## Colchicine

### Erythromycin

Summary: A patient developed severe colchicine toxicity following 2 weeks of concomitant erythromycin administration.

Risk Factors: No specific risk factors known.

Related Drugs: *Troleandomycin (TAO)* or *clarithromycin (Biaxin)* also may inhibit the metabolism of colchicine, provided this interaction is confirmed.

Management Options:

- *Monitor.* Pending further reports of the concomitant usage of erythromycin and colchicine, patients receiving both drugs should be monitored for evidence of colchicine toxicity (fever, gastrointestinal symptoms, leukopenia).

References:

1. Caraco Y et al. Acute colchicine intoxication—possible role of erythromycin administration. J Rheumatol. 1992;19:494.

### Colestipol (Colestid)

### Diclofenac (Voltaren)

Summary: Single dose studies suggest that colestipol moderately reduces the bioavailability of diclofenac; the clinical importance of this effect is not established, but reduced diclofenac effect may occur.

Risk Factors: No specific risk factors known.

Related Drugs: *Cholestyramine (Questran)* also appears to inhibit the absorption of diclofenac, and to a greater extent than colestipol.

Management Options:

- *Circumvent/Minimize.* Give the diclofenac 2 hours before or 6 hours after the colestipol to optimize the absorption of the diclofenac. However, since diclofenac undergoes enterohepatic circulation, reduced diclofenac plasma concentrations may occur even if the doses are separated.
- *Monitor* for reduced diclofenac effect, regardless of how far apart the doses are separated.

References:

1. Al-balla SR et al. The effects of cholestyramine and colestipol on the absorption of diclofenac in man. Int J Clin Pharmacol Ther. 1994;32:441.

### Colestipol (Colestid)

### Furosemide (Lasix)

Summary: Study in healthy subjects suggests that colestipol considerably reduces the bioavailability and diuretic response of furosemide.

Risk Factors: No specific risk factors known.

Related Drugs: *Cholestyramine (Questran)* also substantially reduces the bioavailability of furosemide.

Management Options:

- *Circumvent/Minimize.* Although the ability to circumvent the interaction by separating doses of furosemide from colestipol has not been studied systematically, giving furosemide 2 hours before or 6 hours after the colestipol would be expected to minimize the interaction.

- *Monitor* for altered furosemide response if colestipol therapy is initiated, discontinued, changed in dosage, or if the interval between doses of the two drugs is changed.

References:
1. Neuvonen PJ et al. Effects of resins and activated charcoal on the absorption of digoxin, carbamazepine and furosemide. Br J Clin Pharmacol. 1988;25:229.

### Colestipol (Colestid)
### Gemfibrozil (Lopid)

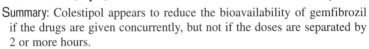

Summary: Colestipol appears to reduce the bioavailability of gemfibrozil if the drugs are given concurrently, but not if the doses are separated by 2 or more hours.

Risk Factors: No specific risk factors known.

Related Drugs: **Cholestyramine (Questran)** probably also inhibits the absorption of gemfibrozil.

Management Options:
- *Circumvent/Minimize.* Until more is known about this interaction, it would be prudent to separate doses of gemfibrozil and colestipol (or cholestyramine) by 2 or more hours.
- *Monitor* for reduced gemfibrozil response if colestipol or cholestyramine is also given.

References:
1. Forland SC et al. Apparent reduced absorption of gemfibrozil when given with colestipol. J Clin Pharmacol. 1990;30:29.

### Colestipol (Colestid)
### Tetracycline

Summary: Colestipol reduces the bioavailability of tetracycline; however, the clinical importance of this interaction is not established.

Risk Factors: No specific risk factors known.

Related Drugs: **Cholestyramine (Questran)** might reduce absorption of tetracycline as well.

Management Options:
- *Circumvent/Minimize.* Until further information is available, patients receiving colestipol and tetracycline should separate the doses in an

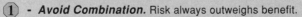

## Significance Classification

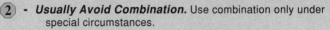

(1) - *Avoid Combination.* Risk always outweighs benefit.

(2) - *Usually Avoid Combination.* Use combination only under special circumstances.

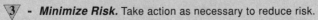

(3) - *Minimize Risk.* Take action as necessary to reduce risk.

attempt to minimize the effect of colestipol on tetracycline absorption. Tetracycline should be administered 2 hours before or at least 3 hours after colestipol.

- *Monitor.* If doses of tetracycline and bile acid binding resin must be administered together, monitor patient for reduced antibiotic effect.

References:

1. Friedman H et al. Impaired absorption of tetracycline by colestipol is not reversed by orange juice. J Clin Pharmacol. 1989;29:748.

## Colestipol (Colestid)

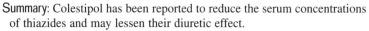

### Thiazides

Summary: Colestipol has been reported to reduce the serum concentrations of thiazides and may lessen their diuretic effect.

Risk Factors: No specific risk factors known.

Related Drugs: Assume that all thiazides interact with colestipol until proved otherwise. ***Cholestyramine (Questran)*** also inhibits thiazide diuretic absorption.

Management Options:

- *Circumvent/Minimize.* Take thiazides at least 2 hr before or 6 hr after the colestipol, and try to maintain a relatively constant interval and sequence of administration of the two drugs.
- *Monitor* for altered thiazide response if colestipol therapy is initiated, discontinued, changed in dosage, or if the interval between doses of the two drugs is changed.

References:

1. Kauffman RE et al. Effect of colestipol on gastrointestinal absorption of chlorothiazide in man. Clin Pharmacol Ther. 1973;14:886.
2. Hunninghake DB et al. The effect of cholestyramine and colestipol on the absorption of hydrochlorothiazide. Int J Clin Pharmacol Ther Toxicol. 1982;20:151.

## Contrast Media

### Propranolol (Inderal)

Summary: Patients taking beta blockers like propranolol are at increased risk for anaphylaxis following the administration of IV contrast media.

Risk Factors:

- *Concurrent Diseases.* Patients with a prior history of anaphylactoid reactions may be at particular risk.

Related Drugs: All beta blockers should be considered to increase the risk of anaphylaxis following contrast media.

Management Options:

- *Circumvent/Minimize.* While the overall incidence of anaphylaxis is low following contrast media, the use of lower osmolality contrast agents or pretreatment with antihistamines and corticosteroids might be considered for patients taking beta blockers.

- *Monitor.* Watch for an increased incidence of anaphylaxis in patients taking beta blockers who receive contrast media.

References:

1. Lang DM et al. Increased risk for anaphylactoid reaction from contrast media in patients on beta-adrenergic blockers or with asthma. Ann Intern Med. 1991;115: 270.
2. Jacobs RL et al. Potentiated anaphylaxis in patients with drug-induced beta-adrenergic blockade. J Allergy Clin Immunol. 1981;68:125.
3. Hannaway PJ et al. Severe anaphylaxis and drug-induced beta-blockade. N Engl J Med. 1983;302:1536.

## Cyclophosphamide (Cytoxan)

### Digoxin (Lanoxin)

Summary: Patients receiving cancer chemotherapy may have impaired absorption of Lanoxin tablets; the magnitude of the reduction appears sufficient to reduce the therapeutic effect of digoxin in some patients. The absorption of digoxin capsules (Lanoxicaps) and digitoxin does not appear to be affected by cytotoxic drugs.

Risk Factors: No specific risk factors known.

Related Drugs: Other cytotoxic drugs also may inhibit the absorption of digoxin. Unlike digoxin, **digitoxin** absorption does not appear to be reduced by cytotoxic drugs.[3]

Management Options:

- *Consider Alternative.* Digoxin capsules (Lanoxicaps) appear less likely to interact with cytotoxic drugs.

- *Monitor.* Be alert for evidence of reduced digoxin response during cytotoxic drug therapy. If oral doses of digoxin are increased to compensate for this effect, it is likely that reductions in digoxin dosage would be required if the cytotoxic drugs are stopped for more than a few days.

References:

1. Kuhlmann J et al. Effects of cytotoxic drugs on plasma level and renal excretion of beta-acetyldigoxin. Clin Pharmacol Ther. 1981;30:518.
2. Bjornsson TD et al. Effects of high-dose cancer chemotherapy on the absorption of digoxin in two different formulations. Clin Pharmacol Ther. 1986;39:25.
3. Kuhlmann J et al. Cytostatic drugs are without significant effect on digitoxin plasma level and renal excretion. Clin Pharmacol Ther. 1982;32:646

## Cyclophosphamide (Cytoxan)

### Succinylcholine (Anectine)

Summary: Cyclophosphamide may prolong the neuromuscular blocking effect of succinylcholine.

Risk Factors: No specific risk factors known.

Related Drugs: No information available.

Management Options:

- *Monitor* for prolonged succinylcholine effect in patients also receiving cyclophosphamide (and probably other antineoplastics). Plasma pseudocholinesterase determinations may be desirable prior to succinylcholine administration. Avoidance of succinylcholine or cyclophosphamide has been recommended if the patient has significantly depressed pseudocholinesterase levels.[1]

References:
1. Walker IR et al. Cyclophosphamide, cholinesterase and anaesthesia. Aust NZ J Med. 1972;2:247.
2. Smith RM Jr et al. Succinylcholine-pantothenyl alcohol: a reappraisal. Anesth Analg Curr Res. 1969;48:205.
3. Zsigmond EK et al. The effect of a series of anticancer drugs on plasma cholinesterase activity. Can Anaesth Soc J. 1972;19:75.

### Cyclophosphamide (Cytoxan)

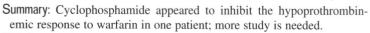

### Warfarin (Coumadin)

Summary: Cyclophosphamide appeared to inhibit the hypoprothrombinemic response to warfarin in one patient; more study is needed.

Risk Factors: No specific risk factors known.

Related Drugs: The effect of cyclophosphamide on oral anticoagulants other than warfarin is not established, but one should be alert for the possibility. Several other cytotoxic drugs have been reported to affect warfarin response.

Management Options:

- *Monitor.* Watch for an alteration in the hypoprothrombinemic response to oral anticoagulants if cyclophosphamide is initiated, discontinued or changed in dosage; adjust oral anticoagulant dosage as needed.

References:
1. Tashima CK. Cyclophosphamide effect on coumarin anticoagulation. South Med J. 1979;72:633.

### Cycloserine (Seromycin)

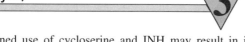

### Isoniazid (INH)

Summary: The combined use of cycloserine and INH may result in increased central nervous system (CNS) toxicity.

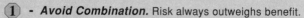

## Significance Classification

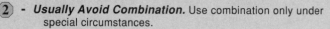

**1** - *Avoid Combination.* Risk always outweighs benefit.

**2** - *Usually Avoid Combination.* Use combination only under special circumstances.

**3** - *Minimize Risk.* Take action as necessary to reduce risk.

Risk Factors: No specific risk factors known.

Related Drugs: No information available.

Management Options:

- *Monitor.* Patients receiving both cycloserine and INH should be monitored more closely for signs of CNS toxicity including dizziness or drowsiness.

References:

1. Mattila MJ et al. Serum levels, urinary excretion, and side-effects of cycloserine in the presence of isoniazid and p-aminosalicyclic acid. Scand J Respir Dis. 1969; 50:291.

## Cyclosporine (Sandimmune)

## Danazol (Danocrine)

Summary: Preliminary case reports suggest that danazol and other androgens can increase serum cyclosporine concentrations and may result in cyclosporine toxicity.

Risk Factors: No specific risk factors known.

Related Drugs: *Tacrolimus (Prograf)*, like cyclosporine, is metabolized by CYP3A4, and its effect also appears to be increased by danazol.[1] Other androgens [e.g., *norethidrone*, *methyltestosterone (Metandren)*] appear to interact similarly.

Management Options:

- *Avoid Unless Benefit Outweighs Risk.* Although this interaction is based upon isolated cases, the potentially severe consequences warrant avoiding the use of anabolic steroids in patients receiving cyclosporine.

- *Monitor.* If anabolic steroids are started in a patient receiving cyclosporine, the patient's cyclosporine response and serum concentrations should be monitored carefully. When cyclosporine therapy is started in a patient who is already taking anabolic steroids, the cyclosporine dose requirements may be lower than expected. In a patient stabilized on both cyclosporine and anabolic steroids, stopping the hormone may cause a fall in cyclosporine blood concentrations; monitor the clinical response of the patient carefully and increase the cyclosporine dose as necessary. Based upon the cases reported as well as theoretical considerations, the changes in cyclosporine concentrations due to such hormones probably occur gradually over several weeks; keep this in mind when monitoring for this interaction.

References:

1. Kramer G et al. Carbamazepine-danazol drug interaction: its mechanism examined by a stable isotope technique. Ther Drug Monit. 1986;8:387.
2. Ross WB et al. Cyclosporine interaction with danazol and noresthisterone. Lancet. 1986;1:330.
3. Shapiro R et al. FK 506 interaction with danazol. Lancet. 1993;341:1344.

## Cyclosporine (Sandimmune)

### Diclofenac (Voltaren)

Summary: Diclofenac has been associated with increased serum concentrations of creatinine and potassium as well as increased blood pressure in a number of patients receiving cyclosporine.

Risk Factors: No specific risk factors known.

Related Drugs: **Sulindac (Clinoril)** was associated with increased serum cyclosporine and serum creatinine concentrations in 1 patient.[3] On the other hand, **indomethacin (Indocin)** and **ketoprofen (Orudis)** appeared *less* likely than diclofenac to interact with cyclosporine in another patient.[1] Given the paucity of data, the relative likelihood of various NSAIDs to increase cyclosporine-induced nephrotoxicity cannot be determined. Assume that all NSAIDs are capable of interacting with cyclosporine until evidence to the contrary is available.

Management Options:
- *Consider Alternative.* Until the clinical importance of this potential interaction is better defined, patients taking cyclosporine should use diclofenac or other NSAIDs only when the expected benefit clearly outweighs the risk of nephrotoxicity.
- *Monitor.* If the combination is used, monitor the patient's renal function carefully and be prepared to discontinue one or both drugs.

References:
1. Branthwaite JP et al. Cyclosporin and diclofenac interaction in rheumatoid arthritis. Lancet. 1991;337:252. Letter.
2. Deray G et al. Enhancement of cyclosporine A nephrotoxicity of diclofenac. Clin Nephrol. 1987;27:213. Letter.
3. Sesin GP et al. Sulindac-induced elevation of serum cyclosporine concentration. Clin Pharm. 1989;8:445.

## Cyclosporine (Sandimmune)

### Digoxin (Lanoxin)

Summary: The administration of cyclosporine to patients stabilized on digoxin may result in increased digoxin serum concentrations and digoxin toxicity.

Risk Factors: No specific risk factors known.

Related Drugs: **Tacrolimus (Prograf)** may produce a similar interaction with digoxin, but data are not available.

Management Options:
- *Circumvent/Minimize.* A reduction in the digoxin dosage may be required. With the discontinuation of cyclosporine, patients may require increased digoxin dosages.
- *Monitor.* Until more data regarding this interaction are available, patients maintained on digoxin should be monitored carefully for digitalis toxicity if cyclosporine is added to their regimen.

References:
1. Dorian P et al. Digoxin-cyclosporine interaction: severe digitalis toxicity after cyclosporine treatment. Clin Invest Med. 1988;11:108.
2. Robieux LC et al. The effect of cardiac transplantation and cyclosporin therapy on digoxin pharmacokinetics. J Clin Pharmacol. 1992;32:338.
3. Okamura N et al. Digoxin-cyclosporin A interaction: modulation of the multidrug transporter P-glycoprotein in the kidney. J Pharmacol Exp Ther. 1993;266:1614.

## Cyclosporine (Sandimmune)
### Diltiazem (Cardizem)

Summary: Cyclosporine blood concentrations are increased by diltiazem; renal toxicity has been reported with the elevated cyclosporine concentrations.

Risk Factors: No specific risk factors known.

Related Drugs: *Nicardipine (Cardene)* and *verapamil (Calan)* inhibit cyclosporine metabolism while *isradipine (DynaCirc)*, *nifedipine (Procardia)*, *amlodipine (Norvasc)*, and *nitrendipine (Baypress)* have minimal effect. Diltiazem may affect *tacrolimus (Prograf)* in a similar manner.

Management Options:
- *Consider Alternative.* Calcium channel blockers that do not appear to alter cyclosporine pharmacokinetics include isradipine,[1] nitrendipine,[2] and amlodipine.[3]
- *Circumvent/Minimize.* Cyclosporine dosage should be reduced and blood concentrations monitored when diltiazem is coadministered.
- *Monitor.* Patients receiving both drugs should be observed for increased cyclosporine concentrations and decreasing renal function.

References:
1. Martinez F et al. No clinically significant interaction between cyclosporin and isradipine. Nephron. 1991;59:658.
2. Copur MS et al. Effects of nitrendipine on blood pressure and blood cyclosporine A level in patients with posttransplant hypertension. Nephron. 1989;52:227.
3. Toupance O et al. Antihypertensive effect of amlodipine and lack of interference with cyclosporine metabolism in renal transplant recipients. Hypertension. 1994; 24:297.

## Cyclosporine (Sandimmune)
### Doxorubicin (Adriamycin)

Summary: A patient receiving cyclosporine and doxorubicin developed central nervous system (CNS) toxicity including coma and seizures; causation has not been established.

Risk Factors: No specific risk factors known.

Related Drugs: The effect of *tacrolimus (Prograf)* on doxorubicin is not established.

Management Options:
- *Monitor.* Until further information is available, patients taking cyclosporine should be observed carefully for changing mental status and CNS toxicity if they receive doxorubicin.

References:
1. Barbui T et al. Neurological symptoms and coma associated with doxorubicin administration during chronic cyclosporine therapy. Lancet. 1992;339:1421. Letter.

### Cyclosporine (Sandimmune)

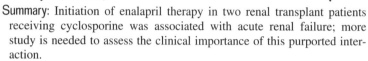

### Enalapril (Vasotec)

Summary: Initiation of enalapril therapy in two renal transplant patients receiving cyclosporine was associated with acute renal failure; more study is needed to assess the clinical importance of this purported interaction.

Risk Factors:
- *Other Drugs.* Diuretic-induced hypovolemia is a possible risk factor.

Related Drugs: Based on the proposed mechanism, expect other ACE inhibitors to interact with cyclosporine in a similar manner.

Management Options:
- *Monitor.* Until further information is available, initiate ACE inhibitors cautiously in patients receiving cyclosporine; monitor renal function carefully.

References:
1. Murray BM et al. Enalapril-associated acute renal failure in renal transplants: possible role of cyclosporine. Am J Kidney Dis. 1990;16:66.
2. Funck-Brentano C et al. Reversible renal failure after combined treatment with enalapril and furosemide in a patient with congestive heart failure. Br Heart J. 1986;55:596.

### Cyclosporine (Sandimmune)

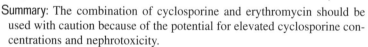

### Erythromycin

Summary: The combination of cyclosporine and erythromycin should be used with caution because of the potential for elevated cyclosporine concentrations and nephrotoxicity.

Risk Factors: No specific risk factors known.

Related Drugs: *Troleandomycin (TAO)* or *clarithromycin (Biaxin)* also may inhibit the metabolism of cyclosporine. *Tacrolimus (Prograf)* is affected similarly by erythromycin administration. *Azithromycin (Zithromax)* does not appear to affect cyclosporine.

## Significance Classification

1. - *Avoid Combination.* Risk always outweighs benefit.

2. - *Usually Avoid Combination.* Use combination only under special circumstances.

3. - *Minimize Risk.* Take action as necessary to reduce risk.

Management Options:
- *Circumvent/Minimize.* Cyclosporine doses may require reduction during erythromycin administration.
- *Monitor.* Renal function and cyclosporine concentrations should be monitored when erythromycin is either added to or deleted from the regimen of patients receiving cyclosporine.

References:
1. Wadhwa NK et al. Interaction between erythromycin and cyclosporine in a kidney and pancreas allograft recipient. Ther Drug Monit. 1987;9:123.
2. Gupta SK et al. Cyclosporin-erythromycin interaction in renal transplant patients. Br J Clin Pharmacol. 1989;27:475.
3. Koselj M et al. Drug interaction between cyclosporine and rifampicin, erythromycin, and azoles in kidney recipients with opportunistic infections. Transplant Proc. 1994;26:2823.

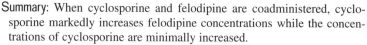

## Cyclosporine (Sandimmune)

### Felodipine (Plendil)

Summary: When cyclosporine and felodipine are coadministered, cyclosporine markedly increases felodipine concentrations while the concentrations of cyclosporine are minimally increased.

Risk Factors:
- *Route of Administration.* The administration of oral cyclosporine would be expected to produce a greater effect on felodipine concentrations than intravenous cyclosporine.

Related Drugs: It is possible that other dihydropyridines that have a large first-pass clearance [e.g., *nitrendipine (Baypress)*] may be similarly affected by concomitant cyclosporine administration. Dihydropyridines that have less first-pass metabolism include *amlodipine (Norvasc)*.

Management Options:
- *Consider Alternative.* Patients receiving cyclosporine could be treated with a dihydropyridine that has less first-pass metabolism than felodipine (see Related Drugs) or a different class of antihypertensive could be selected.
- *Circumvent/Minimize.* Avoid taking felodipine with cyclosporine. Separate the doses by at least two hours.
- *Monitor.* If felodipine and cyclosporine are administered together, watch for excessive hypotensive effects.

References:
1. Madsen JK et al. Pharmacokinetic interaction between cyclosporine and the dihydropyridine calcium antagonist felodipine. Eur J Clin Pharmacol. 1996;50:203.

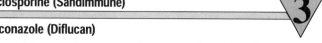

## Cyclosporine (Sandimmune)

### Fluconazole (Diflucan)

Summary: Fluconazole appears to increase cyclosporine plasma concentrations, particularly at higher fluconazole doses; cyclosporine toxicity could result in some patients.

Risk Factors:
- *Dosage Regimen.* Fluconazole doses above 100 mg/day might increase the likelihood of the interaction.

Related Drugs: Fluconazole inhibits **tacrolimus (Prograf)** metabolism. **Ketoconazole (Nizoral)**, **miconazole (Monistat)**, and **itraconazole (Sporanox)** are also inhibitors of cyclosporine metabolism.

Management Options:
- *Monitor.* Until more studies have been done, cyclosporine plasma concentrations and renal function should be monitored when fluconazole is administered. Cyclosporine dosage adjustments may be required in some patients.

References:
1. Lopez-Gill JA. Fluconazole-cyclosporine interaction: a dose-dependent effect? Ann Pharmacother. 1993;27:427.
2. Graves NM et al. Increased cyclosporine levels as a result of simultaneous fluconazole and cyclosporine therapy in renal transplant recipients: a double-blind, randomized pharmacokinetic and safety study. Transplant Proc. 1991;23:1041.
3. Back DJ et al. Comparative effects of the antimycotic drugs ketoconazole, fluconazole, itraconazole and terbinafine on the metabolism of cyclosporin by human liver microsomes. Br J Clin Pharmacol. 1991;32:624.

## Cyclosporine (Sandimmune)

### Gentamicin

Summary: Cyclosporine and gentamicin are both nephrotoxic and produce additive renal damage when administered together.

Risk Factors: No specific risk factors known.

Related Drugs: Other aminoglycosides may produce additive nephrotoxicity with cyclosporine. The effect of aminoglycosides on tacrolimus (Prograf) nephrotoxicity is unknown.

Management Options:
- *Consider Alternative.* If possible, the administration of aminoglycosides should be avoided in patients receiving cyclosporine for immunosuppression after renal transplantation.
- *Monitor.* Patients receiving the combination should be monitored for reduced renal function.

References:
1. Tremeer A et al. Severe nephrotoxicity caused by the combined use of gentamicin and cyclosporine in renal allograft recipients. Transplantation. 1986;42:220.
2. Whiting PH et al. The enhancement of cyclosporine A-induced nephrotoxicity by gentamicin. Biochem Pharmacol. 1983;32:2025.

## Cyclosporine (Sandimmune)

### Glipizide (Glucotrol)

Summary: Glipizide administration appears to increase cyclosporine concentrations; nephrotoxicity could occur.

Risk Factors: No specific risk factors known.

Related Drugs: Other sulfonylureas may affect cyclosporine in a similar manner. It is possible that *tacrolimus (Prograf)* interacts with glipizide.
Management Options:
- *Circumvent/Minimize.* Cyclosporine doses may require adjustment to avoid cyclosporine-induced renal toxicity.
- *Monitor.* Until further information is available, patients stabilized on cyclosporine should be monitored for increased cyclosporine concentrations following the addition of glipizide.

References:
1. Chidester PD et al. Interaction between glipizide and cyclosporine: report of two cases. Transplant Proc. 1993;25:2136.

## Cyclosporine (Sandimmune)

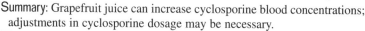

### Grapefruit Juice

Summary: Grapefruit juice can increase cyclosporine blood concentrations; adjustments in cyclosporine dosage may be necessary.
Risk Factors: No specific risk factors known.
Related Drugs: Like cyclosporine, *tacrolimus (Prograf)* also undergoes first-pass metabolism by CYP3A4. Thus, grapefruit juice probably also increases tacrolimus blood concentrations.
Management Options:
- *Consider Alternative.* Orange juice does not appear to interact with cyclosporine.
- *Circumvent/Minimize.* Patients on cyclosporine should be advised to avoid grapefruit juice (unless the combination is being used intentionally to elevate cyclosporine blood levels). Separating doses of grapefruit juice from cyclosporine may not eliminate the interaction completely, since the inhibitory effect of grapefruit juice on CYP3A4 can last for several hours.
- *Monitor.* If grapefruit juice is taken concurrently with cyclosporine, the patient's response to cyclosporine should be monitored carefully, especially if grapefruit juice is initiated, discontinued, or if the interval between the cyclosporine and grapefruit juice is changed.

References:
1. Yee G et al. Effect of grapefruit juice on blood cyclosporin concentration. Lancet. 1995;345:955.
2. Ducharme MP et al. Trough concentrations of cyclosporine in blood following administration with grapefruit juice. Br J Clin Pharmacol. 1993;36:457.
3. Hollander AAMJ et al. The effect of grapefruit juice on cyclosporine and prednisone metabolism in transplant patients. Clin Pharmacol Ther. 1995;57:318.

## Cyclosporine (Sandimmune)

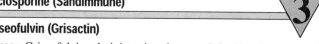

### Griseofulvin (Grisactin)

Summary: Griseofulvin administration decreased the blood concentrations of cyclosporine in one patient; cyclosporine efficacy could be reduced during griseofulvin administration.

Risk Factors: No specific risk factors known.

Related Drugs: Griseofulvin may affect *tacrolimus (Prograf)* similarly. Other antifungal agents [e.g., *ketoconazole (Nizoral)*] may reduce cyclosporine metabolism.

Management Options:
- *Circumvent/Minimize.* Cyclosporine doses may have to be increased during griseofulvin therapy and decreased when griseofulvin is discontinued.
- *Monitor.* Cyclosporine concentrations and signs of transplant rejection should be monitored when griseofulvin is added to or removed from the therapy of a patient receiving cyclosporine.

References:
1. Abu-Romeh SH et al. Cyclosporin A and griseofulvin: another drug interaction. Nephron. 1991;58:237.
2. Klintmalm G et al. High dose methylprednisolone increases plasma cyclosporin levels in renal transplant recipients. Lancet. 1984;1:731.

## Cyclosporine (Sandimmune)

### Imipenem (Primaxin)

Summary: Taking imipenem with cyclosporine resulted in acute central nervous system (CNS) toxicity in one patient.

Risk Factors: No specific risk factors known.

Related Drugs: A similar interaction with *tacrolimus (Prograf)* and imipenem may occur, but data are not available.

Management Options:
- *Monitor.* Until more information about this is available, patients receiving both drugs should be observed carefully for CNS toxic symptoms and altered cyclosporine serum concentrations.

References:
1. Zazgornik J et al. Potentiation of neurotoxic side effects by co-administration of imipenem to cyclosporine therapy in a kidney transplant recipient—synergism of side effects or drug interaction? Clin Nephrol. 1986;26:265.

## Cyclosporine (Sandimmune)

### Indomethacin (Indocin)

Summary: Some nonsteroidal anti-inflammatory drugs may increase the risk of cyclosporine nephrotoxicity, but little clinical information is available for indomethacin.

Risk Factors: No specific risk factors known.

Related Drugs: Another NSAID, *diclofenac (Voltaren)*, has been associated with impaired renal function in a number of patients receiving cyclosporine;[1,2] and *sulindac (Clinoril)* was associated with increased serum cyclosporine and serum creatinine concentrations in 1 patient.[3] However, since little is known regarding the effect of other NSAIDs on cyclosporine response, assume that all NSAIDs are capable of interacting with cyclosporine until evidence to the contrary is available.

Management Options:

- *Consider Alternative.* Even though there is little clinical information available regarding the effect of indomethacin on the response to cyclosporine, all NSAIDs should be used cautiously in patients taking cyclosporine.
- *Monitor.* If the combination is used, monitor the patient's renal function carefully and be prepared to discontinue one or both drugs.

References:

1. Branthwaite JP et al. Cyclosporin and diclofenac interaction in rheumatoid arthritis. Lancet. 1991;337:252. Letter.
2. Deray G et al. Enhancement of cyclosporine A nephrotoxicity of diclofenac. Clin Nephrol. 1987;27:213. Letter.
3. Sesin GP et al. Sulindac-induced elevation of serum cyclosporine concentration. Clin Pharm. 1989;8:445.

## Cyclosporine (Sandimmune)

### Itraconazole (Sporanox)

**Summary:** Itraconazole may increase cyclosporine serum concentrations; nephrotoxicity may result.

**Risk Factors:** No specific risk factors known.

**Related Drugs:** *Ketoconazole (Nizoral)*, *miconazole (Monistat)*, and *fluconazole (Diflucan)* are also inhibitors of cyclosporine metabolism. Itraconazole may affect *tacrolimus (Prograf)* similarly.

Management Options:

- *Monitor.* Cyclosporine concentrations and renal function should be monitored when itraconazole is added to or removed from the therapy of patients taking cyclosporine.

References:

1. Kramer MR et al. Cyclosporin and itraconazole interaction in heart and lung transplant recipients. Ann Intern Med. 1990;113:327.
2. Back DJ et al. Comparative effects of the antimycotic drugs ketoconazole, fluconazole, itraconazole, and terbinafine on the metabolism of cyclosporin by human liver microsomes. Br J Clin Pharmacol. 1991;32:624.
3. Berenguer J et al. Itraconazole for experimental pulmonary aspergillosis: comparison with amphotericin B, interaction with cyclosporine A, and correlation between therapeutic response and itraconazole concentrations in plasma. Antimicrob Agents Chemother. 1994;38:1303.

## Significance Classification

- ① - *Avoid Combination.* Risk always outweighs benefit.
- ② - *Usually Avoid Combination.* Use combination only under special circumstances.
- ③ - *Minimize Risk.* Take action as necessary to reduce risk.

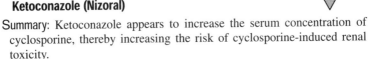

### Cyclosporine (Sandimmune)

### Ketoconazole (Nizoral)

Summary: Ketoconazole appears to increase the serum concentration of cyclosporine, thereby increasing the risk of cyclosporine-induced renal toxicity.

Risk Factors: No specific risk factors known.

Related Drugs: Other antifungal agents [*miconazole (Monistat)*, *itraconazole (Sporanox)*, *fluconazole (Diflucan)*] are likely to increase cyclosporine concentrations. It is likely that *tacrolimus (Prograf)* concentrations will be increased by ketoconazole and other antifungal agents.

Management Options:

- *Circumvent/Minimize.* Cyclosporine dose reduction is usually necessary when administered with ketoconazole.

- *Monitor.* Cyclosporine concentrations and renal function should be monitored when ketoconazole is prescribed during cyclosporine therapy. In patients stabilized on both drugs, large reductions in cyclosporine concentrations may occur when ketoconazole is discontinued.

References:

1. First MR et al. Cyclosporine-ketoconazole interaction. Transplantation. 1993;55: 1000.
2. Back DJ et al. Comparative effects of the antimycotic drugs ketoconazole, fluconazole, itraconazole, and terbinafine on the metabolism of cyclosporin by human liver microsomes. Br J Clin Pharmacol. 1991;32:624.
3. Gomez DY et al. The effects of ketoconazole on the intestinal metabolism and bioavailability of cyclosporine. Clin Pharmacol Ther. 1995;58:15.

### Cyclosporine (Sandimmune)

### Ketoprofen (Orudis)

Summary: Although some nonsteroidal anti-inflammatory drugs (NSAIDs) may increase the risk of cyclosporine nephrotoxicity, little clinical information is available for ketoprofen.

Risk Factors: No specific risk factors known.

Related Drugs: Another NSAID, *diclofenac (Voltaren)*, has been associated with impaired renal function in a number of patients receiving cyclosporine;[1,2] and *sulindac (Clinoril)* was associated with increased serum cyclosporine and serum creatinine concentrations in 1 patient.[3] However, since little is known regarding the effect of other NSAIDs on cyclosporine response, assume that all NSAIDs are capable of interacting with cyclosporine until evidence to the contrary is available.

Management Options:

- *Consider Alternative.* Although little clinical information is available regarding the effect of ketoprofen on the response to cyclo-sporine, all NSAIDs should be used cautiously in patients receiving cyclosporine.

- *Monitor.* If the combination is used, monitor the patient's renal function carefully and be prepared to discontinue one or both drugs.

References:
1. Branthwaite JP et al. Cyclosporin and diclofenac interaction in rheumatoid arthritis. Lancet. 1991;337:252. Letter.
2. Deray G et al. Enhancement of cyclosporine A nephrotoxicity of diclofenac. Clin Nephrol. 1987;27:213. Letter.
3. Sesin GP et al. Sulindac-induced elevation of serum cyclosporine concentration. Clin Pharm. 1989;8:445.

## Cyclosporine (Sandimmune)

### Mefenamic Acid (Ponstel)

Summary: A renal transplant patient rapidly developed nephrotoxicity and an increase in plasma cyclosporine concentration following the use of mefenamic acid, but the clinical importance is not established.

Risk Factors: No specific risk factors known.

Related Drugs: Several NSAIDs [e.g., ***diclofenac (Voltaren), sulindac (Clinoril)***] have been associated with impaired renal function and/or increased cyclosporine blood concentrations. The relative likelihood of various NSAIDs to increase cyclosporine-induced nephrotoxicity is not established, but assume that all NSAIDs are capable of interacting with cyclosporine until evidence to the contrary is available.

Management Options:
- *Consider Alternative.* Until the clinical importance of this potential interaction is better defined, use mefenamic acid (or other NSAIDs) in patients receiving cyclosporine only when the expected benefit clearly outweighs the risk of excessive cyclosporine response and nephrotoxicity.
- *Monitor.* If the combination is used, monitor the patient's renal function and cyclosporine concentrations carefully, and be prepared to discontinue one or both drugs.

References:
1. Agar JWM. Cyclosporin A and mefenamic acid in a renal transplant patient. Aust NZ J Med. 1991;21:784. Letter.

## Cyclosporine (Sandimmune)

### Melphalan (Alkeran)

Summary: Preliminary evidence indicates that melphalan may increase the likelihood of nephrotoxicity in patients receiving cyclosporine.

Risk Factors: No specific risk factors known.

Related Drugs: No information available.

Management Options:
- *Monitor.* Renal function should be monitored carefully in patients receiving concurrent therapy with cyclosporine and melphalan.

References:
1. Morgenstern GR et al. Cyclosporin interaction w ith ketoconazole and melphalan. Lancet. 1982;2:1342.

## Cyclosporine (Sandimmune)

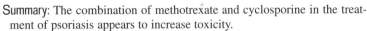

### Methotrexate (Mexate)

Summary: The combination of methotrexate and cyclosporine in the treatment of psoriasis appears to increase toxicity.

Risk Factors: No specific risk factors known.

Related Drugs: No information available.

Management Options:
- *Monitor.* Patients receiving methotrexate and cyclosporine should be monitored carefully for toxicity from both agents. Cyclosporine and methotrexate concentrations should be monitored; the dosage of either drug may require adjustment.

References:
1. Powles AV et al. Cyclosporin toxicity. Lancet. 1990;335:610. Letter.
2. Korstanje MJ et al. Cyclosporine and methotrexate: a dangerous combination. J Am Acad Derm. 1990;23:320.

## Cyclosporine (Sandimmune)

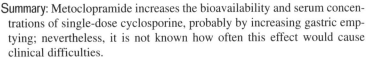

### Metoclopramide (Reglan)

Summary: Metoclopramide increases the bioavailability and serum concentrations of single-dose cyclosporine, probably by increasing gastric emptying; nevertheless, it is not known how often this effect would cause clinical difficulties.

Risk Factors: No specific risk factors known.

Related Drugs: The effect of **cisapride (Propulsid)** on cyclosporine is not established, but caution is in order since both are metabolized by CYP3A4. Competition for metabolism is theoretically possible.

Management Options:
- *Monitor.* Until multiple-dose studies are performed, monitor cyclosporine serum concentrations and responses carefully when metoclopramide is given concurrently. It may be necessary to reduce the cyclosporine dose in some patients.

References:
1. Yee GC et al. Cyclosporine. In: Evans WE et al, eds. Applied Pharmacokinetics: Principles of Therapeutic Drug Monitoring. 3rd ed. Vancouver: Applied Therapeutics, Inc.; 1992:28-1–28-40.
2. Wadhwa NK et al. The effect of oral metoclopramide on the absorption of cyclosporine. Transplantation. 1987;43:211.

## Significance Classification

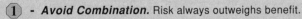

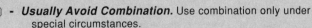

1. - *Avoid Combination.* Risk always outweighs benefit.

2. - *Usually Avoid Combination.* Use combination only under special circumstances.

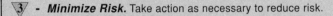

3. - *Minimize Risk.* Take action as necessary to reduce risk.

## Cyclosporine (Sandimmune)

### Miconazole (Monistat)

Summary: Miconazole administration to a patient receiving cyclosporine (CYP3A4) appears to increase cyclosporine concentrations; the clinical significance of this increase is unknown.

Risk Factors: No specific risk factors known.

Related Drugs: Other antifungal agents [*ketoconazole (Nizoral)*, *itraconazole (Sporanox)*, *fluconazole (Diflucan)*] are likely to increase cyclosporine concentrations. Miconazole may produce a similar reaction with *tacrolimus (Prograf)*.

Management Options:
- *Monitor.* Until further studies of this interaction are available, patients stabilized on cyclosporine should be monitored closely for increased concentrations of cyclosporine when miconazole is administered.

References:
1. Horton CM et al. Cyclosporine interactions with miconazole and other azole-antimycotics: a case report and review of the literature. J Heart Lung Transplant. 1992;11:1127.
2. Graves NM et al. Increased cyclosporine levels as a result of simultaneous fluconazole and cyclosporine therapy in renal transplant recipients: a double-blind, randomized pharmacokinetic and safety study. Transplant Proc. 1991;23:1041.

## Cyclosporine (Sandimmune)

### Nafcillin

Summary: Nafcillin therapy reduced cyclosporine blood concentrations during concomitant administration; the clinical significance of this interaction is unknown, but a reduction in cyclosporine activity may be anticipated.

Risk Factors: No specific risk factors known.

Related Drugs: If this interaction is substantiated, *tacrolimus (Prograf)* is likely to be affected similarly.

Management Options:
- *Monitor.* Patients receiving cyclosporine should be monitored for reduced blood concentrations of cyclosporine and evidence of organ rejection during nafcillin administration.

References:
1. Veremis SA et al. Subtherapeutic cyclosporine concentrations during nafcillin therapy. Transplantation. 1987;43:913.

## Cyclosporine (Sandimmune)

### Naproxen (Naprosyn)

Summary: Impaired renal function appears to be greater with naproxen plus cyclosporine than with either drug alone.

Risk Factors: No specific risk factors known.

Related Drugs: In patients receiving cyclosporine, several NSAIDs have been associated with impaired renal function and/or increased cyclosporine blood concentrations.[1-4] The relative likelihood of various NSAIDs [e.g., **sulindac (Clinoril)**] to increase cyclosporine-induced nephrotoxicity is not established, but assume that all NSAIDs are capable of interacting with cyclosporine until evidence to the contrary is available.

Management Options:

- *Consider Alternative.* Until the clinical importance of this potential interaction is better defined, use naproxen (or other NSAIDs) in patients receiving cyclosporine only when the expected benefit clearly outweighs the risk of excessive cyclosporine response and nephrotoxicity.

- *Monitor.* If the combination is used, monitor the patient's renal function carefully and be prepared to discontinue one or both drugs.

References:

1. Sesin GP et al. Sulindac-induced elevation of serum cyclosporine concentrations. Clin Pharm. 1989;8:445.
2. Branthwaite JP et al. Cyclosporin and diclofenac interaction in rheumatoid arthritis. Lancet. 1991;337:252. Letter.
3. Deray G et al. Enhancement of cyclosporine A nephrotoxicity by diclofenac. Clin Nephrol. 1987;27:213. Letter.
4. Altman RD et al. Interaction of cyclosporine A and nonsteroidal anti-inflammatory drugs on renal function in patients with rheumatoid arthritis. Am J Med. 1992; 93:396.

## Cyclosporine (Sandimmune)

## Nicardipine (Cardene)

Summary: Cyclosporine blood concentrations are increased by nicardipine; cyclosporine toxicity could result.

Risk Factors: No specific risk factors known.

Related Drugs: **Diltiazem (Cardizem)** and **verapamil (Calan)** inhibit cyclosporine metabolism while **isradipine (DynaCirc)**, **nifedipine (Procardia)**, **amlodipine (Norvasc)** and **nitrendipine (Baypress)** have minimal effect. Nicardipine may affect **tacrolimus (Prograf)** in a similar manner.

Management Options:

- *Consider Alternative.* Calcium channel blockers that do not appear to alter cyclosporine pharmacokinetics include isradipine,[1] nitrendipine,[2] and amlodipine.[3]

- *Circumvent/Minimize.* Cyclosporine dosage should be reduced and blood concentrations monitored when nicardipine is coadministered.

- *Monitor.* Patients receiving both drugs should be observed for increased cyclosporine concentrations and decreasing renal function.

References:

1. Martinez F et al. No clinically significant interaction between cyclosporin and isradipine. Nephron. 1991;59:658.

2. Coupur MS et al. Effects of nitrendipine on blood pressure and blood cyclosporine A level in patients with posttransplant hypertension. Nephron. 1989;52:227.
3. Toupance O et al. Antihypertensive effect of amlodipine and lack of interference with cyclosporine metabolism in renal transplant recipients. Hypertension. 1994;24:297.

## Cyclosporine (Sandimmune)

### Oral Contraceptives

**Summary:** Isolated case of elevated plasma cyclosporine concentrations have been observed following oral contraceptive use.

**Risk Factors:** No specific risk factors known.

**Related Drugs:** The effect of replacement estrogen therapy on cyclosporine is not established; given the lower doses of estrogen used in replacement therapy, an interaction seems less likely.

**Management Options:**

- *Consider Alternative.* Although this interaction is not well documented, consider using contraception other than oral contraceptives in patients receiving cyclosporine, since the consequences are potentially severe.

- *Monitor.* If oral contraceptives are used, the patient's clinical response and cyclosporine serum concentrations should be monitored carefully. When cyclosporine therapy is started in a patient who is already taking oral contraceptives, the possibility that cyclosporine dosage requirements may be lower than expected should be anticipated. In a patient stabilized on both cyclosporine and an oral contraceptive, discontinuation of the contraceptive may cause a fall in cyclosporine blood concentrations. In both situations, the clinical response of the patient should be monitored carefully and the cyclosporine dose adjusted as necessary. Based on the case reported as well as theoretical considerations, the changes in cyclosporine concentrations due to hormone therapy probably occur gradually over several weeks. Keep this in mind when monitoring patients for this interaction.

**References:**

1. Chambers DM et al. Antipyrine elimination in saliva after low-dose combined or progestogen only oral contraceptive steroids. Br J Clin Pharmacol. 1982;13:229.
2. Deray G. Oral contraceptive interaction with cyclosporine. Lancet. 1987;1:158.
3. Maurer G. Metabolism of cyclosporine. Transplant Proc. 1985;17(Suppl. 1):19.

## Cyclosporine (Sandimmune)

### Phenobarbital

**Summary:** Phenobarbital (and probably other barbiturates) can reduce the effect of cyclosporine; adjustments in cyclosporine dose may be needed.

**Risk Factors:** No specific risk factors known.

Related Drugs: Other barbiturates also should be expected to reduce cyclosporine response until evidence to the contrary appears.

Management Options:

- *Consider Alternative.* If the barbiturate is being used as a sedative-hypnotic, consider using a benzodiazepine in place of the barbiturate.

- *Monitor.* In a patient stabilized on cyclosporine, monitor for altered cyclosporine response if barbiturate therapy is started or stopped or if the barbiturate dose is changed. Note that the enzyme inducing effects of barbiturates tend to have a gradual onset and offset (1–2 weeks or more, depending on the barbiturate). When initiating cyclosporine therapy in a patient receiving a barbiturate, be aware that the cyclosporine dosage requirements may be higher than anticipated.

References:

1. Carstensen H et al. Interaction between cyclosporine A and phenobarbitone. Br J Clin Pharmacol. 1986;21:550.
2. Offermann G et al. Low cyclosporin A blood levels and acute graft rejection in a renal transplant recipient during rifampin treatment. Am J Nephrol. 1985;5:385.
3. Cockburn ITR et al. An appraisal of drug interactions with Sandimmune.® Transplant Proc. 1989;21:3845.

## Cyclosporine (Sandimmune)

## Phenytoin (Dilantin)

Summary: Phenytoin markedly reduces serum cyclosporine concentrations and is likely to increase cyclosporine dosage requirements.

Risk Factors: No specific risk factors known.

Related Drugs: Other enzyme-inducing anticonvulsants also appear to reduce blood cyclosporine concentrations. *Tacrolimus (Prograf)* is probably affected similarly by enzyme inducers.

Management Options:

- *Circumvent/Minimize.* When initiating cyclosporine therapy in a patient receiving phenytoin, be aware that the cyclosporine dosage requirements may be higher than anticipated.

- *Monitor.* In a patient stabilized on cyclosporine, monitor for altered cyclosporine response if phenytoin therapy is started, stopped or if the dose is changed. Starting phenytoin therapy may increase the risk of rejection in patients on cyclosporine.

## Significance Classification

1 - *Avoid Combination.* Risk always outweighs benefit.

2 - *Usually Avoid Combination.* Use combination only under special circumstances.

3 - *Minimize Risk.* Take action as necessary to reduce risk.

References:
1. Freeman DJ et al. Evaluation of cyclosporin-phenytoin interaction with observations of cyclosporin metabolites. Br J Clin Pharmacol. 1984;18:887.
2. Keown PA et al. Interaction between phenytoin and cyclosporine following organ transplantation. Transplantation. 1984;38:304.
3. Rowland M et al. Cyclosporin-phenytoin interaction: re-evaluation using metabolite data. Br J Clin Pharmacol. 1987;24:329.

### Cyclosporine (Sandimmune)
### Prednisolone

Summary: The concurrent use of cyclosporine and methylprednisolone may increase the plasma concentrations of both drugs; isolated case reports indicate that the combination may result in seizures. The clinical importance of these findings is unclear.

Risk Factors: No specific risk factors known.

Related Drugs: There is little evidence of drug interactions when combining cyclosporine with other corticosteroids (e.g., *methylprednisolone*), but it is possible that they interact as well. *Tacrolimus (Prograf)* also may interact with corticosteroids, but little information is available.

Management Options:
- *Monitor.* Although cyclosporine and corticosteroids commonly are used concurrently, be alert for evidence of increased response to both drugs.

References:
1. Boogaerts MA et al. Cyclosporin, methylprednisolone, and convulsions. Lancet. 1982;2:1216.
2. Ost L. Effects of cyclosporin on prednisolone metabolism. Lancet. 1984;1:451.
3. Klintmalm G et al. High dose methylprednisolone increases plasma cyclosporin levels in renal transplant recipients. Lancet. 1984;1:731.

### Cyclosporine (Sandimmune)
### Probucol (Lorelco)

Summary: A preliminary report suggests that probucol slightly reduces blood cyclosporine concentrations, but the clinical importance of this effect is unknown.

Risk Factors: No specific risk factors known.

Related Drugs: No information available.

Management Options:
- *Monitor.* Although the interaction is not well documented, it would be prudent to monitor patients for altered cyclosporine blood levels and response if probucol is initiated or discontinued.

References:
1. Corder CN et al. Interference with steady state cyclosporine levels by probucol. Clin Pharmacol Ther. 1990;47:204. Abstract.
2. Gallego C et al. Interaction between probucol and cyclosporine in renal transplant patients. Ann Pharmacother. 1994;28:940.
3. Sundararajan V et al. Interaction of cyclosporine and probucol in heart transplant patients. Transplant Proc. 1991;23:2028.

### Cyclosporine (Sandimmune)

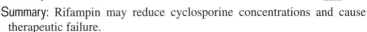

### Rifampin (Rifadin)

**Summary:** Rifampin may reduce cyclosporine concentrations and cause therapeutic failure.

**Risk Factors:** No specific risk factors known.

**Related Drugs:** *Tacrolimus (Prograf)* is likely to be affected similarly by rifampin administration.

**Management Options:**

- *Avoid Unless Benefits Outweigh Risks.* Rifampin and cyclosporine should be coadministered only with careful monitoring of cyclosporine concentrations.

- *Monitor.* Cyclosporine blood concentrations should be monitored when cyclosporine and rifampin are used simultaneously. The addition of rifampin to cyclosporine regimens may require a two- to fourfold increase in cyclosporine dosages to maintain therapeutic blood concentrations. The discontinuation of rifampin may cause cyclosporine concentrations to increase over 5–10 days, possibly resulting in toxicity. Dosage reduction will probably be required, particularly in patients who have had their dosage increased as a result of rifampin administration.

**References:**

1. Hebert MF et al. Bioavailability of cyclosporine with concomitant rifampin administration is markedly less than predicted by hepatic enzyme induction. Clin Pharmacol Ther. 1992;52:453.
2. Combalbert J et al. Metabolism of cyclosporin A. IV. Purification and identification of the rifampicin-inducible human liver cytochrome P-450 (cyclosporin A oxidase) as a product of P450IIIA gene subfamily. Drug Metab Disp. 1989;17:197.
3. Koselj M et al. Drug interaction between cyclosporine and rifampicin, erythromycin, and azoles in kidney recipients with opportunistic infections. Transplant Proc. 1994;26:2823.

### Cyclosporine (Sandimmune)

### Sulindac (Clinoril)

**Summary:** Impaired renal function appears to be greater with sulindac plus cyclosporine than with either drug alone; sulindac has also been reported to increase serum cyclosporine concentrations.

**Risk Factors:** No specific risk factors known.

**Related Drugs:** In patients receiving cyclosporine, several NSAIDs [e.g., *naproxen (Naprosyn)*] have been associated with impaired renal function and/or increased cyclosporine blood concentrations.[1–3] The relative likelihood of various NSAIDs to increase cyclosporine-induced nephrotoxicity is not established, but assume that all NSAIDs are capable of interacting with cyclosporine until evidence to the contrary is available.

Management Options:
- *Consider Alternative.* Until the clinical importance of this potential interaction is better defined, use sulindac (or other NSAIDs) in patients receiving cyclosporine only when the expected benefit clearly outweighs the risk of excessive cyclosporine response and nephrotoxicity.
- *Monitor.* If the combination is used, monitor the patient's renal function carefully and be prepared to discontinue one or both drugs.

References:
1. Branthwaite JP et al. Cyclosporin and diclofenac interaction in rheumatoid arthritis. Lancet. 1991;337:252. Letter.
2. Deray G et al. Enhancement of cyclosporine A nephrotoxicity by diclofenac. Clin Nephrol. 1987;27:213. Letter.
3. Altman RD et al. Interaction of cyclosporine A and nonsteroidal anti-inflammatory drugs on renal function in patients with rheumatoid arthritis. Am J Med. 1992; 93:396.

### Cyclosporine (Sandimmune)

### Sulphadimidine (Sulfamezathine)

Summary: Some sulfonamides can reduce the plasma concentration of cyclosporine, potentially reducing its efficacy.

Risk Factors:
- *Dosage Regimen.* IV administration of sulphadimidine is a probable risk factor.

Related Drugs: *Tacrolimus (Prograf)* concentrations may be reduced in a similar manner.

Management Options:
- *Circumvent/Minimize.* Oral TMP-SMX did not affect cyclosporine plasma concentrations.
- *Monitor.* During the administration of sulfadimidine to patients receiving cyclosporine, plasma cyclosporine concentrations should be monitored.

References:
1. Jones DK et al. Serious interaction between cyclosporine A and sulphadimidine. Br Med J. 1986;292:728.
2. Wallwork H et al. Cyclosporine and intravenous sulphadimidine and trimethoprim therapy. Lancet. 1983;1:366.
3. Spes CH et al. Sulfadiazine therapy for toxoplasmosis in heart transplant recipients decreases cyclosporine concentration. Clin Investig. 1992;70:752.

### Cyclosporine (Sandimmune)

### Ticlopidine (Ticlid)

Summary: A patient with nephrotic syndrome developed a marked reduction in blood cyclosporine concentrations during ticlopidine therapy; a causal relationship was likely in this patient, but more study is needed to assess the clinical importance.

**Risk Factors:** No specific risk factors known.

**Related Drugs:** No information available.

**Management Options:**

- *Monitor.* Until more information is available, monitor cyclosporine blood concentrations and therapeutic response carefully if ticlopidine is initiated or discontinued in patients taking cyclosporine.

**References:**

1. Birmele B et al. Interaction of cyclosporin and ticlopidine. Nephrol Dial Transplant. 1991;6:150. Letter.

## Cyclosporine (Sandimmune)

### Verapamil (Calan)

**Summary:** Cyclosporine blood concentrations are increased by verapamil; cyclosporine toxicity could result.

**Risk Factors:** No specific risk factors known.

**Related Drugs:** *Diltiazem (Cardizem)* and *nicardipine (Cardene)* inhibit cyclosporine metabolism while *isradipine (DynaCirc)*, *nifedipine (Procardia)*, *amlodipine (Norvasc)*, and *nitrendipine (Baypress)* have minimal effect. Verapamil may affect *tacrolimus (Prograf)* in a similar manner.

**Management Options:**

- *Consider Alternative.* Calcium channel blockers that do not appear to alter cyclosporine pharmacokinetics include isradipine,[1] nitrendipine,[2] and amlodipine.[3]
- *Circumvent/Minimize.* Cyclosporine dosage should be reduced and blood concentrations monitored when verapamil is coadministered.
- *Monitor.* Patients receiving both drugs should be observed for increased cyclosporine concentrations and decreasing renal function.

**References:**

1. Martinez F et al. No clinically significant interaction between cyclosporin and isradipine. Nephron. 1991;59:658.
2. Coupur MS et al. Effects of nitrendipine on blood pressure and blood cyclosporine A level in patients with posttransplant hypertension. Nephron. 1989;52:227.
3. Toupance O et al. Antihypertensive effect of amlodipine and lack of interference with cyclosporine metabolism in renal transplant recipients. Hypertension. 1994; 24:297.

## Cyproheptadine (Periactin)

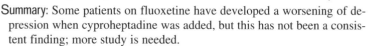

### Fluoxetine (Prozac)

**Summary:** Some patients on fluoxetine have developed a worsening of depression when cyproheptadine was added, but this has not been a consistent finding; more study is needed.

**Risk Factors:** No specific risk factors known.

**Related Drugs:** Theoretically, other selective serotonin reuptake inhibitors would interact similarly with cyproheptadine.

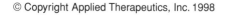

Management Options:
- *Monitor.* Until more information is available, monitor for reduced antidepressant response to fluoxetine if cyproheptadine is started.

References:
1. Feder R. Reversal of antidepressant activity of fluoxetine by cyproheptadine in three patients. J Clin Psychiatry. 1991;52:163.
2. McCormick S et al. Reversal of fluoxetine-induced anorgasmia by cyproheptadine in two patients. J Clin Psychiatry. 1990;51:383.

### Danazol (Danocrine)

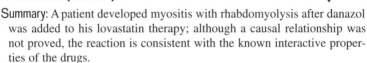

### Lovastatin (Mevacor)

Summary: A patient developed myositis with rhabdomyolysis after danazol was added to his lovastatin therapy; although a causal relationship was not proved, the reaction is consistent with the known interactive properties of the drugs.

Risk Factors: No specific risk factors known.

Related Drugs: It is not known whether androgens other than danazol interact with lovastatin, but consider the possibility. The effect of danazol on other hepatic hydroxymethylglutaryl coenzyme A reductase inhibitors is not established. Since **pravastatin (Pravachol)** and **fluvastatin (Lescol)** appear less likely to interact with cyclosporine than lovastatin, they also may be less likely to interact with danazol.

Management Options:
- *Consider Alternative.* See Related Drugs above.
- *Monitor.* If the combination is used, monitor the patient for evidence of myositis. Patients should be advised to contact their physician if they develop unexpected muscle pain or weakness.

References:
1. Dallaire M et al. Rhabdomyolyse severe ches un patient recevant lovastatine, danazol et doxycyline. Can Med Assoc J. 1994;150:1991.

### Danazol (Danocrine)

### Warfarin (Coumadin)

Summary: Several cases of enhanced hypoprothrombinemic response to warfarin following danazol therapy have been reported.

Risk Factors: No specific risk factors known.

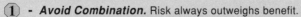
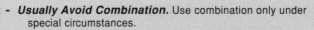

## Significance Classification

1 - *Avoid Combination.* Risk always outweighs benefit.

2 - *Usually Avoid Combination.* Use combination only under special circumstances.

3 - *Minimize Risk.* Take action as necessary to reduce risk.

Related Drugs: Anabolic steroids other than danazol are known to increase the hypoprothrombinemic response to oral anticoagulants. Oral anticoagulants other than warfarin also are likely to interact with danazol.

Management Options:

- *Avoid Unless Benefit Outweighs Risk.* Concomitant therapy with oral anticoagulants and danazol should be avoided if possible.

- *Monitor.* If the combination is used, watch for an alteration in the hypoprothrombinemic response to oral anticoagulants if danazol is initiated, discontinued or changed in dosage; adjust oral anticoagulant dosage as needed. It is possible that danazol, by increasing fibrinolytic activity, increases the bleeding risk in anticoagulated patients even when the warfarin dose has been adjusted to achieve the desired hypoprothrombinemic response. Thus, careful attention should be given to early detection of bleeding.

References:
1. Goulbourne IA et al. An interaction between danazol and warfarin: case report. Br J Obstet Gynaecol. 1981;88:950.
2. Small M et al. Danazol and oral anticoagulants. Scott Med J. 1982;27:331.
3. Meeks ML et al. Danazol increases the anticoagulant effect of warfarin. Ann Pharmacother. 1992;26:641.

## Dapsone (Avlosulfan)

### Didanosine (Videx)

Summary: Dapsone failed to prevent pneumocystis infections in patients being treated with didanosine for human immunodeficiency virus (HIV).

Risk Factors: No specific risk factors known.

Related Drugs: No information available.

Management Options:

- *Circumvent/Minimize.* Dapsone should be administered 2 to 3 hours before didanosine to avoid a reduction in dapsone absorption.

- *Monitor.* Patients receiving the combination should be watched for reduced dapsone efficacy.

References:
1. Metroka CE et al. Failure of prophylaxis with dapsone in patients taking dideoxyinosine. N Engl J Med. 1991;325:737.

## Dapsone (Avlosulfan)

### Probenecid (Benemid)

Summary: Probenecid may increase serum dapsone concentrations, but the clinical importance of this effect is not established.

Risk Factors: No specific risk factors known.

Related Drugs: No information available.

Management Options:

- *Circumvent/Minimize.* The dapsone dose may need to be reduced in some patients taking concomitant probenecid.

- *Monitor.* Patients taking dapsone and probenecid should be monitored for evidence of increased dapsone serum concentrations including hemolytic anemia, methemoglobinemia, and peripheral neuropathy with muscle weakness.

References:
1. Goodwin CS et al. Inhibition of dapsone excretion by probenecid. Lancet. 1969; 2:884.

## Dapsone (Avlosulfan)

### Rifampin (Rifadin)

Summary: Rifampin reduces dapsone serum concentrations; methemoglobin concentrations were increased.

Risk Factors: No specific risk factors known.

Related Drugs: No information available.

Management Options:

- *Circumvent/Minimize.* Dapsone doses may need to be increased during rifampin administration.

- *Monitor* patients for methemoglobin accumulation during rifampin coadministration. Patients being treated for pneumocystis should be observed for reduced efficacy.

References:
1. Pieters FAJM et al. Influence of once-monthly rifampicin and daily clofazimine on the pharmacokinetics of dapsone in leprosy patients in Nigeria. Eur J Clin Pharmacol. 1988;34:73.
2. George J et al. Drug interaction during multidrug regimens for treatment of leprosy. Indian J Med Res. 1988;87:151.
3. Horowitz HW et al. Drug interactions in use of dapsone for Pneumocystis carinii prophylaxis. Lancet. 1992;339:747.

## Dapsone (Avlosulfan)

### Trimethoprim (Proloprim)

Summary: Trimethoprim appears to increase dapsone serum concentrations and effects; dapsone increases trimethoprim concentrations.

Risk Factors: No specific risk factors known.

Related Drugs: ***Trimethoprim-sulfamethoxazole (Bactrim)*** also may produce similar effects.

Management Options:

- *Monitor.* Patients receiving dapsone plus trimethoprim should be monitored (methemoglobin levels) for increased dapsone toxicity.

References:
1. Lee BL et al. Dapsone, trimethoprim, and sulfamethoxazole plasma levels during treatment of pneumocystis pneumonia in patients with the acquired immunodeficiency syndrome (AIDS). Ann Intern Med. 1989;110:606.

### Delavirdine (Rescriptor)
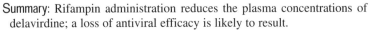
### Rifampin (Rifadin)

Summary: Rifampin administration reduces the plasma concentrations of delavirdine; a loss of antiviral efficacy is likely to result.

Risk Factors: No specific risk factors known.

Related Drugs: **Rifabutin (Mycobutin)** also increases the clearance of delavirdine but to a somewhat lesser (fivefold increase) extent.[2]

Management Options:
- *Consider Alternative.* In view of the magnitude of this interaction, avoiding the use of rifampin in patients taking delavirdine seems prudent.
- *Monitor.* Patients receiving delavirdine should be monitored for loss of efficacy if rifampin or rifabutin are administered.

References:
1. Borin MT et al. Pharmacokinetic study of the interaction between rifampin and delavirdine mesylate. Clin Pharmacol Ther. 1997;61:544–53.
2. Borin MT et al. Effect of rifabutin on delavirdine pharmacokinetics in HIV+ patients. Presented at the 34th Interscience Conference on Antimicrobial Agents and Chemotherapy, Orlando, Florida, 1994. Abstract.

### Desipramine (Norpramin)
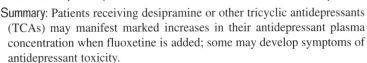
### Fluoxetine (Prozac)

Summary: Patients receiving desipramine or other tricyclic antidepressants (TCAs) may manifest marked increases in their antidepressant plasma concentration when fluoxetine is added; some may develop symptoms of antidepressant toxicity.

Risk Factors: No specific risk factors known.

Related Drugs: Five patients receiving antidepressants including desipramine, **imipramine (Tofranil)**, **nortriptyline (Pamelor)**, and **trazodone (Desyrel)** developed marked increases in their plasma antidepressant concentrations after the addition of fluoxetine.[1] Within 1 or 2 weeks of starting fluoxetine, 3 of the patients developed adverse effects characteristic of the antidepressant they were receiving (e.g., anticholinergic symptoms, sedation). Three other patients developed elevated plasma cyclic concentrations and cyclic toxicity such as seizures and delirium after fluoxetine was added to TCA [desipramine, imipramine, or **doxepin (Sinequan)**] therapy.[2] In 8 depressed patients given fluoxetine plus trazodone, 3 had a good response but 5 experienced intolerable side effects (headaches, dizziness, sedation, fatigue) or did not respond.[3] **Paroxetine (Paxil)** is also a potent inhibitor of CYP2D6 and can increase serum desipramine concentrations substantially.

Management Options:
- *Monitor* patients for increased antidepressant plasma levels and toxicity when fluoxetine is used concurrently; adjustment of the antidepressant dosage is likely to be required. Due to the slow elimination of fluoxetine and its active metabolite, its effect on the metabolism of other antidepressants is likely to dissipate gradually over 2 to 4 weeks.

References:
1. Aranow RB et al. Elevated antidepressant plasma levels after addition of fluoxetine. Am J Psychiatry. 1989;146:911.
2. Preskorn SH et al. Serious adverse effects of combining fluoxetine and tricyclic antidepressants. Am J Psychiatry. 1990;147:532.
3. Nierenberg AA et al. Possible trazodone potentiation of fluoxetine: a case series. J Clin Psychiatry. 1992;53:83.

## Desipramine (Norpramin)

## Guanethidine (Ismelin)

**Summary:** Tricyclic antidepressants (TCAs) consistently inhibit the antihypertensive response to guanethidine.

**Risk Factors:** No specific risk factors known.

**Related Drugs:** In one case report, an interaction between guanethidine and *imipramine (Tofranil)* was implicated in producing cardiac standstill and death.[2] However, a causal relationship was not established. Preliminary reports indicate that doxepin is less potent as an antagonist to guanethidine's antihypertensive effect.[1] Limited clinical evidence indicates that guanethidine's antihypertensive response is unaffected by *mianserin*[3,6] and is only occasionally affected by *maprotiline (Ludiomil)*.[4,5] *Guanadrel* is pharmacologically similar to guanethidine and also may be inhibited by TCAs. *Methyldopa (Aldomet)* may be less likely to interact with tricyclic antidepressants than guanethidine, but more information is needed.

Management Options:
- *Consider Alternative.* Although satisfactory control of hypertension can sometimes be achieved by alteration in guanethidine dosage, it is preferable to avoid the combination when possible. Maprotiline may be less likely to interact with guanethidine than tricyclic antidepressants.

## Significance Classification

- ① - *Avoid Combination.* Risk always outweighs benefit.
- ② - *Usually Avoid Combination.* Use combination only under special circumstances.
- ③ - *Minimize Risk.* Take action as necessary to reduce risk.

• *Monitor.* If the combination is used, monitor patients for rising blood pressures when TCAs are started and for hypotension when cyclics are stopped.

References:

1. Oates JA et al. Effect of doxepin on the norepinephrine pump. A preliminary report. Psychosomatics. 1969;10:12.
2. Williams RB Jr et al. Cardiac complications of tricyclic antidepressant therapy. Ann Intern Med. 1971;74:395.
3. Ghose K et al. Autonomic actions and interactions of mianserin hydrochloride (org. GB 94) and amitriptyline in patients with depressive illness. Psychopharmacology. 1976;49:201.
4. Smith AJ et al. Interaction between postganglionic sympathetic blocking drugs and antidepressants. J Int Med Res. 1975;3(Suppl. 2):55.
5. Briant RH et al. The assessment of potential drug interaction with a new tricyclic antidepressant drug. Br J Clin Pharmacol. 1974;1:113.
6. Burgess CD et al. Cardiovascular responses to mianserin hydrochloride: A comparison with tricyclic antidepressant drugs. Br J Clin Pharmacol. 1978;5:215.

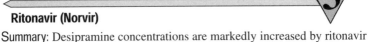

**Desipramine**

**Ritonavir (Norvir)**

Summary: Desipramine concentrations are markedly increased by ritonavir administration; toxicity could result.

Risk Factors: No specific risk factors known.

Related Drugs: Other tricyclic antidepressants may be similarly affected by ritonavir. *Indinavir (Crixivan)* may inhibit the metabolism of tricyclic antidepressants; the magnitude of any inhibition is unknown.

Management Options:

• *Circumvent/Minimize.* Dosage of desipramine may require reduction.

• *Monitor.* Patients stabilized on desipramine and other tricyclic antidepressants should be monitored for cardiac, central nervous system, and anticholinergic side effects.

References:

1. Abbott Laboratories. Norvir prescribing information. 1996.

**Dexfenfluramine (Redux)**

**Fluoxetine (Prozac)**

Summary: Cotherapy with dexfenfluramine and selective serotonin reuptake inhibitors (SSRIs) such as fluoxetine theoretically could result in serotonin syndrome.

Risk Factors: No specific risk factors known.

Related Drugs: Dexfenfluramine also should be avoided in combinations with other SSRIs such as *paroxetine (Paxil)*, *sertraline (Zoloft)*, and *fluvoxamine (Luvox)*. Dexfenfluramine is the S-enantiomer of the racemate *fenfluramine (Pondimin)*, so the two drugs probably interact in a similar way with SSRIs.

Management Options:
- *Avoid Unless Benefit Outweighs Risk.* Patients should avoid the use of SSRIs with either dexfenfluramine or fenfluramine, unless the combinations are found to be safe in well controlled clinical trials. There is also a medicolegal risk in using the combinations, since the manufacturer's information states that cotherapy should be avoided.
- *Monitor.* If the combination is used, be alert for evidence of serotonin syndrome which can result in neurotoxicity (myoclonus, tremors, rigidity, incoordination, restlessness, hyperreflexia, seizures, coma); psychiatric symptoms (agitation, confusion, hypomania); and temperature regulation abnormalities (fever, sweating).

References:
1. Gross AS et al. The influence of the sparteine/debrisoquine genetic polymorphism on the disposition of dexfenfluramine. Br J Clin Pharmacol. 1996;41:311.
2. Redux, Manufacturer's Product Information. Wyeth-Ayerst Laboratories, 1996.

### Dexfenfluramine (Redux)
### Phenelzine (Nardil)

Summary: Cotherapy with dexfenfluramine and nonselective monoamine oxidase inhibitors (MAOIs) such as phenelzine theoretically could result in serotonin syndrome.

Risk Factors: No specific risk factors known.

Related Drugs: Dexfenfluramine also is contraindicated with other nonselective MAOIs such as **tranylcypromine (Parnate)** and **isocarboxazid (Marplan)**. Given that **selegiline (Eldepryl)** can sometimes act as a nonselective MAOI (especially if given in large doses), it also might interact adversely with dexfenfluramine. Dexfenfluramine is the S-enantiomer of the racemate **fenfluramine (Pondimin)**, so the two drugs probably interact in a similar way with nonselective MAOIs.

Management Options:
- *Avoid Combination.* Patients should avoid any combination of a nonselective MAOI with either dexfenfluramine or fenfluramine.

References:
1. Gross AS et al. The influence of the sparteine/debrisoquine genetic polymorphism on the disposition of dexfenfluramine. Br J Clin Pharmacol. 1996;41:311.
2. Redux Manufacturer's Product Information. Wyeth-Ayerst Laboratories, 1996.

### Dextroamphetamine
### Furazolidone (Furoxone)

Summary: Amphetamines may induce a hypertensive response in patients taking furazolidone.

Risk Factors: No specific risk factors known.

Related Drugs: One would expect an enhanced response to other sympathomimetics with indirect activity (e.g., **phenylpropanolamine**, **ephedrine**), but this apparently has not been studied.

Management Options:
- *Consider Alternative.* Patients receiving furazolidone probably should avoid taking amphetamines.
- *Monitor.* Watch for increased blood pressure if amphetamine and furazolidone are coadministered.

References:
1. Pettinger WA et al. Inhibition of monoamine oxidase in man by furazolidone. Clin Pharmacol Ther. 1968;9:442.

## Dextroamphetamine

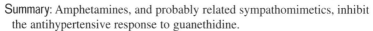

### Guanethidine (Ismelin)

Summary: Amphetamines, and probably related sympathomimetics, inhibit the antihypertensive response to guanethidine.

Risk Factors: No specific risk factors known.

Related Drugs: Although little is known regarding other sympathomimetics, their pharmacologic similarity to amphetamines suggests that they are likely to inhibit guanethidine's effect as well. *Guanadrel (Hylorel)* is similar to guanethidine and also may be inhibited by amphetamines.

Management Options:
- *Consider Alternative.* Consider using an alternative to amphetamine and/or guanethidine.
- *Monitor.* If the combination is used, monitor for inhibition of antihypertensive response to guanethidine or guanadrel.

References:
1. Ober KF et al. Drug interactions with guanethidine. Clin Pharmacol Ther. 1973; 14:190.
2. Gulati OD et al. Antagonism of adrenergic neuron blockade in hypertensive subjects. Clin Pharmacol Ther. 1966;7:510.
3. Starke K. Interactions of guanethidine and indirect-acting sympathomimetic amines. Arch Int Pharmacodyn Ther. 1972;195:309.

## Dextroamphetamine

### Imipramine (Tofranil)

Summary: Theoretically, tricyclic antidepressants (TCAs) such as imipramine would increase the effect of amphetamines, but clinical evidence is lacking.

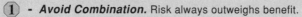
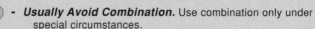

## Significance Classification

(1) - *Avoid Combination.* Risk always outweighs benefit.

(2) - *Usually Avoid Combination.* Use combination only under special circumstances.

(3) - *Minimize Risk.* Take action as necessary to reduce risk.

Risk Factors: No specific risk factors known.

Related Drugs: Other amphetamines may be similarly affected.

Management Options:

- *Circumvent/Minimize.* Patients receiving tricyclic antidepressants should avoid recreational use of amphetamines. The risk of therapeutic use of amphetamines with tricyclic antidepressants is not established.

- *Monitor* for adverse cardiovascular effects in patients on the combination.

References:

1. Raisfeld IH. Cardiovascular complications of antidepressant therapy. Am Heart J. 1972;83:129.
2. Beaumont G. Drug interactions with clomipramine (Anafranil). J Int Med Res. 1973;1:480.

---

### Dextroamphetamine

### Tranylcypromine (Parnate)

Summary: Severe hypertensive reactions have occurred when amphetamines were ingested by patients taking monoamine oxidase inhibitors (MAOIs).

Risk Factors: No specific risk factors known.

Related Drugs: Although **methylphenidate (Ritalin)** has amphetamine-like pharmacologic activity, some evidence indicates that the reactions it causes when used with MAOIs are less severe than those caused by amphetamines. Nevertheless, methylphenidate should be used cautiously in combination with MAOIs.[2,5] All nonselective MAOIs probably interact similarly with amphetamines: **isocarboxazid (Marplan)**, **phenelzine (Nardil)**, tranylcypromine (Parnate). **Furazolidone (Furoxone)**, another MAOI, has been shown to increase pressor sensitivity to amphetamines.[3,4] **Selegiline (Eldepryl)** has been reported to enhance the pressor effect of tyramine, particularly following doses >10 mg/day; it could theoretically interact with amphetamines as well.[6] Type B MAOIs (e.g., selegiline) should be less likely than the type A MAOIs (e.g., moclobemide) to interact with drugs that release catecholamines (e.g., amphetamines). Nevertheless, little is known regarding drug interactions with type B MAOIs, and they should be used cautiously until more data are available.

Management Options:

- *Avoid Combination.* Amphetamines should not be given to patients receiving a nonselective MAOI. Phentolamine (Regitine) appears to be the logical therapy for severe hypertension resulting from this interaction, since it blocks the alpha effects of the released norepinephrine.[1] Remember that the effects of nonselective MAOIs should be assumed to persist for 2 weeks after they are discontinued.

References:

1. Goldberg LI. Monoamine oxidase inhibitors. Adverse reactions and possible mechanisms. JAMA. 1964;190:456.

2. Sjoqvist F. Psychotropic drugs (2). Interaction between monoamine oxidase (MAO) inhibitors and other substances. Proc R Soc Med. 1965;58:967.
3. Pettinger WA et al. Inhibition of monoamine oxidase in man by furazolidone. Clin Pharmacol Ther. 1968;9:442.
4. Pettinger WA et al. Supersensitivity to tyramine during monoamine oxidase inhibition in man. Mechanism at the level of the adrenergic neuron. Clin Pharmacol Ther. 1968;9:341.
5. Dexedrine product information. Physician's Desk Reference. 44th ed. Oradell: Medical Economics Data; 1990.
6. Schulz R et al. Tyramine kinetics and pressor sensitivity during monoamine oxidase inhibition by selegiline. Clin Pharmacol Ther. 1989;46:528.

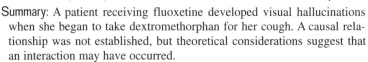

## Dextromethorphan (Robitussin-DM)

## Fluoxetine (Prozac)

Summary: A patient receiving fluoxetine developed visual hallucinations when she began to take dextromethorphan for her cough. A causal relationship was not established, but theoretical considerations suggest that an interaction may have occurred.

Risk Factors: No specific risk factors known.

Related Drugs: A patient on *paroxetine (Paxil)* developed symptoms of serotonin syndrome after taking dextromethorphan, but a causal relationship was not established. *Sertraline (Zoloft)* and *fluvoxamine (Luvox)* appear to have less effect on CYP2D6 than fluoxetine and paroxetine, but little is known regarding their use with dextromethorphan. When considering codeine as an alternative to dextromethorphan, keep in mind that inhibitors of CYP2D6 may reduce the *analgesic* effect of codeine by inhibiting its conversion to morphine. The extent to which the antitussive effect of codeine is affected by inhibitors of CYP2D6 is not established.

Management Options:

- *Consider Alternative.* Although clinical data are very limited, there are theoretical reasons for limiting the use of dextromethorphan in patients taking fluoxetine (or other selective serotonin reuptake inhibitors). Moreover, the limited therapeutic usefulness of dextromethorphan in many patients is another reason for avoiding it in patients receiving fluoxetine, even though the risk of the combination is not established.

- *Monitor.* If the combination is used, monitor for evidence of serotonin syndrome which can result in neurologic findings (e.g., dizziness, tremor, myoclonus, rigidity, seizures, incoordination and coma), psychiatric symptoms (e.g., agitation, confusion, hypomania) and disorders of temperature regulation (e.g., fever, sweating, shivering); severe cases can be fatal.

References:

1. Achamallah NS. Visual hallucinations after combining fluoxetine and dextromethorphan. Am J Med. 1992;149:1406. Letter.
2. Crewe HK et al. The effect of selective serotonin re-uptake inhibitors on cytochrome P4052D6 (CYP2D6) activity in human liver microsomes. Br J Clin Pharmacol. 1992;34:262.

### Dextromethorphan (Robitussin-DM)

### Moclobemide

Summary: Since dextromethorphan can cause serotonin syndrome when administered with nonselective monoamine oxidase inhibitors (MAOIs), cotherapy of dextromethorphan with moclobemide or other MAO-A inhibitors would theoretically produce the same effect.

Risk Factors: No specific risk factors known.

Related Drugs: Since serotonin is metabolized by MAO-A, one would expect all type A monoamine oxidase inhibitors to interact with dextromethorphan.

Management Options:
- *Avoid Combination.* Dextromethorphan is contraindicated in patients receiving nonselective or type A MAO inhibitors.

References:
1. Sovner R et al. Interaction between dextromethorphan and monoamine oxidase inhibitor therapy with isocarboxazid. N Engl J Med. 1988;319:1671. Letter.
2. Nierenberg DW et al. The central nervous system serotonin syndrome. Clin Pharmacol Ther. 1993;53:84.
3. Amrein R et al. Interactions of moclobemide with concomitantly administered medication: evidence from pharmacological and clinical studies. Psychopharmacology. 1992;106:S24.

### Dextromethorphan (Robitussin-DM)

### Phenelzine (Nardil)

Summary: Dextromethorphan may cause serotonin syndrome (agitation, confusion, hypomania, myoclonus, rigidity, hyperreflexia, tremor, incoordination, sweating, shivering, seizures, coma) when administered with monoamine oxidase (MAO) inhibitors.

Risk Factors: No specific risk factors known.

Related Drugs: In one case, a patient taking *isocarboxazid (Marplan)* 30 mg/day developed dizziness, muscle tremor, and urinary retention within one hour of ingesting 15 mg of dextromethorphan.[2] *Tranylcypromine (Parnate)* also should be assumed to produce serotonin syndrome with dextromethorphan.

Management Options:
- *Avoid Combination.* Dextromethorphan is contraindicated in patients receiving nonselective MAO inhibitors. Remember that the effects of nonselective MAO inhibitors can persist for 2 weeks after they are discontinued.

References:
1. Rivers N et al. Possible lethal reaction between Nardil and dextromethorphan. Can Med Assoc J. 1970;103:85. Letter.
2. Sovner R et al. Interaction between dextromethorphan and monoamine oxidase inhibitor therapy with isocarboxazid. N Engl J Med. 1988;319:1671. Letter.
3. Nierenberg DW et al. The central nervous system serotonin syndrome. Clin Pharmacol Ther. 1993;53:84.

### Dextromethorphan (Robitussin-DM)

### Quinidine

Summary: Dextromethorphan concentrations may be increased to toxic levels during quinidine coadministration.

Risk Factors:
- *Pharmacogenetics.* Rapid metabolizers of dextromethorphan are at risk.

Related Drugs: No information available.

Management Options:
- *Circumvent/Minimize.* Caution patients taking quinidine to avoid dextromethorphan-containing medications. Dextromethorphan dosage reduction should be considered if it is administered with quinidine. Codeine may not be a suitable alternative since quinidine inhibits its conversion to morphine and may thus limit its antitussive effects.
- *Monitor.* If dextromethorphan is administered with quinidine, patients should be monitored for side effects (nausea, headache, nervousness, insomnia, tremors, or confusion).

References:
1. Zhang Y et al. Dextromethorphan: enhancing its systemic availability by way of low-dose quinidine-mediated inhibition of cytochrome P4502D6. Clin Pharmacol Ther. 1992;51:647.

### Dextromethorphan (Robitussin-DM)

### Selegiline (Eldepryl)

Summary: Since dextromethorphan can cause serotonin syndrome when administered with nonselective monoamine oxidase inhibitors (MAOIs), selegiline (especially in large doses) theoretically could produce the same effect.

Risk Factors:
- *Dosage Regimen.* Selegiline doses of 10 mg/day can have some inhibitory effect on MAO-A, and this effect increases as the daily dose is increased.

## Significance Classification

 - ***Avoid Combination.*** Risk always outweighs benefit.

 - ***Usually Avoid Combination.*** Use combination only under special circumstances.

 - ***Minimize Risk.*** Take action as necessary to reduce risk.

Related Drugs: **Meperidine (Demerol)** interacts similarly with selegiline. Other nonselective MAOIs also interact similarly with selegiline.

Management Options:

- *Avoid Unless Benefit Outweighs Risk.* Although dextromethorphan is contraindicated in patients receiving nonselective or type A MAO inhibitors, little is known about the use of type B MAO inhibitors such as selegiline with dextromethorphan. Nonetheless, it would be prudent to avoid concomitant use until more data are available.
- *Monitor.* If the combination is used, monitor for evidence of serotonin syndrome (agitation, confusion, hypomania, myoclonus, rigidity, hyperreflexia, tremor, incoordination, sweating, shivering, seizures, coma).

References:

1. Sovner R et al. Interaction between dextromethorphan and monoamine oxidase inhibitor therapy with isocarboxazid. N Engl J Med. 1988;319:1671. Letter.
2. Nierenberg DW et al. The central nervous system serotonin syndrome. Clin Pharmacol Ther. 1993;53:84.
3. Zornberg GL et al. Severe adverse interaction between pethidine and selegiline. Lancet. 1991;337:246.

## Dextrothyroxine

## Warfarin (Coumadin)

**2**

Summary: Dextrothyroxine consistently increases the hypoprothrombinemic response to warfarin and probably other oral anticoagulants. Adjustments in oral anticoagulant dosage are likely to be needed when dextrothyroxine therapy is initiated or discontinued.

Risk Factors: No specific risk factors known.

Related Drugs: All combinations of thyroid and oral anticoagulants are likely to interact.

Management Options:

- *Avoid Unless Benefit Outweighs Risk.* Concomitant therapy with dextrothyroxine and oral anticoagulants should be avoided if possible. If oral anticoagulant therapy is begun in a patient receiving dextrothyroxine, use conservative doses until the maintenance dose is established.
- *Monitor.* Initiation or discontinuation of dextrothyroxine therapy in a patient stabilized on an oral anticoagulant is likely to necessitate a change in the maintenance anticoagulant dose.

References:

1. Weintraub M et al. The effects of dextrothyroxine on the kinetics of prothrombin activity: proposed mechanism of the potentiation of warfarin by D-thyroxine. J Lab Clin Med. 1973;81:273.
2. Schrogie JJ et al. The anticoagulant response to bishydroxycoumarin II: the effect of D-thyroxine, clofibrate, and norethandrolone. Clin Pharmacol Ther. 1967;8:70.
3. Solomon HM et al. Change in receptor site affinity: a proposed explanation for the potentiating effect of D-thyroxine on the anticoagulant response to warfarin. Clin Pharmacol Ther. 1967;8:797.

## Diazepam (Valium)

### Disulfiram (Antabuse)

**Summary:** Disulfiram may increase serum concentrations of diazepam and benzodiazepines that undergo oxidative metabolism, but the frequency of excessive benzodiazepine response is unknown.

**Risk Factors:** No specific risk factors known.

**Related Drugs:** *Chlordiazepoxide (Librium)* affects disulfiram similarly.[1] Other benzodiazepines that undergo oxidative metabolism [*clonazepam (Klonopin), clorazepate (Tranxene), flurazepam (Dalmane), halazepam (Paxipam), prazepam (Centrax),* and *triazolam (Halcion)*] also might be affected by disulfiram treatment, but studies are not available. In 11 alcoholic patients undergoing withdrawal, disulfiram 0.5 gm/day for 14 days did not appear to affect the pharmacokinetics of *alprazolam (Xanax)*;[3] however, poor compliance with the disulfiram therapy and the alcohol withdrawal process may have affected the results of this study. *Oxazepam (Serax)* and *lorazepam (Ativan)* are converted to inactive glucuronides, a process that does not appear to be affected by disulfiram.[1,2] *Temazepam (Restoril)* also undergoes glucuronide conjugation and would not be expected to be affected by disulfiram.

**Management Options:**

- *Monitor.* Be alert for evidence of enhanced benzodiazepine response in patients receiving disulfiram. Some patients may require a reduction in benzodiazepine dosage during concurrent disulfiram use.

**References:**

1. MacLeod SM et al. Interaction of disulfiram with benzodiazepines. Clin Pharmacol Ther. 1978;24:583.
2. Sellers EM et al. Differential effects of benzodiazepine disposition by disulfiram and ethanol. Arzneimittelforschung. 1980;30:882.
3. Diquet B et al. Lack of interaction between disulfiram and alprazolam in alcoholic patients. Eur J Clin Pharmacol. 1990;38:157.

## Diazepam (Valium)

### Ethanol (Ethyl Alcohol)

**Summary:** Ethanol may enhance the adverse psychomotor effects of benzodiazepines like diazepam; combined use may be dangerous in patients performing tasks requiring alertness.

**Risk Factors:** No specific risk factors known.

**Related Drugs:** *Nitrazepam (Mogadon), bromazepam,* and *lorazepam (Ativan)*[10,11] appear to have a similar effect when given with ethanol. *Chlordiazepoxide (Librium)* may be less likely than diazepam to enhance the adverse psychomotor effects of alcohol,[1,3–8] but it seems likely that such enhancement would occur with sufficient doses of chlordiazepoxide. Ethanol also seems less likely to affect the hepatic metabolism of *oxazepam (Serax)* than diazepam,[9] but additive central nervous system

(CNS) depression would be expected in either case. All benzodiazepines should be expected to result in additive CNS depression with alcohol.[2]

Management Options:

- *Circumvent/Minimize.* Patients receiving benzodiazepines should be warned against ingestion of moderate to large amounts of ethanol. Occasional ingestion of small amounts of ethanol (especially if taken with food) probably causes little difficulty unless alertness is required (as in driving) or the patient has a disease or condition that makes him sensitive to CNS depression.
- *Monitor* for excessive CNS depression if the combination is used.

References:

1. Reggiani G et al. Some aspects of the experimental and clinical toxicology of chlordiazepoxide. In: Toxicity and Side-Effects of Psychotropic Drugs. Amsterdam: Excerpta Medica Foundation; 1968:79–97.
2. Rosinga WM. Interaction of drugs and alcohol in relation to traffic safety. In: Meyer L, Peck HM eds. Drug Induced Disease. Vol. 3. Amsterdam: Excerpta Medica Foundation; 1968:295–306.
3. Hughes FW et al. Comparative effect in human subjects of chlordiazepoxide, diazepam, and placebo on mental and physical performance. Clin Pharmacol Ther. 1965;6:139.
4. Hoffer A. Lack of potentiation by chlordiazepoxide (Librium) of depression or excitation due to alcohol. Can Med Assoc J. 1962;87:920.
5. Betts TA et al. Effect of four commonly-used tranquilizers on low-speed driving performance tests. Br Med J. 1972;4:580.
6. Dundee JW et al. Alcohol and the benzodiazepines. The interaction between intravenous ethanol and chlordiazepoxide and diazepam. Q J Stud Alcohol. 1971; 32:960.
7. Goldberg L. Behavioral and physiological effects of alcohol on man. Psychosom Med. 1966;28:570.
8. Miller AI et al. Effects of combined chlordiazepoxide and alcohol in man. Q J Stud Alcohol. 1963;24:9.
9. Sellers EM et al. Different effects on benzodiazepine disposition by disulfiram and ethanol. Arzneimittelforschung. 1980;30:882.
10. Mattila MJ et al. Acute effects of buspirone and alcohol on psychomotor skills. J Clin Psychiatry. 1982;43:56.
11. Linnoila M et al. Effect of adinazolam and diazepam, alone and in combination with ethanol, on psychomotor and cognitive performance and on autonomic nervous system reactivity in healthy volunteers. Eur J Clin Pharmacol. 1990;38:371.

## Diazepam (Valium)

## Fluoxetine (Prozac)

Summary: A study in healthy subjects suggests that fluoxetine increases plasma diazepam concentrations and reduces the plasma concentration of its active metabolite, desmethyldiazepam. Fluoxetine may increase modestly the psychomotor impairment produced by diazepam in some patients, but the clinical importance of this effect is not established.

Risk Factors:

- *Age.* The elderly are known to be more sensitive to diazepam and may be more sensitive to this interaction.

Related Drugs: Preliminary evidence suggests that **sertraline (Zoloft)** slightly reduces diazepam elimination. The effect of other selective serotonin reuptake inhibitors other than fluoxetine on diazepam is not established, but **fluvoxamine (Luvox)** is known to inhibit CYP3A4, an isozyme important in the metabolism of diazepam. Fluoxetine also inhibits the metabolism of **alprazolam (Xanax)**.

Management Options:

- *Circumvent/Minimize.* It would be prudent to use conservative doses of diazepam in the presence of fluoxetine until patient response is assessed. Advise patients receiving combined therapy to watch for excessive sedation.

- *Monitor* for altered diazepam effect if fluoxetine is initiated, discontinued, or changed in dosage; adjust diazepam dose as needed.

References:

1. Lemberger L et al. The effect of fluoxetine on the pharmacokinetics and psychomotor responses of diazepam. Clin Pharmacol Ther. 1988;43:412.
2. Moskowitz H et al. The effects on performance of two antidepressants, alone and in combination with diazepam. Prog Neuropsychopharmacol Biol Psychiatry. 1988;12:783.

## Diazepam (Valium)

### Isoniazid (INH)

Summary: Isoniazid may increase diazepam serum concentrations; the clinical significance is not known.

Risk Factors: No specific risk factors known.

Related Drugs: The effect of isoniazid on other benzodiazepines is unknown. Isoniazid may affect other benzodiazepines [e.g., **triazolam (Halcion)**] in a similar manner.

Management Options:

- *Monitor.* Watch for evidence of altered diazepam effects when isoniazid is initiated or discontinued.

References:

1. Ochs HR et al. Diazepam interaction with antituberculosis drugs. Clin Pharmacol Ther. 1981;29:671.

## Diazepam (Valium)

### Itraconazole (Sporanox)

Summary: Itraconazole administration increases the serum concentration of diazepam; diazepam toxicity could result.

Risk Factors: No specific risk factors known.

Related Drugs: Itraconazole is known to inhibit **triazolam (Halcion)** and **temazepam (Restoril)** metabolism. It also is likely to reduce the metabolism of **chlordiazepoxide (Librium)** and **midazolam (Versed)**. **Lorazepam (Ativan)**, a benzodiazepine not metabolized by CYP3A4, may be less likely to interact. Other antifungal agents such as **ketoconazole (Nizoral)** and **fluconazole (Diflucan)** would be likely to inhibit the metabolism of diazepam.

Management Options:
- *Consider Alternative.* A benzodiazepine such as lorazepam (Ativan) that is not metabolized by CYP3A4 would be a potential alternative anxiolytic agent.
- *Monitor* for increased diazepam effects (e.g., sedation, ataxia, and mental confusion) when itraconazole is administered concomitantly with diazepam.

References:
1. Ahonen J et al. The effects of the antimycotic itraconazole on the pharmacokinetics and pharmacodynamics of diazepam. Fundam Clin Pharmacol. 1996;10:314.

### Diazepam (Valium)

### Levodopa (Larodopa)

Summary: Diazepam appeared to exacerbate parkinsonism in a few patients receiving levodopa, but a causal relationship was not established.

Risk Factors: No specific risk factors known.

Related Drugs: Another patient well controlled on levodopa, benztropine, and diphenhydramine developed an acute exacerbation of parkinsonism following administration of **chlordiazepoxide (Librium)**; control returned 5 days after the chlordiazepoxide was discontinued.[3] These case reports suggest that benzodiazepines are capable of inhibiting the antiparkinsonian effects of levodopa, but little is known regarding the incidence of the interaction between these drugs or the factors that make it more likely to occur. The effect of other benzodiazepines on levodopa is not established.

Management Options:
- *Monitor* for evidence of a reduced antiparkinsonian effect of levodopa in the presence of benzodiazepine therapy. If one suspects that this interaction may be occurring, the benzodiazepine probably should be discontinued and the patient monitored to determine whether improvement occurs.

References:
1. Wodak J et al. Review of 12 months' treatment with L-DOPA in Parkinson's disease, with remarks on unusual side effects. Med J Aust. 1972;2:1277.
2. Hunter KR et al. Use of levodopa with other drugs. Lancet. 1970;2:1283.
3. Yosselson-Superstine S et al. Chlordiazepoxide interaction with levodopa. Ann Intern Med. 1982;96:259.

## Significance Classification

(1) - *Avoid Combination.* Risk always outweighs benefit.

(2) - *Usually Avoid Combination.* Use combination only under special circumstances.

(3) - *Minimize Risk.* Take action as necessary to reduce risk.

### Diazepam (Valium)

### Metoprolol (Lopressor)

Summary: Metoprolol may slightly reduce the metabolism of diazepam, but it does not affect the metabolism of lorazepam (Ativan) or alprazolam (Xanax). Metoprolol may increase the pharmacodynamic effects of some benzodiazepines.

Risk Factors: No specific risk factors known.

Related Drugs: *Atenolol (Tenormin)* had no effect on diazepam pharmacokinetics or pharmacodynamics.[2] *Propranolol (Inderal)* and *labetalol (Normodyne)* increased the pharmacodynamic effects of *oxazepam (Serax)* without affecting its pharmacokinetics.[3] Propranolol produces a small reduction in diazepam clearance. Metoprolol increased *bromazepam* AUC 35%.[1] *Lorazepam (Ativan)* and *alprazolam (Xanax)* metabolisms are unaffected by metoprolol.

Management Options:
- *Monitor.* Patients receiving diazepam and metoprolol or propranolol should be monitored for increased central nervous system depression.

References:
1. Scott AK et al. Interaction of metoprolol with lorazepam and bromazepam. Eur J Clin Pharmacol. 1991;40:405.
2. Hawksorth G et al. Diazepam/beta-adrenoceptor antagonist interactions. Br J Clin Pharmacol. 1984;17:69S.
3. Sonne J et al. Single dose pharmacokinetics and pharmacodynamics of oral oxazepam during concomitant administration of propranolol and labetalol. Br J Clin Pharmacol. 1990;29:33.

### Diazepam (Valium)

### Omeprazole (Prilosec)

Summary: Omeprazole increases plasma diazepam concentrations considerably after single doses of diazepam in healthy subjects; the effect of this interaction on diazepam response is not established.

Risk Factors: No specific risk factors known.

Related Drugs: The effect of omeprazole on other benzodiazepines is unknown, but it would be most likely to affect benzodiazepines that undergo phase I metabolism [e.g., agents *other than* *lorazepam (Ativan)*, *oxazepam (Serax)*, and *temazepam (Restoril)*]. The effect of *lansoprazole (Prevacid)* on benzodiazepines needs further study, but it generally has less effect on hepatic drug metabolism than omeprazole.

Management Options:
- *Monitor.* Until data on the pharmacodynamics of this interaction are available, monitor for enhanced diazepam response if omeprazole is given concurrently.

References:
1. Henry DA et al. Omeprazole: effects on oxidative drug metabolism. Br J Clin Pharmacol. 1984;18:195.

2. Jensen JC et al. Inhibition of human liver cytochrome P-450 by omeprazole. Br J Clin Pharmacol. 1986;21:328.
3. Gugler R et al. Omeprazole inhibits oxidative drug metabolism: studies with diazepam and phenytoin *in vivo* and 7-ethoxycoumarin *in vitro*. Gastroenterology. 1985;89:1235.

## Diazepam (Valium)
### Rifampin (Rifadin)

Summary: Rifampin appears to reduce the serum concentration of diazepam and perhaps other benzodiazepines.

Risk Factors: No specific risk factors known.

Related Drugs: Rifampin did not significantly increase the clearance of *temazepam (Restoril)*.[3] Rifampin increased *nitrazepam (Mogadon)* clearance significantly. Rifampin also may reduce the effect of those benzodiazepines metabolized to desmethyldiazepam, such as *halazepam (Paxipam)*, *clorazepate (Tranxene)*, and *prazepam (Centrax)*.

Management Options:
- *Monitor.* Patients should be monitored for evidence of reduced diazepam and nitrazepam effect when rifampin is given concurrently. The response to halazepam, clorazepate, and prazepam also may be reduced by rifampin.

References:
1. Ochs HR et al. Diazepam interaction with antituberculosis drugs. Clin Pharmacol Ther. 1981;29:671.
2. Ohnhaus EE et al. The effect of antipyrine and rifampin on the metabolism of diazepam. Clin Pharmacol Ther. 1987;42:148.
3. Brockmeyer NH et al. Comparative effects of rifampin and/or probenecid on the pharmacokinetics of temazepam and nitrazepam. Int J Clin Pharmacol Ther Toxicol. 1990;28:387.

## Diclofenac (Voltaren)
### Lithium (Eskalith)

Summary: A study in healthy subjects suggests that diclofenac, like most nonsteroidal anti-inflammatory drugs (NSAIDs), increases plasma lithium concentrations; one would expect this to increase the risks of lithium toxicity.

Risk Factors: No specific risk factors known.

Related Drugs: Most NSAIDs increase lithium serum concentrations, but *sulindac (Clinoril)* and *aspirin* appear to have minimal effects.

Management Options:
- *Consider Alternative.* If appropriate for the patient, consider using an anti-inflammatory agent that is less likely to affect lithium, such as sulindac or aspirin.
- *Monitor.* If diclofenac therapy is initiated in a patient taking lithium, monitor serum lithium concentrations for evidence of lithium toxicity (e.g., nausea, vomiting, diarrhea, anorexia, coarse tremor, slurred speech, vertigo, confusion, lethargy; in severe cases, seizures, stu-

por, coma, and cardiovascular collapse). In a patient stabilized on lithium and an NSAID, discontinuation of the NSAID may result in inadequate serum lithium concentrations.

References:
1. Reimann IW et al. Effects of diclofenac on lithium kinetics. Clin Pharmacol Ther. 1981;30:348.
2. Ragheb M et al. Ibuprofen can increase serum lithium level in lithium-treated patients. J Clin Psychiatry. 1987;48:161.

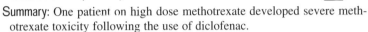

### Diclofenac (Voltaren)

### Methotrexate (Mexate)

**Summary:** One patient on high dose methotrexate developed severe methotrexate toxicity following the use of diclofenac.

**Risk Factors:**
- *Dosage Regimen.* The risk of adverse effects from this interaction is primarily in patients receiving antineoplastic doses of methotrexate, rather than the lower doses used to treat rheumatoid arthritis, psoriasis, and related diseases.
- *Concurrent Diseases.* Particular caution is suggested in patients with pre-existing renal impairment [who may be more susceptible to nonsteroidal anti-inflammatory drug (NSAID)-induced renal failure].

**Related Drugs:** Other NSAIDS appear to interact similarly with methotrexate, but the relative risk of one NSAID versus another is not established.

**Management Options:**
- *Avoid Unless Benefit Outweighs Risk.* Until more information is available on this interaction, it would be prudent to avoid diclofenac (as well as other NSAIDs) in patients receiving antineoplastic doses of methotrexate. Particular caution is suggested in patients with pre-existing renal impairment, who may be more susceptible to NSAID-induced renal failure.
- *Monitor.* If the combination is used, monitor for methotrexate toxicity. Findings in methotrexate toxicity can include stomatitis, severe gastrointestinal symptoms (nausea, diarrhea, vomiting), bone marrow suppression, fever, bleeding, skin rashes, nephrotoxicity, and hepatotoxicity. Although decreasing the methotrexate dosage would be expected to reduce the likelihood of toxicity, the magnitude of the required reduction in methotrexate dosage has not been established.

## Significance Classification

(1) - **Avoid Combination.** Risk always outweighs benefit.

(2) - **Usually Avoid Combination.** Use combination only under special circumstances.

(3) - **Minimize Risk.** Take action as necessary to reduce risk.

References:

1. Furst DE et al. Effect of aspirin and sulindac on methotrexate clearance. J Pharm Sci. 1990;79:782.
2. Dupuis LL et al. Methotrexate-nonsteroidal anti-inflammatory drug interaction in children with arthritis. J Rheumatol. 1990;17:1469.
3. Skeith KJ et al. Lack of significant interaction between low dose methotrexate and ibuprofen or flurbiprofen in patients with arthritis. J Rheumatol. 1990;17:1008.

## Diclofenac (Voltaren)

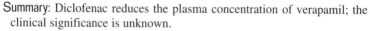

## Verapamil (Calan)

Summary: Diclofenac reduces the plasma concentration of verapamil; the clinical significance is unknown.

Risk Factors: No specific risk factors known.

Related Drugs: **Naproxen (Naprosyn)** coadministration appears to have no effect on verapamil concentrations. The effects of other NSAIDs on verapamil are unknown. Diclofenac 50 mg administered once increased **isradipine (DynaCirc)** peak concentration by 20% but did not change its area under the concentration-time curve.[3] The clinical effects of this change would be minimal.

Management Options:

- *Consider Alternative.* Naproxen should be considered for patients taking verapamil.

- *Monitor.* Until more information is available, patients stabilized on verapamil should be monitored for reduced efficacy during concomitant therapy with diclofenac.

References:

1. Peterson MS et al. Differential effects of naproxen and diclofenac on verapamil pharmacokinetics. Clin Pharmacol Ther. 1991;49:129. Abstract.
2. Houston MC et al. The effects of nonsteroidal anti-inflammatory drugs on blood pressures of patients with hypertension controlled by verapamil. Arch Intern Med. 1995;155:1049.
3. Sommers DK et al. Effects of diclofenac on isradipine pharmacokinetics and platelet aggregation in volunteers. Eur J Clin Pharmacol. 1993;44:391.

## Diclofenac (Voltaren)

## Warfarin (Coumadin)

Summary: A preliminary study indicates that diclofenac does not affect the hypoprothrombinemic response to oral anticoagulants; nonetheless, co-therapy requires caution because of possible detrimental effects of diclofenac on the gastric mucosa and platelet function.

Risk Factors:

- *Concurrent Diseases.* Patients with peptic ulcer disease or a history of gastrointestinal (GI) bleeding are probably at greater risk.

Related Drugs: All NSAIDs inhibit platelet function, cause gastric erosions, and appear to have an additive effect with oral anticoagulants in increasing the risk of GI bleeding.

Management Options:
- *Avoid Unless Benefit Outweighs Risk.* Since all NSAIDs probably increase the risk of GI bleeding in patients on oral anticoagulants, use the combination only after careful consideration of the benefit versus risk. If the diclofenac is being used as an analgesic or antipyretic, acetaminophen is probably safer to use with oral anticoagulants. Nonacetylated salicylates (e.g., choline salicylate, magnesium salicylate, salsalate, sodium salicylate) also are probably safer with oral anticoagulants than diclofenac since they have minimal effects on platelet function and the gastric mucosa.
- *Monitor.* If any NSAID is used with an oral anticoagulant, one should carefully monitor the prothrombin time and watch for evidence of bleeding, especially from the GI tract.

References:
1. Michot F et al. A double-blind clinical trial to determine if an interaction exists between diclofenac sodium and the oral anticoagulant acenocoumarol (Nicoamalone). J Int Med Res. 1975;3:153.
2. Shorr RI et al. Concurrent use of nonsteroidal anti-inflammatory drugs and oral anticoagulants places elderly persons at high risk for hemorrhagic peptic ulcer disease. Arch Intern Med. 1993;153:1665.

### Didanosine (Videx)

### Ganciclovir (Cytovene)

Summary: Didanosine concentrations are increased during coadministration with ganciclovir; didanosine toxicity could occur in some patients.
Risk Factors: No specific risk factors known.
Related Drugs: No information available.
Management Options:
- *Monitor.* Until further information regarding this interaction is available, patients receiving didanosine should be monitored carefully for toxicity, including peripheral neuropathy and pancreatitis, if ganciclovir is added.

References:
1. Trapnell MD et al. Altered didanosine pharmacokinetics with concomitant oral ganciclovir. Clin Pharmacol Ther. 1994;55:193. Abstract.

### Didanosine (Videx)
### Itraconazole (Sporanox)

Summary: Didanosine administration can significantly reduce the absorption of itraconazole; loss of antifungal efficacy may result.
Risk Factors: No specific risk factors known.
Related Drugs: A preliminary report noted a similar interaction between **ketoconazole (Nizoral)** and didanosine. Other drugs that alkalinize the

stomach might be expected to cause a similar interaction with itraconazole. *Fluconazole (Diflucan)* absorption does not appear to be affected by didanosine.

Management Options:

- *Circumvent/Minimize.* Administration of itraconazole at least two hours before didanosine will minimize this interaction.
- *Monitor.* If itraconazole and didanosine are coadministered, watch the patient for loss of antifungal activity.

References:

1. May DB et al. Effect of simultaneous didanosine administration on itraconazole absorption in healthy volunteers. Pharmacotherapy. 1994;14:509.
2. Moreno R et al. Itraconazole-didanosine excipient interaction. JAMA. 1993;269: 1508. Letter.

### Didanosine (Videx)

### Ketoconazole (Nizoral)

Summary: Buffers contained in oral formulations of didanosine may reduce serum concentrations of ketoconazole.

Risk Factors: No specific risk factors known.

Related Drugs: Concentrations of other antifungal agents [e.g., *itraconazole (Sporanox)*] are likely to be decreased by didanosine administration. *Fluconazole (Diflucan)* absorption does not appear to be affected by didanosine.

Management Options:

- *Circumvent/Minimize.* Ketoconazole should be administered at least 2 hours before didanosine to avoid interaction with the buffers in the didanosine.
- *Monitor.* If didanosine is coadministered with ketoconazole, watch for reduced antifungal efficacy.

References:

1. Knupp CA et al. Pharmacokinetics of didanosine and ketoconazole after coadministration to patients seropositive for the human immunodeficiency virus. J Clin Pharmacol. 1993;33:912.

### Diflunisal (Dolobid)

### Warfarin (Coumadin)

Summary: Limited data indicate the diflunisal may enhance the hypoprothrombinemic response to oral anticoagulants in some patients; caution during cotherapy with these drugs also is required because of the detrimental effects of diflunisal on the gastric mucosa and platelet function.

Risk Factors:

- *Concurrent Diseases.* Patients with peptic ulcer disease or a history of gastrointestinal bleeding (GI) are probably at greater risk.

Related Drugs: All NSAIDs inhibit platelet function, cause gastric erosions, and probably increase the risk of GI bleeding. Some NSAIDs, however, such as **ibuprofen (Advil), naproxen (Naprosyn)**, or **diclofenac (Voltaren)** may be less likely to increase oral anticoagulant-induced hypoprothrombinemia than other NSAIDs. **Acenocoumarol** appears to interact with diflunisal similarly.

Management Options:

- *Avoid Unless Benefit Outweighs Risk.* Since all NSAIDs probably increase the risk of GI bleeding in patients on oral anticoagulants, use the combination only after careful consideration of the benefit versus risk. If an NSAID must be used with an oral anticoagulant, it would be prudent to use NSAIDs that are unlikely to affect the hypoprothrombinemic response to oral anticoagulants. (See Related Drugs above.) If the NSAID is being used as an analgesic or antipyretic, acetaminophen is probably safer to use with oral anticoagulants. Nonacetylated salicylates (e.g., choline salicylate, magnesium salicylate, salsalate, sodium salicylate) are probably also safer with oral anticoagulants than NSAIDs, since such salicylates have minimal effects on platelet function and the gastric mucosa.

- *Monitor.* If any NSAID is used with an oral anticoagulant, one should carefully monitor the prothrombin time and watch for evidence of bleeding, especially from the GI tract.

References:

1. Davies RO. Review of the animal and clinical pharmacology of diflunisal. Pharmacotherapy. 1983;2(Suppl. 1):9S.
2. Rider JA. Comparison of fecal blood loss after use of aspirin and diflunisal. Pharmacotherapy. 1983;3(Suppl. 1):61S.
3. Shorr RI et al. Concurrent use of nonsteroidal anti-inflammatory drugs and oral anticoagulants places elderly persons at high risk for hemorrhagic peptic ulcer disease. Arch Intern Med. 1993;153:1665.

**Digitoxin (Crystodigin)**

**Phenobarbital**

Summary: Phenobarbital administration may reduce digitoxin serum concentrations, but it is unknown how often this decreases the therapeutic response to digitoxin.

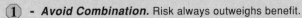

## Significance Classification

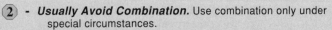

(1) - *Avoid Combination.* Risk always outweighs benefit.

(2) - *Usually Avoid Combination.* Use combination only under special circumstances.

(3) - *Minimize Risk.* Take action as necessary to reduce risk.

Risk Factors: No specific risk factors known.

Related Drugs: *Digoxin (Lanoxin)* elimination is not likely to be affected by barbiturates to the same degree as digitoxin since it primarily is excreted renally.

Management Options:

- *Consider Alternative.* Digoxin would seem less likely to be affected by enzyme induction and may be preferable to digitoxin in patients taking chronic phenobarbital or other barbiturates.
- *Monitor.* Until further information is available, patients receiving both digitoxin and a barbiturate should be evaluated for underdigitalization, and the digitoxin dose should be increased if necessary.

References:

1. Jelliffe RW et al. Effect of phenobarbital on digitoxin metabolism. Clin Res. 1966; 14:160.
2. Solomon HM et al. Interactions between digitoxin and other drugs in man. Am Heart J. 1972;83:277.
3. Kaldor A et al. Interaction of heart glycosides and phenobarbital. Int J Clin Pharmacol. 1975;12:403.

## Digitoxin (Crystodigin)

## Rifampin (Rifadin)

Summary: Rifampin reduces the serum concentration of digoxin and digitoxin.

Risk Factors: No specific risk factors known.

Related Drugs: *Digoxin (Lanoxin)* is affected similarly by rifampin.

Management Options:

- *Circumvent/Minimize.* Dosage adjustments of digitalis glycosides (especially digitoxin) likely will be necessary when rifampin is added to or removed from a patient's regimen.
- *Monitor.* When rifampin and digitalis glycosides are used concomitantly, be alert for reduced digoxin and digitoxin efficacy.

References:

1. Poor DM et al. Interaction of rifampin and digitoxin. Arch Intern Med. 1983; 143:599.
2. Gault H et al. Digoxin-rifampin interaction. Clin Pharmacol Ther. 1984;35:750.
3. Novi C et al. Rifampin and digoxin: possible drug interaction in a dialysis patient. JAMA. 1980;244:2521.

## Digoxin (Lanoxin)

## Diltiazem (Cardizem)

Summary: Diltiazem increases digoxin serum concentrations; digoxin toxicity may result.

Risk Factors: No specific risk factors known.

Related Drugs: *Verapamil (Calan)*, *bepridil (Vascor)*, and *nitrendipine (Baypress)* appear to reduce digoxin elimination. *Digitoxin (Crystodigin)* is likely to be affected similarly. *Nifedipine (Procardia)*,[1–4,6] *isradipine (DynaCirc)*,[7] *nicardipine (Cardene)*,[8] *felodipine (Plendil)*,[5] and *amlodipine (Norvasc)*[7] do not appear to increase digoxin concentration.

Management Options:

- *Consider Alternative.* Nifedipine, isradipine, nicardipine, felodipine, and amlodipine do not appear to increase digoxin concentration and may be possible alternatives.
- *Circumvent/Minimize.* Digoxin dosages may need to be reduced when diltiazem is added to a patient stabilized on digoxin.
- *Monitor.* Patients should be monitored for evidence of increased serum digitalis effects (e.g., bradycardia, heart block, gastrointestinal upset, mental changes) in the presence of calcium channel blocker therapy.

References:

1. Belz GG et al. Digoxin plasma concentrations and nifedipine. Lancet. 1981;1:844.
2. Rameis H et al. The diltiazem-digoxin interaction. Clin Pharmacol Ther. 1984; 36:183.
3. Clarke WR et al. Potentially serious drug interactions secondary to high-dose diltiazem used in the treatment of pulmonary hypertension. Pharmacotherapy. 1993; 13:402.
4. Schwartz JB et al. Effect of nifedipine on serum digoxin concentration and renal digoxin clearance. Clin Pharmacol Ther. 1984;36:19.
5. Kirch W et al. The felodipine/digoxin interaction. A placebo-controlled study in patients with heart failure. Br J Clin Pharmacol. 1988;26:644P. Abstract.
6. Hutt HJ et al. Dose-dependence of the nifedipine/digoxin interaction? Arch Toxicol. 1986;9(Suppl.):209.
7. Rodin SM et al. Comparative effects of verapamil and isradipine on steady-state digoxin kinetics. Clin Pharmacol Ther. 1988;43:668.
8. Debruyne D et al. Nicardipine does not significantly affect serum digoxin concentrations at the steady state of patients with congestive heart failure. Int J Clin Pharmacol. 1989;9:15.

### Digoxin (Lanoxin)

### Erythromycin

Summary: Erythromycin can reduce bacterial gastrointestinal (GI) flora and increase digoxin concentrations in a minority of patients.

Risk Factors: No specific risk factors known.

Related Drugs: It is possible that other oral broad-spectrum antibiotics could affect digoxin in a similar manner.

Management Options:

- *Consider Alternative.* Several penicillins [amoxicillin (Amoxil), flucloxacillin, penicillin] have been shown to cause no change in digoxin concentrations.[3] The effect of other antibiotics is unknown.
- *Monitor.* In the 1 patient in 10 who metabolizes substantial amounts of digoxin in the GI tract, concomitant antibiotic therapy can increase serum digoxin concentration. Monitor for potential increases

in the response to digoxin (e.g., bradycardia, nausea, anorexia, or heart block) and reduce digoxin dosage as needed.

References:

1. Morton MR et al. Erythromycin-induced digoxin toxicity. DICP, Ann Pharmacother. 1989;23:668.
2. Norregaard-Hansen K et al. The significance of the enterohepatic circulation on the metabolism of digoxin in patients with the ability of intestinal conversion of the drug. Acta Med Scand. 1986;220:89.
3. Rhodes KM et al. Do the penicillin antibiotics interact with digoxin? Eur J Clin Pharmacol. 1994;46:479.

## Digoxin (Lanoxin)

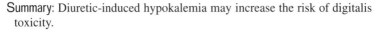

## Furosemide (Lasix)

Summary: Diuretic-induced hypokalemia may increase the risk of digitalis toxicity.

Risk Factors: No specific risk factors known.

Related Drugs: *Ethacrynic acid (Edecrin)*, *bumetanide (Bumex)*, *chlorthalidone (Hygroton)*, *metolazone (Zaroxolyn)*, and *thiazides* interact similarly. *Torsemide (Demadex)* may produce a similar increased risk of digoxin toxicity. Patients taking *digitoxin (Crystodigin)* also would be at risk.

Management Options:

- *Consider Alternative.* Potassium-sparing diuretics could be considered as alternatives to potassium-wasting agents; however, note the interactions with amiloride (Midamor) and spironolactone (Aldactone).

- *Monitor.* The potassium and magnesium status of patients on concomitant diuretic-digitalis therapy should be monitored. Replacement potassium or magnesium therapy should be undertaken if needed. Be alert for increased digoxin effects.

References:

1. Young IS et al. Magnesium status and digoxin toxicity. Br J Clin Pharmacol. 1991; 32:717.
2. Steines E. Suppression of renal excretion of digoxin in hypokalemic patients. Clin Pharmacol Ther. 1978;23:511.
3. Tsutsumi E et al. Effect of furosemide on serum clearance and renal excretion of digoxin. J Clin Pharmacol. 1979;19:200.

## Digoxin (Lanoxin)

## Hydroxychloroquine (Plaquenil)

Summary: Hydroxychloroquine may increase serum digoxin concentrations, but the degree to which this increases the risk of digoxin toxicity is unknown.

Risk Factors: No specific risk factors known.

Related Drugs: No information available.

Management Options:

- *Monitor.* Digoxin concentration should be monitored and patients observed for toxicity (e.g., nausea, arrhythmia) when hydroxychloroquine is started in a patient receiving digoxin. Digoxin dosage may need to be altered.

References:
1. Leden I. Digoxin-hydroxychloroquine interaction? Acta Med Scand. 1982;211:411.

### Digoxin (Lanoxin)

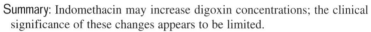

### Indomethacin (Indocin)

Summary: Indomethacin may increase digoxin concentrations; the clinical significance of these changes appears to be limited.

Risk Factors: No specific risk factors known.

Related Drugs: The clinical significance of the interactions between non-steroidal anti-inflammatory drugs (NSAIDs) and digoxin appears to be limited in magnitude and frequency. In 12 patients stabilized on digoxin, the addition of *ibuprofen (Advil)* ≥1600 mg/day resulted in approximately a 60% increase in serum digoxin after 1 week. However, the increase was highly variable from patient to patient and was not detectable after about a month of ibuprofen treatment.[2] Another study in patients on chronic digoxin taking ibuprofen 600 mg TID found no change in digoxin concentrations.[1] The pharmacokinetics of a single IV dose of digoxin were not altered by *aspirin* 975 mg TID.[3] *Phenylbutazone (Butazolidin)* may reduce serum concentrations of digoxin.

Management Options:

- *Monitor.* Patients stabilized on digoxin should be monitored for altered digoxin effect when an NSAID is initiated (increased concentration, electrocardiogram changes) or discontinued (reduced digoxin efficacy).

References:
1. Jorgensen HS et al. Interaction between digoxin and indomethacin or ibuprofen. Br J Clin Pharmacol. 1991;31:108.
2. Quattrocchi FP et al. The effects of ibuprofen on serum digoxin concentrations. Drug Intell Clin Pharm. 1983;17:286.
3. Fenster PE et al. Kinetics of the digoxin-aspirin combination. Clin Pharmacol Ther. 1982;32:429.

### Digoxin (Lanoxin)

### Itraconazole (Sporanox)

Summary: An increase in digoxin serum concentration following itraconazole administration was noted in several patients. The clinical significance of this interaction is unclear, but some patients may experience digoxin toxicity.

Risk Factors: No specific risk factors known.

Related Drugs: Other azole antifungal agents also might increase digoxin serum concentrations, but little information is available.

Management Options:

- *Monitor.* Until further information is available, patients stabilized on digoxin should be monitored for altered digoxin concentrations when itraconazole is added to or removed from their drug regimens.

References:
1. Rex J. Itraconazole-digoxin interaction. Ann Intern Med. 1992;116:525.
2. Sachs MK et al. Interaction of itraconazole and digoxin. Clin Infect Dis. 1993;16:400.
3. McClean KL et al. Interaction between itraconazole and digoxin. Clin Infect Dis. 1994;18:259. Letter.

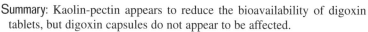

### Digoxin (Lanoxin)

### Kaolin-Pectin

Summary: Kaolin-pectin appears to reduce the bioavailability of digoxin tablets, but digoxin capsules do not appear to be affected.

Risk Factors:

- *Dosage Form.* Digoxin tablets (but not capsules) appear to be affected by kaolin-pectin.

Related Drugs: Kaolin-pectin may be expected to affect **digitoxin (Crystodigin)** in a similar manner.

Management Options:

- *Circumvent/Minimize.* Administer digoxin 2 hours before the kaolin-pectin to minimize the interaction. The use of digoxin capsules may help minimize the interaction.
- *Monitor.* Patients receiving digoxin and kaolin-pectin should be monitored for reduced digoxin concentrations and effect.

References:
1. Albert KS et al. Influence of kaolin-pectin suspension on digoxin bioavailability. J Pharm Sci. 1978;67:1582.
2. Allen MD et al. Effect of magnesium-aluminum hydroxide and kaolin-pectin on absorption of digoxin from tablets and capsules. J Clin Pharmacol. 1981;21:26.
3. Albert KS et al. Influence of kaolin-pectin suspension on steady-state plasma digoxin levels. J Clin Pharmacol. 1982;21:449.

## Significance Classification

(1) - *Avoid Combination.* Risk always outweighs benefit.

(2) - *Usually Avoid Combination.* Use combination only under special circumstances.

(3) - *Minimize Risk.* Take action as necessary to reduce risk.

**Digoxin (Lanoxin)**

**Mibefradil (Posicor)**

Summary: Mibefradil produces a dose-dependent increase in digoxin concentrations; increased digoxin side effects may occur at high mibefradil doses.

Risk Factors:
* *Dosage Regimen.* Mibefradil doses above 100 mg/day may increase the risk of interaction.

Related Drugs: Other calcium channel blockers including **verapamil (Calan)** and **diltiazem (Cardizem)** are known to increase digoxin concentrations and may produce similar effects on cardiac conduction.

Management Options:
* *Monitor.* Observe patients taking digoxin and mibefradil, particularly if mibefradil doses exceed 100 mg/day, for evidence of increased digoxin concentrations or heart block.

References:
1. Siepmann M et al. The interaction of the calcium antagonist RO 40-5967 with digoxin. Br J Clin Pharmacol. 1995;39:491.

**Digoxin (Lanoxin)**

**Omeprazole (Prilosec)**

Summary: Omeprazole increases the serum concentration of digoxin. Digoxin effects may be increased, but the clinical importance is not established.

Risk Factors: No specific risk factors known.

Related Drugs: **Pentagastrin (Peptavlon)** may reduce digoxin response. **Lansoprazole (Prevacid)** may produce similar effects on digoxin.

Management Options:
* *Monitor.* Until further information is available, patients receiving digoxin should be monitored for elevated digoxin concentrations and symptoms of toxicity if omeprazole is added and diminished effect if omeprazole is deleted from their regimen.

References:
1. Cohen AF et al. Influence of gastric acidity on the bioavailability of digoxin. Ann Intern Med. 1991;115:540.
2. Cohen AF et al. Effects of gastric acidity on the bioavailability of digoxin. Evidence for a new mechanism for interactions with omeprazole. Br J Clin Pharmacol. 1991;31:565P. Abstract.
3. Oosterhuis B et al. Minor effect of multiple dose omeprazole on the pharmacokinetics of digoxin after a single oral dose. Br J Clin Pharmacol. 1991;32:569.

**Digoxin (Lanoxin)**

**Penicillamine (Cuprimine)**

Summary: Penicillamine has been reported to reduce digoxin serum concentrations, but the clinical importance of the effect is not established.

Risk Factors: No specific risk factors known.

Related Drugs: No information available.

Management Options:

- *Monitor.* Patients should be monitored for evidence of reduced digoxin concentration and effect when penicillamine is initiated. The digoxin dosage should be adjusted as necessary.

References:

1. Moezzi B et al. The effect of penicillamine on serum digoxin levels. Jpn Heart J. 1978;19:366.

### Digoxin (Lanoxin)

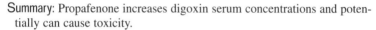

### Propafenone (Rythmol)

Summary: Propafenone increases digoxin serum concentrations and potentially can cause toxicity.

Risk Factors: No specific risk factors known.

Related Drugs: A similar effect may be seen with ***digitoxin (Crystodigin)***, but data are lacking.

Management Options:

- *Circumvent/Minimize.* The digoxin dosage may need to be reduced during concomitant propafenone administration.

- *Monitor.* Since propafenone may increase digoxin serum concentrations by 30% to 60%, some patients maintained on digoxin could develop toxicity following its addition. Digoxin concentrations and response should be monitored when propafenone is initiated or discontinued in a patient taking digoxin.

References:

1. Calvo MV et al. Interaction between digoxin and propafenone. Ther Drug Monit. 1989;11:10.
2. Bigot MC et al. Serum digoxin levels related to plasma propafenone levels during concomitant treatment. J Clin Pharmacol. 1991;31:521.
3. Zalzstein E et al. Interaction between digoxin and propafenone in children. J Pediatr. 1990;116:310.

### Digoxin (Lanoxin)

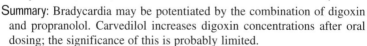

### Propranolol (Inderal)

Summary: Bradycardia may be potentiated by the combination of digoxin and propranolol. Carvedilol increases digoxin concentrations after oral dosing; the significance of this is probably limited.

Risk Factors:

- *Concurrent Diseases.* Patients with concomitant myocardial conduction delays or those with renal dysfunction who have elevated digoxin concentrations are at risk.

Related Drugs: In both acute and chronic dosing studies, ***carvedilol (Coreg)*** 25 mg administered concomitantly with oral digoxin resulted in a significant increase in digoxin peak serum concentrations and area under the concentration-time curve.[1,2] The clinical significance of these changes is likely to be small. No change in digoxin pharmacokinetics was noted following IV digoxin or oral digitoxin and carvedilol.[1,3] Most beta blockers would be expected to have the potential for bradycardia when used with digoxin. Although specific data are lacking, beta blockers with partial agonist activity [e.g., **pindolol (Visken)**] may be less likely to produce bradycardia at rest. A similar interaction would be expected with **digitoxin (Crystodigin)**.

Management Options:
- *Monitor.* All patients receiving beta blockers and digoxin or digitoxin should be monitored for reduced heart rate.

References:
1. De May C et al. Carvedilol increases the systemic bioavailability of oral digoxin. Br J Clin Pharmacol. 1990;29:486.
2. Wermeling DP et al. Effects of long-term oral carvedilol on the steady-state pharmacokinetics of oral digoxin in patients with mild to moderate hypertension. Pharmacotherapy. 1994;14:600.
3. Harder S et al. Lack of a pharmacokinetic interaction between carvedilol and digitoxin or phenprocoumon. J Clin Pharmacol. 1993;44:583.

**Digoxin (Lanoxin)**

**Quinidine**

Summary: Quinidine increases the serum concentration of digoxin and digitoxin sufficiently to lead to digitalis toxicity in some patients.

Risk Factors:
- *Dosage Regimen.* Quinidine doses above 500 mg/day may increase digoxin serum concentration.

Related Drugs: The effect of quinidine on **digitoxin (Crystodigin)** disposition has been disputed, but the bulk of the evidence indicates that quinidine does increase serum digitoxin concentrations to a clinically significant degree.[1-3] Quinidine appears to reduce digitoxin nonrenal clearance but causes less change in its renal clearance and no change in the volume of distribution of digitoxin.

Management Options:
- *Circumvent/Minimize.* A reduction in digoxin dose when quinidine is started will reduce the likelihood of digoxin toxicity. However,

## Significance Classification

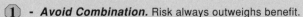 - ***Avoid Combination.*** Risk always outweighs benefit.

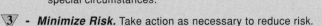 - ***Usually Avoid Combination.*** Use combination only under special circumstances.

- ***Minimize Risk.*** Take action as necessary to reduce risk.

because the magnitude of the interaction varies considerably from patient to patient, further adjustments in digoxin dose are likely to be necessary.

- *Monitor.* During the first 7 to 10 days of combined therapy, the patient should be monitored carefully for symptoms and electrocardiogram evidence of digoxin toxicity. In general, these precautions also would apply to the concurrent use of quinidine and digitoxin, although it may take longer to achieve a new steady-state serum digitoxin level after starting quinidine therapy.

References:

1. Ochs HR et al. Noninteraction of digitoxin and quinidine. N Engl J Med. 1980; 303:672.
2. Kuhlmann J et al. Effects of quinidine on pharmacokinetics and pharmacodynamics of digitoxin achieving steady-state conditions. Clin Pharmacol Ther. 1986; 39:288.
3. Kuhlmann J. Effects of quinidine, verapamil and nifedipine on the pharmacokinetics and pharmacodynamics of digitoxin during steady state conditions. Arzneimittelforschung. 1987;37:545.

## Digoxin (Lanoxin)

## Quinine

Summary: Quinine potentially could increase digoxin concentrations, particularly when it is administered in high doses.

Risk Factors:

- *Dosage Regimen.* Quinine doses of ≥600 mg/day could increase digoxin concentrations.

Related Drugs: **Digitoxin (Crystodigin)** also may be affected by large doses of quinine.

Management Options:

- *Monitor.* No digoxin dosage adjustment is likely to be required when quinine is administered in low doses. If large quinine doses are administered, monitor the patient for increased digoxin concentrations and signs of digoxin toxicity (nausea, anorexia, arrhythmia).

References:

1. Wandell M et al. Effect of quinine on digoxin kinetics. Clin Pharmacol Ther. 1980;28:425.

## Digoxin (Lanoxin)

## Spironolactone (Aldactone)

Summary: Substantial evidence indicates that spironolactone may interfere with certain serum digoxin assays. More limited evidence suggests that spironolactone may produce a true increase in serum digoxin concentrations.

Risk Factors: No specific risk factors known.

Related Drugs: No information available.

Management Options:
- *Monitor.* In patients receiving digoxin and spironolactone, monitor the digoxin response by means other than serum digoxin concentrations, unless the digoxin assay used has been proven not to be affected by spironolactone therapy. Since there is some evidence that spironolactone may produce a small increase in serum digoxin concentration, watch for evidence of enhanced digoxin effect such as nausea or arrhythmia.

References:
1. Morris RG et al. The effect of renal and hepatic impairment and of spironolactone on digoxin immunoassays. Eur J Clin Pharmacol. 1988;34:233.
2. Morris RG et al. Spironolactone as a source of interference in commercial digoxin immunoassays. Ther Drug Monit. 1987;9:208.
3. Hedman A et al. Digoxin-interactions in man: spironolactone reduced renal but not biliary digoxin clearance. Eur J Clin Pharmacol. 1992;42:481.

### Digoxin (Lanoxin)
### Sulfasalazine (Azulfidine)

Summary: Sulfasalazine can reduce digoxin serum concentrations.
Risk Factors:
- *Dosage Regimen.* Sulfasalazine doses >2 gm/day can reduce digoxin serum concentrations.

Related Drugs: **Digitoxin (Crystodigin)** may be less likely to interact with sulfasalazine.
Management Options:
- *Consider Alternative.* Digitoxin may be preferable in sulfasalazine-treated patients.
- *Monitor.* It does not seem necessary to avoid the concomitant use of digoxin and sulfasalazine, but patients should be monitored for a decreased or inadequate therapeutic response to digoxin. Based on the response of one patient, separation of the doses of digoxin and sulfasalazine did not circumvent the interaction.

References:
1. Juhl RP et al. Effect of sulfasalazine on digoxin bioavailability. Clin Pharmacol Ther. 1976;20:387.

### Digoxin (Lanoxin)
### Tetracycline

Summary: Tetracycline can reduce bacterial gastrointestinal (GI) flora and increase digoxin concentrations in a minority of patients.
Risk Factors: No specific risk factors known.
Related Drugs: No information available.
Management Options:
- *Monitor.* In the 1 patient in 10 who metabolizes substantial amount of digoxin in the GI tract, concomitant tetracycline therapy can

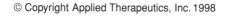

increase serum digoxin concentrations. Monitor for digoxin toxicity (e.g., nausea, anorexia, arrhythmia) and reduce the dosage as needed.

References:
1. Lindenbaum J et al. Inactivation of digoxin by the gut flora: reversal by antibiotic therapy. N Engl J Med. 1981;305:789.
2. Norregaard-Hansen K et al. The significance of the enterohepatic circulation on the metabolism of digoxin in patients with the ability of intestinal conversion of the drug. Acta Med Scand. 1986;220:89.

## Digoxin (Lanoxin)
## Verapamil (Calan)

Summary: Verapamil increases digoxin serum concentrations; digoxin toxicity may result.

Risk Factors:
- *Dosage Regimen.* Verapamil doses >160 mg/day produce larger increases in digoxin concentrations.[2]

Related Drugs: **Diltiazem (Cardizem)**, **bepridil (Vascor)** and **nitrendipine (Baypress)** appear to reduce digoxin elimination. **Digitoxin (Crystodigin)** is likely to be affected similarly. **Nifedipine (Procardia)**,[1,3,4,7] **isradipine (DynaCirc)**,[8] **nicardipine (Cardene)**,[9] **felodipine (Plendil)**,[5] and **amlodipine (Norvasc)**[6] do not appear to increase digoxin concentrations.

Management Options:
- *Consider Alternative.* Nifedipine, isradipine, nicardipine, felodipine, and amlodipine do not appear to increase digoxin concentrations and may be suitable alternatives.
- *Circumvent/Minimize.* Digoxin dosages may need to be reduced when verapamil is added to a patient stabilized on digoxin.
- *Monitor.* Patients should be monitored for evidence of increased serum digitalis effects (e.g., bradycardia, heart block, gastrointestinal upset, mental changes) in the presence of verapamil therapy.

References:
1. Belz GG et al. Digoxin plasma concentrations and nifedipine. Lancet. 1981;1:844.
2. Klein HO et al. The influence of verapamil on serum digoxin concentration. Circulation. 1982;65:998.
3. Kuhlmann J. Effects of nifedipine and diltiazem on plasma levels and renal excretion of beta-acetyldigoxin. Clin Pharmacol Ther. 1985;37:150.
4. Schwartz JB et al. Effect of nifedipine on serum digoxin concentration and renal digoxin clearance. Clin Pharmacol Ther. 1984;36:19.
5. Kirch W et al. The felodipine/digoxin interaction. A placebo-controlled study in patients with heart failure. Br J Clin Pharmacol. 1988;26:644P. Abstract.
6. Schwartz JB. Effects of amlodipine on steady-state digoxin concentrations and renal digoxin clearance. J Cardiovasc Pharmacol. 1988;12:1.
7. Hutt HJ et al. Dose-dependence of the nifedipine/digoxin interaction? Arch Toxicol. 1986;(Suppl. 9):209.
8. Rodin SM et al. Comparative effects of verapamil and isradipine on steady-state digoxin kinetics. Clin Pharmacol Ther. 1988;43:668.
9. Debruyne D et al. Nicardipine does not significantly affect serum digoxin concentrations at the steady state of patients with congestive heart failure. Int J Clin Pharmacol. 1989;9:15.

### Diltiazem (Cardizem)

### Encainide (Enkaid)

Summary: Diltiazem substantially increases serum encainide concentrations, but the clinical importance of this interaction is not established.

Risk Factors:
- *Pharmacogenetics.* Rapid encainide metabolizers are at risk.

Related Drugs: The effect of other calcium channel blockers on encainide metabolism has not been studied; however, **verapamil (Calan)** might produce similar effects because of its effects on drug metabolism.

Management Options:
- *Monitor.* Patients maintained on encainide should be monitored for possible toxicity (arrhythmia, dizziness) or increased encainide concentrations when diltiazem is administered concurrently.

References:
1. Kazierad DJ et al. Effects of diltiazem on the disposition of encainide and its active metabolites. Clin Pharmacol Ther. 1989;46:668.

### Diltiazem (Cardizem)

### Lovastatin (Mevacor)

Summary: Diltiazem administration produces a marked increase in lovastatin concentrations; increased toxicity may result.

Risk Factors: No specific risk factors known.

Related Drugs: **Simvastatin (Zocor)** is likely to be affected by diltiazem in a similar manner. **Verapamil (Isoptin)** and **mibefradil (Posicor)** would be likely to produce similar changes in lovastatin concentrations. Dihydropyridine calcium channel antagonists would be less likely to alter lovastatin pharmacokinetics, although **isradipine (DynaCirc)** was reported to decrease lovastatin concentrations.[2] **Pravastatin (Pravachol)** metabolism is not altered by diltiazem. The effect of diltiazem on other HMG-CoA reductase inhibitors is unknown.

Management Options:
- *Consider Alternative.* Pravastatin would be a good alternative for patients taking calcium channel blockers that inhibit CYP3A4 activity (e.g., diltiazem, verapamil, and mibefradil).

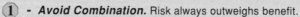

## Significance Classification

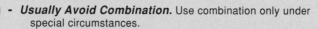

(1) - *Avoid Combination.* Risk always outweighs benefit.

(2) - *Usually Avoid Combination.* Use combination only under special circumstances.

(3) - *Minimize Risk.* Take action as necessary to reduce risk.

- *Monitor.* Patients taking lovastatin or simvastatin who receive diltiazem, verapamil, or mibefradil should be carefully monitored for evidence of myositis.

References:
1. Agbim NE et al. Interaction of diltiazem with lovastatin and pravastatin. Clin Pharmacol Ther. 1997;61:201. Abstract.
2. Zhou L-X et al. Pharmacokinetic interaction between isradipine and lovastatin in normal, female and male volunteers. J Pharmacol Exper Ther. 1995;273:121.

## Diltiazem (Cardizem)

### Midazolam (Versed)

Summary: Diltiazem increases midazolam plasma concentrations and may prolong sedation and respiratory depression.

Risk Factors: No specific risk factors known.

Related Drugs: Diltiazem has been noted to increase the concentrations of *triazolam (Halcion).*[2,3] *Verapamil (Isoptin)* may affect midazolam in a similar manner.[1] *Mibefradil (Posicor)* also would be expected to inhibit midazolam metabolism.

Management Options:
- *Consider Alternative.* The use of a dihydropyridine calcium channel blocker would probably avoid the interaction. Selection of a benzodiazepine such as lorazepam (Ativan) or temazepam (Restoril) that is not metabolized by CYP3A4 would prevent an interaction with diltiazem.
- *Monitor.* Patients receiving diltiazem and midazolam should be monitored for prolonged sedation and respiratory depression.

References:
1. Backman JT et al. Dose of midazolam should be reduced during diltiazem and verapamil treatments. Br J Clin Pharmacol. 1994;55:481.
2. Kosuge K et al. Enhanced effect of triazolam with diltiazem. Br J Clin Pharmacol. 1997;43:367.
3. Varhe A et al. Diltiazem enhances the effects of triazolam by inhibiting its metabolism. Clin Pharmacol Ther. 1996;59:369.

## Diltiazem (Cardizem)

### Nifedipine (Procardia)

Summary: Diltiazem increases the serum concentration of nifedipine; nifedipine increases the serum concentration of diltiazem. Increased pharmacodynamic effects could occur.

Risk Factors:
- *Dosage Regimen.* Patients with daily diltiazem doses of greater than 270 mg are at particular risk.

Related Drugs: The combination of *nitrendipine (Baypress)* and diltiazem produced greater hypotensive effects than each drug alone; no pharmacokinetic data were evaluated.[3] The combination of amlodipine (Norvasc) and verapamil (Calan) produced a greater increase in forearm blood flow than amlodipine alone.[1] Since the drugs were infused into the brachial artery for 3 minutes, this effect is likely due to combined vasodilation.

Management Options:
- *Monitor.* Patients receiving both nifedipine and diltiazem should be monitored for increased nifedipine effects such as hypotension or headache and increased diltiazem effects including bradycardia.

References:
1. Kiowski W et al. Arterial vasodilator effects of the dihydropyridine calcium antagonist amlodipine alone and in combination with verapamil in systemic hypertension. Am J Cardiol. 1990;66:1469.
2. Ohashi K et al. The influence of pretreatment periods with diltiazem on nifedipine kinetics. J Clin Pharmacol. 1993;33:222.
3. Andreyev N et al. Comparison of diltiazem, nitrendipine, and their combination for systemic hypertension and stable angina pectoris. J Cardiovasc Pharmacol. 1991;18(Suppl. 9):S73.

### Diltiazem (Cardizem)

### Nitroprusside (Nipride)

Summary: Diltiazem administration reduces the dose of nitroprusside required to produce hypotension and may enhance nitroprusside-induced hypotension.

Risk Factors: No specific risk factors known.

Related Drugs: Other calcium channel blockers may produce similar interactions with nitroprusside.

Management Options:
- *Monitor.* Patients stabilized on diltiazem may require reduced doses of nitroprusside to produce a controlled hypotension. This interaction could be advantageous in that the reduced thiocyanate formation could decrease the risk of cyanide toxicity in patients who require long-term infusions. Additional data are needed to assess this interaction over longer administration times.

References:
1. Bernard J-M et al. Diltiazem reduces the nitroprusside doses for deliberate hypotension. Anesthesiology. 1992;77:A427. Abstract.

### Diltiazem (Cardizem)

### Propranolol (Inderal)

Summary: Diltiazem increases the plasma concentrations of propranolol and metoprolol. Although the interaction may be used to advantage, some predisposed patients may experience adverse effects.

Risk Factors: No specific risk factors known.

Related Drugs: Diltiazem had no effect on **atenolol (Tenormin)** serum concentrations. **Verapamil (Calan)** reduces the metabolism of several beta blockers, including **metoprolol (Lopressor)**.

Management Options:
- *Circumvent/Minimize.* The use of beta blockers that are not metabolized (e.g., atenolol) should minimize pharmacokinetic (but not pharmacodynamic) interactions with diltiazem.
- *Monitor.* Patients receiving therapy with beta blockers and diltiazem should be monitored for enhanced effects, particularly AV conduction slowing, resulting from pharmacokinetic or pharmacodynamic interactions.

References:
1. Dimmett DC et al. Pharmacokinetics of cardizem and propranolol when administered alone and in combination. Biopharm Drug Dispos. 1991;12:515.
2. Hunt BA et al. Effects of calcium channel blockers on the pharmacokinetics of propranolol stereoisomers. Clin Pharmacol Ther. 1990;47:584.
3. Tateishi T et al. The influence of diltiazem versus cimetidine on propranolol metabolism. J Clin Pharmacol. 1992;32:1099.

### Diltiazem (Cardizem)

### Rifampin (Rifadin)

Summary: Rifampin decreases diltiazem plasma concentrations; loss of therapeutic effect may result.

Risk Factors:
- *Route of Administration.* Administration of oral diltiazem will lead to a greater effect.

Related Drugs: Rifampin probably affects other calcium channel blockers in a similar manner.

Management Options:
- *Consider Alternative.* Because this interaction is likely to reduce the efficacy of diltiazem, one should consider an alternative to diltiazem. Other calcium channel blockers also may be affected. A therapeutic substitution to a different class of agent (noncalcium blocker) may be required.
- *Circumvent/Minimize.* Larger doses of calcium channel blocker (particularly those administered orally) may be required when rifampin is coadministered.
- *Monitor.* Patients taking calcium channel blockers should be monitored for a reduction in efficacy when rifampin is given.

References:
1. Drda KD et al. Effects of debrisoquine hydroxylation phenotype and enzyme induction with rifampin on diltiazem pharmacokinetics and pharmacodynamics. Pharmacotherapy. 1991;11:278.

### Disopyramide (Norpace)

### Erythromycin

Summary: In isolated case reports, erythromycin administration appeared to increase the serum disopyramide concentration, resulting in cardiac arrhythmias.

Risk Factors: No specific risk factors known.

Related Drugs: Other macrolides [e.g., **troleandomycin (TAO)**, **clarithromycin (Biaxin)**] may affect disopyramide similarly. **Azithromycin (Zithromax)** and **dirithromycin (Dynabac)** would be unlikely to inhibit disopyramide elimination.

Management Options:
- *Monitor.* Patients taking disopyramide should be monitored for the development of arrhythmias if erythromycin is added to their regimen.

References:
1. Ragosta M et al. Potentially fatal interaction between erythromycin and disopyramide. Am J Med. 1989;86:465.
2. Echizen H et al. A potent inhibitory effect of erythromycin and other macrolide antibiotics on the mono-N-dealkylation metabolism of disopyramide with human liver microsomes. J Pharmacol Exper Ther. 1993;264:1425.

### Disopyramide (Norpace)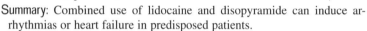

### Lidocaine (Xylocaine)

Summary: Combined use of lidocaine and disopyramide can induce arrhythmias or heart failure in predisposed patients.

Risk Factors: No specific risk factors known.

Related Drugs: No information available.

Management Options:
- *Monitor.* Patients receiving combined therapy with disopyramide and lidocaine should be monitored closely for arrhythmias and heart failure.

References:
1. Ellrodt G et al. Adverse effects of disopyramide (Norpace): toxic interactions with other antiarrhythmic agents. Heart Lung. 1980;9:469.

### Disopyramide (Norpace)

### Phenobarbital

Summary: Phenobarbital appears to reduce the serum concentrations of disopyramide, perhaps to subtherapeutic levels.

Risk Factors: No specific risk factors known.

Related Drugs: Other barbiturates probably have a similar effect on disopyramide, but little clinical evidence is available.

## Significance Classification

1 - **Avoid Combination.** Risk always outweighs benefit.

2 - **Usually Avoid Combination.** Use combination only under special circumstances.

3 - **Minimize Risk.** Take action as necessary to reduce risk.

Management Options:
  • *Monitor.* The changes in disopyramide clearance and half-life observed after phenobarbital administration could result in loss of arrhythmia control in some patients. Disopyramide serum concentrations should be monitored when phenobarbital is added to or removed from the drug regimen. Watch for dry mouth and urinary retention due to increased metabolite serum concentrations.

References:
  1. Kapil RP et al. Disopyramide pharmacokinetics and metabolism: effect of inducers. Br J Clin Pharmacol. 1987;24:781.

### Disopyramide (Norpace)

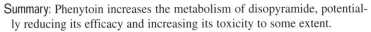

### Phenytoin (Dilantin)

Summary: Phenytoin increases the metabolism of disopyramide, potentially reducing its efficacy and increasing its toxicity to some extent.

Risk Factors: No specific risk factors known.

Related Drugs: No information available.

Management Options:
  • *Monitor.* Disopyramide serum concentrations and patient response (e.g., control of arrhythmia) should be monitored closely when phenytoin therapy is added to or removed from disopyramide therapy. Be alert for reduced antiarrhythmic efficacy and increased anticholinergic side effects such as dry mouth or urinary retention.

References:
  1. Kessler JM et al. Disopyramide and phenytoin interaction. Clin Pharm. 1982;1:263.
  2. Matos JA et al. Disopyramide-phenytoin interaction. Clin Res. 1981;29:655A.
  3. Nightingale J et al. Effect of phenytoin on serum disopyramide concentrations. Clin Pharm. 1987;6:46.

### Disopyramide (Norpace)

### Rifampin (Rifadin)

Summary: Rifampin can lower serum disopyramide concentrations to subtherapeutic levels; loss of efficacy may result.

Risk Factors: No specific risk factors known.

Related Drugs: No information available.

Management Options:
  • *Monitor.* Patients should be monitored for re-emergence of arrhythmias when rifampin is added to disopyramide and disopyramide toxicity if rifampin is discontinued. Serum disopyramide concentrations would be useful to monitor this interaction.

References:
  1. Aitio ML et al. The effect of enzyme induction on the metabolism of disopyramide in man. Br J Clin Pharmacol. 1981;11:279.
  2. Staum JM et al. Enzyme induction: rifampin-disopyramide interaction. DICP, Ann Pharmacother. 1990;24:701.

### Disulfiram (Antabuse)

### Ethanol (Ethyl Alcohol)

Summary: Disulfiram results in severe ethanol intolerance; patients must be warned to avoid all forms of ethanol.

Risk Factors: No specific risk factors known.

Related Drugs: No information available.

Management Options:

- *Avoid Combination*. Warn patients about ethanol in foods and pharmaceuticals, as well as beverages. Advise patients receiving disulfiram to avoid oral liquid pharmaceuticals unless they are known to be ethanol-free.

References:

1. Kitson TM. The disulfiram-ethanol reaction: a review. J Stud Alcohol. 1977;38:96.
2. Syed J et al. An unusual presentation of a disulfiram-alcohol reaction. Del Med J. 1995;67:183.
3. Johansson B et al. Dose-effect relationship of disulfiram in human volunteers. II. A study of the relation between the disulfiram-alcohol reaction and plasma concentrations of acetaldehyde, diethyldithiocarbamic acid methyl ester, and erythrocyte aldehyde dehydrogenase activity. Pharmacol Toxicol. 1991;68:166.

### Disulfiram (Antabuse)

### Isoniazid (INH)

Summary: The combined use of disulfiram and INH may result in adverse CNS effects.

Risk Factors: No specific risk factors known.

Related Drugs: No information available.

Management Options:

- *Avoid Unless Benefit Outweighs Risk*. Although evidence is somewhat limited, enough has been presented to warrant caution in the concomitant use of INH and disulfiram. It would be wise in most cases to avoid the use of disulfiram in patients receiving INH until more information is known about the interaction.
- *Monitor.* If combined use is necessary, monitor patients for adverse central nervous system effects (altered mood, behavioral changes, ataxia).

References:

1. Rothstein E. Rifampin with disulfiram. JAMA. 1972;219:1216. Letter.
2. Whittington HG et al. Possible interaction between disulfiram and isoniazid. Am J Psychiatry. 1969;125:1725.

### Disulfiram (Antabuse)

### Metronidazole (Flagyl)

Summary: The combined use of disulfiram and metronidazole may produce central nervous system toxicity.

Risk Factors: No specific risk factors known.

Related Drugs: No information available.

Management Options:

- *Consider Alternative.* Until the potential interaction between metronidazole and disulfiram is better described, it would be wise to avoid concomitant use of these drugs.
- *Monitor.* If the drugs are coadministered, watch for behavioral toxicity and confusion.

References:

1. Rothstein E et al. Toxicity of disulfiram combined with metronidazole. N Engl J Med. 1969;280:1006.
2. Goodhue WW Jr. Disulfiram-metronidazole (well identified) toxicity. N Engl J Med. 1969;280:1482.
3. Scher JM. Psychotic reaction to disulfiram. JAMA. 1967;201:1051. Letter.

## Disulfiram (Antabuse)

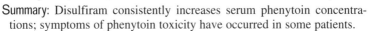

### Phenytoin (Dilantin)

Summary: Disulfiram consistently increases serum phenytoin concentrations; symptoms of phenytoin toxicity have occurred in some patients.

Risk Factors: No specific risk factors known.

Related Drugs: No information available.

Management Options:

- *Consider Alternative:* Consider using alternative treatment for alcohol abuse.
- *Circumvent/Minimize:* Reduction of the phenytoin dose may be necessary.
- *Monitor.* Patients receiving phenytoin and disulfiram should be monitored for evidence of phenytoin toxicity (e.g., ataxia, nystagmus, mental impairment). Serum phenytoin determinations are useful to detect an interaction between these drugs. Monitor patients for a reduced phenytoin response when disulfiram therapy is discontinued.

References:

1. Olesen OV. The influence of disulfiram and calcium carbamide on the serum diphenylhydantoin. Arch Neurol. 1967;16:642.
2. Svendsen TL et al. The influence of disulfiram on the half-life and metabolic clearance rate of diphenylhydantoin and tolbutamide in man. Eur J Clin Pharmacol. 1976;9:439.
3. Taylor JW et al. Mathematical analysis of a phenytoin-disulfiram interaction. Am J Hosp Pharm. 1981;38:93.

## Disulfiram (Antabuse)

### Theophylline

Summary: Disulfiram increases serum theophylline concentrations; the magnitude of the effect appears sufficient to produce theophylline toxicity in at least some patients.

Risk Factors: No specific risk factors known.

Related Drugs: No information available.

Management Options:
- *Monitor* for altered theophylline effect if disulfiram therapy is initiated, discontinued, or if the disulfiram dosage is changed. Patients receiving disulfiram therapy may require lower theophylline dosages.

References:
1. Loi CM et al. Dose-dependent inhibition of theophylline metabolism by disulfiram in recovering alcoholics. Clin Pharmacol Ther. 1989;45:476.

### Disulfiram (Antabuse)

### Tranylcypromine (Parnate)

**Summary:** A patient on disulfiram developed delirium following the addition of tranylcypromine, but a causal relationship was not established.

**Risk Factors:** No specific risk factors known.

**Related Drugs:** The effect of combining other nonselective monoamine oxidase inhibitors (MAOIs) with disulfiram is not established; assume that they may interact until proven otherwise.

Management Options:
- *Monitor.* Although data are limited, monitor for evidence of delirium if tranylcypromine or other nonselective MAOIs are used with disulfiram.

References:
1. Blansjaar BA et al. Delirium in a patient treated with disulfiram and tranylcypromine. Am J Psychiatry. 1995;152:296.

### Disulfiram (Antabuse)

### Warfarin (Coumadin)

**Summary:** Disulfiram increases the hypoprothrombinemic response to warfarin in most patients receiving both drugs concurrently.

**Risk Factors:** No specific risk factors known.

**Related Drugs:** Although little is known regarding the effect of disulfiram on oral anticoagulants other than warfarin, one should assume that they interact until evidence to the contrary is available.

Management Options:
- *Avoid Unless Benefit Outweighs Risk.* Concomitant use of disulfiram and oral anticoagulants should be avoided if possible. If oral anticoagulant therapy is begun in the patient receiving disulfiram, use conservative doses until the maintenance dose is established.

- *Monitor.* Patients receiving oral anticoagulants should be monitored for altered anticoagulant effect when disulfiram is started or stopped.

References:
1. O'Reilly RA. Dynamic interaction between disulfiram and separated enantiomorphs of racemic warfarin. Clin Pharmacol Ther. 1981;29:332.

2. Rothstein E. Warfarin effect enhanced by disulfiram (Antabuse). JAMA. 1972; 22:1052. Letter.
3. O'Reilly RA. Potentiation of anticoagulant effect by disulfiram. Clin Res. 1971; 19:180.

## Dopamine (Intropin)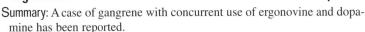

### Ergonovine

Summary: A case of gangrene with concurrent use of ergonovine and dopamine has been reported.

Risk Factors: No specific risk factors known.

Related Drugs: The effect of other combinations of ergot alkaloids and vasoconstricting sympathomimetics is unknown, but excessive vasoconstriction might occur.

Management Options:
- *Monitor.* The concurrent use of dopamine and ergot alkaloids such as ergonovine should be undertaken with caution; monitor for evidence of excessive vasoconstriction in the extremities (e.g., cold, pale skin, pain).

References:
1. Buchanan N et al. Symmetrical gangrene of the extremities associated with the use of dopamine subsequent to ergometrine administration. Intensive Care Med. 1977; 3:55.

## Dopamine (Intropin)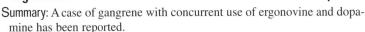

### Phenytoin (Dilantin)

Summary: Case reports and animal studies indicate that patients receiving dopamine may be more susceptible to hypotension following IV phenytoin.

Risk Factors: No specific risk factors known.

Related Drugs: No information available.

Management Options:
- *Monitor.* In patients receiving IV dopamine, IV phenytoin should be administered only with careful monitoring of the cardiovascular status.

References:
1. Bivins BA et al. Dopamine-phenytoin interaction. Arch Surg. 1978;113:245.

## Significance Classification

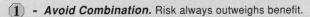 **1** - *Avoid Combination.* Risk always outweighs benefit.

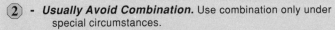 **2** - *Usually Avoid Combination.* Use combination only under special circumstances.

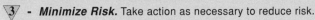 **3** - *Minimize Risk.* Take action as necessary to reduce risk.

### Doxazosin (Cardura)
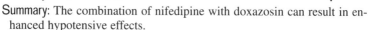

### Nifedipine (Procardia)

Summary: The combination of nifedipine with doxazosin can result in enhanced hypotensive effects.

Risk Factors: No specific risk factors known.

Related Drugs: Other calcium channel blockers may have additive hypotensive effects when administered with doxazosin or other alpha blockers.

Management Options:
- *Monitor.* The combination of nifedipine and doxazosin appears to produce an increased antihypertensive effect. Patients stabilized on one of these drugs should be monitored for hypotension during the institution of the second drug.

References:
1. Donnelly R et al. The pharmacodynamics and pharmacokinetics of the combination of nifedipine and doxazosin. Eur J Clin Pharmacol. 1993;44:279.

### Doxepin (Sinequan)
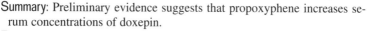

### Propoxyphene (Darvocet-N)

Summary: Preliminary evidence suggests that propoxyphene increases serum concentrations of doxepin.

Risk Factors: No specific risk factors known.

Related Drugs: It is not known whether tricyclic antidepressants other than doxepin would be affected by propoxyphene, but it certainly seems possible. Propoxyphene impairs the hepatic metabolism of ***carbamazepine (Tegretol)***.

Management Options:
- *Monitor* for altered doxepin effect if propoxyphene is initiated, discontinued, or changed in dosage; adjust doxepin dose as needed.

References:
1. Abernethy DR et al. Impairment of hepatic drug oxidation by propoxyphene. Ann Intern Med. 1982;97:223.

### Doxepin (Sinequan)

### Tolazamide (Tolinase)

Summary: Doxepin may enhance the hypoglycemic effects of tolazamide or insulin.

Risk Factors: No specific risk factors known.

Related Drugs: A patient who had been maintained on ***chlorpropamide (Diabinese)*** 250 mg/day was found to have a blood glucose of 50 mg/dL four days after the initiation of ***nortriptyline (Pamelor)***. Chlorpropamide was discontinued, and the patient remained normoglycemic. Nortriptyline has been reported to increase insulin sensitivity and lower blood glucose.[1] In other case reports, patients with diabetes developed hypoglycemia following the addition of *amitriptyline (Elavil)*,[2] *imipramine (Tofranil)*,[3] and *maprotiline (Ludiomil)*.[4]

Management Options:

- *Monitor.* Pending prospective evaluation of this interaction, diabetic patients should monitor their blood glucose daily when cyclic antidepressants are initiated or discontinued.

References:

1. Grof E et al. Effects of lithium, nortriptyline and dexamethasone on insulin sensitivity. Prog Neuropsychopharmacol Biol Psychiatry. 1984;8:687.
2. Sherman KE et al. Amitriptyline and asymptomatic hypoglycemia. Ann Intern Med. 1988;109:683.
3. Shrivastava RK et al. Hypoglycemia associated with imipramine. Biol Psychiatry. 1983;18:1509.
4. Zogno MG et al. Hypoglycemia caused by maprotiline in a patient taking oral antidiabetics. Ann Pharmacother. 1994;28:406. Letter.

## Doxorubicin (Adriamycin)

## Verapamil (Calan)

Summary: Verapamil appears to increase doxorubicin serum concentrations.

Risk Factors: No specific risk factors known.

Related Drugs: The effect of calcium channel blockers other than verapamil on doxorubicin is not established.

Management Options:

- *Monitor* for altered doxorubicin effect if verapamil is initiated, discontinued, or changed in dosage; adjust doxorubicin dose as needed.

References:

1. Kerr DJ et al. The effect of verapamil on the pharmacokinetics of Adriamycin. Cancer Chemother Pharmacol. 1986;18:239.

## Doxycycline (Vibramycin)

## Phenobarbital

Summary: Doxycycline serum concentrations may be reduced by the administration of phenobarbital.

Risk Factors: No specific risk factors known.

Related Drugs: Other barbiturates may affect doxycycline in a similar manner. Theoretically, other tetracyclines should not be affected by barbiturates like phenobarbital.

Management Options:

- *Consider Alternative.* Tetracyclines other than doxycycline, theoretically, should not be affected by barbiturates, since hepatic metabolism is not an important route of elimination.

- *Monitor.* If barbiturates cannot be avoided in patients receiving doxycycline, the clinical response to doxycycline should be monitored closely.

References:

1. Neuvonen PJ et al. Interaction between doxycycline and barbiturates. Br Med J. 1974;1:535.

### Doxycycline (Vibramycin)

### Phenytoin (Dilantin)

Summary: Phenytoin reduces doxycycline serum concentrations, but other tetracyclines do not appear to be affected.

Risk Factors: No specific risk factors known.

Related Drugs: **Chlortetracycline (Aureomycin), demeclocycline (Declomycin), methacycline**, and **oxytetracycline (Terramycin)** do not appear to be affected by phenytoin administration. Theoretically, tetracycline also should be unaffected by phenytoin.

Management Options:

- *Consider Alternative.* If possible, use a tetracycline other than doxycycline in patients receiving phenytoin. (See Related Drugs.)
- *Monitor.* If doxycycline is used with phenytoin, watch for reduced doxycycline efficacy and consider using larger doses of doxycycline.

References:

1. Penttila O et al. Interaction between doxycycline and some antiepileptic drugs. Br Med J. 1974;2:470.
2. Neuvonen PJ et al. Interaction between doxycycline and barbiturates. Br Med J. 1974;1:535.
3. Neuvonen PJ et al. Effect of antiepileptic drugs on the elimination of various tetracycline derivatives. Eur J Clin Pharmacol. 1975;9:147.

### Doxycycline (Vibramycin)

### Warfarin (Coumadin)

Summary: Although doxycycline theoretically may increase the hypoprothrombinemic response to oral anticoagulants like warfarin, clinical evidence is limited.

## Significance Classification

 - *Avoid Combination.* Risk always outweighs benefit.

 - *Usually Avoid Combination.* Use combination only under special circumstances.

 - *Minimize Risk.* Take action as necessary to reduce risk.

Risk Factors:
- *Concurrent Diseases.* The hypoprothrombinemic response to doxycycline may be larger in patients with deficient vitamin K intake.

Related Drugs: Other tetracyclines may produce similar effects on oral anticoagulants.

Management Options:
- *Monitor.* Although the clinical evidence for an interaction between doxycycline and oral anticoagulants is limited, monitor patients for an enhanced anticoagulant effect when these drugs are used concurrently.

References:
1. Westfall LK et al. Potentiation of warfarin by tetracycline. Am J Hosp Pharm. 1980;37:1620.
2. Messinger WJ et al. The effect of bowel sterilizing antibiotic on blood coagulation mechanism. Angiology. 1965;16:29.
3. Caraco Y et al. Enhanced anticoagulant effect of coumarin derivatives induced by doxycycline coadministration. Ann Pharmacother. 1992;26:1084.

## Dyphylline (Lufyllin)

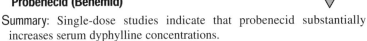

## Probenecid (Benemid)

Summary: Single-dose studies indicate that probenecid substantially increases serum dyphylline concentrations.

Risk Factors: No specific risk factors known.

Related Drugs: Unlike dyphylline, theophylline does not appear to interact with probenecid.[2] (Also see Allopurinol/Theophylline; consult index for page number.)

Management Options:
- *Consider Alternative.* Theophylline does not appear to interact with probenecid and may be a suitable alternative.
- *Monitor* for evidence of altered dyphylline effect if probenecid therapy is initiated, discontinued, or changed in dosage.

References:
1. May DC et al. Effect of probenecid on dyphylline elimination. Clin Pharmacol Ther. 1983;33:822.
2. Chen TWD et al. Effect of probenecid on the pharmacokinetics of aminophylline. Drug Intell Clin Pharm. 1983;17:465.

## Echothiophate Iodide (Phosphate Iodide)

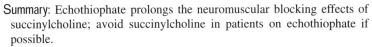

## Succinylcholine (Anectine)

Summary: Echothiophate prolongs the neuromuscular blocking effects of succinylcholine; avoid succinylcholine in patients on echothiophate if possible.

Risk Factors: No specific risk factors known.

Related Drugs: No information available.

Management Options:
- *Avoid Unless Benefit Outweighs Risk.* A neuromuscular blocker other than succinylcholine is preferred in most patients on echothiophate.
- *Monitor.* If succinylcholine is used, monitor carefully for prolonged neuromuscular blockade. Serum pseudocholinesterase determinations would be useful to determine which patients are at highest risk.

References:
1. Kinyon GE. Anticholinesterase eye drops—need for caution. N Engl J Med. 1969;280:53.
2. Lipson ML et al. Oral administration of pralidoxime chloride in echothiophate iodide therapy. Arch Ophthalmol. 1969;82:830.
3. Cohen PJ et al. A simple test for abnormal pseudocholinesterase. Anesthesiology. 1970;32:281.

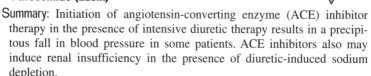

## Enalapril (Vasotec)

## Furosemide (Lasix)

Summary: Initiation of angiotensin-converting enzyme (ACE) inhibitor therapy in the presence of intensive diuretic therapy results in a precipitous fall in blood pressure in some patients. ACE inhibitors also may induce renal insufficiency in the presence of diuretic-induced sodium depletion.

Risk Factors:
- *Dosage Regimen.* Hypovolemia due to diuretic therapy may predispose hypotensive reactions or acute renal failure.[1,2,4]
- *Concurrent Diseases.* Very high pre-existing blood pressure, secondary hypertension, high circulating levels of renin and angiotensin II, and congestive heart failure (CHF) may increase the risk of acute hypotensive episodes.[3,4,6]

Related Drugs: Other loop diuretics such as **bumetanide (Bumex)**, **torsemide (Demadex)**, and **ethacrynic acid (Edecrin)** probably interact with ACE inhibitors such as enalapril in the same way as furosemide. It is likely that all ACE inhibitors interact in a similar way with diuretics.

Management Options:
- *Circumvent/Minimize.* Some have recommended that congestive heart failure patients on furosemide should be kept supine for 3 hours after the first dose of ACE inhibitors; this especially refers to the elderly.[5]
- *Monitor.* Initiation of therapy with ACE inhibitors should be undertaken cautiously in patients receiving diuretics, especially if there is evidence of hypovolemia. Monitor blood pressure carefully for at least 3 hours after the ACE inhibitor is given. In some patients it may be desirable to withdraw the diuretic temporarily before starting the ACE inhibitor.

References:
1. Atkinson AB et al. Captopril in a hyponatremic hypertensive: need for caution in initiating therapy. Lancet. 1979;1:557.

2. Vlasses PH et al. Captopril: clinical pharmacology and benefit-to-risk ratio in hypertension and congestive heart failure. Pharmacotherapy. 1982;2:1.
3. Hodsman GP et al. Factors related to first dose hypotensive effect of captopril: prediction and treatment. Br Med J. 1983;286:832.
4. Mandal AK et al. Diuretics potentiate angiotensin converting enzyme inhibitor-induced acute renal failure. Clin Nephrol. 1994;42:170.
5. Mets T et al. First-dose hypotension, ACE inhibitors, and heart failure in the elderly. Lancet. 1992;339:1487. Letter.
6. MacFayden RJ. The response to the first dose of an ACE inhibitor in essential hypertension: a placebo controlled study utilizing ambulatory blood pressure recording. Br J Clin Pharmacol. 1991;31:568P. Abstract.

## Enalapril (Vasotec)

### Iron

Summary: Three patients on enalapril developed systemic reactions (gastrointestinal symptoms, hypotension) following intravenous iron; more study is needed to establish a causal relationship.

Risk Factors:
- *Route of Administration.* Intravenous administration of iron appears more likely to interact than oral.

Related Drugs: Oral iron has not been associated with these reactions in patients receiving other ACE inhibitors.

Management Options:
- *Consider Alternative.* Although this potential interaction is not well established, given the severity of the reactions it would be prudent to consider alternatives to either the intravenous iron or the ACE inhibitor.
- *Monitor.* If intravenous iron is given to a patient on an ACE inhibitor, monitor for systemic reactions and be prepared to treat anaphylaxis.

References:
1. Rolla G et al. Systemic reactions to intravenous iron therapy in patients receiving angiotension-converting enzyme inhibitor. J Allergy Clin Immunol. 1994;93:1074.

## Encainide (Enkaid)

### Quinidine

Summary: Quinidine can substantially increase encainide serum concentrations in patients who are extensive (rapid) encainide metabolizers. However, because of the opposing effects of quinidine on the serum concentrations of encainide and its active metabolites, the clinical outcome is likely to be limited.

Risk Factors:
- *Pharmacogenetics.* Rapid encainide metabolizers are at greater risk.

Related Drugs: No information available.

Management Options:
- *Monitor.* Patients maintained on encainide should be monitored for changes in antiarrhythmic efficacy when quinidine is added or deleted.

References:
1. Funck-Brentano C et al. Effect of low dose quinidine on encainide pharmacokinetics and pharmacodynamics. Influence of genetic polymorphism. J Pharmacol Exp Ther. 1989;249:134.
2. Turgeon J et al. Genetically determined steady-state interaction between encainide and quinidine in patients with arrhythmias. J Pharmacol Exp Ther. 1990;255:642.
3. Turgeon J et al. Genetically determined stereoselective excretion of encainide in humans and electrophysiologic effects of its enantiomers in canine cardiac purkinje fibers. Clin Pharmacol Ther. 1991;49:488.

### Enoxacin (Penetrex)
### Ranitidine (Zantac)

Summary: Ranitidine administration reduces the plasma concentrations of enoxacin; failure of antibiotic efficacy could result.

Risk Factors: No specific risk factors known.

Related Drugs: While cimetidine (Tagamet) is known to increase enoxacin concentrations, the effects to other $H_2$-receptor antagonist [e.g., *famotidine (Pepcid)*, *nizatidine (Axid)*] or proton pump inhibitors [e.g., *lansoprazole (Prevacid)*, *omeprazole (Prilosec)*] on orally administered enoxacin are unknown. However, they all would be expected to have effects similar to those of ranitidine. The effect of ranitidine on other quinolones is unknown.

Management Options:
- *Consider Alternative.* Separation of the doses of ranitidine and oral enoxacin will probably have little effect on this interaction since the pH tends to stay somewhat elevated during therapy with $H_2$-receptor antagonists or omeprazole. The administration of IV enoxacin or an alternative antibiotic may be necessary in patients requiring gastric acid suppression.
- *Monitor.* Patients receiving enoxacin and drugs that alkalinize the gut should be observed for loss of antibiotic efficacy.

References:
1. Lebsack ME et al. Effect of gastric acidity on enoxacin absorption. Clin Pharmacol Ther. 1992;52:252.
2. Grasela TH et al. Inhibition of enoxacin absorption by antacids or ranitidine. Antimicrob Agents Chemother. 1989;33:615.

### Enoxacin (Penetrex)
### Tacrine (Cognex)

Summary: *In vitro* studies suggest that enoxacin is a potent inhibitor of tacrine metabolism. Given the major effect that enoxacin has on theophylline metabolism [which is metabolized by the same enzyme (CYP1A2) as tacrine], it seems likely that enoxacin has a similar effect on tacrine.

Risk Factors: No specific risk factors known.

Related Drugs: One might expect the various quinolones to affect tacrine metabolism in a manner similar to their effects on theophylline. If that proves to be true, enoxacin would have a marked effect on tacrine metabolism, *ciprofloxacin (Cipro)* a moderate effect, and *norfloxacin (Noroxin)* a small effect. Theoretically, quinolones such as *lomefloxacin (Maxquin)* and *ofloxacin (Floxin)* would be less likely to interact with tacrine.

Management Options:
- *Consider Alternative.* Consider using a quinolone which is less likely to interact (e.g., lomefoxacin, ofloxacin).
- *Monitor.* If quinolones and tacrine are used together, monitor for tacrine toxicity (e.g., nausea, vomiting, anorexia, diarrhea, abdominal pain). However, some evidence suggests that tacrine hepatotoxicity results from reactive tacrine metabolites.[1] Thus, if quinolones are found to inhibit tacrine metabolism clinically, the effect actually might be expected to *reduce* the risk of hepatotoxicity.

References:
1. Madden S et al. An investigation into the formation of stable, protein-reactive and cytotoxic metabolites from tacrine *in vitro*. Studies with human and rat liver microsomes. Biochem Pharmacol. 1993;46:13.

### Enoxacin (Penetrex)

### Theophylline

Summary: Enoxacin markedly increases the serum concentrations of theophylline and may result in the development of theophylline toxicity.

Risk Factors:
- *Dosage Regimen.* Higher doses of enoxacin produce a greater risk.

Related Drugs: Quinolones reported to inhibit the metabolism of drugs include *ciprofloxacin (Cipro)*, enoxacin (Penetrex), *norfloxacin (Noroxin)*, *pipemidic acid*, and *pefloxacin*. Quinolones reported to produce no or minor changes in theophylline pharmacokinetics include *fleroxacin*, *flosequinan*, *lomefloxacin (Maxquin)*, *ofloxacin (Floxin)*, *rufloxacin*, *sparfloxacin*, and *temafloxacin*.

Management Options:
- *Use Alternative.* Enoxacin should not be administered with theophylline. Use a quinolone known to have no or minor effect on theophylline pharmacokinetics (e.g., fleroxacin, flosequinan, lomefloxacin, ofloxacin, rufloxacin, sparfloxacin, temafloxacin).

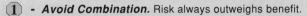

## Significance Classification

(1) - *Avoid Combination.* Risk always outweighs benefit.

(2) - *Usually Avoid Combination.* Use combination only under special circumstances.

 - *Minimize Risk.* Take action as necessary to reduce risk.

References:

1. Koup JR et al. Theophylline dosage adjustment during enoxacin coadministration. Anitmicrob Agents Chemother. 1990;34:803.
2. Rogge MC et al. The theophylline-enoxacin interaction: I. Effect of enoxacin dose size on theophylline disposition. Clin Pharmacol Ther. 1988;44:579.
3. Sarkar M et al. *In vitro* effect of fluoroquinolones of theophylline metabolism in human liver microsomes. Antimicrob Agents Chemother. 1990;34:594.

## Enprostil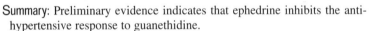

### Ethanol (Ethyl Alcohol)

Summary: Enprostil appears to increase instead of decrease the gastric mucosal damage produced by ethanol.

Risk Factors: No specific risk factors known.

Related Drugs: The effect of ethanol combined with prostaglandins other than enprostil is not established.

Management Options:

- *Circumvent/Minimize.* Until more information is available, it would be prudent for patients taking enprostil (and possibly other prostaglandins) to minimize their alcohol intake.

- *Monitor* for evidence of gastrointestinal intolerance if the combination is used.

References:

1. Cohen MM et al. Human antral damage induced by alcohol is potentiated by enprostil. Gastroenterology. 1990;99:45.

## Ephedrine

### Guanethidine (Ismelin)

Summary: Preliminary evidence indicates that ephedrine inhibits the antihypertensive response to guanethidine.

Risk Factors: No specific risk factors known.

Related Drugs: Theoretically, one would expect **guanadrel**, a drug pharmacologically similar to guanethidine, to be similarly affected by ephedrine.

Management Options:

- *Monitor.* If ephedrine must be used in a patient receiving guanethidine, the patient should be watched closely for rising blood pressure. If the guanethidine dosage is increased to compensate for this effect, watch for hypotension when ephedrine is discontinued.

References:

1. Starr KJ et al. Drug interactions in patients on long-term oral anticoagulant and antihypertensive adrenergic neuron-blocking drugs. Br Med J. 1972;4:133.
2. Day MD et al. Antagonism of guanethidine and bretylium by various agents. Lancet. 1962;2:1282. Letter.
3. Gulati OD et al. Antagonism of adrenergic neuron blockade in hypertensive subjects. Clin Pharmacol Ther. 1966;7:510.

## Ephedrine

## Moclobemide

Summary: Moclobemide substantially enhances the pressor response to ephedrine, and increases the risk of palpitations, headache, and lightheadedness.

Risk Factors: No specific risk factors known.

Related Drugs: Theoretically, the pressor response to other sympathomimetics with significant indirect activity (e.g., ***phenylpropanolamine, pseudoephedrine***) also would be increased in patients receiving moclobemide.

Management Options:

- *Use Alternative.* Based upon available data, ephedrine should be avoided in patients receiving moclobemide. Until safety data are available, one also should avoid other indirect acting sympathomimetics (e.g., phenylpropanolamine, pseudoephedrine) with agents that inhibit MAO-A.

References:

1. Dingemanse J. An update of recent moclobemide interaction data. Int Clin Psychopharmacol. 1993;7:167.

## Epinephrine (Adrenalin)

## Imipramine (Tofranil)

Summary: The pressor response to IV epinephrine may be markedly enhanced in patients receiving tricyclic antidepressants (TCAs) like imipramine.

Risk Factors: No specific risk factors known.

Related Drugs: ***Protriptyline (Vivactil)*** affects epinephrine similarly. Little is known about the use of epinephrine with other TCAs; assume they interact until proved otherwise.

Management Options:

- *Avoid Unless Benefit Outweighs Risk.* Patients receiving TCAs should be given IV epinephrine only with close monitoring of blood pressure. Some caution should also be exercised if the epinephrine is administered by other routes. When epinephrine is used to prevent or treat anaphylaxis, however, consider the real possibility that the benefit of giving epinephrine will outweigh the risks in such patients.

- *Monitor.* If IV epinephrine is given to patients receiving TCAs, monitor blood pressure carefully and adjust epinephrine dose as needed.

References:

1. Boakes AJ et al. Interactions between sympathomimetic amines and antidepressant agents in man. Br Med J. 1973;1:311.

2. Svedmyr N. The influence of a tricyclic antidepressant agent (protriptyline) on some of the circulatory effects of noradrenaline and adrenaline in man. Life Sci. 1968;7:77.

3. Boakes AJ. Sympathomimetic amines and antidepressant agents. Br Med J. 1973; 2:114. Letter.

## Epinephrine (Adrenalin)

## Propranolol (Inderal)

**Summary:** Noncardioselective beta blockers enhance the pressor response to epinephrine, resulting in hypertension and bradycardia.

**Risk Factors:** No specific risk factors known.

**Related Drugs:** Other nonspecific beta blockers [e.g., *alprenolol*, *nadolol (Corgard)*, *pindolol (Visken)*, *timolol (Blocadren)*] would produce a similar effect. *Labetalol (Normodyne)* (which is a nonspecific beta blocker as well as an $\alpha_1$-blocker) increases the diastolic pressure and slows the heart rate during epinephrine infusions,[4] but acute hypertensive reactions appear unlikely.[5] *Metoprolol (Lopressor)* (and perhaps other cardioselective beta blockers) has minimal effects on the pressor response to epinephrine even at doses of 200 to 300 mg/day.[1–3]

**Management Options:**

- *Consider Alternative.* Selective beta$_1$-blockers (e.g., metoprolol) may be less likely than propranolol to result in hypertension and bradycardia when epinephrine is administered or when endogenous epinephrine is released.

- *Monitor.* In patients receiving propranolol or other non-selective beta blockers, epinephrine should be administered with caution, and blood pressure should be monitored carefully. If the epinephrine is used to treat anaphylaxis, the response to epinephrine may be poor, and vigorous supportive care (e.g., volume replacement) may be needed.

**References:**

1. Houben H et al. Effect of low-dose epinephrine infusion on hemodynamics after selective and nonselective beta blockade in hypertension. Clin Pharmacol Ther. 1982;31:685.

## Significance Classification

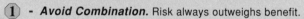 **1** - *Avoid Combination.* Risk always outweighs benefit.

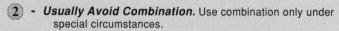 **2** - *Usually Avoid Combination.* Use combination only under special circumstances.

**3** - *Minimize Risk.* Take action as necessary to reduce risk.

2. Houben H et al. Influence of selective and nonselective beta-adrenoreceptor blockade on the haemodynamic effect of adrenaline during combined antihypertensive drug therapy. Clin Sci. 1979;57:397S.
3. Van Herwaarden CLA et al. Haemodynamic effects of adrenaline during treatment of hypertensive patients with propranolol and metoprolol. Eur J Clin Pharmacol. 1977;12:397.
4. Richards DA et al. Circulatory effects of noradrenaline and adrenaline before and after labetalol. Br J Clin Pharmacol. 1979;7:371.
5. Doshi BS et al. Effects of labetalol and propranolol on responses to adrenaline infusion in healthy volunteers. Int J Clin Pharmacol Res. 1984;4:29.

## Ergotamine (Ergostat)

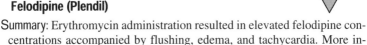

### Nitroglycerin

Summary: Ergotamine may oppose the coronary vasodilation of nitrates.

Risk Factors: No specific risk factors known.

Related Drugs: No information available.

Management Options:

- *Avoid Unless Benefit Outweighs Risk.* Patients receiving nitroglycerin for angina pectoris should avoid ergotamine if at all possible.

- *Monitor.* If the combination is used, patients should be monitored for enhanced ergotamine effect, the ergot dosage lowered as needed.

References:
1. Bobik A et al. Low oral bioavailability of dihydroergotamine and first-pass extraction in patients with orthostatic hypotension. Clin Pharmacol Ther. 1981;30:673.

## Erythromycin

### Felodipine (Plendil)

Summary: Erythromycin administration resulted in elevated felodipine concentrations accompanied by flushing, edema, and tachycardia. More information is needed to establish a causal relationship.

Risk Factors: No specific risk factors known.

Related Drugs: **Troleandomycin (TAO)** also may inhibit the metabolism of calcium channel blockers. Since other calcium channel blockers are metabolized similarly to felodipine, erythromycin also may affect their metabolism.

Management Options:

- *Monitor.* Until further information is available, patients taking felodipine, and perhaps other calcium channel blockers, should be observed for adverse effects (hypotension, headache, arrythmias) during the concomitant administration of erythromycin.

References:
1. Liedholm H et al. Erythromycin-felodipine interaction. DICP Ann Pharmacother. 1991;25:1007.

## Erythromycin

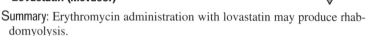

### Lovastatin (Mevacor)

Summary: Erythromycin administration with lovastatin may produce rhabdomyolysis.

Risk Factors: No specific risk factors known.

Related Drugs: Other macrolides [e.g., *troleandomycin (TAO)*, *clarithromycin (Biaxin)*] could affect lovastatin in a similar manner. *Azithromycin (Zithromax)* and *dirithromycin (Dynabac)* would not likely inhibit the metabolism of lovastatin.

Management Options:
- *Monitor.* Until further information is available, patients maintained on lovastatin should be watched for symptoms of rhabdomyolysis (e.g., muscle pain and myoglobinuria) when erythromycin is administered concurrently.

References:
1. Ayanian JZ et al. Lovastatin and rhabdomyolysis. Ann Intern Med. 1988;109:682. Letter.
2. East C et al. Rhabdomyolysis in patients receiving lovastatin after cardiac transplantation. N Engl J Med. 1988;318:47.

## Erythromycin

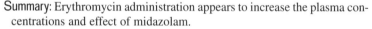

### Midazolam (Versed)

Summary: Erythromycin administration appears to increase the plasma concentrations and effect of midazolam.

Risk Factors:
- *Route of Administration.* Oral midazolam is much more affected than parenteral.

Related Drugs: Three days erythromycin administration reduced the clearance of *triazolam (Halcion)* by 52%.[1] Triazolam is metabolized by the same cytochrome P450 isozyme as midazolam.[3] *Troleandomycin (TAO)* and *clarithromycin (Biaxin)* also may inhibit the metabolism of midazolam and triazolam. Other benzodiazepines also may be affected by erythromycin, clarithromycin or TAO. *Azithromycin (Zithromax)* and *dirithromycin (Dynabac)* would be less likely to affect midazolam metabolism.

Management Options:
- *Monitor.* Until further information is available, patients taking erythromycin should be monitored for increased response (sedation, drowsiness) to midazolam and triazolam.

References:
1. Philips JP et al. A pharmacokinetic drug interaction between erythromycin and triazolam. J Clin Psychopharmacol. 1986;6:297.
2. Olkkola KT et al. A potentially hazardous interaction between erythromycin and midazolam. Clin Pharmacol Ther. 1993;53:298.
3. Kronbach T et al. Oxidation of midazolam and triazolam by human liver cytochrome P450IIIA4. Mol Pharmacol. 1989;36:89.

## Erythromycin

### Quinidine

**Summary:** Erythromycin increased quinidine concentrations; cardiac arrhythmias could result.

**Risk Factors:**
- *Concurrent Diseases.* Patients with pre-existing cardiac disease are at greater risk.

**Related Drugs:** Other macrolides that inhibit CYP3A4 [e.g., *troleandomycin (TAO)*, *clarithromycin (Biaxin)*] also may inhibit quinidine metabolism. *Azithromycin (Zithromax)* and *dirithromycin (Dynabac)* are unlikely to affect quinidine concentrations.

**Management Options:**
- *Consider Alternative.* The use of azithromycin or a non-macrolide antibiotic would likely avoid the interaction with quinidine.
- *Monitor.* If quinidine and erythromycin are coadministered, monitor for signs of quinidine cardiac toxicity (prolonged QRS and QT intervals).

**References:**
1. Spinler SA et al. Possible inhibition of hepatic metabolism of quinidine by erythromycin. Clin Pharmacol Ther. 1995;57:89.

## Erythromycin

### Ritonavir (Norvir)

**Summary:** Ritonavir may inhibit erythromycin metabolism; erythromycin may inhibit ritonavir metabolism. The clinical significance of this potential interaction is unknown.

**Risk Factors:** No specific risk factors known.

**Related Drugs:** *Clarithromycin (Biaxin)* serum concentrations are increased by ritonavir and clarithromycin produces a small increase in ritonavir concentrations.[1] Other protease inhibitors such as *indinavir (Crixivan)*, *saquinavir (Invirase)*, and *nelfinavir (Viracept)* may affect erythromycin in a similar manner. Since *azithromycin (Zithromax)* is not metabolized and is not a CYP3A4 inhibitor, ritonavir would not be expected to interact with azithromycin. Ritonavir concentrations are increased by clarithromycin, and *troleandomycin (TAO)* would be expected to have a similar effect. *Dirithromycin (Dynabac)* would not be expected to have much effect on ritonavir although it could reduce ritonavir concentrations. The effect of ritonavir on dirithromycin concentrations is unknown.

**Management Options:**
- *Consider Alternative.* Azithromycin would probably be a noninteracting alternative to erythromycin for patients receiving ritonavir.
- *Monitor* for evidence of erythromycin or ritonavir toxicity when the two drugs are coadministered.

**References:**
1. Abbott Laboratories. Ritonavir (Norvir) package insert. 1996.

### Erythromycin

### Tacrolimus (Prograf)

Summary: Patients receiving tacrolimus developed increased concentrations and nephrotoxicity following coadministration with erythromycin.

Risk Factors: No specific risk factors known.

Related Drugs: Erythromycin also is known to inhibit **cyclosporine (Sandimmune)** metabolism. The effects of other macrolides on tacrolimus concentration are unknown, but **troleandomycin (TAO)** and **clarithromycin (Biaxin)** might produce similar changes in tacrolimus. While no data is available, **azithromycin (Zithromax)** would appear to be less likely to interact with tacrolimus.

Management Options:
- *Monitor.* Pending further investigation of this interaction, patients should have their tacrolimus and creatinine serum concentrations monitored if they are concurrently administered erythromycin.

References:
1. Shaeffer MS et al. Interaction between FK506 and erythromycin. Ann Pharmacother. 1994;28:280. Letter.
2. Jensen C et al. Interaction between tacrolimus and erythromycin. Lancet. 1994; 344:825.
3. Furlan V et al. Interactions between FK506 and rifampicin or erythromycin in pediatric liver recipients. Transplantation. 1995;59:1217.

### Erythromycin

### Terfenadine (Seldane)

Summary: Erythromycin administration may cause cardiac arrythmias in patients taking terfenadine.

Risk Factors: No specific risk factors known.

Related Drugs: The manufacturer of terfenadine has received case reports of an interaction between **troleandomycin (TAO)** and terfenadine that resulted in cardiac arrhythmias.

Management Options:
- *Avoid Combination.* Patients taking terfenadine should avoid concomitant use of erythromycin or troleandomycin. Until further data are available, careful observation is warranted during the administration of terfenadine and other macrolides. Loratadine (Claritin) or citirazine (Zyrtec) may be acceptable alternatives for terfenadine.

References:
1. Biglin KE et al. Drug-induced torsades de pointes: a possible interaction of terfenadine and erythromycin. Ann Pharmacother. 1994;28:282. Letter.
2. Eller M et al. Effect of erythromycin on terfenadine metabolite pharmacokinetics. Clin Pharmacol Ther. 1993;53:161. Abstract.
3. Honig PK et al. Comparison of the effect of the macrolide antibiotics erythromycin, clarithromycin and azithromycin on terfenadine steady-state pharmacokinetics and electrocardiographic parameters. Drug Invest. 1994;7:148.

## Erythromycin

### Theophylline

Summary: Erythromycin can increase theophylline serum concentrations and may produce toxicity; theophylline can reduce the concentration of erythromycin.

Risk Factors: No specific risk factors known.

Related Drugs: *Troleandomycin (TAO)* and *clarithromycin (Biaxin)* also may inhibit the metabolism of theophylline.

Management Options:
- *Consider Alternative.* Azithromycin (Zithromax) does not appear to alter theophylline concentrations.
- *Monitor.* Patients should be closely monitored when erythromycin therapy is initiated. Although some clinicians suggest lowering the dose of theophylline by 25% when erythromycin is initiated, this precaution may excessively complicate the management of low-risk patients (i.e., those likely to have a low serum theophylline concentration). Be aware that a reduction in erythromycin serum concentration by theophylline may also be observed.

References:
1. Pasic J et al. The interaction between chronic oral slow-release theophylline and single-dose intravenous erythromycin. Xenobiotica. 1987;17:493.
2. Paulsen O et al. The interaction of erythromycin with theophylline. Eur J Clin Pharmacol. 1987;32:493.
3. Paulsen O et al. The interaction of erythromycin with theophylline. Eur J Clin Pharmacol. 1987;32:493.

## Erythromycin

### Triazolam (Halcion)

Summary: Erythromycin causes considerable increases in triazolam plasma concentrations.

Risk Factors: No specific risk factors known.

Related Drugs: *Troleandomycin (TAO)* and *clarithromycin (Biaxin)* also may inhibit the metabolism of triazolam; theoretically, *azithromycin (Zithromax)* would be unlikely to interact. Other benzodiazepines that undergo oxidative metabolism are likely to be affected similarly.

## Significance Classification

① - *Avoid Combination.* Risk always outweighs benefit.

② - *Usually Avoid Combination.* Use combination only under special circumstances.

③ - *Minimize Risk.* Take action as necessary to reduce risk.

Management Options:
> • *Monitor.* Patients receiving triazolam who are prescribed erythromycin should be observed carefully for enhanced triazolam effects. Several days may be required for the maximum effect of erythromycin to become evident, and triazolam dosages may require adjustment after addition of the antibiotic and again when it is discontinued.

References:
1. Philips JP et al. A pharmacokinetic drug interaction between erythromycin and triazolam. J Clin Psychopharmacol. 1986;6:297.

## Erythromycin

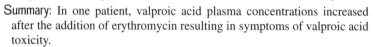

### Valproic Acid (Depakene)

Summary: In one patient, valproic acid plasma concentrations increased after the addition of erythromycin resulting in symptoms of valproic acid toxicity.

Risk Factors: No specific risk factors known.

Related Drugs: *Troleandomycin (TAO)* and *clarithromycin (Biaxin)* also may inhibit the metabolism of valproic acid.

Management Options:
> • *Monitor.* Patients should be monitored for altered responses to valproic acid when erythromycin is initiated, discontinued, or changed in dosage.

References:
1. Redington K. Erythromycin and valproate interaction. Ann Intern Med. 1992; 116:877.

## Erythromycin

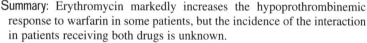

### Warfarin (Coumadin)

Summary: Erythromycin markedly increases the hypoprothrombinemic response to warfarin in some patients, but the incidence of the interaction in patients receiving both drugs is unknown.

Risk Factors:
> • *Concurrent Diseases.* Fever may enhance the catabolism of clotting factors.
> • *Diet/Food.* A diet low in vitamin K may contribute to the risk of this interaction.

Related Drugs: Little is known regarding the effect of erythromycin on oral anticoagulants other than warfarin. A study in 6 healthy subjects found no effect of *ponsinomycin* on the pharmacokinetics of a single dose of acenocoumarol. *Troleandomycin (TAO)* or *clarithromycin (Biaxin)* may alter warfarin elimination, but specific information is not available.

Management Options:
> • *Consider Alternative.* Early evidence suggests that azithromycin (Zithromax) is not likely to be an enzyme inhibitor, and the manu-

facturer states that it did not affect the hypoprothrombinemic response to a single dose of warfarin.

- *Monitor.* Be alert for evidence of an increased response to oral anticoagulants when erythromycin therapy is initiated and the converse when erythromycin is discontinued. The anticoagulant dose may need to be adjusted.

References:
1. Grau E et al. Erythromycin-oral anticoagulant interaction. Arch Intern Med. 1986; 146:1639.
2. Weibert RT et al. Effect of erythromycin in patients receiving long-term warfarin therapy. Clin Pharmacol Ther. 1987;41:224.
3. Couet W et al. Lack of effect of ponsinomycin on the pharmacokinetics of nicoumalone enantiomers. Br J Clin Pharmacol. 1990;30:616.

### Erythromycin

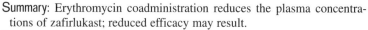

### Zafirlukast (Accolate)

Summary: Erythromycin coadministration reduces the plasma concentrations of zafirlukast; reduced efficacy may result.

Risk Factors: No specific risk factors known.

Related Drugs: The effect of other macrolides on zafirlukast is unknown.

Management Options:
- *Monitor.* Be alert for reduced zafirlukast efficacy when it is administered with erythromycin.

References:
1. Zeneca Pharmaceuticals. Zafirlukast (Accolate) package insert. 1997.

### Ethacrynic Acid (Edecrin)

### Gentamicin (Garamycin)

Summary: The risk of ototoxicity increases when ethacrynic acid and aminoglycosides are coadministered.

Risk Factors:
- *Concurrent Diseases.* Impaired renal function increases the risk of interaction.

Related Drugs: **Furosemide (Lasix)**, **torsemide (Demadex)**, or **bumetanide (Bumex)** are less likely to produce an increase in nephrotoxicity when used with an aminoglycoside. Other aminoglycosides, such as **kanamycin (Kantrex)**, **neomycin**, and **streptomycin**, are likely to produce ototoxicity with ethacrynic acid.

Management Options:
- *Use Alternative.* Select an alternative diuretic such as furosemide, torsemide, or bumetanide which are less likely to produce increased nephrotoxicity when coadministered with an aminoglycoside.

References:
1. Mathog RH et al. Ototoxicity of ethacrynic acid and aminoglycoside antibiotics in uremia. N Engl J Med. 1969;280:1223.

2. Pillay VKG et al. Transient and permanent deafness following treatment with ethacrynic acid in renal failure. Lancet. 1969;1:77.
3. Meriwether WD et al. Deafness following standard intravenous dose of ethacrynic acid. JAMA. 1971;216:795.

## Ethanol (Ethyl Alcohol)

### Furazolidone (Furoxone)

Summary: A disulfiram-like reaction may occur when patients taking furazolidone ingest alcohol.

Risk Factors: No specific risk factors known.

Related Drugs: No information available.

Management Options:
- *Monitor.* Patients on furazolidone should be warned that a disulfiram-like reaction (e.g., flushing, nausea, sweating) may occur following ethanol ingestion.

References:
1. Todd RG, ed. Extra Pharmacopoeia-Martindale. 25th ed. London: The Pharmaceutical Press; 1967:844–45.
2. Kolodny AL. Side-effects produced by alcohol in a patient receiving furazolidone. Maryland State Med J. 1962;11:248.
3. Calesnick B. Antihypertensive action of the antimicrobial agent furazolidone. Am J Med Sci. 1958;236:736.

## Ethanol (Ethyl Alcohol)

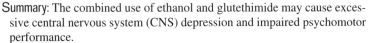

### Glutethimide

Summary: The combined use of ethanol and glutethimide may cause excessive central nervous system (CNS) depression and impaired psychomotor performance.

Risk Factors: No specific risk factors known.

Related Drugs: Alcohol would be expected to increase the CNS depression of all sedative-hypnotic drugs.

Management Options:
- *Circumvent/Minimize.* Patients on glutethimide should limit their intake of ethanol to avoid excessive CNS depression.
- *Monitor* for excessive CNS depression if the combination is used.

References:
1. Mould GP et al. Interaction of glutethimide and phenobarbitone with ethanol in man. J Pharm Pharmacol. 1972;24:894.

## Ethanol (Ethyl Alcohol)

### Isoniazid (INH)

Summary: Alcoholics have a higher incidence of INH-induced hepatitis.

Risk Factors:
- *Dosage Regimen.* Daily alcohol consumption can increase the risk of interaction.

Related Drugs: No information available.
Management Options:
- *Circumvent/Minimize.* Avoiding the combination of alcohol and INH would be prudent, but since alcoholism and tuberculosis often co-exist, it may not be possible in some cases.
- *Monitor.* Alcoholic patients should be monitored carefully for INH hepatitis if they are administered isoniazid.

References:
1. Physicians' Desk Reference. 50th ed. Oradell: Medical Economics Data; 1996: 1530.

### Ethanol (Ethyl Alcohol)

### Ketoconazole (Nizoral)

Summary: Ethanol consumption during ketoconazole therapy may result in a disulfiram-like reaction.
Risk Factors: No specific risk factors known.
Related Drugs: No information available.
Management Options:
- *Circumvent/Minimize.* Advise patients taking ketoconazole to minimize their alcohol intake.
- *Monitor.* Patients taking ketoconazole should be counseled that ethanol consumption might cause flushing, nausea, and headache and should avoid ethanol while taking ketoconazole.

References:
1. Magnasco AJ et al. Interaction of ketoconazole and ethanol. Clin Pharm. 1986; 5:522.

### Ethanol (Ethyl Alcohol)

### Meperidine (Demerol)

Summary: Ethanol and narcotic analgesics are likely to exhibit additive central nervous system (CNS) depressant effects. Ethanol also may affect the distribution of meperidine, but the clinical importance of this effect is not established.
Risk Factors: No specific risk factors known.

## Significance Classification

 - *Avoid Combination.* Risk always outweighs benefit.

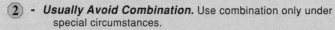 - *Usually Avoid Combination.* Use combination only under special circumstances.

 - *Minimize Risk.* Take action as necessary to reduce risk.

Related Drugs: Ethanol also would be expected to add to the CNS depressant effects of narcotic analgesics other than meperidine.

Management Options:

- *Circumvent/Minimize.* Patients taking narcotic analgesics should limit their use of alcohol, especially if performing tasks requiring alertness.

- *Monitor* for excessive CNS depression in patients receiving the combination.

References:

1. Linnoila M et al. Effects of diazepam and codeine, alone and in combination with alcohol, on simulated driving. Clin Pharmacol Ther. 1974;15:368.
2. Mather LE et al. Meperidine kinetics in man. Intravenous injection in surgical patients and volunteers. Clin Pharmacol Ther. 1975;17:21.

### Ethanol (Ethyl Alcohol)

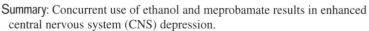

### Meprobamate (Equanil)

Summary: Concurrent use of ethanol and meprobamate results in enhanced central nervous system (CNS) depression.

Risk Factors: No specific risk factors known.

Related Drugs: Alcohol would be expected to increase the CNS depression of all sedative-hypnotics.

Management Options:

- *Circumvent/Minimize.* Patients should be made aware that the combined use of ethanol and meprobamate can cause excessive CNS depression. Patients on meprobamate should avoid ingesting moderate to large amounts of ethanol.

- *Monitor* for excessive CNS depression in patients receiving the combination.

References:

1. Ashford JR et al. Drug interactions. The effects of alcohol and meprobamate applied singly and jointly in human subjects. III. J Stud Alcohol.1975;7(Suppl.): 140.
2. Cobby JM et al. Drug interactions. The effect of alcohol and meprobamate applied singly and jointly in human subjects. IV. J Stud Alcohol. 1975;7(Suppl.):162.
3. Ashford JR et al. Drug interactions. The effects of alcohol and meprobamate applied singly and jointly in human subjects. V. J Stud Alcohol. 1975;7(Suppl.): 177.

### Ethanol (Ethyl Alcohol)

### Methotrexate (Mexate)

Summary: Some evidence indicates that ethanol may increase the likelihood of methotrexate-induced liver injury, but a causal relationship has not been established.

Risk Factors: No specific risk factors known.

Related Drugs: No information available.

Management Options:
- *Avoid Combination.* Some feel strongly that ethanol should be avoided by patients receiving methotrexate,[1] and the manufacturer of methotrexate also recommends the avoidance of ethanol.[3] Even though the evidence for additive hepatotoxic effects is not conclusive, alcohol restriction probably is appropriate for most patients receiving methotrexate.

References:
1. Pai SH et al. Severe liver damage caused by treatment of psoriasis with methotrexate. NY State J Med. 1973;73:2585.
2. Methotrexate. Product Information. Wayne, NJ: Lederle Laboratories; 1988.
3. Glassner J. Methotrexate and psoriasis. JAMA. 1970;210:1925. Letter.

## Ethanol (Ethyl Alcohol)

## Metoclopramide (Reglan)

Summary: Metoclopramide may enhance the sedative effects of ethanol, but the clinical importance of this effect is not established.

Risk Factors: No specific risk factors known.

Related Drugs: No information available.

Management Options:
- *Circumvent/Minimize.* Until more is known about this purported interaction, patients taking metoclopramide should be advised that alcohol may have a greater than expected effect.
- *Monitor* for excessive central nervous system depression in patients receiving the combination.

References:
1. Bateman DN et al. Pharmacokinetic and concentration-effect studies with intravenous metoclopramide. Br J Clin Pharmacol. 1978;6:401.
2. Gibbons DO et al. Effects of intravenous and oral propantheline and metoclopramide on ethanol absorption. Clin Pharmacol Ther. 1975;17:578.

## Ethanol (Ethyl Alcohol)

## Metronidazole (Flagyl)

Summary: Alcohol ingestion during metronidazole therapy may lead to a disulfiram-like reaction in some patients.

Risk Factors: No specific risk factors known.

Related Drugs: The coadministration of metronidazole and other IV drugs containing ethanol [e.g., **phenytoin (Dilantin), trimethoprim-sulfamethoxazole (Bactrim), phenobarbital, diazepam (Valium)**, and **nitroglycerin**] may result in flushing and vomiting.

Management Options:
- *Circumvent/Minimize.* Patients receiving metronidazole should be warned about the possibility of reactions following ethanol ingestion and avoid ethanol or ethanol-containing drugs.

• *Monitor.* If ethanol is taken by a patient receiving metronidazole, watch for flushing, nausea, and vomiting.

References:
1. Edwards DL et al. Disulfiram-like reaction associated with intravenous trimethoprim-sulfamethoxazole and metronidazole. Clin Pharm. 1986;5:999.

## Ethanol (Ethyl Alcohol)

### Phenelzine (Nardil)

Summary: Alcoholic beverages containing tyramine may induce a severe hypertensive response in patients taking nonselective monoamine oxidase inhibitors (MAOIs).

Risk Factors: No specific risk factors known.

Related Drugs: All nonselective MAOIs including *isocarboxazid* and *tranylcypromine (Parnate)* interact with tyramine-containing alcoholic beverages.

Management Options:
• *Avoid Combination.* Since it is difficult to assess the tyramine content of a given drink (especially drinks with many ingredients), patients receiving MAOIs probably should be advised to avoid all alcoholic beverages. If alcohol is ingested, the patient should use products that are unlikely to contain significant amounts of tyramine (e.g., vodka, white wine) and ingest small amounts initially.[3] Remember that the effects of nonselective monoamine oxidase inhibitors should be assumed to persist for 2 weeks after they are discontinued.

References:
1. Ellis J et al. Modification by monoamine oxidase inhibitors of the effect of some sympathomimetics on blood pressure. Br Med J. 1967;2:75.
2. MacLeod I. Fatal reaction to phenelzine. Br Med J. 1965;1:1554.
3. Shulman KI et al. Dietary restriction, tyramine, and the use of monoamine oxidase inhibitors. J Clin Psychopharmacol. 1989;9:397.

## Ethanol (Ethyl Alcohol)

### Phenobarbital

Summary: Ethanol and barbiturates like phenobarbital have additive depressant effects on the central nervous system (CNS); combined use is dangerous in patients performing tasks requiring alertness and may be fatal in overdose.

Risk Factors: No specific risk factors known.

Related Drugs: All barbiturates are likely to result in additive CNS depressant effects with ethanol. Acute ethanol intoxication appears to inhibit *pentobarbital* metabolism.

Management Options:
• *Circumvent/Minimize.* Patients receiving barbiturates should be warned that the combined use of ethanol can lead to excessive CNS depression.

- *Monitor* for excessive CNS depression in patients receiving the combination.

References:
1. Lieber CS. Hepatic and metabolic effects of alcohol (1966 to 1973). Gastroenterology. 1973;65:821.
2. Mezey E et al. Effects of phenobarbital administration on rates of ethanol clearance and on ethanol-oxidizing enzymes in man. Gastroenterology. 1974;66:248.
3. Stead AH et al. Quantification of the interaction between barbiturates and alcohol and interpretation of fatal blood concentrations. Hum Toxicol. 1983;2:5.

## Ethanol (Ethyl Alcohol)
## Phenytoin (Dilantin)

Summary: Chronic ethanol abuse may reduce serum phenytoin concentrations, but the clinical importance of this effect is not established.
Risk Factors: No specific risk factors known.
Related Drugs: No information available.
Management Options:
- *Monitor.* Epileptic patients receiving phenytoin who also drink heavily should be monitored for a decreased anticonvulsant effect.

References:
1. Kater RMH et al. Increased rate of clearance of drugs from the circulation of alcoholics. Am J Med Sci. 1969;258:35.
2. Finer MJ. Diphenylhydantoin in alcohol withdrawal. JAMA. 1971;217:211. Letter.

## Ethanol (Ethyl Alcohol)
## Procarbazine (Matulane)

Summary: Ingestion of ethanol by patients receiving procarbazine may result in a disulfiram-like reaction: flushing, headache, nausea, and hypotension.
Risk Factors: No specific risk factors known.
Related Drugs: No information available.
Management Options:
- *Avoid Combination.* Advise patients receiving procarbazine to avoid alcohol.

References:
1. Vasiliou V et al. The mechanism of alcohol intolerance produced by various therapeutic agents. Acta Pharmacol et Toxicol. 1986;58:305.

## Significance Classification

1 - *Avoid Combination.* Risk always outweighs benefit.
2 - *Usually Avoid Combination.* Use combination only under special circumstances.
3 - *Minimize Risk.* Take action as necessary to reduce risk.

2. Math G et al. Methyl-hydrazine in treatment of Hodgkin's disease and various forms of haematosarcoma and leukaemia. Lancet. 1963;2:1077.

3. Todd IDH. Natulan in management of late Hodgkin's disease, other lymphoreticular neoplasms, and malignant melanoma. Br Med J. 1965;628.

## Ethanol (Ethyl Alcohol)

### Propoxyphene (Darvocet-N)

**Summary:** Overdoses of propoxyphene combined with ethanol have been associated with fatal reactions, but there is little evidence of danger when alcohol is combined with therapeutic doses of propoxyphene.

**Risk Factors:**
- *Dosage Regimen.* The danger of this interaction occurs primarily when large amounts of alcohol are ingested.

**Related Drugs:** No information available.

**Management Options:**
- *Circumvent/Minimize.* It does not appear that patients taking propoxyphene need to abstain from alcohol, but they certainly should be warned to avoid acute alcohol intoxication.
- *Monitor* for excessive central nervous system depression in patients receiving the combination.

**References:**
1. Girre C et al. Enhancement of propoxyphene bioavailability by ethanol: relation to psychomotor and cognitive function in healthy volunteers. Eur J Clin Pharmacol. 1991;41:147.
2. Sellers EM et al. Pharmacokinetic interaction of propoxyphene with ethanol. Br J Clin Pharmacol. 1985;19:398.
3. Finkle BS et al. A national assessment of propoxyphene in post-mortem medicolegal investigation 1972–1975. J Forensic Sci. 1976;21:706.

## Ethanol (Ethyl Alcohol)

### Tolbutamide (Orinase)

**Summary:** Excessive ethanol intake may lead to altered glycemic control, most commonly hypoglycemia. An "Antabuse"-like reaction may occur in patients taking sulfonylureas.

**Risk Factors:** No specific risk factors known.

**Related Drugs:** Excessive ethanol produce hypoglycemia in patients taking insulin or other oral hypoglycemic agents. Two patients receiving chlorpropamide for diabetes insipidus developed polyuria and polydipsia following ethanol intake, presumably due to ethanol inhibition of chlorpropamide-induced antidiuresis.[3] Ethanol ingestion may contribute to lactic acidosis in patients receiving phenformin.[1,2]

**Management Options:**
- *Avoid Combination.* Since an "Antabuse reaction" may occur following ethanol ingestion in patients receiving sulfonylureas, patients should be informed of this possibility when therapy is initiated. Ingestion of moderate-to-large amounts of ethanol probably

should be avoided by patients on antidiabetics because of the possible adverse effects of alcohol on diabetic control.

References:

1. Johnson HK et al. Relationship of alcohol and hyperlactatemia in diabetic subjects treated with phenformin. Am J Med. 1968;45:98.
2. Kreisberg RA et al. Hyperlacticacidemia in man: ethanol-phenformin synergism. J Clin Endocrinol. 1972;34:29.
3. Yamamoto LT. Diabetes insipidus and drinking alcohol. N Engl J Med. 1976;294:55. Letter.

## Ethanol (Ethyl Alcohol)

## Verapamil (Calan)

**Summary:** Consumption of ethanol following the chronic administration of verapamil results in increased ethanol concentrations with the possibility of prolonged and increased levels of intoxication.

**Risk Factors:** No specific risk factors known.

**Related Drugs:** Ethanol was reported to increase the hypotensive response of a 5 mg dose of *felodipine (Plendil)* in 10 hypertensive patients.[1] The ethanol was administered in double-strength grapefruit juice which has been demonstrated to increase felodipine concentrations.[2] Therefore, it is uncertain whether ethanol affects felodipine or if the changes were due to an interaction between grapefruit juice and felodipine. Ethanol administration resulted in a 53% increase in *nifedipine (Procardia)* area under the concentration-time curve in healthy subjects; nifedipine-induced blood pressure changes were not affected by ethanol.[3]

**Management Options:**

- *Avoid Unless Benefit Outweighs Risk.* Ethanol intake should be avoided or reduced while taking verapamil. Verapamil may enhance the psychomotor effects of ethanol.

- *Monitor.* Patients taking verapamil should be cautioned regarding the consumption of ethanol. Serum ethanol concentrations may be higher than normally experienced when the patient is not taking verapamil.

References:

1. Bailey DG et al. Ethanol enhances the hemodynamic effect of felodipine. Clin Invest Med. 1989;12:357.
2. Bailey DG et al. Interaction of citrus juices with felodipine and nifedipine. Lancet. 1991;337:268.
3. Qureshi S et al. Effect of an acute dose of alcohol on the pharmacokinetics of oral nifedipine in humans. Pharm Res. 1992;9:683.

## Ethanol (Ethyl Alcohol)

## Warfarin (Coumadin)

**Summary:** Enhanced hypoprothrombinemic response to oral anticoagulants has been reported following acute ethanol intoxication.

Risk Factors:
- *Dosage Regimen.* Enhanced anticoagulant effect appears to occur primarily with acute alcohol intoxication; small amounts of ethanol (e.g., 2 drinks per day or less) seem to have little effect in most patients.

Related Drugs: Until we have evidence to the contrary, expect all oral anticoagulants to be affected by alcohol intoxication. In another study, 80 gm of ethanol did not affect the hypoprothrombinemic response in healthy subjects maintained on **phenprocoumon**.[1] Additional study in patients with coronary disease indicated a slight increase in hypoprothrombinemic response to phenprocoumon in some patients following administration of moderate amounts of ethanol.

Management Options:
- *Circumvent/Minimize.* Patients on oral anticoagulants should avoid large amounts of ethanol, but two or three drinks/day or less are unlikely to affect warfarin response.
- *Monitor* for altered hypoprothrombinemic response if patient takes >3 drinks/day or if alcohol intake changes considerably.

References:
1. Waris E. Effect of ethyl alcohol on some coagulation factors in man during anticoagulant therapy. Ann Med Exp Biol Fenn. 1963;41:45.
2. O'Reilly RA. Lack of effect of mealtime wine on the hypoprothrombinemia of oral anticoagulants. Am J Med Sci. 1979;277:189.
3. O'Reilly RA. Lack of effect of fortified wine ingested during fasting and anticoagulant therapy. Arch Intern Med. 1981;141:458.

---

**Etodolac (Lodine)**

**Warfarin (Coumadin)**

**2**

Summary: Preliminary data suggest that etodolac does not affect the hypoprothrombinemic response to warfarin, but cotherapy requires caution because of possible detrimental effects of etodolac on the gastric mucosa and platelet function.

Risk Factors:
- *Concurrent Diseases.* Patients with peptic ulcer disease (PUD) or a history of gastrointestinal (GI) bleeding probably are at greater risk.

Related Drugs: All NSAIDs inhibit platelet function, cause gastric erosions, and probably increase the risk of GI bleeding.

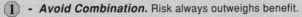

## Significance Classification

(1) - **Avoid Combination.** Risk always outweighs benefit.

(2) - **Usually Avoid Combination.** Use combination only under special circumstances.

(3) - **Minimize Risk.** Take action as necessary to reduce risk.

Management Options:

- *Avoid Unless Benefit Outweighs Risk.* Since all NSAIDs probably increase the risk of GI bleeding in patients on oral anticoagulants, use the combination only after careful consideration of the benefit versus risk. If the NSAID is being used as an analgesic or antipyretic, acetaminophen (Tylenol) probably is safer to use with oral anticoagulants. Nonacetylated salicylates (e.g., choline salicylate, magnesium salicylate, salsalate, sodium salicylate) probably also are safer with oral anticoagulants than NSAIDs since they have minimal effects on platelet function and the gastric mucosa.
- *Monitor.* If any NSAID is used with an oral anticoagulant, one should carefully monitor the prothrombin time and watch for evidence of bleeding, especially from the GI tract.

References:

1. Ermer JC et al. Concomitant etodolac affects neither the unbound clearance nor the pharmacologic effect of warfarin. Clin Pharmacol Ther. 1994;55:305.
2. Shorr RI et al. Concurrent use of nonsteroidal anti-inflammatory drugs and oral anticoagulants places elderly persons at high risk for hemorrhagic peptic ulcer disease. Arch Intern Med. 1993;153:1665.

## Etretinate (Tegison)

## Methotrexate (Mexate)

Summary: Concurrent use of etretinate with methotrexate may be associated with an increased incidence of hepatotoxicity.

Risk Factors: No specific risk factors known.

Related Drugs: No information available.

Management Options:

- *Avoid Unless Benefit Outweighs Risk.* Until adequate trials of methotrexate and etretinate have been conducted to determine the true nature of this interaction, this combination should be reserved for patients with severe, refractory disease.
- *Monitor.* Patients should be warned to notify their physician if icterus, dark urine, light-colored stools, or flu-like symptoms occur.

References:

1. Larsen FG et al. Interaction of etretinate with methotrexate pharmacokinetics in psoriatic patients. J Clin Pharmacol. 1990;30:802.
2. Zachariae H. Methotrexate and etretinate as concurrent therapies in the treatment of psoriasis. Arch Dermatol. 1984;120:155.
3. Beck HI et al. Toxic hepatitis due to combination therapy with methotrexate and etretinate in psoriasis. Dermatologica. 1983;167:94.

## Felbamate (Felbatol)

## Phenobarbital

Summary: Felbamate increases phenobarbital concentrations and may result in toxicity.

Risk Factors: No specific risk factors known.

Related Drugs: No information available.

Management Options:
- *Consider Alternative.* Given the serious toxicity that has been reported with felbamate, it is reserved for carefully selected patients. Thus, alternatives to felbamate should be used if possible, whether or not the patient is on interacting drugs.
- *Circumvent/Minimize.* Since patients may manifest an increase in serum phenobarbital concentrations when felbamate therapy is added, consider reducing the phenobarbital dose by 20% to 25% when felbamate is added. Conversely, an increase in phenobarbital dosage may be required if felbamate is discontinued. It is not clear whether an alteration in felbamate dosage is needed when phenobarbital therapy is initiated or discontinued.
- *Monitor* symptoms of phenobarbital toxicity for at least 1 month after felbamate is added.

References:
1. Gidal B et al. Potential pharmacokinetic interaction between felbamate and phenobarbital. Ann Pharmacother. 1994;28:455.
2. Reidenberg P et al. Effects of felbamate on the pharmacokinetics of phenobarbital. Clin Pharmacol Ther. 1995;58:279.

## Felbamate (Felbatol)

## Phenytoin (Dilantin)

**Summary:** Felbamate consistently increases serum phenytoin concentrations; phenytoin toxicity may occur in some patients. Phenytoin appears to decrease serum felbamate concentrations, but the clinical importance of this effect is not established.

**Risk Factors:** No specific risk factors known.

**Related Drugs:** No information available.

**Management Options:**
- *Consider Alternative.* Given the serious toxicity that has been reported with felbamate, it is reserved for carefully selected patients. Thus, alternatives to felbamate should be used if possible, whether or not the patient is on interacting drugs.
- *Circumvent/Minimize.* Since almost all patients appear to manifest an increase in serum phenytoin concentrations when felbamate therapy is added, consider reducing the phenytoin dose by 25% when felbamate is added. Conversely, an increase in phenytoin dosage may be required if felbamate is discontinued. It is not clear whether an alteration in felbamate dosage is needed when phenytoin therapy is initiated or discontinued.
- *Monitor.* When the 2 agents are used together, monitor for symptoms of phenytoin toxicity.

References:
1. Graves NM et al. Effects of felbamate on phenytoin and carbamazepine serum concentrations. Epilepsia. 1989;30:488.

2. Fuerst RH et al. Felbamate increases phenytoin and decreases carbamazepine concentrations. Epilepsia. 1988;29:488.
3. Wagner ML et al. Discontinuation of phenytoin and carbamazepine in patients receiving felbamate. Epilepsia. 1991;32:398.

## Felbamate (Felbatol)

## Valproic Acid (Depakene)

Summary: Preliminary evidence suggests that felbamate consistently increases serum valproic acid concentrations, but the magnitude of the effect varies from patient to patient.

Risk Factors: No specific risk factors known.

Related Drugs: No information available.

Management Options:

- *Consider Alternative.* Given the serious toxicity that has been reported with felbamate, it is reserved for carefully selected patients. Thus, alternatives to felbamate should be used if possible, whether or not the patient is on interacting drugs.

- *Circumvent/Minimize.* In patients stabilized on valproic acid, titrating felbamate slowly may reduce the risk of adverse effects. If felbamate is rapidly added to valproic acid, it may be necessary to reduce valproic acid doses. Also be aware that *discontinuing* felbamate may affect valproic acid requirements.

- *Monitor* for symptoms of valproic toxicity such as tremor, confusion, irritability, and restlessness.

References:
1. Wagner ML et al. The effect of felbamate on valproic acid disposition. Clin Pharmacol Ther. 1994;56:494.

## Felodipine (Plendil)

## Itraconazole (Sporanox)

Summary: Itraconazole increases felodipine concentrations and enhances its vasodilatory effects; excessive hypotensive response could result.

Risk Factors: No specific risk factors known.

Related Drugs: The bioavailability and metabolism of other calcium channel blockers that undergo CYP3A4 metabolism are likely to be affected by itraconazole. Other azole antifungal agents such as **ketoconazole (Nizoral)**, **miconazole (Monistat)**, and **fluconazole (Diflucan)** would also be expected to reduce the metabolism of felodipine. **Terbinafine (Lamisil)** may be less likely to affect felodipine clearance.

Management Options:

- *Consider Alternative.* Although there are no specific data, terbinafine may be less likely to affect felodipine clearance. Since most calcium channel blockers will likely be affected to some extent, the use of a non-calcium blocker may be appropriate during treatment with an azole antifungal agent.

- *Circumvent/Minimize.* A reduction in the dose of felodipine may be necessary to avoid excessive pharmacologic effects.
- *Monitor.* Patients receiving the combination of itraconazole and felodipine should be carefully monitored for excessive hypotension.

References:
1. Jalava K-M et al. Itraconazole greatly increases plasma concentrations and effects of felodipine. Clin Pharmacol Ther. 1997;61:410.

### Fenfluramine (Pondimin)

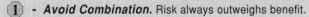

### Fluoxetine (Prozac)

Summary: Cotherapy with fenfluramine and selective serotonin reuptake inhibitors (SSRIs) such as fluoxetine theoretically could result in serotonin syndrome.

Risk Factors: No specific factors known.

Related Drugs: **Dexfenfluramine (Redux)** also should be avoided in combination with other SSRIs such as **paroxetine (Paxil)**, **sertraline (Zoloft)**, and **fluvoxamine (Luvox)**.

Management Options:
- *Avoid Unless Benefit Outweighs Risk.* Patients should avoid the use of SSRIs with either fenfluramine or dexfenfluramine, unless the combinations are found to be safe in well controlled clinical trials. There is also a medicolegal risk in using the combinations, since the manufacturer's information states that cotherapy should be avoided.
- *Monitor.* If the combination is used, be alert for evidence of serotonin syndrome, which can result in neurotoxicity (myoclonus, tremors, rigidity, incoordination, restlessness, hyperreflexia, seizures, coma); psychiatric symptoms (agitation, confusion, hypomania); and temperature regulation abnormalities (fever, sweating).

References:
1. Gross AS et al. The influence of the sparteine/debrisoquine genetic polymorphism on the disposition of dexfenfluramine. Br J Clin Pharmacol. 1996;41:311.
2. Redux Manufacturer's Product Information. Wyeth-Ayerst Laboratories, 1996.

## Significance Classification

① - **Avoid Combination.** Risk always outweighs benefit.

② - **Usually Avoid Combination.** Use combination only under special circumstances.

③ - **Minimize Risk.** Take action as necessary to reduce risk.

### Fenfluramine (Pondimin)

### Phenelzine (Nardil)

Summary: Cotherapy with fenfluramine and nonselective monamine oxidase inhibitors (MAOIs) such as phenelzine theoretically could result in serotonin syndrome.

Risk Factors: No specific factors known.

Related Drugs: Fenfluramine also is contraindicated with other nonselective MAOIs such as *tranylcypromine (Parnate)* and *isocarboxazid (Marplan)*. Given that *selegiline (Eldepryl)* also can act as a nonselective MAOI (especially if given in large doses), it also might interact adversely with fenfluramine. Dexfenfluramine is the S-enantiomer of the racemate fenfluramine, so the two drugs probably interact in a similar way with nonselective MAOIs.

Management Options:
- *Avoid Combination.* Patients should avoid any combination of a nonselective MAO inhibitor with either fenfluramine or dexfenfluramine.

References:
1. Gross AS et al. The influence of the sparteine/debrisoquine genetic polymorphism on the disposition of dexfenfluramine. Br J Clin Pharmacol. 1996;41:311.
2. Pondimin Manufacturer's Product Information. A. H. Robins Company, 1996.

### Fenoprofen (Nalfon)

### Warfarin (Coumadin)

Summary: Although little is known regarding the effect of fenoprofen on the hypoprothrombinemic response to oral anticoagulants, cotherapy requires caution because of possible detrimental effects of fenoprofen on the gastric mucosa and platelet function.

Risk Factors:
- *Concurrent Diseases.* Patients with peptic ulcer disease (PUD) or a history of gastrointestinal (GI) bleeding probably are at greater risk.

Related Drugs: All NSAIDs inhibit platelet function, cause gastric erosions, and probably increase the risk of GI bleeding. Some NSAIDs, however, such as *ibuprofen (Advil)*, *naproxen (Anaprox)*, or *diclofenac (Voltaren)* may be less likely to increase oral anticoagulant-induced hypoprothrombinemia than other NSAIDs.

Management Options:
- *Avoid Unless Benefit Outweighs Risk.* Since all NSAIDs probably increase the risk of GI bleeding in patients on oral anticoagulants, use the combination only after careful consideration of the benefit versus risk. If an NSAID must be used with an oral anticoagulant, it would be prudent to use NSAIDs that are unlikely to affect the hypoprothrombinemic response to oral anticoagulants. If the NSAID is being used as an analgesic or antipyretic, acetaminophen probably is safer to use with oral anticoagulants. Nonacetylated sa-

licylates (e.g., choline salicylate, magnesium salicylate, salsalate, sodium salicylate) probably also are safer with oral anticoagulants than NSAIDs, since such salicylates have minimal effects on platelet function and the gastric mucosa.

- *Monitor.* If any NSAID is used with an oral anticoagulant, one should carefully monitor the prothrombin time and watch for evidence of bleeding, especially from the GI tract.

References:
1. Rubin A et al. Physiological disposition of fenoprofen in man. J Pharmacol Exp Ther. 1972;183:449.
2. Shorr RI et al. Concurrent use of nonsteroidal anti-inflammatory drugs and oral anticoagulants places elderly persons at high risk for hemorrhagic peptic ulcer disease. Arch Intern Med. 1993;153:1665.

### Flecainide (Tambocor)

### Propranolol (Inderal)

Summary: Flecainide increases the serum concentration of propranolol; propranolol increases the concentration of flecainide. Concomitant administration of these drugs produces additive negative inotropic effects.

Risk Factors: No specific risk factors known.

Related Drugs: It is probable that other beta blockers also will exert additive negative inotropic effects with flecainide, but little is known regarding pharmacokinetic interaction between flecainide and other beta blockers.

Management Options:
- *Monitor.* Patients taking both propranolol and flecainide should be monitored for increased effects of both drugs and additive negative inotropic effects on the heart.

References:
1. Holtzman JL et al. The pharmacodynamic and pharmacokinetic interaction of flecainide acetate with propranolol: effects on cardiac function and drug clearance. Eur J Clin Pharmacol. 1987;33:97.

### Flecainide (Tambocor)
### Sotalol (Betapace)

Summary: A case report notes sinus bradycardia, atrioventricular (AV) block, and cardiac arrest following a switch from flecainide to sotalol therapy for ventricular arrhythmia, but a causal relationship was not established.

Risk Factors: No specific risk factors known.

Related Drugs: *Propranolol (Inderal)* and other beta blockers may cause similar reactions with flecainide.

Management Options:
- *Circumvent/Minimize.* It may be prudent to avoid the administration of sotalol for several days to patients previously receiving drugs that depress myocardial conduction.

- *Monitor.* Until further information is available, patients receiving sotalol and flecainide should be monitored carefully for reduced myocardial conduction (bradycardia).

References:
1. Warren R et al. Serious interactions of sotalol with amiodarone and flecainide. Med J Aust. 1990;152:227. Letter.

## Fluconazole (Diflucan)

## Losartan (Cozaar)

Summary: Fluconazole reduces the concentration of losartan's active metabolite; reduction of losartan's antihypertensive efficacy may result.

Risk Factors: No specific risk factors known.

Related Drugs: Antifungal agents that do not inhibit CYP2C9 [e.g., *terbinafine (Lamisil)*] are unlikely to interact. The effect of other antifungal agents on losartan is unknown but is likely to be less than the effect seen with fluconazole. The effects of fluconazole on other angiotensin receptor antagonists are unknown.

Management Options:
- *Consider Alternative.* An antifungal agent that does not inhibit CYP2C9 could be selected for patients stabilized on losartan. Patients taking fluconazole could be treated with an angiotensin-converting enzyme inhibitor.
- *Monitor* patients stabilized on losartan for a reduction in their blood pressure control if fluconazole is administered.

References:
1. Kazierad DJ et al. Fluconazole significantly alters the pharmacokinetics of losartan but not eprosartan. Clin Pharmacol Ther. 1997;61:203. Abstract.

## Fluconazole (Diflucan)

## Midazolam (Versed)

Summary: Fluconazole administration appears to increase the concentrations and effects of midazolam.

Risk Factors: No specific risk factors known.

Related Drugs: *Ketoconazole (Nizoral)* and *itraconazole (Sporanox)* also may inhibit midazolam metabolism. Other benzodiazepines including *diazepam (Valium)* and *triazolam (Halcion)* are likely to be affected in a similar manner by fluconazole.

Management Options:
- *Monitor.* Patients requiring midazolam and fluconazole should be monitored for increased sedation.

References:
1. Mattila MJ et al. Fluconazole moderately increases midazolam effects on performance. Br J Clin Pharmacol. 1995;39:567P. Abstract.

## Fluconazole (Diflucan)

### Phenytoin (Dilantin)

Summary: Fluconazole may increase plasma phenytoin concentrations substantially, resulting in phenytoin toxicity in some patients.

Risk Factors: No specific risk factors known.

Related Drugs: Available evidence suggests that *ketoconazole (Nizoral)* does not affect phenytoin pharmacokinetics.

Management Options:

- *Monitor* patients carefully for phenytoin toxicity (e.g., nystagmus, ataxia, confusion, dizziness, slurred speech, involuntary muscular movements) when fluconazole is started in the presence of phenytoin therapy. Serum phenytoin determinations would also be useful. When fluconazole therapy is stopped in the presence of phenytoin therapy, monitor the patient for a reduced phenytoin effect.

References:

1. Cadle RM et al. Fluconazole induced symptomatic phenytoin toxicity. Ann Pharmacother. 1994;28:191.
2. Blum RA et al. Effect of fluconazole on the disposition of phenytoin. Clin Pharmacol Ther. 1991;49:420.
3. Touchette M et al. Contrasting effects of fluconazole and ketoconazole on phenytoin and testosterone disposition in man. Br J Clin Pharmacol. 1992;34:75.

## Fluconazole (Diflucan)

### Rifampin (Rifadin)

Summary: Chronic rifampin administration reduces fluconazole plasma concentrations; the clinical significance of this interaction is unknown.

Risk Factors: No specific risk factors known.

Related Drugs: Rifampin reduces the concentration of fluconazole (Diflucan), *itraconazole (Sporanox)*, and *ketoconazole (Nizoral)*. *Rifabutin (Mycobutin)* does not affect fluconazole.

Management Options:

- *Circumvent/Minimize.* A limited increase in fluconazole dose may be warranted in patients requiring high fluconazole concentrations.
- *Monitor.* Until further information is available, practitioners should be aware of potentially reduced fluconazole plasma concentrations when rifampin is coadministered.

## Significance Classification

(1) - *Avoid Combination.* Risk always outweighs benefit.

(2) - *Usually Avoid Combination.* Use combination only under special circumstances.

(3) - *Minimize Risk.* Take action as necessary to reduce risk.

References:

1. Apseloff G et al. Induction of fluconazole metabolism by rifampin: *in vivo* study in humans. J Clin Pharmacol. 1991;31:358.
2. Coker RJ et al. Interaction between fluconazole and rifampicin. Br Med J. 1990;301:818. Letter.

## Fluconazole (Diflucan)

## Tacrolimus (Prograf)

Summary: Fluconazole administration significantly increases tacrolimus concentrations and can increase the risk of nephrotoxicity.

Risk Factors:

• *Dosage Regimen.* Fluconazole doses >100 mg/day will increase the risk of an interaction.

Related Drugs: Fluconazole also inhibits **cyclosporine (Sandimmune)** metabolism. Other oral antifungal agents [e.g., **ketoconazole (Nizoral)**, **itraconazole (Sporanox)**] also may inhibit tacrolimus metabolism.

Management Options:

• *Monitor.* Patients receiving tacrolimus should have their plasma concentrations monitored during the coadministration of fluconazole. A reduction in the dose of tacrolimus is likely to be necessary to avoid nephrotoxicity.

References:

1. Manez R et al. Fluconazole therapy in transplant recipients receiving FK506. Transplantation. 1994;57:1521.
2. Assan R et al. FK 506/fluconazole interaction enhances FK 506 nephrotoxicity. Diabetes Metab. 1994;20:49.

## Fluconazole (Diflucan)

## Terfenadine (Seldane)

Summary: The plasma concentration of terfenadine is increased by large doses of fluconazole; the concentration of the active, carboxylic acid metabolite of terfenadine is increased, but this is without apparent significance.

Risk Factors:

• *Dosage Regimen.* Fluconazole doses above 200 mg/day may lead to terfenadine accumulation.

Related Drugs: **Ketoconazole (Nizoral)** and **itraconazole (Sporanox)** also inhibit the metabolism of terfenadine. **Loratadine (Claritin)**, **fexofenadine**, and **cetirizine (Zyrtec)** would be less likely to interact with fluconazole and cause toxicity.

Management Options:

• *Circumvent/Minimize.* Until additional studies of the interaction between fluconazole and terfenadine are available, it would be prudent to avoid giving the two drugs together. The use of sedating antihistamines or perhaps loratadine or cetirizine instead of terfenadine would seem to be preferred in patients taking fluconazole or other oral antifungal agents.

• *Monitor.* Watch for cardiotoxicity in patients receiving terfenadine and fluconazole.

References:
1. Honig PK et al. The effect of fluconazole on the steady-state pharmacokinetics and electrocardiographic pharmacodynamics of terfenadine in humans. Clin Pharmacol Ther. 1993;53:630.
2. Cantilena LR et al. Fluconazole alters terfenadine pharmacokinetics and electrocardiographic pharmacodynamics. Clin Pharmacol Ther. 1995;57:185. Abstract.

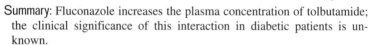

**Fluconazole (Diflucan)**

**Tolbutamide (Orinase)**

Summary: Fluconazole increases the plasma concentration of tolbutamide; the clinical significance of this interaction in diabetic patients is unknown.

Risk Factors: No specific risk factors known.

Related Drugs: Fluconazole 50 mg/day for 14 days did not affect the glycosylated hemoglobin or fructosamine concentrations in 14 diabetic women taking **glipizide** or **glyburide**.[2] Although glycosylated hemoglobin concentrations may not reflect short-term changes in blood glucose, no patient had symptoms of hypoglycemia. No pharmacokinetic data were presented; higher fluconazole doses may alter glipizide or glyburide pharmacokinetics. Other azole antifungal agents [e.g., **ketoconazole (Nizoral)**, **miconazole (Monistat)**, **itraconazole (Sporanox)**] may inhibit the metabolism of tolbutamide.

Management Options:
• *Monitor.* Until further information is available, patients maintained on tolbutamide should be observed for reduced glucose concentrations when fluconazole is started or increased glucose when fluconazole is discontinued.

References:
1. Lazar J et al. Drug interactions with fluconazole. Rev Infect Dis. 1990;12(Suppl. 3):S327.
2. Rowe BR et al. Safety of fluconazole in women taking oral hypoglycemic agents. Lancet. 1992;339:255. Letter.

**Fluconazole (Diflucan)**

**Triazolam (Halcion)**

Summary: Fluconazole increases the serum concentration of triazolam and may increase its pharmacodynamic effects such as sedation.

Risk Factors:
- *Dosage Regimen.* While the authors did not do a dose response study, fluconazole is known to produce a greater magnitude of metabolic inhibition when administered in doses above 100 mg/day.

Related Drugs: Fluconazole inhibits the metabolism of **midazolam (Versed)** (also see Fluconazole/Midazolam monograph) and could affect **diazepam (Valium)** in a similar manner. A benzodiazepine such as **lorazepam (Ativan)** which is not metabolized by CYP3A4 may be less likely to interact. Other antifungal agents such as ketoconazole (Nizoral) or itraconazole (Sporanox) similarly inhibit the metabolism of triazolam; however, terbinafine does not appear to inhibit triazolam metabolism.

Management Options:
- *Use Alternative.* The combination of fluconazole and triazolam should be avoided. A benzodiazepine such as lorazepam that is not metabolized by CYP3A4 would be a potential alternative anxiolytic agent. The antifungal agent terbinafine does not appear to inhibit the metabolism of triazolam.

References:
1. Varhe A et al. Fluconazole, but not terbinafine, enhances the effects of triazolam by inhibiting its metabolism. Br J Clin Pharmacol. 1996;41:319.

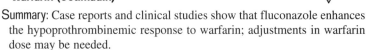

## Fluconazole (Diflucan)

## Warfarin (Coumadin)

Summary: Case reports and clinical studies show that fluconazole enhances the hypoprothrombinemic response to warfarin; adjustments in warfarin dose may be needed.

Risk Factors:
- *Dosage Regimen.* Although the ability of fluconazole to inhibit drug metabolism by CYP3A4 has been shown to require large doses of fluconazole, doses of 100 mg/day can inhibit warfarin metabolism (metabolized by CYP2C9).

Related Drugs: The effect of fluconazole on oral anticoagulants other than warfarin is unknown, but one should consider the possibility. **Phenprocoumon**, however, is metabolized primarily by glucuronidation and, theoretically, would be less likely to interact with cytochrome P450 inhibitors such as fluconazole. **Ketoconazole (Nizoral)** and **itraconazole (Sporanox)** also may increase the effect of oral anticoagulants.

Management Options:
- *Monitor* for altered oral anticoagulant effect if fluconazole is initiated, discontinued, or changed in dosage. Adjust the anticoagulant dose as needed.

References:
1. Gericke KR. Possible interaction between warfarin and fluconazole. Pharmacotherapy. 1993;13:508.
2. Kerr HD. Case report: potentiation of warfarin by fluconazole. Am J Med Sci. 1993;305:164.
3. Crussel-Porter LL et al. Low-dose fluconazole therapy potentiates the hypoprothrombinemic response of warfarin sodium. Arch Intern Med. 1993;153:102.

## Fluorouracil (5-FU)

## Metronidazole (Flagyl)

Summary: Metronidazole enhances the toxicity of fluorouracil (FU) without increasing its efficacy.

Risk Factors: No specific risk factors known.

Related Drugs: No information available.

Management Options:
- *Avoid Unless Benefit Outweighs Risk.* Patients taking FU should generally avoid metronidazole administration.
- *Monitor.* Patients should be monitored for enhanced toxicity when metronidazole is concomitantly administered.

References:
1. Bardakji Z et al. 5-fluorouracil-metronidazole combination therapy in metastatic colorectal cancer. Cancer Chemother Pharmacol. 1986;18:140.

## Fluorouracil (5-FU)

## Warfarin (Coumadin)

Summary: Case reports suggest that fluorouracil may increase the hypoprothrombinemic response to warfarin; more study is needed to establish a causal relationship.

Risk Factors: No specific risk factors known.

Related Drugs: The effect of fluorouracil on oral anticoagulants other than warfarin is not established, but one should assume that they interact until proven otherwise.

Management Options:
- *Monitor* for altered warfarin effect if fluorouracil is initiated, discontinued, or changed in dosage; adjustments of warfarin dosage

---

# Significance Classification

1. - *Avoid Combination.* Risk always outweighs benefit.
2. - *Usually Avoid Combination.* Use combination only under special circumstances.
3. - *Minimize Risk.* Take action as necessary to reduce risk.

may be needed. If warfarin is initiated in the presence of fluorouracil therapy, it would be prudent to begin with conservative doses of warfarin.

References:

1. Scarfe MA et al. Possible drug interaction between warfarin and combination of levamisole and fluorouracil. Ann Pharmacother. 1994;28:464.
2. Wajima T et al. Possible interaction between warfarin and 5-fluorouracil. Am J Hematol. 1992;40:238.

### Fluoxetine (Prozac)

### Furosemide (Lasix)

Summary: Two patients receiving fluoxetine and furosemide died unexpectedly, and it was proposed that the combination of these two drugs may have contributed to their death. A causal relationship, however, was not established.

Risk Factors: No specific risk factors known.

Related Drugs: If the furosemide-fluoxetine combination did, in fact, contribute to the fatal reactions, one would expect other loop diuretics such as **bumetanide (Bumex)** and **torsemide (Demadex)** to produce the same effect. Little is known regarding the ability of other selective serotonin reuptake inhibitors (SSRIs) to produce SIADH. **Sertraline (Zoloft)** has been reported to produce hyponatremia due to SIADH in one 73-year-old man,[2] and cases of **paroxetine (Paxil)**-induced hyponatremia have been reported to the manufacturer.[3] It is possible that other SSRIs have a similar effect.

Management Options:

• *Monitor* for evidence of hyponatremia if fluoxetine is used in patients undergoing vigorous diuresis or others at risk of hyponatremia. The relative likelihood of SIADH in patients receiving fluoxetine versus other SSRIs or tricyclic antidepressants is not established. Thus, it is not known if any of them would be preferable to fluoxetine in a patient prone to hyponatremia.

References:

1. Spier SA et al. Unexpected deaths in depressed medical inpatients treated with fluoxetine. J Clin Psychiatry. 1991;52:377.
2. Crews JR et al. Hyponatremia in a patient treated with sertraline. Am J Psychiatry. 1993;150:1564. Letter.
3. Smith Kline Beecham. Paxil Product Information. 1993.

### Fluoxetine (Prozac)

### Haloperidol (Haldol)

Summary: A woman on haloperidol developed severe extrapyramidal symptoms after starting fluoxetine, but a causal relationship was not established.

Risk Factors: No specific risk factors known.

Related Drugs: The effect of fluoxetine on other neuroleptics is not established. **Paroxetine (Paxil)** also is a potent inhibitor of CYP2D6 and also might inhibit haloperidol metabolism. **Sertraline (Zoloft)** appears to be a less potent CYP2D6 inhibitor, but it may have some effect.

Management Options:

- *Monitor.* Until more information is available, monitor patients for extrapyramidal symptoms if fluoxetine is used concomitantly with haloperidol (and possibly other neuroleptics).

References:

1. Tate JOL. Extrapyramidal symptoms in a patient taking haloperidol and fluoxetine. Am J Psychiatry. 1989;146:399. Letter.

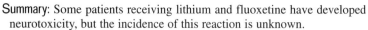

### Fluoxetine (Prozac)

### Lithium (Eskalith)

Summary: Some patients receiving lithium and fluoxetine have developed neurotoxicity, but the incidence of this reaction is unknown.

Risk Factors: No specific risk factors known.

Related Drugs: Theoretically, other selective serotonin reuptake inhibitors would interact with lithium in a similar manner.

Management Options:

- *Monitor.* Until additional information is available, monitor for evidence of neurotoxicity in patients receiving lithium and fluoxetine. Symptoms have included tremor, confusion, ataxia, dizziness, dysarthria, and absence seizures. If symptoms occur, consider trying a tricyclic antidepressant (e.g., nortriptyline, imipramine) with the lithium.

References:

1. Austin LS et al. Toxicity resulting from lithium augmentation of antidepressant treatment in elderly patients. J Clin Psychiatry. 1990;51: 344.
2. Salama AA et al. A case of severe lithium toxicity induced by combined fluoxetine and lithium carbonate. Am J Psychiatry. 1989;146: 278. Letter.
3. Pope HG et al. Possible synergism between fluoxetine and lithium in refractory depression. Am J Psychiatry. 1988;145:1292.

### Fluoxetine (Prozac)

### Phenytoin (Dilantin)

Summary: Several case reports have appeared describing phenytoin toxicity with concurrent use of fluoxetine.

Risk Factors: No specific risk factors known.

Related Drugs: The effect of selective serotonin reuptake inhibitors other than fluoxetine on phenytoin is not established.

Management Options:

- *Monitor* patients carefully for phenytoin toxicity (e.g., nystagmus, ataxia, confusion, dizziness, slurred speech, involuntary muscular movements) when fluoxetine is started. Serum phenytoin determinations also would be useful. Monitor the patient for a reduced phenytoin effect when fluoxetine therapy is stopped in the presence of phenytoin therapy.

References:

1. Woods DJ et al. Interaction of phenytoin and fluoxetine. N Z Med J. 1994;107:19.
2. Jalis P. Toxic reaction following the combined administration of fluoxetine and phenytoin: two case reports. J Neurol Neurosurg Psychiatry. 1992;55:412.

### Fluoxetine (Prozac)

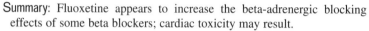

### Propranolol (Inderal)

Summary: Fluoxetine appears to increase the beta-adrenergic blocking effects of some beta blockers; cardiac toxicity may result.

Risk Factors: No specific risk factors known.

Related Drugs: *Metoprolol (Lopressor)* interacts similarly with fluoxetine, while *sotalol (Betapace)* appears unaffected. While the effects of other selective serotonin reuptake inhibitors on beta blocker clearance is not known, *fluvoxamine (Floxyfral)* and *sertraline (Zoloft)* appear to be less potent inhibitors of CYP2D6 than fluoxetine.

Management Options:

- *Consider Alternative.* Although specific data are lacking, beta blockers that are renally eliminated [e.g., atenolol (Tenormin)] may be a safer choice.

- *Monitor.* Patients stabilized on propranolol or metoprolol should be monitored for toxicity (e.g., bradycardia, conduction defects, hypotension, heart failure, central nervous system disturbances) if fluoxetine is coadministered. The long half-life of fluoxetine (24 hours) and its metabolite norfluoxetine (half-life 7 days and also known to be a metabolic inhibitor) explains why this interaction may take several weeks to reach its maximum effect. Caution also should be exercised when administering a beta blocker to a patient who has stopped taking fluoxetine within the past two weeks.

References:

1. Otton AV et al. Inhibition by fluoxetine of cytochrome P4502D6 activity. Clin Pharmacol Ther. 1993;53:401.
2. Drake WM et al. Heart block in a patient on propranolol and fluoxetine. Lancet. 1994;343:425. Letter.
3. Walley T et al. Interaction of fluoxetine and metoprolol. Lancet. 1993;341:967.

### Fluoxetine (Prozac)

### Selegiline (Eldepryl)

Summary: Isolated cases suggest that combined therapy with selegiline and fluoxetine may result in mania or hypertension, but a causal relationship has not been established.

Risk Factors: No specific risk factors known.

Related Drugs: The manufacturer of selegiline recommends that it not be used with SSRIs, including fluoxetine, *paroxetine (Paxil)*, *sertraline (Zoloft)*, and *fluvoxamine (Luvox)*.[2]

Management Options:
- *Avoid Unless Benefit Outweighs Risk.* Although the risk of combined use is not established, the potential adverse effects are severe.
- *Monitor* for evidence of hypertension or mania if the combination is used.

References:
1. Suchowersky O et al. Interaction of fluoxetine and selegiline. Can J Psychiatry. 1990;35:571. Letter.
2. Solvay Pharmaceuticals. Eldepryl prescribing information. 1996.

### Fluoxetine (Prozac)
### Terfenadine (Seldane)

Summary: A patient receiving fluoxetine and terfenadine developed possible cardiac rhythm disturbances, but a causal relationship was not established.

Risk Factors: No specific risk factors known.

Related Drugs: *Astemizole (Hismanal)*, like terfenadine, is metabolized by CYP3A4 and can cause ventricular arrhythmias; its interactions appear similar to terfenadine. *Loratadine (Claritin)*, *fexofenadine (Allegra)*, and *cetirizine (Zyrtec)* do not appear to produce cardiotoxicity and thus probably would be safer in patients on fluoxetine. *Fluvoxamine (Luvox)* is known to inhibit CYP3A4 and is contraindicated with terfenadine or astemizole (Hismanal).

Management Options:
- *Avoid Unless Benefit Outweighs Risk.* Although evidence for an interaction between terfenadine and fluoxetine is scanty, it would be prudent to avoid concurrent use until more information is available.
- *Monitor.* If the combination is used, monitor for evidence of cardiac arrhythmias (e.g., palpitations, fainting, shortness of breath).

References:
1. Swims MP. Potential terfenadine-fluoxetine interaction. Ann Pharmacother. 1993; 27:1404. Letter.

### Fluoxetine (Prozac)
### Tranylcypromine (Parnate)

Summary: Severe or fatal reactions have been reported when nonselective monoamine oxidase inhibitors (MAOIs) are coadministered with selective serotonin reuptake inhibitors (SSRIs) such as fluoxetine; the combination should be avoided.

Risk Factors: No specific risk factors known.

Related Drugs: All combinations of nonselective MAOIs [e.g., *phenelzine (Nardil)*, *isocarboxazid*] and SSRIs [e.g., *fluvoxamine (Luvox)*, *paroxetine (Paxil)*, *sertraline (Zoloft)*] are contraindicated.

Management Options:

- *Avoid Combination.* The combined use of fluoxetine and MAOIs should be avoided. Wait at least 2 weeks after stopping an MAOI before starting fluoxetine or any other SSRI and 5 weeks after stopping fluoxetine before starting an MAOI.

References:

1. Kline SS et al. Serotonin syndrome versus neuroleptic malignant syndrome as cause of death. Clin Pharm. 1989;8:510.
2. Sternbach H. Danger of MAOI therapy after fluoxetine withdrawal. Lancet. 1988;2:850.
3. Feighner JP et al. Adverse consequences of fluoxetine-MAOI combination therapy. J Clin Psychiatry. 1990;51:222.

## Fluoxetine (Prozac)

### Tryptophan

Summary: Several patients on fluoxetine developed symptoms of agitation, restlessness, poor concentration, and nausea when tryptophan was added to their therapy; the symptoms resolved when the tryptophan was discontinued.

Risk Factors: No specific risk factors known.

Related Drugs: Pending additional study, assume that all selective serotonin reuptake inhibitors (SSRIs) interact with tryptophan.

Management Options:

- *Avoid Unless Benefit Outweighs Risk.* Until more information on safety and efficacy is available, it would be prudent to avoid concurrent use of fluoxetine or other SSRIs with tryptophan.

- *Monitor.* If the combination is used, monitor patients for the symptoms previously described and for a reduced therapeutic response to fluoxetine. It may be necessary to discontinue tryptophan if the reaction occurs.

References:

1. Steiner W et al. Toxic reaction following the combined administration of fluoxetine and L-tryptophan: five case reports. Biol Psychiatry. 1986;21:1067.

## Significance Classification

 - *Avoid Combination.* Risk always outweighs benefit.

 - *Usually Avoid Combination.* Use combination only under special circumstances.

 - *Minimize Risk.* Take action as necessary to reduce risk.

## Fluoxetine (Prozac)

### Warfarin (Coumadin)

**Summary:** Limited clinical evidence suggests that fluoxetine does not affect the hypoprothrombinemic response to warfarin, but more study is needed. Isolated reports suggest that fluoxetine alone can increase the risk of bleeding in some patients.

**Risk Factors:** No specific risk factors known.

**Related Drugs:** Although little is known regarding the use of fluoxetine with oral anticoagulants other than warfarin, the same precautions would apply until data are available. Based on limited data, other selective serotonin reuptake inhibitors may also increase the risk of bleeding in patients receiving oral anticoagulants.

**Management Options:**

- *Monitor.* Although evidence for a fluoxetine-induced increase in the hypoprothrombinemic response to warfarin is scanty, monitor for altered warfarin effect if fluoxetine is initiated, discontinued, or changed in dosage. Adjust warfarin dose as needed. Keep in mind that the risk of bleeding might be increased even if the hypoprothrombinemic response is in the desired range.

**References:**

1. Rowe H et al. The effects of fluoxetine on warfarin metabolism in the rat and man. Life Sciences. 1978;23:807.
2. Aranth J et al. Bleeding, a side effect of fluoxetine. Am J Psychiatry. 1992;149:412.
3. Alderman CP et al. Abnormal platelet aggregation associated with fluoxetine therapy. Ann Pharmacother. 1992;26:1517.

## Fluphenazine Decanoate (Prolixin)

### Imipramine (Tofranil)

**Summary:** Phenothiazines may increase serum concentrations of some tricyclic antidepressants (TCAs), and TCAs may increase neuroleptic serum concentrations. These changes would be expected to increase both the therapeutic and toxic effects of each drug, but the degree to which these interactions alter the therapeutic and toxic responses to each drug is not well established.

**Risk Factors:** No specific risk factors known.

**Related Drugs:** *Desipramine (Norpramin)* interacts with *trifluoperizine (Stelazine)*, *chlorpromazine (Thorazine)*, and *butaperazine*. *Nortriptyline (Pamelor)* interacts with fluphenazine and *perphenazine*. See **Hansten and Horn's Drug Interactions Analysis and Management** page 299 for more information.

**Management Options:**

- *Monitor.* In patients receiving combined therapy with neuroleptics and TCAs, be alert for evidence of increased toxicity and altered therapeutic response.

References:
1. Conrad CD et al. Symptom exacerbation in psychotically depressed adolescents due to high desipramine plasma concentrations. J Clin Psychopharmacol. 1986; 6:161.
2. Bock JL et al. Desipramine hydroxylation: variability and effect of antipsychotic drugs. Clin Pharmacol Ther. 1983;33:322.
3. Wilens TE et al. Adverse cardiac effects of combined neuroleptic ingestion and tricyclic antidepressant overdose. J Clin Psychopharmacol. 1990;10:51.

## Flurbiprofen (Ansaid)
## Methotrexate (Mexate)

Summary: A case report suggested flurbiprofen increased methotrexate toxicity; prospective study failed to demonstrate an interaction.

Risk Factors: No specific risk factors known.

Related Drugs: Several nonsteroidal anti-inflammatory drugs and aspirin have been shown to increase methotrexate plasma concentrations. *Acetaminophen (Tylenol)* has not been shown to affect methotrexate response.

Management Options:
- *Consider Alternative.* Until more information is available on this interaction, it is preferable to avoid flurbiprofen (as well as other NSAIDs) in patients receiving antineoplastic doses of methotrexate. If possible, use a non-NSAID analgesic instead.
- *Monitor.* If the combination is used, observe the patient for signs of methotrexate toxicity including mucosal ulceration, renal dysfunction, and blood dyscrasias. Decreasing the methotrexate dosage may be required.

References:
1. Frenia ML et al. Methotrexate and nonsteroidal anti-inflammatory drug interactions. Ann Pharmacother. 1992;26:234.
2. Skeith KJ et al. Lack of significant interaction between low dose methotrexate and ibuprofen or flurbiprofen in patients with arthritis. J Rheumatol. 1990;17:1008.

## Flurbiprofen (Ansaid)
## Phenprocoumon

Summary: Some patients receiving oral anticoagulants have developed excessive hypoprothrombinemia and bleeding after flurbiprofen was initiated.

Risk Factors:
- *Concurrent Disease.* Patients with peptic ulcer disease (PUD) or a history of gastrointestinal (GI) bleeding are probably at greater risk.

Related Drugs: All nonsteroidal anti-inflammatory drugs inhibit platelet function, cause gastric erosions, and probably increase the risk of GI bleeding. Some NSAIDs, however, such as *ibuprofen (Advil)*, *naproxen (Naprosyn)*, or *diclofenac (Voltaren)* may be less likely to increase oral anticoagulant-induced hypoprothrombinemia than other NSAIDs. The degree to which **warfarin** interacts with flurbiprofen has not been established, but one should assume that an interaction will occur until evidence to the contrary is available. In a retrospective cohort study, hospitalizations for hemorrhagic PUD were about 13 times higher in patients receiving warfarin plus an NSAID than in patients receiving neither drug.[3] **Acenocoumarol** interacts similarly.

Management Options:
- *Avoid Unless Benefit Outweighs Risk.* Since all NSAIDs probably increase the risk of GI bleeding in patients on oral anticoagulants, use the combination only after careful consideration of the benefit versus risk. If an NSAID must be used with an oral anticoagulant, it would be prudent to use NSAIDs that are unlikely to affect the hypoprothrombinemic response to oral anticoagulants. (See Related Drugs above). If the NSAID is being used as an analgesic or antipyretic, acetaminophen is probably safer to use with oral anticoagulants. Non-acetylated salicylates (e.g., choline salicylate, magnesium salicylate, salsalate, sodium salicylate) also are probably safer with oral anticoagulants than NSAIDs, since such salicylates have minimal effects on platelet function and the gastric mucosa.
- *Monitor.* If any NSAID is used with an oral anticoagulant, one should monitor carefully the prothrombin time and watch for evidence of bleeding, especially from the GI tract.

References:
1. Marbet GA et al. Interaction study between phenoprocoumon and flurbiprofen. Curr Med Res Opin. 1977;5:26.
2. Stricker BHC et al. Interaction between flurbiprofen and coumarins. Br Med J. 1982;285:812.
3. Shorr RI et al. Concurrent use of nonsteroidal anti-inflammatory drugs and oral anticoagulants places elderly persons at high risk for hemorrhagic peptic ulcer disease. Arch Intern Med. 1993;153:1665.

**Fluvoxamine (Luvox)**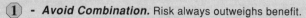

**Lithium (Eskalith)**

Summary: Isolated cases of adverse neurological effects have been reported in patients receiving fluvoxamine and lithium, but a causal relationship is not established.

## Significance Classification

1. - *Avoid Combination.* Risk always outweighs benefit.
2. - *Usually Avoid Combination.* Use combination only under special circumstances.
3. - *Minimize Risk.* Take action as necessary to reduce risk.

Risk Factors: No specific risk factors known.

Related Drugs: Other SSRIs may interact with lithium is a similar manner.

Management Options:
- *Monitor.* Until more information is available, monitor patients for adverse neurologic effects if fluvoxamine and lithium are used concurrently.

References:
1. Evans M et al. Fluvoxamine and lithium: an unusual interaction. Br J Psychiatry. 1990;156:286. Letter.

## Fluvoxamine (Luvox)
## Tacrine (Cognex)

Summary: Fluvoxamine markedly increases tacrine serum concentrations and may increase tacrine adverse effects; avoid the combination if possible.

Risk Factors: No specific risk factors known.

Related Drugs: The effect of other selective serotonin reuptake inhibitors such as **fluoxetine (Prozac)**, **paroxetine (Paxil)**, and **sertraline (Zoloft)** on tacrine is not established, but none of these drugs is known to inhibit CYP1A2. The effect of fluvoxamine on **donepezil (Aricept)** is not established.

Management Options:
- *Use Alternative.* Until more data are available, it would be preferable to use an alternative selective serotonin reuptake inhibitor such as fluoxetine, paroxetine, or sertraline in patients on tacrine. If the combination is used, monitor for adverse tacrine gastrointestinal effects and for tacrine-induced hepatotoxicity.

References:
1. Becquemont L et al. Influence of the CYP1A2 inhibitor fluvoxamine on tacrine pharmacokinetics in humans. Clin Pharmacol Ther. 1997;61:619.

## Fluvoxamine (Floxyfral)
## Terfenadine (Seldane)

Summary: Fluvoxamine appears to inhibit the enzyme that metabolizes terfenadine, which theoretically could result in increased unchanged serum terfenadine concentrations and cardiac arrhythmias; the combination should be avoided.

Risk Factors: No specific risk factors known.

Related Drugs: **Astemizole (Hismanal)** is also metabolized by CYP3A4 and can cause the same types of cardiac arrhythmias when combined with CYP3A4 inhibitors; thus it also may interact adversely with fluvoxamine. **Loratadine (Claritin)** also may be metabolized by CYP3A4, but it does not appear to produce cardiotoxicity when given with drugs that inhibit its metabolism.

Management Options:
- *Avoid Combination.* Although this interaction is based largely upon theoretical considerations, the combination of terfenadine and fluvoxamine generally should be avoided.[2] The potential adverse effects of the interaction can be life-threatening, and terfenadine is generally used for symptomatic relief of allergic disorders. Theoretically, loratadine would be a safer nonsedating antihistamine in the presence of fluvoxamine.

References:
1. Fleishaker JC et al. A pharmacokinetic and pharmacodynamic evaluation of the combined administration of alprazolam and fluvoxamine. Eur J Clin Pharmacol. 1994;46:35.
2. Solvay Pharmaceuticals. Luvox prescribing information. 1996.

## Fluvoxamine (Floxyfral)

## Theophylline

**2**

Summary: Several cases of theophylline toxicity due to fluvoxamine have been reported. Although more study is needed to establish a causal relationship, the interaction is consistent with the interactive properties of the two drugs.

Risk Factors: No specific risk factors known.

Related Drugs: Based on *in vitro* studies in human hepatic microsomes, other selective serotonin reuptake inhibitors (SSRIs) such as **citalopram**, **fluoxetine (Prozac)**, **paroxetine (Paxil)**, and **sertraline (Zoloft)** would be less likely to interact with theophylline.[1]

Management Options:
- *Use Alternative.* Given the magnitude of the interaction, and the potential toxicity of theophylline, it would be prudent to use an alternative to fluvoxamine, (e.g., citlopram, fluoxetine, paroxetine, sertraline). Until clinical evidence is available, however, be alert for evidence of theophylline toxicity when therapy with any SSRI is started. If the combination is used, monitor for altered serum theophylline concentrations and clinical evidence of theophylline toxicity if fluvoxamine is initiated, discontinued, or changed in dosage. Evidence of theophylline toxicity includes nausea, vomiting, diarrhea, restlessness, irritability, and insomnia. Higher serum concentrations can result in cardiac arrhythmias or seizures. Permanent brain damage and death have been reported in severe cases. Note that nausea is also a common side effect of fluvoxamine,[5] so measuring the theophylline serum concentration may be needed to determine whether nausea is due to fluvoxamine or theophylline toxicity.

References:
1. Brosen K et al. Fluvoxamine is a potent inhibitor of cytochrome P4501A2. Biochem Pharmacol. 1993;45:1211.

2. Sperber AD. Toxic interaction between fluvoxamine and sustained release theophylline in an 11-year-old boy. Drug Safety. 1991;6:460.

3. Thomson AH et al. Interaction between fluvoxamine and theophylline. Pharmaceutical J. 1992;249:137.

## Fluvoxamine (Floxyfral)

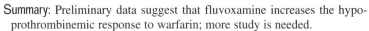

## Warfarin (Coumadin)

**Summary:** Preliminary data suggest that fluvoxamine increases the hypoprothrombinemic response to warfarin; more study is needed.

**Risk Factors:** No specific risk factors known.

**Related Drugs:** The effect of fluvoxamine on the response to other oral anticoagulants is not established. Some evidence suggests that other selective serotonin reuptake inhibitors (SSRIs) also may increase the bleeding risk from warfarin, in some cases without affecting the hypoprothrombinemic response.

**Management Options:**

- *Monitor.* Although data are scanty, one should be alert for evidence of altered hypoprothrombinemic response to warfarin (or other anticoagulants) if fluvoxamine is initiated, discontinued, or changed in dosage. Although not reported for fluvoxamine, some SSRIs may impair hemostasis; thus one should be alert for evidence of bleeding even if the hypoprothrombinemic response is in the desired range.

**References:**

1. Benfield P et al. Fluvoxamine: a review of its pharmacodynamic and pharmacokinetic properties, and therapeutic efficacy in depressive illness. Drugs. 1986;32:313.

## Folic Acid (Folvite)

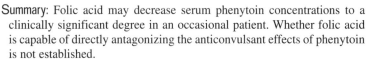

## Phenytoin (Dilantin)

**Summary:** Folic acid may decrease serum phenytoin concentrations to a clinically significant degree in an occasional patient. Whether folic acid is capable of directly antagonizing the anticonvulsant effects of phenytoin is not established.

**Risk Factors:**

- *Dosage Regimen.* Small amounts of folic acid found in multiple vitamins are not likely to have much effect.

**Related Drugs:** No information available.

**Management Options:**

- *Monitor.* When folic acid is given to patients receiving phenytoin, they should be watched for decreased seizure control (although most patients are probably not significantly affected).

**References:**

1. Poppell TD et al. Effect of folic acid on recurrence of phenytoin-induced gingival overgrowth following gingivectomy. J Clin Periodontol. 1991;18:134.

2. Inoue F. Clinical implications of anticonvulsant-induced folate deficiency. Clin Pharm. 1982;1:372.
3. MacCosbe PE et al. Interaction of phenytoin and folic acid. Clin Pharm. 1983; 2:362.

## Folic Acid (Folvite)

### Pyrimethamine (Daraprim)

**Summary:** Folic acid potentially can interfere with the efficacy of pyrimethamine.

**Risk Factors:** No specific risk factors known.

**Related Drugs:** No information available.

**Management Options:**

- *Avoid Unless Benefit Outweighs Risk.* Until more information is available, folic acid should not be administered to patients receiving pyrimethamine for treatment of toxoplasmosis or in patients with leukemia.
- *Monitor.* If folic acid is used, monitor for loss of efficacy of pyrimethamine.

**References:**

1. Tong MJ et al. Supplemental folates in the therapy of Plasmodium falciparum malaria. JAMA. 1970;214:2330.

## Furosemide (Lasix)

### Indomethacin (Indocin)

**Summary:** Indomethacin administration reduces the diuretic and antihypertensive efficacy of furosemide.

**Risk Factors:**

- *Concurrent Diseases.* Patients with hyponatremia may be at greatest risk for reduced glomerular filtration when nonsteroidal anti-inflammatory drugs (NSAIDs) are administered.

**Related Drugs:** Some evidence indicates that other NSAIDs, including *naproxen (Naprosyn), ibuprofen (Advil), piroxicam (Feldene), flurbiprofen (Ansaid), sulindac (Clinoril),* and large doses of salicylates have similar effects.[1,6-8] Some clinical evidence suggests that sulindac may be less

## Significance Classification

(1) - *Avoid Combination.* Risk always outweighs benefit.

(2) - *Usually Avoid Combination.* Use combination only under special circumstances.

(3) - *Minimize Risk.* Take action as necessary to reduce risk.

likely than other NSAIDs to interfere with the response to furosemide,[2–4,8] but the difference may be only relative.[5–7]

Management Options:

- *Monitor.* Patients should be monitored for evidence of reduced response to furosemide when indomethacin or another NSAID is coadministered. If increasing the dose of furosemide does not achieve the desired response, a different NSAID such as sulindac or salicylates, which may not affect furosemide to the same degree, should be considered.

References:

1. Rawles JM. Antagonism between non-steroidal anti-inflammatory drugs and diuretics. Scott Med J. 1982;27:37.
2. Ciabattoni G et al. Renal effects of anti-inflammatory drugs. Eur J Rheumatol Inflamm. 1980;3:210.
3. Bunning RD et al. Sulindac: a potentially renal-sparing nonsteroidal anti-inflammatory drug. JAMA. 1982;248:2864.
4. Wong DG et al. Non-steroidal antiinflammatory drugs (NSAIDs) vs placebo in hypertension treated with diuretic and beta-blocker. Clin Pharmacol Ther. 1984; 35:284.
5. Roberts DG et al. Comparative effects of sulindac and indomethacin in humans. Clin Pharmacol Ther. 1984;35:269.
6. Wilkins MR et al. The effects of selective and nonselective inhibition of cyclo-oxygenase on furosemide-stimulated natriuresis. Int J Clin Pharmacol Ther Toxicol. 1986;24:55.
7. Brater DC et al. Sulindac does not spare the kidney. Clin Pharmacol Ther. 1984; 35:258.
8. Eriksson L-O et al. Renal function and tubular transport effects of sulindac and naproxen in chronic heart failure. Clin Pharmacol Ther. 1987;42:646.

## Furosemide (Lasix)

### Phenytoin (Dilantin)

**Summary:** Studies in patients and healthy subjects indicate that phenytoin may reduce the diuretic response to furosemide.

**Risk Factors:** No specific risk factors known.

**Related Drugs:** The effect of phenytoin on other loop diuretics is not established. **Phenobarbital** affects furosemide similarly.

Management Options:

- *Monitor.* In patients taking phenytoin, be alert for an impaired diuretic response to furosemide; larger furosemide doses may be required. It is not known if separating the doses of the drugs would minimize the interaction.

References:

1. Ahmad S. Renal insensitivity to furosemide caused by chronic anticonvulsant therapy. Br Med J. 1974;3:657.
2. Fine A et al. Malabsorption of furosemide caused by phenytoin. Br Med J. 1977; 4:1061.

### Furosemide (Lasix)

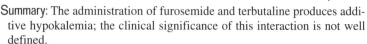

### Terbutaline (Brethaire)

Summary: The administration of furosemide and terbutaline produces additive hypokalemia; the clinical significance of this interaction is not well defined.

Risk Factors:

- *Concurrent Diseases.* Patients with low basal serum potassium may be at increased risk for arrhythmia when treated with combinations of furosemide and terbutaline.
- *Other Drugs.* Patients taking potassium-depleting corticosteroids may be more prone to hypokalemia from this interaction.

Related Drugs: It is likely that other combinations of potassium-wasting diuretics and beta$_2$-agonists also would tend to reduce serum potassium concentrations.

Management Options:

- *Circumvent/Minimize.* In patients who appear predisposed to hypokalemia, triamterene or potassium supplementation may be given to prevent excessive reduction in serum potassium concentrations.
- *Monitor.* Patients treated with combinations of potassium-wasting diuretics and beta$_2$-agonists should be monitored for signs of hypokalemia including ECG changes, fatigue, and muscle pains.

References:
1. Newnham DM et al. The effects of furosemide and terbutaline on the hypokalemic and electrocardiographic responses to inhaled terbutaline. Br J Clin Pharmacol. 1991;32:630.

### Gamma Globulin

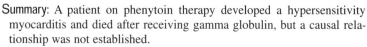

### Phenytoin (Dilantin)

Summary: A patient on phenytoin therapy developed a hypersensitivity myocarditis and died after receiving gamma globulin, but a causal relationship was not established.

Risk Factors: No specific risk factors known.

Related Drugs: No information available.

Management Options:

- *Consider Alternative.* Although a causal relationship between hypersensitivity myocarditis and combined phenytoin-gamma globulin therapy is not established, the severity of the reaction dictates that the benefit-risk of using this combination be considered carefully.
- *Monitor.* If gamma globulin is given in the presence of phenytoin therapy, be alert for evidence of hypersensitivity (e.g., fever, skin rash, eosinophilia) and cardiac findings (e.g., tachycardia, ECG changes, enzyme elevations).

References:
1. Keohler PJ et al. Lethal hypersensitivity myocarditis associated with the use of intravenous gamma globulin for Guillain-Barré syndrome, in combination with phenytoin. J Neurol. 1996;243:366.

## Ganciclovir (Cytovene)

## Zidovudine (Retrovir)

Summary: Combination therapy with ganciclovir and zidovudine in the treatment of cytomegalovirus (CMV) disease increases hematological toxicity.

Risk Factors: No specific risk factors known.

Related Drugs: No information available.

Management Options:
- *Avoid Combination*. Until more information is available, this combination of drugs should be avoided. Foscarnet (Foscavir) may be a reasonable alternative to ganciclovir for the treatment of CMV retinitis in patients treated with zidovudine.[2]

References:
1. Hochster H et al. Toxicity of combined ganciclovir and zidovudine for cytomegalovirus disease associated with AIDS. Ann Intern Med. 1990;113:111.
2. Jacobson MA et al. Foscarnet therapy for ganciclovir-resistant cytomegalovirus retinitis in patients with AIDS. J Infect Dis. 1991;163:1348.
3. Burger DM et al. Pharmacokinetic variability of zidovudine in HIV-infected individuals: subgroup analysis and drug interactions. AIDS. 1994;8:1683.

## Gemfibrozil (Lopid)

## Glyburide (DiaBeta)

Summary: Gemfibrozil appeared to cause hypoglycemia in a patient receiving glyburide; a causal relationship is likely in this patient, but more study is needed.

Risk Factors: No specific risk factors known.

Related Drugs: It is possible that other sulfonylureas would be affected similarly by gemfibrozil.

Management Options:
- *Circumvent/Minimize*. The glyburide dose may need to be reduced during concomitant gemfibrozil and glyburide therapy.
- *Monitor*. Patients receiving gemfibrozil and glyburide should be monitored for symptoms of hypoglycemia (e.g., tachycardia, sweating, tremor).

References:
1. Ahmad S. Gemfibrozil: interaction with glyburide. South Med J.1991;84:102.

## Gemfibrozil (Lopid)

## Lovastatin (Mevacor)

Summary: Case reports suggest that gemfibrozil increases the likelihood of lovastatin-induced myopathy, but the incidence of the reaction is not established.

Risk Factors: No specific risk factors known.

Related Drugs: Available evidence suggests that *pravastatin (Pravachol)* is less likely to cause myopathy than lovastatin, either when given alone or when combined with other drugs such as gemfibrozil.[1] Nonetheless, comparative "head-to-head" studies will be required to confirm these findings. Little is known regarding the likelihood of myopathy with **simvastatin (Zocor)** plus gemfibrozil (or clofibrate), but assume that it is similar to lovastatin plus gemfibrozil until information is available. Although little is known regarding the safety of combined use of lovastatin and **clofibrate (Atromid)**, apply the same precautions as with lovastatin plus gemfibrozil.

Management Options:
- *Avoid Unless Benefit Outweighs Risk.* Some experts recommend against using combined therapy with lovastatin and gemfibrozil, and the manufacturer suggests that the benefits of combined therapy are not likely to outweigh the risk of myopathy and rhabdomyolysis.[2]
- *Monitor.* If the combination is used, patients should be alert for muscular symptoms such as pain, tenderness, or weakness; CK should be measured in patients with such symptoms. Early recognition of this disorder is important since it may progress to acute renal failure in some patients if the drugs are not discontinued promptly. The same precautions should apply to combined use of lovastatin and clofibrate.

References:
1. East C et al. Rhabdomyolysis in patients receiving lovastatin after cardiac transplantation. N Engl J Med. 1988;318:47. Letter.
2. Merck Sharp & Dohme. Mevacor, Product Information. West Point, PA: 1993.
3. Wirebaugh SR et al. A retrospective review of the use of lipid-lowering agents in combination, specifically, gemfibrozil and lovastatin. Pharmacotherapy. 1992; 12:445.

### Gemfibrozil (Lopid)
### Pravastatin (Pravachol)

▷ 3 ▽

Summary: Most patients appear to tolerate the combined use of pravastatin and gemfibrozil well, but it is possible that an occasional patient might develop myopathy (as has been reported with lovastatin and gemfibrozil).

Risk Factors: No specific risk factors known.

Related Drugs: Available evidence suggests that pravastatin is less likely to cause myopathy than **lovastatin (Mevacor)**, either when given alone or when combined with other drugs such as gemfibrozil.[2] Nonetheless, com-

## Significance Classification

(1) - *Avoid Combination.* Risk always outweighs benefit.

(2) - *Usually Avoid Combination.* Use combination only under special circumstances.

(3) - *Minimize Risk.* Take action as necessary to reduce risk.

parative "head-to-head" studies will be required to confirm these findings. Little is known regarding the likelihood of myopathy with **simvastatin (Zocor)** plus gemfibrozil, but assume that it is similar to lovastatin plus gemfibrozil until information is available. One patient developed myopathy when **clofibrate (Atromid)** was added to well-tolerated pravastatin therapy; the myopathy resolved when the clofibrate was discontinued with continued pravastatin therapy.

Management Options:

- *Consider Alternative.* Although the combination of pravastatin and gemfibrozil is well tolerated in most patients, the routine use of this combination generally should be avoided until more evidence of safety is available.[1,3]

- *Monitor.* If the combination is used, patients should be alert for muscular symptoms such as pain, tenderness, or weakness; creatine kinase should be measured in patients with such symptoms.

References:

1. Wiklund O et al. Pravastatin and gemfibrozil alone and in combination for the treatment of hypercholesterolemia. Am J Med. 1993;94:13.

2. Jungnickel PW et al. Pravastatin: a new drug for the treatment of hypercholesterolemia. Clin Pharm. 1992;11:677.

3. Bristol-Myers Squibb. Pravastatin, Product Information. Princeton, NJ: 1993.

### Gemfibrozil (Lopid)

### Warfarin (Coumadin)

Summary: Gemfibrozil appeared to increase the hypoprothrombinemic response to warfarin in one patient, but more study is needed to confirm this effect.

Risk Factors: No specific risk factors known.

Related Drugs: The effect of gemfibrozil on oral anticoagulants other than warfarin is not established, but one should consider the possibility of an interaction until clinical studies are performed. **Clofibrate (Atromid)**, **lovastatin (Mevacor)**, and **simvastatin (Zocor)** also may increase the effect of oral anticoagulants, while **cholestyramine (Questran)** and **colestipol (Colestid)** may reduce their effect.

Management Options:

- *Avoid Unless Benefit Outweighs Risk.* Concomitant therapy with gemfibrozil and oral anticoagulants should be avoided if possible. If oral anticoagulant therapy is begun in a patient receiving gemfibrozil, anticoagulant doses probably should be conservative until the maintenance dose is established.

- *Monitor* for altered oral anticoagulant effect if gemfibrozil is initiated, discontinued, or changed in dosage.

References:

1. Ahmad S. Gemfibrozil interaction with warfarin sodium (Coumadin). Chest. 1990; 98:1041. Letter.

2. Parke-Davis, Lopid product information. Morris Plains, NJ: 1993.

### Gentamicin (Garamycin)

### Indomethacin (Indocin)

Summary: Indomethacin appears to reduce the renal clearance of gentamicin and amikacin in premature infants, resulting in increased gentamicin serum concentrations.

Risk Factors:
- *Age.* The glomerular filtration rate for preterm newborns is only 0.7–0.8 mL/min compared to 2–4 mL/min or10–20 mL/min/1.73 $m^2$ for full-term newborns.

Related Drugs: *Amikacin (Amikin)* interacts similarly. Other aminoglycosides may be affected by indomethacin. Other nonsteroidal anti-inflammatory drugs also may reduce the renal clearance of aminoglycosides.

Management Options:
- *Monitor.* If aminoglycosides and indomethacin are administered to infants, monitor plasma antibiotic concentrations and renal function. The potential for this interaction in adults is unknown.

References:
1. Gagliardi L. Possible indomethacin-aminoglycoside interaction in preterm infants. J Pediatr. 1985;106:991. Letter.
2. Zarfin Y et al. Possible indomethacin-aminoglycoside interaction in preterm infants. J Pediatr. 1985;106:511.

### Gentamicin (Garamycin)

### Vancomycin (Vancocin)

Summary: The combination of vancomycin and aminoglycosides may lead to increased nephrotoxicity in some patients.

Risk Factors:
- *Dosage Regimen.* Individuals with increased antibiotic concentrations, undergoing prolonged therapy, or receiving other nephrotoxic drugs are at increased risk.
- *Concurrent Diseases.* Individuals with pre-existing renal failure are at risk.

Related Drugs: Other aminoglycosides administered with vancomycin may increase the risk of nephrotoxicity.

Management Options:
- *Monitor.* If aminoglycosides and vancomycin are administered concurrently, monitor renal function and maintain antibiotic concentrations in the normal range.

References:
1. Pauly DJ et al. Risk of nephrotoxicity with combination vancomycin-aminoglycoside therapy. Pharmacotherapy. 1990;10:378.
2. Rybak MJ et al. Nephrotoxicity of vancomycin, alone and with an aminoglycoside. J Antimicrob Chemother. 1990;25:679.
3. Munar MY et al. The effect of tobramycin on the renal handling of vancomycin. J Clin Pharmacol. 1991;31:618.

## Glipizide (Glucotrol)

## Ranitidine (Zantac)

Summary: Ranitidine may increase the serum concentration of glipizide and enhance its hypoglycemic effects. Ranitidine may have independent effects on serum glucose.

Risk Factors: No specific risk factors known.

Related Drugs: Ranitidine does not alter *tolbutamide (Orinase)*[1,4] or *glyburide (DiaBeta)*[2] pharmacokinetics. *Cimetidine (Tagamet)* increases the concentrations of tolbutamide, glipizide, and glyburide. The effect of *famotidine (Pepcid)* and *nizatidine (Axid)* on sulfonylurea pharmacokinetics is unknown, but they may interact if increased gastric pH is involved in the observed changes with cimetidine and ranitidine. Proton pump inhibitors [e.g., *omeprazole (Prilosec)*, *lansoprazole (Pevacid)*] may affect glipizide in a similar manner.

Management Options:
- *Consider Alternative.* Sucralfate (Carafate) may be a good alternative therapy for the treatment of ulcer disease in diabetics because it appears unlikely to alter glycemic control to a clinically significant degree.[3]
- *Monitor.* Diabetics stabilized on any hypoglycemic therapy (and especially glipizide) in whom H$_2$-receptor antagonist therapy is initiated or discontinued should be observed for altered glycemic responses.

References:
1. Catt EW et al. Inhibition of tolbutamide elimination by cimetidine but not ranitidine. J Clin Pharmacol. 1986;26:372.
2. Kubacka RT et al. The paradoxical effect of cimetidine and ranitidine on glibenclamide pharmacokinetics and pharmacodynamics. Br J Clin Pharmacol. 1987; 23:743.
3. Letendre PW et al. Effect of sucralfate on the absorption and pharmacokinetics of chlorpropamide. J Clin Pharmacol. 1986;26:622.
4. Toon S et al. Effects of cimetidine, ranitidine and omeprazole on tolbutamide pharmacokinetics. J Pharm Pharmacol. 1995;47:85.

## Glucagon

## Warfarin (Coumadin)

Summary: Glucagon appears to enhance the hypoprothrombinemic response to warfarin, and possibly other oral anticoagulants, causing bleeding in some patients. Adjustment of the oral anticoagulant dose may be needed in patients receiving both drugs.

Risk Factors: No specific risk factors known.

Related Drugs: Little is known regarding the effect of glucagon on oral anticoagulants other than warfarin: assume that an interaction occurs until information to the contrary appears. A potentiating effect of *acenocoumarol (Sintrom)* by glucagon has been demonstrated in animals.[2]

Management Options:
- *Monitor* for altered oral anticoagulant effect if glucagon is given concurrently. Adjust the anticoagulant dose as needed.

References:
1. Koch-Weser J. Potentiation by glucagon of the hypoprothrombinemic action of warfarin. Ann Intern Med. 1970;72:331.
2. Weiner M et al. The effect of glucagon and insulin on the prothrombin response to coumarin anticoagulants. Proc Soc Exp Biol Med. 1968;127:761.

## Glutethimide (Doriden)

**2**

## Warfarin (Coumadin)

Summary: Glutethimide inhibits the hypoprothrombinemic response to warfarin, and probably other oral anticoagulants; the dose of the oral anticoagulant may have to be increased during coadministration of these drugs.

Risk Factors:
- *Dosage Regimen.* Since the onset and offset of enzyme induction is gradual, this interaction would be expected to take place over a week or more and to continue for a week or more after glutethimide is stopped.

Related Drugs: Although little is known regarding the effect of glutethimide on oral anticoagulants other than warfarin, assume that an interaction exists until information to the contrary appears.

Management Options:
- *Use Alternative.* Benzodiazepines such as flurazepam (Dalmane), temazepam (Restoril), and triazolam (Halcion) are preferable to glutethimide in patients on oral anticoagulants. If glutethimide is used, monitor for altered oral anticoagulant effect if glutethimide is initiated, discontinued, or changed in dosage. Adjust the anticoagulant dose as needed. Note that it may take up to 2 weeks or more for the maximal effect of glutethimide on warfarin to develop, and a similar time for the effect to fully dissipate.

References:
1. Corn M. Effect of phenobarbital and glutethimide on biological half-life of warfarin. Thromb Diath Haemorrh. 1966;16:606.
2. MacDonald MG et al. The effects of phenobarbital, chloral betaine, and glutethimide administration on warfarin plasma levels and hypoprothrombinemic responses in man. Clin Pharmacol Ther. 1969;10:80.
3. Udall JA. Clinical implications of warfarin interactions with five sedatives. Am J Cardiol. 1975;35:67.

## Glyburide (DiaBeta)

**3**

## Warfarin (Coumadin)

Summary: A patient on warfarin developed a marked increase in warfarin response and bleeding after starting glyburide, but a causal relationship was not established.

Risk Factors: No specific risk factors known.

Related Drugs: It does not seem likely that oral anticoagulants would interact with insulin.

Management Options:

- *Monitor.* Although this interaction is poorly documented, the potential severity of the adverse outcome suggests that warfarin response should be monitored if glyburide is initiated, discontinued, or changed in dosage.

References:

1. Jassal SV. Warfarin potentiated by proguanil. Br Med J. 1991;28:789.
2. Heine P et al. The influence of hypoglycaemic sulphonylureas on elimination and efficacy of phenprocoumon following a single oral dose in diabetic patients. Eur J Clin Pharmacol. 1976;10:31.

## Grapefruit Juice

### Nifedipine (Procardia)

Summary: Grapefruit juice increases the serum concentrations of several dihydropyridine calcium channel blockers; increased toxicity could occur in some patients.

Risk Factors:

- *Dosage Regimen.* Double strength grapefruit juice (i.e., diluted with half the usual amount of water) increased the risk of toxicity.

Related Drugs: Grapefruit juice increases the AUC of *felodipine (Plendil)*. Orange juice had no effect on felodipine.[1] A single dose of grapefruit juice caused a 40% increase in the AUC of *nitrendipine (Baypress)*,[3] while multiple doses produced a 106% increase in the AUC.[2] The combination of *nisoldipine (Sular)* and grapefruit juice produced a twofold increase in nisoldipine AUC and nearly a fourfold increase in its peak concentration.[4] Other dihydropyridine calcium channel blockers may be affected similarly by grapefruit juice.

Management Options:

- *Consider Alternative.* Patients should avoid taking calcium channel blockers with grapefruit juice. Orange juice does not affect calcium channel blocker metabolism.

- *Monitor.* Patients who drink grapefruit juice while taking calcium channel blockers should be monitored for increased response to the calcium channel blocker.

## Significance Classification

- (1) - *Avoid Combination.* Risk always outweighs benefit.
- (2) - *Usually Avoid Combination.* Use combination only under special circumstances.
- (3) - *Minimize Risk.* Take action as necessary to reduce risk.

References:
1. Bailey DG et al. Interaction of citrus juices with felodipine and nifedipine. Lancet. 1991;337:268.
2. Soons PA et al. Grapefruit juice and cimetidine inhibit stereoselective metabolism of nitrendipine in humans. Clin Pharmacol Ther. 1991;50:394.
3. Bailey DG et al. Grapefruit juice and naringin interaction with nitrendipine. Clin Pharmacol Ther. 1992;51:156.
4. Bailey DG et al. Effect of grapefruit juice and naringin on nisoldipine pharmacokinetics. Clin Pharmacol Ther. 1993;54:589.

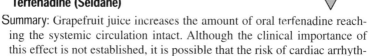

## Grapefruit Juice

### Terfenadine (Seldane)

Summary: Grapefruit juice increases the amount of oral terfenadine reaching the systemic circulation intact. Although the clinical importance of this effect is not established, it is possible that the risk of cardiac arrhythmias is increased in predisposed individuals.

Risk Factors: No specific risk factors known.

Related Drugs: ***Astemizole (Hismanal)*** is likely to interact with grapefruit juice in a similar manner, but one would not expect adverse effects with grapefruit juice given with the nonsedating antihistamines, ***loratadine (Claritin)*** and ***fexofenadine (Allegra)***, or the low-sedating agent, ***cetirizine (Zyrtec)***.

Management Options:
- *Circumvent/Minimize.* Although the clinical significance of this interaction is not established, given the potentially serious nature of the adverse effect, it would be prudent to warn patients to avoid grapefruit products while taking terfenadine or astemizole.
- *Monitor.* If terfenadine or astemizole is taken with grapefruit, monitor for evidence of ventricular arrhythmias (e.g., syncope, palpitations).

References:
1. Benton RE et al. Grapefruit juice alters terfenadine pharmacokinetics, resulting in prolongation of repolarization on the electrocardiogram. Clin Pharmacol Ther. 1996;59:383.
2. Honig PK et al. Grapefruit juice alters the systemic bioavailability and cardiac repolarization of terfenadine in poor metabolizers of terfenadine. J Clin Pharmacol. 1996;36:345.

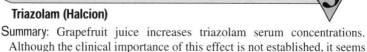

## Grapefruit Juice

### Triazolam (Halcion)

Summary: Grapefruit juice increases triazolam serum concentrations. Although the clinical importance of this effect is not established, it seems likely that some patients would be adversely affected.

Risk Factors:
- *Age.* The elderly are known to be more sensitive to triazolam and are likely to be at greater risk from this interaction.

Related Drugs: ***Alprazolam (Xanax)*** and ***midazolam (Versed)*** are also metabolized by CYP3A4. When given orally, they would also be expected to interact with grapefruit juice. ***Diazepam (Valium)*** is partially metabolized by CYP3A4, but would not be expected to interact to the same degree. Most other benzodiazepines are metabolized primarily by enzymes other than CYP3A4 and would not be expected to interact.

Management Options:

- *Consider Alternative.* Orange juice does not appear to inhibit CYP3A4 and would not be expected to interact with triazolam. Also, one could use a benzodiazepine other than triazolam, alprazolam, or midazolam such as diazepam.

- *Circumvent/Minimize.* Patients on triazolam should be warned to avoid taking it with or within several hours after grapefruit. Ingesting grapefruit in the morning and taking the triazolam in the evening theoretically would minimize the interaction, but there may still be a small effect.

- *Monitor.* If the combination is used, be alert for excessive triazolam effect (e.g., drowsiness).

References:
1. Hukkinen SK et al. Plasma concentrations of triazolam are increased by concomitant ingestion of grapefruit juice. Clin Pharmacol Ther. 1995;58:127.
2. Vanakoski J et al. Grapefruit juice does not enhance the effects of midazolam and triazolam in man. Eur J Clin Pharmacol. 1996;50:501.

### Griseofulvin (Grisactin)
### Oral Contraceptives

Summary: Griseofulvin may induce menstrual irregularities or increase the risk of pregnancy in women taking oral contraceptives.

Risk Factors: No specific risk factors known.

Related Drugs: Other antifungal agents may affect oral contraceptives similarly.

Management Options:

- *Circumvent/Minimize.* Patients on low-estrogen oral contraceptives may need a contraceptive with a higher estrogen dose when taking griseofulvin.

- *Monitor.* Women taking oral contraceptives should consider using additional contraceptives during and for 1 cycle after griseofulvin therapy. The development of menstrual irregularities (e.g., spotting, breakthrough bleeding) may indicate that the interaction is occurring and warrants particular caution.

References:
1. van Dijke CPH et al. Interaction between oral contraceptives and griseofulvin. Br Med J. 1984;228:1125.
2. McDaniel PA et al. Oral contraceptives and griseofulvin interaction. Drug Intell Clin Pharm. 1986;20:384.

### Griseofulvin (Grisactin)

### Phenobarbital

Summary: Phenobarbital may reduce the serum concentration of griseofulvin, but the clinical significance of this effect is not established.

Risk Factors: No specific risk factors known.

Related Drugs: Other barbiturates may produce a similar reaction with griseofulvin or other antifungal agents.

Management Options:

- *Circumvent/Minimize.* It has been suggested that divided griseofulvin doses (e.g., TID) may be absorbed better than larger doses taken less often.[1]

- *Monitor.* Until further information is available, monitor patients for lack of griseofulvin efficacy. Whether an increase in the daily dosage of griseofulvin is warranted when phenobarbital is coadministered requires further study.

References:

1. Riegelman S et al. Griseofulvin-phenobarbital interaction in man. JAMA. 1970; 213:426.
2. Busfield D et al. An effect of phenobarbitone on blood levels of griseofulvin in man. Lancet. 1963;2:1042.
3. Lorenc E. A new factor in griseofulvin treatment failures. Missouri Med. 1967; 64:32.

### Griseofulvin (Grisactin)

### Warfarin (Coumadin)

Summary: Griseofulvin appears to inhibit the hypoprothrombinemic response to warfarin and possibly other oral anticoagulants. An adjustment in the oral anticoagulant dose may be required in patients receiving both drugs.

Risk Factors:

- *Dosage Regimen.* Some evidence suggests that the effect of griseofulvin on warfarin is very gradual, so it may take several weeks or longer for the maximal effect to be seen.

Related Drugs: Little is known regarding the effect of griseofulvin on oral anticoagulants other than warfarin; however, one should assume that an interaction exists until information to the contrary appears.

## Significance Classification

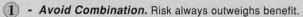
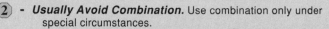

1 - *Avoid Combination.* Risk always outweighs benefit.

2 - *Usually Avoid Combination.* Use combination only under special circumstances.

3 - *Minimize Risk.* Take action as necessary to reduce risk.

Management Options:
- *Monitor* for altered oral anticoagulant effect if griseofulvin is initiated, discontinued, or changed in dosage. Since the effect of griseofulvin may be very gradual, monitor the hypoprothrombinemic response until it is stable, adjusting the anticoagulant dose as needed.

References:
1. Cullen SI et al. Griseofulvin-warfarin antagonism. JAMA. 1967;199:582.
2. Okino K et al. Warfarin-griseofulvin interaction. Drug Intell Clin Pharm. 1986; 20:291.
3. Udall JA. Drug interference with warfarin therapy. Clin Med. 1970;77:20.

### Guanethidine (Ismelin)

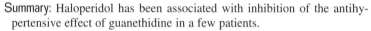

### Haloperidol (Haldol)

Summary: Haloperidol has been associated with inhibition of the antihypertensive effect of guanethidine in a few patients.

Risk Factors: No specific risk factors known.

Related Drugs: *Guanadrel (Hylorel)* is pharmacologically similar to guanethidine and also may be inhibited by haloperidol.

Management Options:
- *Consider Alternative.* Consider using an antihypertensive other than guanethidine (or drugs related to guanethidine such as guanadrel).
- *Monitor.* If the combination is used, monitor blood pressure for inhibition of antihypertensive effect. Increasing the guanethidine dose may overcome the interaction.[1]

References:
1. Janowsky DS et al. Antagonism of guanethidine by chlorpromazine. Am J Psychiatry. 1973;130:808.

### Guanethidine (Ismelin)

### Methylphenidate (Ritalin)

Summary: Methylphenidate appears to inhibit the antihypertensive effect of guanethidine.

Risk Factors: No specific risk factors known.

Related Drugs: *Guanadrel (Hylorel)* is pharmacologically similar to guanethidine and also may be inhibited by methylphenidate.

Management Options:
- *Consider Alternative.* Consider using antihypertensive agents other than guanethidine or guanadrel in patients who require methylphenidate therapy.
- *Monitor.* If the combination is used, monitor blood pressure and heart rate.

References:
1. Day MD et al. Antagonism of guanethidine and bretylium by various agents. Lancet. 1962;2:1282. Letter.

2. Gulati OD et al. Antagonism of adrenergic neuron blockade in hypertensive subjects. Clin Pharmacol Ther. 1966;7:510.
3. Deshmankar BS et al. Ventricular tachycardia associated with the administration of methylphenidate during guanethidine therapy. Can Med Assoc J. 1967;97:1166.

## Guanethidine (Ismelin)

## Norepinephrine (Levarterenol)

Summary: Patients on guanethidine have an exaggerated pressor response to norepinephrine.

Risk Factors: No specific risk factors known.

Related Drugs: *Guanadrel (Hylorel)* is pharmacologically similar to guanethidine and also may enhance the pressor response to norepinephrine.

Management Options:
- *Monitor.* In patients receiving guanethidine or guanadrel, use conservative doses of norepinephrine (and other sympathomimetics); monitor blood pressure carefully.

References:
1. Muelheims GH et al. Increased sensitivity of the heart to catecholamine-induced arrhythmias following guanethidine. Clin Pharmacol Ther. 1965;6:757.
2. Dollery CT. Physiological and pharmacological interactions of antihypertensive drugs. Proc R Soc Med. 1965;58:983.

## Guanethidine (Ismelin)

## Phenelzine (Nardil)

Summary: Monoamine oxidase inhibitors (MAOIs) may inhibit the antihypertensive response to guanethidine.

Risk Factors: No specific risk factors known.

Related Drugs: All nonselective MAOIs including *isocarboxazid (Marplan)* and *tranylcypromine (Parnate)* would be expected to inhibit guanethidine effect. *Guanadrel (Hylorel)* is pharmacologically similar to guanethidine and also may be inhibited by MAOIs.

Management Options:
- *Monitor.* Until more information is available, patients receiving guanethidine should be watched for hypertension if an MAOI is administered. Patients receiving MAOI therapy should be watched for a pressor response upon initiation of guanethidine therapy. The effects of nonselective MAOIs should be assumed to persist for 2 weeks after they are discontinued.

References:
1. Gulati OD et al. Antagonism of adrenergic neuron blockade in hypertensive subjects. Clin Pharmacol Ther. 1966;7:510.
2. Goldberg LI. Monoamine oxidase inhibitors: adverse reactions and possible mechanisms. JAMA. 1964;190:456.
3. Esbenshade JH Jr et al. A long-term evaluation of pargyline hydrochloride in hypertension. Am J Med Sci. 1966;251:119.

## Guanethidine (Ismelin)

## Phenylephrine (Neo-Synephrine)

Summary: Guanethidine enhances the pupillary response to phenylephrine; other phenylephrine effects also might be enhanced.

Risk Factors: No specific risk factors known.

Related Drugs: *Guanadrel (Hylorel)* is pharmacologically similar to guanethidine and also may interact with phenylephrine.

Management Options:
* *Monitor* for excessive phenylephrine response in patients receiving guanethidine; adjust phenylephrine dose as needed.

References:
1. Jablonski J. Guanethidine (Ismelin) as an adjuvant in pharmacological mydriasis. Ophthalmologica. 1974;168:27.
2. Sneddon JM et al. The interactions of local guanethidine and sympathomimetic amines in the human eye. Arch Ophthalmol. 1969;81:622.
3. Cooper B. Neo-Synephrine (10%) eye drops. Med J Aust. 1968;2:420. Letter.

## Guanethidine (Ismelin)

## Thiothixene (Navane)

Summary: Thiothixene appeared to substantially inhibit the anti-hypertensive response to guanethidine in one patient; other neuroleptics may have a similar effect.

Risk Factors: No specific risk factors known.

Related Drugs: The effect of another thioxanthine, *chlorprothixene (Taractan)*, on guanethidine is not established, but it may interact in a similar way. *Guanadrel (Hylorel)* is pharmacologically similar to guanethidine and also may be inhibited by thiothixene.

Management Options:
* *Monitor.* Although evidence for an interaction is scanty at present, patients on guanethidine therapy might be watched more closely for a decreased antihypertensive response if thioxanthines also are prescribed.

References:
1. Janowsky DS et al. Antagonism of guanethidine by chlorpromazine. Am J Psychiatry. 1973;130:808.

## Haloperidol (Haldol)

## Lithium (Eskalith)

Summary: A number of patients have developed severe neurotoxic extrapyramidal symptoms while receiving lithium and haloperidol, but many other patients have received the combination without such adverse effects.

Risk Factors:
- *Dosage Regimen.* Large doses of one or both drugs and failure to discontinue drugs when adverse effects occur can increase the risk of an interaction.
- *Concurrent Diseases.* Presence of acute mania; pre-existing brain damage; the presence of other physiologic disturbances such as infection, fever, or dehydration; and/or a history of extrapyramidal symptoms with neuroleptic therapy alone can increase the risk of an interaction occurring.
- *Other Drugs.* Concurrent use of anticholinergic antiparkinsonian drugs can increase the risk.

Related Drugs: No information available.

Management Options:
- *Circumvent/Minimize.* It has been recommended that neuroleptics such as haloperidol be used alone for initial control of acute mania symptoms and that lithium be added as the neuroleptic dosage is reduced.[1,3] Avoid excessive doses of either agent.
- *Monitor.* If haloperidol and lithium are used concomitantly, monitor carefully for signs of neurotoxicity, particularly in the presence of one or more of the risk factors described above.

References:
1. Kamlana SH et al. Lithium: some drug interactions. Practitioner. 1980;224:1291.
2. Thomas C et al. Lithium/haloperidol combinations and brain damage. Lancet. 1982;1:626.
3. Tupin JP et al. Lithium and haloperidol incompatibility reviewed. Psychiat J Univ Ottawa. 1978;3:245.

## Haloperidol (Haldol)

### Quinidine

Summary: Quinidine administration increases haloperidol concentrations, potentially increasing the risk of haloperidol toxicity.

Risk Factors: No specific risk factors known.

Related Drugs: No information available.

## Significance Classification

 - *Avoid Combination.* Risk always outweighs benefit.

 - *Usually Avoid Combination.* Use combination only under special circumstances.

 - *Minimize Risk.* Take action as necessary to reduce risk.

Management Options:
  • *Monitor.* Until further studies are available, patients taking haloperidol should be monitored for extrapyramidal symptoms, sedation, and hypotension if quinidine is coadministered.

References:
  1. Young D et al. Effect of quinidine on the interconversion kinetics between haloperidol and reduced haloperidol in humans: implications for the involvement of cytochrome P450IID6. Eur J Clin Pharmacol. 1993;44:433.

## Heparin

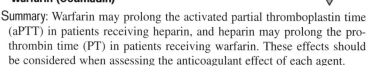

### Warfarin (Coumadin)

Summary: Warfarin may prolong the activated partial thromboplastin time (aPTT) in patients receiving heparin, and heparin may prolong the prothrombin time (PT) in patients receiving warfarin. These effects should be considered when assessing the anticoagulant effect of each agent.

Risk Factors: No specific risk factors known.

Related Drugs: All oral anticoagulants probably interact with heparin in a similar way.

Management Options:
  • *Monitor.* In patients receiving both heparin and an oral anticoagulant, monitor for oral anticoagulant-induced increases in aPTT. To minimize the interference of heparin with PT determinations, blood samples for PTs should not be drawn within about 5 or 6 hours of bolus IV heparin administration.

References:
  1. Moser KM et al. Effect of heparin on the one-stage prothrombin time: source of artifactual "resistance" to prothrombinopenic therapy. Ann Intern Med. 1967;66:1207.
  2. Mungall D et al. Bayesian forecasting of APTT response to continuously infused heparin with and without warfarin administration. J Clin Pharmacol. 1989;29:1043.
  3. Hauser VM et al. Effect of warfarin on the activated partial thromboplastin time. Drug Intell Clin Pharm. 1986;2:964.

### Hydralazine (Apresoline)

### Indomethacin (Indocin)

Summary: Indomethacin has been shown to inhibit the antihypertensive response to hydralazine in normal subjects.

Risk Factors: No specific risk factors known.

Related Drugs: Nonsteroidal anti-inflammatory drugs (NSAIDs) other than indomethacin would be expected to produce a similar effect.

Management Options:
  • *Monitor* for a reduced antihypertensive response when indomethacin or other NSAIDs are given with hydralazine.

References:
1. Cinquegrani MP et al. Indomethacin attenuates the hypotensive action of hydralazine. Clin Pharmacol Ther. 1986;39:564.
2. Jackson SHD et al. Indomethacin does not attenuate the effects of hydralazine in normal subjects. Eur J Clin Pharmacol. 1983;25:303.

## Ibuprofen (Advil)

## Lithium (Eskalith)

Summary: Ibuprofen increases lithium serum concentrations and may increase the risk of lithium toxicity; the magnitude of the effect appears to vary considerably from patient to patient.

Risk Factors:
- *Age.* It has been proposed that older patients may be more susceptible to the interaction;[1] if that is true, it may explain the difference in the magnitude of the interaction noted in the studies.

Related Drugs: Most NSAIDs increase lithium serum concentrations, but **sulindac (Clinoril)** and **aspirin** appear to have minimal effects.

Management Options:
- *Consider Alternative.* If appropriate for the patient, consider using an anti-inflammatory agent that is less likely to affect lithium, such as sulindac or aspirin.
- *Circumvent/Minimize.* Advise patients receiving lithium to avoid ibuprofen-containing products unless approved by the prescriber.
- *Monitor.* If ibuprofen therapy is initiated, monitor for lithium toxicity (e.g., nausea, vomiting, diarrhea, anorexia, coarse tremor, slurred speech, vertigo, confusion, lethargy; in severe cases, seizures, stupor, coma, and cardiovascular collapse) and elevated serum lithium concentrations. In a patient stabilized on lithium and an NSAID, discontinuation of the NSAID may result in inadequate serum lithium concentrations.

References:
1. Ragheb M et al. Ibuprofen can increase serum lithium level in lithium-treated patients. J Clin Psychiatry. 1987;48:161.
2. Kristoff CA et al. Effect of ibuprofen on lithium plasma and red blood cell concentrations. Clin Pharm. 1986;5:51.
3. Ragheb M et al. Interaction of indomethacin and ibuprofen with lithium in manic patients under a steady-state lithium level. J Clin Psychiatry. 1980;41:397.

## Ibuprofen (Advil)

## Methotrexate (Mexate)

Summary: Ibuprofen has been reported to increase the serum concentrations of methotrexate, but this has not been a consistent finding. It is not known how often this would result in adverse effects.

Risk Factors: No specific risk factors known.

Related Drugs: Several NSAIDs and *aspirin* have been shown to increase methotrexate plasma concentrations. *Acetaminophen (Tylenol)* has not been shown to affect methotrexate response.

Management Options:

- *Consider Alternative.* Until more information is available on this interaction, it would be prudent to avoid ibuprofen (as well as other NSAIDs) in patients receiving antineoplastic doses of methotrexate.
- *Monitor.* If methotrexate and ibuprofen are used concurrently, observe the patient for signs of methotrexate toxicity including mucosal ulceration, renal dysfunction, and blood dyscrasias. Decreasing the methotrexate dosage may be required.

References:

1. Tracy TS et al. The effect of NSAIDs on methotrexate disposition in patients with rheumatoid arthritis. Clin Pharmacol Ther. 1990;47:138. Abstract.
2. Skeith KJ et al. Lack of significant interaction between low dose methotrexate and ibuprofen or flurbiprofen in patients with arthritis. J Rheumatol. 1990;17:1008.

---

**Ibuprofen (Advil)**

**Warfarin (Coumadin)**

Summary: Ibuprofen does not appear to affect the hypoprothrombinemic response to warfarin or phenprocoumon, but cotherapy requires caution because of possible detrimental effects of ibuprofen on the gastric mucosa and platelet function.

Risk Factors:

- *Concurrent Diseases.* Patients with peptic ulcer disease (PUD) or a history of gastrointestinal (GI) bleeding are probably at greater risk for this interaction.

Related Drugs: *Phenprocoumon* interacts similarly. All NSAIDs inhibit platelet function, cause gastric erosions, and probably increase the risk of GI bleeding.

Management Options:

- *Avoid Unless Benefit Outweighs Risk.* Since all NSAIDs probably increase the risk of GI bleeding in patients on oral anticoagulants, use the combination only after careful consideration of the benefit versus risk. If the NSAID is being used as an analgesic or antipyretic, acetaminophen is probably safer to use with oral anticoagulants. Nonacetylated salicylates (e.g., choline salicylate, magnesium salicylate, salsalate, sodium salicylate) also are probably safer with oral anticoagulants than NSAIDs since they have minimal effects on platelet function and the gastric mucosa.
- *Monitor.* If any NSAID is used with an oral anticoagulant, one should monitor the prothrombin time carefully and watch for evidence of bleeding, especially from the GI tract.

References:
1. Penner JA et al. Lack of interaction between ibuprofen and warfarin. Curr Ther Res. 1975;18:862.
2. McQueen EG. New Zealand committee on adverse drug reactions: tenth annual report, 1975. NZ Med J. 1975;82:308.
3. Shorr RI et al. Concurrent use of nonsteroidal anti-inflammatory drugs and oral anticoagulants places elderly persons at high risk for hemorrhagic peptic ulcer disease. Arch Intern Med. 1993;153:1665.

## Imipenem (Primaxin)

### Theophylline

Summary: Several patients receiving theophylline developed generalized seizures following the addition of imipenem, but more study is needed to establish a causal relationship.

Risk Factors: No specific risk factors known.

Related Drugs: No information available.

Management Options:

- *Circumvent/Minimize.* Patients with reduced renal function should have appropriate imipenem dosage adjustments to avoid potentially toxic concentrations.

- *Monitor.* Until more information is known about this interaction, practitioners should monitor patients for appropriate theophylline and imipenem dosage. Be alert for signs of CNS stimulation or seizures.

References:
1. Semel JD et al. Seizures in patients simultaneously receiving theophylline and imipenem or ciprofloxacin or metronidazole. South Med J. 1991;84:465.

## Imipramine (Tofranil)

### Norepinephrine (Levarterenol)

Summary: Imipramine and other tricyclic antidepressants can markedly enhance the pressor response to norepinephrine.

Risk Factors: No specific risk factors known.

Related Drugs: *Desipramine (Norpramin), amitriptyline (Elavil)*, and *protriptyline (Vivactil)* interact similarly. Assume that all TCAs will interact with norepinephrine until proven otherwise.

## Significance Classification

(1) - *Avoid Combination.* Risk always outweighs benefit.

(2) - *Usually Avoid Combination.* Use combination only under special circumstances.

(3) - *Minimize Risk.* Take action as necessary to reduce risk.

Management Options:
- *Avoid Unless Benefit Outweighs Risk.* If IV norepinephrine is used, begin with conservative doses.
- *Monitor* blood pressure carefully if the combination is used.

References:
1. Boakes AJ et al. Interactions between sympathomimetic amines and antidepressant agents in man. Br Med J. 1973;1:311.
2. Mitchell JR et al. Guanethidine and related agents. III. Antagonism by drugs which inhibit the norepinephrine pump in man. J Clin Invest. 1970;49:1596.
3. Ghose K. Sympathomimetic amines and tricyclic antidepressant drugs. Neuropharmacology. 1980;19:1251.

## Imipramine (Tofranil)

## Phenelzine (Nardil)

**2**

Summary: Severe reactions have occurred in patients receiving combined therapy with tricyclic antidepressants (TCAs) and phenelzine or other nonselective monoamine oxidase inhibitors (MAOIs), but some combinations can be used safely with appropriate precautions.

Risk Factors:
- *Dosage Regimen.* Large doses of one or both drugs appear to increase the risk.
- *Order of Administration.* Most reactions occurred when the cyclic agent was added to established MAOI therapy.

Related Drugs: Antidepressants that inhibit serotonin reuptake such as **clomipramine (Anafranil)**, **amitriptyline (Elavil)**, **desipramine (Norpramin)**, and **trazodone (Desyrel)** may be more likely to result in serotonin syndrome than other tricyclic antidepressants.

Management Options:
- *Avoid Unless Benefit Outweighs Risk.* Some MAOIs and some tricyclics can be used together; however, when cotherapy is contemplated, any possible benefit of the combination should be weighed against the potential hazards. Moreover, it should be noted that the product information for both MAOIs and TCAs states that concurrent use is contraindicated, which may have medicolegal implications. Finally, be aware that a potentially lethal combination (in overdose) will be at the disposal of suicide-prone patients.
- *Monitor.* If the combination is used, monitor for evidence of excitation, fever, mania, seizures, or other unexpected adverse effects.

References:
1. De La Fuente RJ et al. Mania induced by tricyclic-MAOI combination therapy in bipolar treatment-resistant disorder: case reports. J Clin Psychiatry. 1986;47:40.
2. White K et al. The combined use of MAOIs and tricyclics. J Clin Psychiatry. 1984; 45:67.
3. Tackley RM et al. Fatal disseminated intravascular coagulation following a monoamine oxidase inhibitor/tricyclic interaction. Anaesthesia. 1987;42:760.

### Imipramine (Tofranil)

### Phenylephrine (Neo-Synephrine)

Summary: Imipramine and possibly other tricyclic antidepressants (TCAs) may enhance the pressor response to intravenous (IV) phenylephrine; the effect on oral or nasal phenylephrine is not established.

Risk Factors: No specific risk factors known.

Related Drugs: Until additional information is available, assume that other TCAs would produce a similar effect if combined with IV phenylephrine.

Management Options:
- *Monitor.* Patients receiving TCAs should be given parenteral phenylephrine only with caution and careful monitoring of the blood pressure. Until additional information is available, also be alert for enhanced pressor responses to oral phenylephrine.

References:
1. Boakes AJ et al. Interactions between sympathomimetic amines and antidepressant agents in man. Br Med J. 1973;1:311.
2. Boakes AJ. Sympathomimetic amines and antidepressant agents. Br Med J. 1973;2: 114. Letter.

### Imipramine (Tofranil)

### Quinidine

Summary: Quinidine markedly increases imipramine and desipramine serum concentrations; toxicity may result.

Risk Factors:
- *Pharmacogenetics.* Extensive metabolizers of the antidepressants are at greater risk.[2]

Related Drugs: **Desipramine (Norpramin)** and **nortriptyline (Pamelor)** concentrations are increased by quinidine. Other cyclic antidepressants also may be affected by this interaction but little clinical information is available.

Management Options:
- *Monitor.* Patients maintained on cyclic antidepressants should be monitored for increased side effects (sedation, arrhythmia, confusion) if quinidine is added to their drug therapy.

References:
1. Brosen K et al. Quinidine inhibits the 2-hydroxylation of imipramine and desipramine but not the demethylation of imipramine. Eur J Clin Pharmacol. 1989; 37:155.
2. Steiner E et al. Inhibition of desipramine 2-hydroxylation by quinidine and quinine. Clin Pharmacol Ther. 1988;43:577.
3. Pfandl B et al. Stereoselective inhibition of nortriptyline hydroxylation in man by quinidine. Xenobiotica. 1992;22:721.

### Imipramine (Tofranil)

### Verapamil (Calan)

Summary: Verapamil and diltiazem appear to increase imipramine serum concentrations; the clinical significance is unknown.

Risk Factors: No specific risk factors known.

Related Drugs: Verapamil and *diltiazem (Cardizem)* likely would affect other cyclic antidepressants in a similar manner. The effects of other calcium channel blockers on cyclic antidepressants are unknown.

Management Options:

• *Monitor.* Patients maintained on imipramine should be monitored for increased serum imipramine concentrations (e.g., sedation, dry mouth, tachycardia) if either verapamil or diltiazem is initiated concurrently.

References:

1. Krol TF et al. Comparison of verapamil, diltiazem, and labetalol on the bioavailability and metabolism of imipramine. J Clin Pharmacol. 1992;32:176.

## Indinavir (Crixivan)

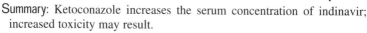

## Ketoconazole (Nizoral)

Summary: Ketoconazole increases the serum concentration of indinavir; increased toxicity may result.

Risk Factors: No specific risk factors known.

Related Drugs: Other protease inhibitors including *ritonavir (Norvir)*, *saquinavir (Invirase)*, and *nelfinavir (Viracept)* may be affected by ketoconazole in a similar manner. *Itraconazole (Sporanox)*, *miconazole (Monistat)*, and *fluconazole (Diflucan)* are also likely to inhibit the metabolism of indinavir. *Terbinafine (Lamisil)* does not appear to affect CYP3A4 activity and may be less likely to affect indinavir metabolism.

Management Options:

• *Circumvent/Minimize.* Pending further clinical studies, the dose or dosing interval of indinavir may need to be altered. The manufacturer has suggested a regimen of 600 mg Q 8 hr during concomitant ketoconazole administration.

• *Monitor.* Watch for indinavir toxicity (e.g., nephrolithiasis, hyperbilirubinemia, nausea).

References:

1. Merck & Company, Inc. Indinavir (Crixivan) package insert. 1996.

## Indinavir (Crixivan)

## Rifabutin (Mycobutin)

Summary: Indinavir markedly increases rifabutin serum concentrations while rifabutin lowers indinavir serum concentrations. Rifabutin toxicity and reduction of indinavir efficacy may result.

Risk Factors: No specific risk factors known.

Related Drugs: Rifabutin decreases the AUC of *saquinavir (Invirase)* and would be expected to affect *ritonavir (Norvir)* similarly. Ritonavir increases rifabutin concentrations. *Rifampin (Rifadin)* may affect saquinavir in a similar manner.

Management Options:
- *Circumvent/Minimize.* The dose of rifabutin may require reduction to avoid toxicity, and the dose of indinavir may require an increase to maintain efficacy.
- *Monitor* for rifabutin toxicity (gastrointestinal upset, skin rash) and loss of indinavir efficacy.

References:
1. Merck and Co., Inc. Crixivan prescribing information. 1996.

## Indomethacin (Indocin)    ▽ 3

## Lithium (Eskalith)

Summary: Indomethacin may increase plasma lithium concentrations.
Risk Factors: No specific risk factors known.
Related Drugs: Most NSAIDs increase lithium serum concentrations, but **sulindac (Clinoril)** and **aspirin** appear to have minimal effects.
Management Options:
- *Consider Alternative.* If appropriate for the patient, consider using an anti-inflammatory agent that is less likely to affect lithium, such as sulindac or aspirin.
- *Monitor* plasma lithium concentrations carefully if indomethacin (or another NSAID) is initiated or discontinued in patients on lithium therapy. Monitor also for lithium toxicity (e.g., nausea, vomiting, diarrhea, anorexia, coarse tremor, slurred speech, vertigo, confusion, lethargy; in severe cases, seizures, stupor, coma, and cardiovascular collapse).

References:
1. Frolich JC et al. Indomethacin increases plasma lithium. Br Med J. 1978;1:1115.
2. Ragheb M et al. Interaction of indomethacin and ibuprofen with lithium in manic patients under a steady-state lithium level. J Clin Psychiatry. 1980;41:397.

## Indomethacin (Indocin)    *2*

## Methotrexate (Mexate)

Summary: Isolated cases indicate that indomethacin may increase the toxicity of antineoplastic doses of methotrexate.

## Significance Classification

① - ***Avoid Combination.*** Risk always outweighs benefit.

② - ***Usually Avoid Combination.*** Use combination only under special circumstances.

▽ - ***Minimize Risk.*** Take action as necessary to reduce risk.

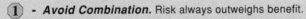

Risk Factors:
- *Dosage Regimen.* The risk of adverse effects from this interaction is primarily in patients receiving antineoplastic doses of methotrexate rather than the lower doses used to treat rheumatoid arthritis, psoriasis, and related diseases.
- *Concurrent Diseases.* Particular caution is suggested in patients with pre-existing renal impairment [who may be more susceptible to nonsteroidal anti-inflammatory drug (NSAID)-induced renal failure].

Related Drugs: Although a causal relationship has not been established, similar reactions have been reported following the concomitant administration of indomethacin and other NSAIDs.

Management Options:
- *Avoid Unless Benefit Outweighs Risk.* Until more information is available on this interaction, it would be prudent to avoid indomethacin (as well as other NSAIDs) in patients receiving antineoplastic doses of methotrexate. Particular caution is suggested in patients with pre-existing renal impairment who may be more susceptible to NSAID-induced renal failure.
- *Monitor.* If the combination is used, monitor for methotrexate toxicity. Findings in methotrexate toxicity can include stomatitis, severe gastrointestinal symptoms (nausea, diarrhea, vomiting), bone marrow suppression, fever, bleeding, skin rashes, nephrotoxicity, and hepatotoxicity. Although decreasing the methotrexate dosage would be expected to reduce the likelihood of toxicity, the magnitude of the required reduction in methotrexate dosage has not been established.

References:
1. Furst DE et al. Effect of aspirin and sulindac on methotrexate clearance. J Pharm Sci. 1990;79:782.
2. Dupuis LL et al. Methotrexate-nonsteroidal antiinflammatory drug interaction in children with arthritis. J Rheumatol. 1990;17:1469.
3. Skeith KJ et al. Lack of significant interaction between low dose methotrexate and ibuprofen or flurbiprofen in patients with arthritis. J Rheumatol. 1990;17:1008.

## Indomethacin (Indocin)

### Phenylpropanolamine

Summary: A patient receiving phenylpropanolamine developed an acute hypertensive reaction on two occasions following single doses of indomethacin, but the interaction was not confirmed in a study of healthy subjects.

Risk Factors: No specific risk factors known. It is possible that the interaction only occurs in certain predisposed individuals (e.g., those in whom prostaglandins are playing an important role in counteracting hypertensive stimuli).

Related Drugs: The effect of phenylpropanolamine with other nonsteroidal anti-inflammatory drugs in not established.

Management Options:
- *Monitor.* Until more information is available, blood pressure should be monitored in patients receiving concurrent therapy with sympathomimetics (such as phenylpropanolamine) and prostaglandin inhibitors (such as indomethacin).

References:
1. Lee KY et al. Severe hypertension after ingestion of an appetite suppressant (phenylpropanolamine) with indomethacin. Lancet. 1979;1:1110.
2. McKenney JM et al. The effect of phenylpropanolamine on 24-hour blood pressure in normotensive subjects administered indomethacin. Ann Pharmacother, DICP. 1991;25:234.

## Indomethacin (Indocin)

### Prazosin (Minipress)

Summary: In some patients indomethacin may inhibit the antihypertensive response to prazosin; the effect of other nonsteroidal anti-inflammatory drugs (NSAIDs) is not known, but they may produce a similar effect.

Risk Factors: No specific risk factors known.

Related Drugs: The effect of other NSAIDs on prazosin has not been studied, but they probably produce a similar response. *Ibuprofen (Advil)* in a dose of 400 mg TID for 3 weeks has been shown to increase the mean blood pressure by about 5 to 7 mm Hg in a parallel trial of 45 hypertensive patients receiving a variety of antihypertensive drugs.[2] *Doxazosin (Cardura)* and *terazosin (Hytrin)* probably interact with NSAIDs in a similar manner.

Management Options:
- *Consider Alternative.* Sulindac (Clinoril) appears less likely than other NSAIDs to inhibit the anithypertensive response to beta blockers, captopril (Capoten), and thiazides. It is possible that it also would have less effect on prazosin.
- *Monitor* for reduced hypotensive response to prazosin (or other antihypertensive agents) when NSAIDs are given concurrently. If blood pressure increases, alteration in antihypertensive drug dosage and/or the use of alternative antihypertensive agents may be required.

References:
1. Rubin P et al. Studies on the clinical pharmacology of prazosin. II. The influence of indomethacin and of propranolol on the action and disposition of prazosin. Br J Clin Pharmacol. 1980;10:33.
2. Radack KL et al. Ibuprofen interferes with the efficacy of antihypertensive drugs: a randomized, double-blind, placebo-controlled trial of ibuprofen compared with acetaminophen. Ann Intern Med. 1987; 107:628.

## Indomethacin (Indocin)

### Prednisone

Summary: The combined effects of prednisone and indomethacin may result in an increased incidence and/or severity of gastrointestinal (GI) ulceration; other combinations of nonsteroidal anti-inflammatory drugs (NSAIDs) and corticosteroids probably produce a similar effect.

Risk Factors: No specific risk factors known.

Related Drugs: If indomethacin does increase GI toxicity of corticosteroids, other NSAIDs would be expected to act similarly.

Management Options:
- *Circumvent/Minimize.* Consider the concurrent use of misoprostol (Cytotec).
- *Monitor.* Be particularly alert for evidence of GI ulceration and bleeding in patients receiving combinations of NSAIDs and corticosteroids.

References:
1. Emmanuel JH et al. Gastric ulcer and the antiarthritic drugs. Postgrad Med J. 1971;47:227.
2. Hvidberg E et al. Influence of indomethacin on the distribution of cortisol in man. Eur J Clin Pharmacol. 1971;3:102.

### Indomethacin (Indocin)
### Propranolol (Inderal)

Summary: Indomethacin and many other nonsteroidal anti-inflammatory drugs (NSAIDs) can reduce the hypotensive effect of propranolol and other beta blockers.

Risk Factors:
- *Dosage Regimen.* Chronic administration of an NSAID may inhibit antihypertensive response.

Related Drugs: Other beta blockers [e.g., **pindolol (Visken), labetalol (Normodyne), atenolol (Tenormin)**, and **oxprenolol**] may be affected similarly. Other NSAIDs [e.g., **sulfinpyrazone (Anturane), piroxicam (Feldene)**, and **naproxen (Naprosyn)**] probably produce a similar effect, but there may be differences in the magnitude of the interaction with different NSAIDs. **Sulindac (Clinoril)** appears least likely to interfere with beta blockers' antihypertensive effects.

Management Options:
- *Circumvent/Minimize.* Using the shortest duration of NSAID therapy will minimize the magnitude of the interaction. Using an antihypertensive other than a beta blocker may not circumvent the interaction because NSAIDs generally tend to inhibit the effect of antihypertensives.
- *Monitor.* Patients should be monitored for altered antihypertensive or antianginal response to beta blockers when indomethacin is initiated or discontinued. Short-term NSAID use requires no special precautions.

References:
1. Sugimoto K et al. Influence of indomethacin on a reduction in forearm blood flow induced by propranolol in healthy subjects. J Clin Pharmacol. 1989;29:307.

2. Abate MA et al. Interaction of indomethacin and sulindac with labetalol. Br J Clin Pharmacol. 1991;31:363.
3. Schuna AA et al. Lack of interaction between sulindac or naproxen and propranolol in hypertensive patients. J Clin Pharmacol. 1989; 29:524.

## Indomethacin (Indocin)

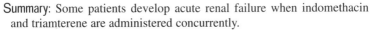

## Triamterene (Dyrenium)

Summary: Some patients develop acute renal failure when indomethacin and triamterene are administered concurrently.

Risk Factors: No specific risk factors known.

Related Drugs: Nephrotoxicity was not seen when indomethacin was combined with *furosemide (Lasix)*, *hydrochlorothiazide (Dyazide)*, or *spironolactone (Aldactone)*.[1] Cases of reduced renal function have been reported with triamterene combined with other nonsteroidal anti-inflammatory drugs (NSAIDs), one involving *diclofenac (Voltaren)* and triamterene[2] and one involving *ibuprofen (Advil)* and triamterene.[3] Other NSAIDs also may interact, but little information is available.

Management Options:
- *Consider Alternative.* It is possible that spironolactone and amiloride are less likely than triamterene to interact adversely with indomethacin, but this has not been established clinically.
- *Monitor.* Carefully monitor renal function in patients on combined therapy with triamterene and indomethacin (or other NSAIDs).

References:
1. Favre L et al. Reversible acute renal failure from combined triamterene and indomethacin: a study in healthy subjects. Ann Intern Med. 1982;96:317.
2. Harkonen M et al. Reversible deterioration of renal function after diclofenac in patient receiving triamterene. Br Med J. 1986;293:698.
3. Gehr TWB et al. Interaction of triamterene-hydrochlorothiazide and ibuprofen. Clin Pharmacol Ther. 1990;47:200. Abstract.

## Indomethacin (Indocin)

## Vancomycin (Vancocin)

Summary: Indomethacin administration may increase the concentration of vancomycin in neonates; vancomycin toxicity may result.

Risk Factors: No specific risk factors known.

Related Drugs: Other nonsteroidal anti-inflammatory drugs may affect vancomycin in a similar manner.

Management Options:
- *Circumvent/Minimize.* Vancomycin dosage may need to be reduced during indomethacin coadministration.
- *Monitor.* Vancomycin concentrations should be monitored in neonates receiving indomethacin.

References:
1. Spivey MJ et al. Vancomycin pharmacokinetics in neonates. Am J Dis Child. 1986;149:859. Letter.

## Indomethacin (Indocin)

## Warfarin (Coumadin)

**2**

**Summary:** Although isolated case reports of indomethacin-induced increases in the hypoprothrombinemic response to warfarin have appeared, most patients do not manifest an enhanced anticoagulant effect. Nonetheless, caution is indicated during cotherapy with these drugs because of possible detrimental effects of indomethacin on the gastric mucosa and platelet function.

**Risk Factors:**
- *Concurrent Diseases.* Patients with peptic ulcer disease (PUD) or a history of gastrointestinal (GI) bleeding are probably at greater risk.

**Related Drugs:** All NSAIDs inhibit platelet function, cause gastric erosions, and probably increase the risk of GI bleeding. Some NSAIDs, however, such as ***ibuprofen (Advil)***, ***naproxen (Naprosyn)***, or ***diclofenac (Voltaren)*** may be less likely to increase oral anticoagulant-induced hypoprothrombinemia than other NSAIDs. One should assume that ***phenprocoumon*** interacts similarly.

**Management Options:**
- *Avoid Unless Benefit Outweighs Risk.* Since all NSAIDs probably increase the risk of GI bleeding in patients on oral anticoagulants, use the combination only after careful consideration of the benefit versus risk. If an NSAID must be used with an oral anticoagulant, it would be prudent to use NSAIDs that are unlikely to affect the hypoprothrombinemic response to oral anticoagulants. If the NSAID is being used as an analgesic or antipyretic, acetaminophen is probably safer to use with oral anticoagulants. Non-acetylated salicylates (e.g., choline salicylate, magnesium salicylate, salsalate, sodium salicylate) also are probably safer with oral anticoagulants than NSAIDs since such salicylates have minimal effects on platelet function and the gastric mucosa.
- *Monitor.* If any NSAID is used with an oral anticoagulant, one should carefully monitor the prothrombin time and watch for evidence of bleeding, especially from the GI tract.

**References:**
1. Shorr RI et al. Concurrent use of nonsteroidal anti-inflammatory drugs and oral anticoagulants places elderly persons at high risk hemorrhagic peptic ulcer disease. Arch Intern Med. 1993;153:1665.

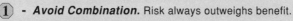

## Significance Classification

 **1** - ***Avoid Combination.*** Risk always outweighs benefit.

**2** - ***Usually Avoid Combination.*** Use combination only under special circumstances.

**3** - ***Minimize Risk.*** Take action as necessary to reduce risk.

2. Chan TYK et al. Adverse interaction between warfarin and indomethacin. Drug Safety. 1994;10:267.
3. Day R et al. Adverse interaction between warfarin and indomethacin. Drug Safety. 1994;1:213.

## Influenza Vaccine

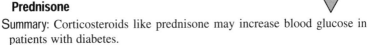

### Phenytoin (Dilantin)

Summary: Some patients appear to develop an increase in total serum phenytoin concentrations following vaccination, but reductions in free serum phenytoin concentrations also have been reported. The clinical importance of these findings is not established.

Risk Factors: No specific risk factors known.

Related Drugs: No information available.

Management Options:

• *Monitor.* Although patients should be monitored for evidence of phenytoin toxicity following influenza vaccination, an adjustment in phenytoin dosage rarely is needed. If the phenytoin dose is changed, additional adjustments should be anticipated as the effect of the vaccine dissipates (this has taken as little as 2 weeks but may take much longer).

References:

1. Levine M et al. Phenytoin therapy and immune response to influenza vaccine. Clin Pharm. 1985;4:191.
2. Jann MW et al. Effect of influenza vaccine on serum anticonvulsant concentrations. Clin Pharm. 1986;5:817.
3. Smith CD et al. Effect of influenza vaccine on serum concentrations of total and free phenytoin. Clin Pharm. 1988;7:828.

## Insulin

### Prednisone

Summary: Corticosteroids like prednisone may increase blood glucose in patients with diabetes.

Risk Factors:

• *Dosage Regimen.* Chronic administration of corticosteroids can increase glucose concentrations.

Related Drugs: All corticosteroids can increase glucose concentrations during chronic dosing.

Management Options:

• *Monitor.* Patients should be observed for evidence of altered diabetic control when corticosteroids are initiated, discontinued or changed in dosage.

References:

1. Gomez EC et al. Induction of glycosuria and hyperglycemia by topical corticosteroid therapy. Arch Dermatol. 1976;112:1559.

2. Hunder GG et al. Daily and alternate-day corticosteroid regimens in treatment of giant cell arteritis. Comparison in a prospective study. Ann Intern Med. 1975; 82:613.
3. McMahon M et al. Effects of glucocorticoids on carbohydrate metabolism. Diabetes Metab Rev. 1988;4:17.

## Insulin

### Propranolol (Inderal)

Summary: Propranolol and other beta blockers may alter the response to hypoglycemia by prolonging the recovery of normoglycemia, causing hypertension and blocking tachycardia. They also may increase blood glucose concentrations and impair peripheral circulation.

Risk Factors: No specific risk factors known.

Related Drugs: Nonselective beta blockers [e.g., *timolol (Blocadren)*, *alprenolol*, *nadolol (Corgard)*] would be expected to produce results similar to propranolol when administered to patients taking insulin. Oral hypoglycemic agents [e.g., *tolbutamide (Orinase)*] may interact with the nonselective beta blockers but, since they are less likely to produce hypoglycemia than insulin, the incidence and magnitude of reactions associated with hypoglycemic episodes will be reduced.

Management Options:

- *Consider Alternative.* Cardioselective beta blockers [e.g., *metoprolol (Lopressor)*, *acebutolol (Sectral)*, *penbutolol (Levatol)*, and *atenolol (Tenormin)*] are preferable in diabetic patients, especially if the patient is prone to hypoglycemic episodes. The increased safety of cardioselective agents is only relative, as they may exhibit nonselective beta blockade at higher doses.

- *Monitor.* Diabetic patients receiving beta blockers should be aware that hypoglycemic episodes may not result in the expected tachycardia, but hypoglycemic-induced sweating will occur or even may be increased.

References:

1. Mills GA et al. Beta-blockers and glucose control. Drug Intell Clin Pharm. 1985; 19:246.
2. Pollare T et al. Sensitivity to insulin during treatment with atenolol and metoprolol; a randomized, double blind study of effects of carbohydrate and lipoprotein metabolism in hypertensive patients. Br Med J. 1989;298:1152.
3. Reeves RL et al. The effect of metoprolol and propranolol on pancreatic insulin release. Clin Pharmacol Ther. 1982;31:262.

## Insulin

### Thiazides

Summary: Thiazides tend to increase blood glucose and may increase the dosage requirements of antidiabetic drugs.

Risk Factors:
- *Dosage.* Thiazide dosage above 50 mg daily may increase blood glucose.

Related Drugs: Thiazides may inhibit the hypoglycemic effect of *chlorpropamide (Diabinese)* and other oral hypoglycemic agents.

Management Options:
- *Monitor.* Watch for decreased diabetic control when thiazide therapy is started in a patient receiving any diabetic drug.

References:
1. Grunfeld C et al. Hypokalemia and diabetes mellitus. Am J Med. 1983;75:553.
2. Helderman JN et al. Prevention of the glucose intolerance of thiazide diuretics by maintenance of body potassium. Diabetes. 1983;32:106.
3. Lowder NK et al. Clinically significant diuretic-induced glucose intolerance. Drug Intell Clin Pharm. 1988;22:969.

## Insulin

## Tranylcypromine (Parnate)

Summary: Excessive hypoglycemia may occur when tranylcypromine, and other monoamine oxidase inhibitors (MAOIs), are administered to patients with diabetes.

Risk Factors: No specific risk factors known.

Related Drugs: Sulfonylureas such as *chlorpropamide (Diabinase)* and *tolbutamide (Orinase)* interact with type A MAOIs like tranylcypromine similarly. While it is likely that all Type A MAOIs will interact in a similar manner, the effect of Type B MAOIs [e.g., selegiline (Eldepryl)] on glucose tolerance is not established.

Management Options:
- *Monitor.* Until further information on this interaction is available, diabetic patients should be warned about possible hypoglycemic reactions when MAOI therapy is started. Be alert for deterioration of glycemic control when MAOI therapy is discontinued.

References:
1. Cooper AJ et al. Modification of insulin and sulfonylurea hypoglycemia by monoamine-oxidase inhibitor drugs. Diabetes. 1967;16:272.
2. Bressler R et al. Tranylcypromine: a potent insulin secretagogue and hypoglycemic agent. Diabetes. 1968;17:617.
3. Adnitt PI. Hypoglycemic action of monoamine oxidase inhibitors (MAOI's). Diabetes. 1968;17:628.

## Interferon (Roferon A)

## Theophylline

Summary: Interferon alpha may increase theophylline plasma concentrations, especially in patients with high pre-existing theophylline clearance (i.e., smokers); the degree to which this increases the risk of theophylline toxicity is not known.

Risk Factors:
- *Habits.* Limited evidence suggests that the reduction in theophylline clearance by interferon is greater in patients who have high pre-existing theophylline clearance due to smoking.[3]

Related Drugs: *Interferon-α2b (Intron A)* and theophylline interact similarly. Aminophylline and interferon interact similarly.

Management Options:
- *Monitor* for excessive theophylline response if interferon is given, especially in theophylline-treated patients who are smokers or other patients in whom theophylline clearance may be high [e.g., those on enzyme inducers such as barbiturates, carbamazepine (Tegretol), phenytoin (Dilantin), primidone (Mysoline), and rifampin (Rifadin)]. The effect of interferon on theophylline elimination appears to occur rapidly, so expect to see increased plasma theophylline concentrations within a day or two of interferon administration.

References:
1. Okuno H et al. Depression of drug metabolizing activity in the human liver by interferon-alpha. Eur J Clin Pharmacol. 1990;39:365.
2. Jonkman JHG et al. Effects of alpha-interferon on theophylline pharmacokinetics and metabolism. Br J Clin Pharmacol. 1989;27:795.
3. Williams SJ et al. Inhibition of theophylline metabolism by interferon. Lancet. 1987;2:939.

---

### Interferon (Betaseron)

### Zidovudine (Retrovir)

Summary: Beta interferon markedly increases the plasma concentrations of zidovudine.

Risk Factors: No specific risk factors known.

Related Drugs: *Interleukin-2 (IL-2)* interacts similarly.

Management Options:
- *Circumvent/Minimize.* Patients taking zidovudine who are given beta interferon should be given reduced doses of zidovudine. If additional studies substantiate the large degree of metabolic inhibition, zidovudine doses could be reduced by 75% or more.

---

## Significance Classification

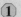 - *Avoid Combination.* Risk always outweighs benefit.

 - *Usually Avoid Combination.* Use combination only under special circumstances.

 - *Minimize Risk.* Take action as necessary to reduce risk.

• *Monitor* for altered zidovudine effect if beta interferon is initiated, discontinued or changed in dosage; adjust zidovudine dose as needed.

References:

1. Nolta M et al. Molecular interaction of recombinant beta interferon and zidovudine (AZT): alternations of AZT pharmacokinetics in HIV-infected patients. Fifth International Conference on AIDS. Quebec; 1989:278. Abstract.
2. Skinner MH et al. IL-2 does not alter zidovudine kinetics. Clin Pharmacol Ther. 1989;45:128. Abstract.

**Iron**

**Levodopa (Larodopa)**

Summary: Oral iron reduced levodopa bioavailability by half in a single-dose study of normal subjects; the importance of this interaction in parkinsonian patients on chronic levodopa therapy is not established.

Risk Factors: No specific risk factors known.

Related Drugs: Theoretically, other oral iron preparations also would be expected to reduce levodopa absorption; however, the small amounts of iron found in most vitamin-mineral products probably are insufficient to produce much interaction.

Management Options:

• *Circumvent/Minimize.* Until more information is available, separate the doses of iron and levodopa as much as possible, and monitor the patient for inadequate levodopa response.

• *Monitor* for reduced levodopa response if the combination is used.

References:

1. Campbell NRC et al. Ferrous sulfate reduces levodopa bioavailability: chelation as a possible mechanism. Clin Pharmacol Ther. 1989;45:220.

**Iron**

**Methyldopa (Aldomet)**

Summary: Pharmacokinetic studies in healthy subjects and blood pressure measurements in hypertensive patients both indicate that oral iron may inhibit the antihypertensive response to methyldopa.

Risk Factors No specific risk factors known.

Related Drugs: Although the effect of oral iron salts other than ferrous sulfate and ferrous gluconate on methyldopa is not known, assume that they interact until proven otherwise. The amount of iron in most multivitamins may not be sufficient to inhibit methyldopa absorption, but clinical studies are needed to confirm this. Parenteral iron would not be expected to interact, but this has not been studied. Little is known regarding the effect of iron on antihypertensives other than methyldopa.

Management Options:

• *Consider Alternative.* Methyldopa has disadvantages compared to many other antihypertensives; consider alternative therapy.

- *Circumvent/Minimize.* Give methyldopa 2 hours before or 6 hours after oral iron.
- *Monitor* for reduced antihypertensive response when oral iron and methyldopa are used concurrently.

References:
1. Campbell N et al. Alteration of methyldopa absorption, metabolism and blood pressure control caused by ferrous sulfate and ferrous gluconate. Clin Pharmacol Ther. 1988;43:381.

## Iron

### Norfloxacin (Noroxin)

Summary: The administration of iron salts with norfloxacin lowers the antibiotic serum concentration and may lead to therapeutic failure.

Risk Factors: No specific risk factors known.

Related Drugs: Other quinolones [e.g. *ciprofloxacin (Cipro)*] have been reported to be affected similarly by iron.[1-3,5] *Ofloxacin (Floxin)* absorption may be less affected by iron.[2,5]

Management Options:
- *Consider Alternative.* Patients taking norfloxacin should not take oral iron concurrently since serum norfloxacin concentrations may be subtherapeutic.
- *Circumvent/Minimize.* The administration of norfloxacin at least 2 hours before oral iron would theoretically reduce the magnitude of the interaction. IV iron could be used to avoid the interaction.
- *Monitor.* If the drugs are used together, watch for lessened antibiotic effect.

References:
1. Polk RE et al. Effect of ferrous sulfate and multivitamins with zinc on absorption of ciprofloxacin in normal volunteers. Antimicrob Agents Chemother. 1989;33:1841.
2. Akerele JO et al. Influence of oral co-administered metallic drug on ofloxacin pharmacokinetics. J Antimicrob Chemother. 1991;28:87.
3. Kara M et al. Clinical and chemical interactions between iron preparations and ciprofloxacin. Br J Clin Pharmacol. 1991;31:257.
4. Campbell NCR et al. Norfloxacin interactions with antacids and minerals. Br J Clin Pharmacol. 1992;33:115.
5. Lehto P et al. The effect of ferrous sulphate on the absorption of norfloxacin, ciprofloxacin and ofloxacin. Br J Clin Pharmacol. 1994; 37:82.

## Iron

### Penicillamine (Cuprimine)

Summary: Oral iron may reduce plasma penicillamine concentrations substantially; reduced therapeutic response to penicillamine may occur in some patients.

Risk Factors: No specific risk factors known.

Related Drugs: No information available.

Management Options:
- *Circumvent/Minimize.* Patients receiving penicillamine (e.g., for rheumatoid arthritis) should separate penicillamine ingestion from oral iron to minimize mixing in the gastrointestinal tract. Theoretically, giving the penicillamine a few hours *before* the iron would minimize the interaction.
- *Monitor.* Be alert for evidence of reduced penicillamine response, and adjust the penicillamine dosage as needed.

References:
1. Lyle WH. Penicillamine and iron. Lancet. 1976;2:420. Letter.
2. Osman MA et al. Reduction in oral penicillamine absorption by food, antacid, and ferrous sulfate. Clin Pharmacol Ther. 1983;33:465.

## Iron
### Tetracycline

Summary: Oral iron products may reduce the serum concentrations and, possibly, the antibacterial efficacy of tetracycline.

Risk Factors: No specific risk factors known.

Related Drugs: **Oxytetracycline (Terramycin)**, **methacycline (Rondomycin)**, and **doxycycline (Vibramycin)** interact similarly with oral iron products.

Management Options:
- *Consider Alternative.* On the basis of current evidence, iron preparations should not be administered simultaneously with oral tetracyclines. When possible, a different antibiotic should be chosen if iron is administered.
- *Circumvent/Minimize.* If both need to be given to a patient, ferrous sulfate should be administered 3 hours before or 2 hours after tetracycline to minimize the interaction between them.[1] However, the separation of doses may not circumvent interactions between doxycycline and iron preparations.
- *Monitor.* If tetracycline and iron are coadministered, be alert for reduced antibiotic effects.

## Significance Classification

1. - *Avoid Combination.* Risk always outweighs benefit.
2. - *Usually Avoid Combination.* Use combination only under special circumstances.
3. - *Minimize Risk.* Take action as necessary to reduce risk.

References:
1. Mattila MJ et al. Interference of iron preparations and milk with the absorption of tetracyclines. In: Exerpta Medica International Congress Series No. 254. Amsterdam: Exerpta Medica; 1972:128–33.
2. Neuvonen P et al. Interference of iron with the absorption of tetracyclines in man. Br Med J. 1970;4:532.
3. Neuvonen PJ et al. Effect of oral ferrous sulphate on the half-life of doxycycline in man. Eur J Clin Pharmacol. 1974;7:361.

## Iron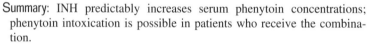

## Vitamin E

**Summary:** Vitamin E may impair the hematologic response to iron therapy in children with iron-deficiency anemia.

**Risk Factors:** No specific risk factors known.

**Related Drugs:** No information available.

**Management Options:**

- *Monitor.* Patients with iron-deficiency anemia who are receiving iron therapy should be observed for impaired hematologic response if vitamin E is given concomitantly.

References:
1. Melhorn DK et al. Relationships between iron-dextran and vitamin E in an iron deficiency anemia in children. J Lab Clin Med. 1969;74:789.

## Isoniazid (INH)

## Phenytoin (Dilantin)

**Summary:** INH predictably increases serum phenytoin concentrations; phenytoin intoxication is possible in patients who receive the combination.

**Risk Factors:**

- *Pharmacogenetics.* Patients who are slow metabolizers of INH are at increased risk for the interaction.

**Related Drugs:** No information available.

**Management Options:**

- *Monitor.* Patients receiving both INH and phenytoin should be watched closely for signs of phenytoin toxicity (e.g., ataxia, nystagmus, mental impairment, involuntary muscular movements, seizures); the phenytoin dose should be decreased if necessary. If INH is discontinued, monitor the patient for a decreased therapeutic response to phenytoin and increase the dose as needed.

References:
1. Kutt H et al. Diphenylhydantoin intoxication. A complication of isoniazid therapy. Am Rev Respir Dis. 1970;101:377.

2. Brennan RW et al. Diphenylhydantoin intoxication attendant to slow inactivation of isoniazid. Neurology. 1970;20:687.
3. Miller RR et al. Clinical importance of the interaction of phenytoin and isoniazid. Chest. 1979;75:356.

## Isoniazid (INH)
### Prednisolone (Prelone)

Summary: Prednisolone may reduce the plasma concentrations of INH.
Risk Factors:
- *Pharmacogenetics.* Patients who are rapid INH acetylators are at increased risk for the interaction.

Related Drugs: Other corticosteroids might be similarly affected.
Management Options:
- *Monitor.* In patients receiving concurrent INH and corticosteroids, watch for evidence of reduced INH effect and enhanced corticosteroid effect.

References:
1. Sarma GR et al. Effect of prednisone and rifampin on isoniazid metabolism in slow and rapid inactivators of isoniazid. Antimicrob Agents Chemother. 1980;18:661.
2. Brodie MJ et al. Effect of isoniazid on vitamin D metabolism and hepatic monooxygenase activity. Clin Pharmacol Ther. 1981;30:363.

## Isoniazid (INH)
### Rifampin (Rifadin)

Summary: Although rifampin may increase the hepatic toxicity of INH in certain predisposed patients, the combination does not cause hepatotoxicity in the vast majority of patients.
Risk Factors:
- *Pharmacogenetics.* Patients who are slow INH acetylators are at increased risk for the interaction.
- *Concurrent Diseases.* Patients with pre-existing liver disease and those having recently undergone general anesthesia are at increased risk of the interaction.

Related Drugs: No information available.
Management Options:
- *Monitor.* Patients receiving INH and rifampin should be monitored for evidence of hepatotoxicity, especially if they are known to be slow acetylators of INH and/or have pre-existing liver disease.

References:
1. Beever IW et al. Circulating hydrazine during treatment with isoniazid and rifampicin in man. Br J Clin Pharmacol. 1982;13:599.
2. Sarma GR et al. Rifampin-induced release of hydrazine from isoniazid. Am Rev Resp Dis. 1986;133:1072.
3. Steele MA et al. Toxic hepatitis with isoniazid and rifampin. A meta-analysis. Chest. 1991;99:465.

## Isoniazid (INH)

### Theophylline

Summary: Theophylline plasma concentrations increased following several weeks of INH administration; some patients may develop theophylline toxicity.

Risk Factors: No specific risk factors known.

Related Drugs: No information available.

Management Options:

- *Monitor.* Patients stabilized on theophylline should be monitored for increased theophylline concentrations when INH is administered. The interaction may require several weeks to reach its full potential.

References:

1. Torrent J et al. Theophylline-isoniazid interaction. DICP, Ann Pharmacother. 1989; 23:143.
2. Dal Nergo R et al. Rifampicin-isoniazid and delayed elimination of theophylline: a case report. Int J Clin Pharm Res. 1988;8:275.
3. Samigun M et al. Lowering of theophylline clearance by isoniazid in slow and rapid acetylators. Br J Clin Pharmacol. 1990;29:570.

## Isoniazid (INH)

### Triazolam (Halcion)

Summary: INH may increase triazolam serum concentrations; the clinical significance is unknown.

Risk Factors: No specific risk factors known.

Related Drugs: INH inhibits the metabolism of *diazepam (Valium)*.

Management Options:

- *Monitor.* Watch for evidence of increased sedation when triazolam is administered with INH.

References:

1. Ochs HR et al. Interaction of triazolam with ethanol and isoniazid. Clin Pharmacol Ther. 1983;33:241.

## Isoniazid (INH)

### Valproic Acid (Depakene)

Summary: In 1 patient, valproic acid plasma concentrations increased after the addition of INH resulting in symptoms of valproic acid toxicity.

Risk Factors:

- *Pharmacogenetics.* Patients who are slow acetylators of INH are at increased risk for the interaction.

Related Drugs: No information available.

Management Options:

- *Monitor.* Patients should be monitored for changes in response to valproic acid when INH is started (nausea, sedation) or stopped (reduced seizure control).

References:
1. Jonville AP et al. Interaction between isoniazid and valproate: a case of valproate overdosage. Eur J Clin Pharmacol. 1991;40:197.

## Isoniazid (INH)

## Warfarin (Coumadin)

Summary: Isolated case reports and theoretical considerations indicate that INH may enhance the effect of oral anticoagulants such as warfarin, but the incidence and clinical significance of this interaction are unknown.

Risk Factors: No specific risk factors known.

Related Drugs: Other oral anticoagulants may be similarly affected.

Management Options:
- *Monitor.* Patients stabilized on oral anticoagulants should be monitored for increased hypoprothrombinemic response when INH therapy is initiated and decreased response when it is discontinued. Initiation of oral anticoagulant therapy in a patient already on chronic INH should not pose difficulties because the patient can be titrated to the proper dose of anticoagulant.

References:
1. Rosenthal AR et al. Interaction of isoniazid and warfarin. JAMA. 1977;238:2177.
2. Otis PT et al. An acquired inhibitor of fibrin stabilization associated with isoniazid therapy: clinical and biochemical observations. Blood. 1974;44:771.

## Isradipine (DynaCirc)
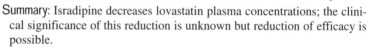

## Lovastatin (Mevacor)

Summary: Isradipine decreases lovastatin plasma concentrations; the clinical significance of this reduction is unknown but reduction of efficacy is possible.

Risk Factors: No specific risk factors known.

Related Drugs: The effect of isradipine on other HMG-CoA inhibitors is unknown, but they may be similarly affected.

Management Options:
- *Monitor.* Until more information is available, patients taking lovastatin should be monitored for reduced effects during isradipine coadministration.

References:
1. Holtzman JL et al. Interaction between isradipine and lovastatin in normal male volunteers. Clin Pharmacol Ther. 1993;53:164. Abstract.
2. Zhou L-X et al. Pharmacokinetic interaction between isradipine and lovastatin in normal, female and male volunteers. J Pharmacol Exper Ther. 1995;273:121.

## Itraconazole (Sporanox)

## Lovastatin (Mevacor)

Summary: Itraconazole administration produces a very large increase in lovastatin concentrations; toxicity including rhabdomyolysis may occur. Avoid concurrent use.

Risk Factors: No specific risk factors known.

Related Drugs: *Simvastatin (Zocor)* and *atorvastatin (Lipitor)* are metabolized in a similar manner to lovastatin and their metabolism probably would be inhibited by itraconazole. *Pravastatin (Pravachol)* may not be as dependent on CYP3A4 metabolism and therefore may not be inhibited to the same extent by itraconazole. The safety of *fluvastatin (Lescol)* has not been established. *Ketoconazole (Nizoral), miconazole (Monistat),* and *fluconazole (Diflucan)* would be expected to inhibit the metabolism of some HMG-CoA reductase inhibitors. *Terbinafine (Lamisil)* may have minimal effect on the metabolism of HMG-CoA reductase inhibitors.

Management Options:

- *Use Alternative.* Pending further studies on other HMG-CoA reductase inhibitors, lovastatin and probably simvastatin should not be administered with itraconazole or other inhibitors of CYP3A4. The safety of pravastatin or fluvastatin when combined with itraconazole has not been established. Terbinafine may have minimal effect on the metabolism of the HMG-CoA reductase inhibitors since it does not appear to inhibit CYP3A4 activity. Patients receiving HMG-CoA reductase inhibitors, especially lovastatin or simvastatin, should be monitored carefully for muscle pain or weakness when any drug known to inhibit the activity of CYP3A4 is administered.

References:

1. Lees RS et al. Rhabdomyolysis from the coadministration of lovastatin and the antifungal agent itraconazole. N Engl J Med. 1995;333:664.
2. Neuvonen PJ et al. Itraconazole drastically increases plasma concentrations of lovastatin and lovastatin acid. Clin Pharmacol Ther. 1996;60:54.

### Itraconazole (Sporanox)

### Midazolam (Versed)

Summary: Itraconazole administration causes a large increase in oral midazolam plasma concentrations and pharmacodynamic effects; increased side effects are likely.

Risk Factors:

- *Route of Administration.* Plasma midazolam concentrations will increase to a greater extent following oral administration than after intravenous midazolam dosing.

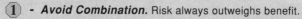

## Significance Classification

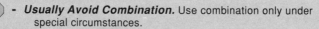

(1) - *Avoid Combination.* Risk always outweighs benefit.

(2) - *Usually Avoid Combination.* Use combination only under special circumstances.

(3) - *Minimize Risk.* Take action as necessary to reduce risk.

Related Drugs: **Ketoconazole (Nizoral)** and **fluconazole (Diflucan)** also reduce the metabolism of midazolam. **Terbinafine (Lamisil)** does not affect midazolam pharmacokinetics. Other benzodiazepines metabolized by CYP3A4 also will be affected by itraconazole, including **alprazolam (Xanax)** and **triazolam (Halcion)**. Benzodiazepines that are metabolized by glucoronidation [e.g., **oxazepam (Serax), lorazepam (Ativan), temazepam (Restoril)**] will likely be minimally affected by itraconazole.

Management Options:

- *Consider Alternative.* Patients maintained on itraconazole should be prescribed an oral benzodiazepine that is not metabolized via the CYP3A4 enzyme. (See Related Drugs.) Patients stabilized on midazolam requiring antifungal therapy might be candidates for terbinafine.

- *Monitor.* Patients receiving both oral midazolam and itraconazole should be carefully monitored for increased sedation and reduced psychomotor performance.

References:

1. Ahonen J et al. Effect of itraconazole and terbinafine on the pharmacokinetics and pharmacodynamics of midazolam in healthy volunteers. Br J Clin Pharmacol. 1995;40:270.
2. Olkkola KT et al. Midazolam should be avoided in patients receiving the systemic antimycotics ketoconazole and itraconazole. Clin Pharmacol Ther. 1994;55:481.
3. Olkkola KT et al. The effect of the systemic antimycotics, itraconazole and fluconazole, on the pharmacokinetics and pharmacodynamics of intravenous and oral midazolam. Anesth Analg. 1996;82:511.

**Itraconazole (Sporanox)**

**Phenytoin (Dilantin)**

**2**

Summary: Phenytoin dramatically reduces itraconazole serum concentrations and is likely to reduce its therapeutic response.

Risk Factors: No specific risk factors known.

Related Drugs: Enzyme inducers other than phenytoin also have been shown to reduce itraconazole serum concentrations.

Management Options:

- *Use Alternative.* Given the marked reduction in itraconazole serum concentrations, it would be prudent to use an alternative antifungal agent in patients receiving phenytoin. Ketoconazole (Nizoral) metabolism also is increased by enzyme inducers and probably would not be a suitable alternative. Phenytoin is not likely to substantially affect fluconazole (Diflucan) (eliminated primarily unchanged by the kidneys), but fluconazole can inhibit phenytoin metabolism (via inhibition of CYP2C9). Thus, if fluconazole is used, monitor for increased phenytoin effect.

References:

1. Ducharme MP et al. Itraconazole and hydroxyitraconazole serum concentrations are reduced more than tenfold by phenytoin. Clin Pharmacol Ther. 1995;58:617.

## Itraconazole (Sporanox)

## Rifampin (Rifadin)

Summary: Rifampin appears to reduce itraconazole plasma concentrations; the interaction may reduce the efficacy of itraconazole.

Risk Factors: No specific risk factors known.

Related Drugs: Rifampin also reduces the concentration of *fluconazole (Diflucan)* and *ketoconazole (Nizoral)*.

Management Options:

- *Monitor.* Until further information is available, patients should be observed for reduced itraconazole concentrations and response when they are receiving rifampin.

References:

1. Blomley M et al. Itraconazole and anti-tuberculosis drugs. Lancet. 1990;336:1255. Letter.
2. Tucker RM et al. Interaction of azoles with rifampin, phenytoin, and carbamazepine: In vitro and clinical observations. Clin Infect Dis. 1992;14:165.
3. Drayton J et al. Coadministration of rifampin and itraconazole leads to undetectable levels of serum itraconazole. Clin Infect Dis. 1994;18:266. Letter.

## Itraconazole (Sporanox)

## Terfenadine (Seldane)

Summary: Itraconazole administration produces elevated plasma concentrations of terfenadine that can lead to prolonged QTc intervals and ventricular arrhythmias. Terfenadine should not be taken by patients requiring itraconazole for antifungal therapy.

Risk Factors: No specific risk factors known.

Related Drugs: Other antifungal agents, including *ketoconazole (Nizoral)* and *fluconazole (Diflucan)*, have been noted to increase terfenadine concentrations. *Astemizole (Hismanal)* concentrations have been noted to increase when it is administered with antifungal agents. *Cetirizine (Zyrtec)* and *loratadine (Claritin)* appear to be less likely to interact with itraconazole and produce cardiotoxicity.

Management Options:

- *Avoid Combination.* Until more information on the interaction between itraconazole and terfenadine is available, it would be prudent to avoid giving the 2 drugs together. The use of sedating antihistamines or perhaps loratadine instead of terfenadine would seem to be preferred in patients taking itraconazole or other oral antifungal agents.

References:

1. Honig PK et al. Itraconazole affects single-dose terfenadine pharmacokinetics and cardiac repolarization pharmacodynamics. J Clin Pharmacol. 1993;33:1201.
2. Crane JK et al. Syncope and cardiac arrhythmia due to an interaction between itraconazole and terfenadine. Am J Med. 1993;95:445.

3. Pohjola-Sintonen S et al. Itraconazole prevents terfenadine metabolism and increases risk of torsades de pointes ventricular tachycardia. Eur J Clin Pharmacol. 1993;45:191.

### Itraconazole (Sporanox)

### Triazolam (Halcion)

Summary: Itraconazole administration produces large increases in triazolam concentrations and pharmacologic effects.

Risk Factors:
- *Route of Administration.* Oral administration of triazolam increases the risk for the interaction.

Related Drugs: **Midazolam (Versed)** and **diazepam (Valium)** concentrations are likely to be increased by itraconazole. **Ketoconazole (Nizoral)** or **fluconazole (Diflucan)** administration may result in increased triazolam concentrations.

Management Options:
- *Avoid Unless Benefit Outweighs Risk.* The concomitant administration of triazolam and itraconazole should be avoided.
- *Monitor.* Patients receiving triazolam and itraconazole should be monitored for increased triazolam effects including drowsiness and prolonged amnesia. Reduced doses of triazolam should be considered in patients taking itraconazole.

References:
1. Varhe A et al. Oral triazolam is potentially hazardous to patients receiving systemic antimycotics ketoconazole or itraconazole. Clin Pharmacol Ther. 1994;56:601.

### Itraconazole (Sporanox)

### Warfarin (Coumadin)

Summary: A patient stabilized on warfarin developed excessive hypoprothrombinemia and severe bleeding after itraconazole was added to her regimen.

Risk Factors: No specific risk factors known.

Related Drugs: Other azole antifungal agents such as **fluconazole (Diflucan)**, **ketoconazole (Nizoral)**, and **miconazole (Monistat)** also have been reported to increase the hypoprothrombinemic response to warfarin. The effect of itraconazole on oral anticoagulants other than warfarin is unknown, but theoretically **phenprocoumon** would be less likely to interact.

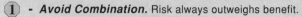

## Significance Classification

①  -  *Avoid Combination.* Risk always outweighs benefit.

②  -  *Usually Avoid Combination.* Use combination only under special circumstances.

③  -  *Minimize Risk.* Take action as necessary to reduce risk.

Management Options:
- *Monitor* for altered oral anticoagulant effect if itraconazole is initiated, discontinued, or changed in dosage. Adjust the anticoagulant dose as needed.

References:
1. Yeh J et al. Potentiation of action of warfarin by itraconazole. Br Med J. 1990; 301:669.

## Kaolin-Pectin
## Lincomycin (Lincocin)

Summary: Kaolin-pectin mixtures may reduce the antibacterial efficacy of lincomycin.

Risk Factors: No specific risk factors known.

Related Drugs: *Clindamycin (Cleocin)* may be similarly affected by kaolin-pectin.

Management Options:
- *Avoid Unless Benefit Outweighs Risk.* Kaolin-pectin should generally not be administered to patients taking lincomycin.
- *Monitor* for reduced lincomycin efficacy if administered with kaolin-pectin.

References:
1. Wagner JG. Pharmacokinetics 1. Definitions, modeling and reasons for measuring blood levels and urinary excretion. Drug Intell Clin Pharm. 1968;2:38.
2. McCall CE et al. Lincomycin: activity *in vitro* and absorption and excretion in normal young men. Am J Med Sci. 1967;254:144.
3. McGehee RF Jr et al. Comparative studies of antibacterial activity *in vitro* and absorption and excretion of lincomycin and clindamycin. Am J Med Sci. 1968; 256:279.

## Kaolin-Pectin
## Quinidine

Summary: Kaolin-pectin reduces quinidine plasma concentrations when the 2 drugs are administered concurrently.

Risk Factors: No specific risk factors known.

Related Drugs: No information available.

Management Options:
- *Circumvent/Minimize.* Although no data are available on the effect of separating the doses of quinidine and kaolin-pectin, it would be prudent to administer kaolin-pectin suspension several hours after quinidine to minimize this interaction.
- *Monitor.* Quinidine concentrations and diminished antiarrhythmic efficacy should be monitored if kaolin-pectin is coadministered.

References:
1. Moustafa MA et al. Decreased bioavailability of quinidine sulphate due to interactions with adsorbent antacids and antidiarrheal mixtures. Int J Pharm. 1987;34:207.

### Ketoconazole (Nizoral)

### Loratadine (Claritin)

Summary: Ketoconazole administration increases loratadine plasma concentrations; the clinical significance of this effect is unknown.

Risk Factors: No specific risk factors known.

Related Drugs: Other antifungal agents [*miconazole (Monistat)*, *itraconazole (Sporanox)*, *fluconazole (Diflucan)*] are likely to increase loratadine concentrations.

Management Options:
- *Monitor.* Patients receiving ketoconazole and loratadine should be monitored for increased loratadine effects.

References:
1. Brannan MD et al. Effects of various cytochrome p450 inhibitors on the metabolism of loratadine. Clin Pharmacol Ther. 1995;57:193. Abstract.

### Ketoconazole (Nizoral)

### Lovastatin (Mevacor)

Summary: Like itraconazole, ketoconazole administration may produce very large increases in lovastatin concentrations; toxicity including rhabdomyolysis may occur. Avoid concurrent use.

Risk Factors: No specific risk factors known.

Related Drugs: *Simvastatin (Zocor)* and *atorvastatin (Lipitor)* are metabolized in a similar manner to lovastatin and their metabolism probably would be inhibited by ketoconazole. *Pravastatin (Pravachol)* may not be as dependent on CYP3A4 metabolism and therefore may not be inhibited to the same extent by ketoconazole. The safety of *fluvastatin (Lescol)* has not been established. *Itraconazole (Sporanox)*, *miconazole (Monistat)*, and *flucon-azole (Diflucan)* would be expected to inhibit the metabolism of some HMG-CoA reductase inhibitors. *Terbinafine (Lamisil)* may have minimal effect on the metabolism of HMG-CoA reductase inhibitors.

Management Options:
- *Use Alternative.* Pending studies on other HMG-CoA reductase inhibitors, lovastatin and probably simvastatin should not be administered with ketoconazole or other inhibitors of CYP3A4. The safety of pravastatin or fluvastatin when combined with ketoconazole has not been established. Terbinafine may have minimal effect on the metabolism of the HMG-CoA reductase inhibitors since it does not appear to inhibit CYP3A4 activity. Patients receiving HMG-CoA reductase inhibitors, especially lovastatin or simvastatin, should be monitored carefully for muscle pain or weakness when any drug known to inhibit the activity of CYP3A4 is administered.

References:
1. Neuvonen PJ et al. Itraconazole drastically increases plasma concentrations of lovastatin and lovastatin acid. Clin Pharmacol Ther. 1996;60:54.

## Ketoconazole (Nizoral)

### Methylprednisolone (Medrol)

Summary: Ketoconazole increases methylprednisolone concentrations and enhances methylprednisolone-induced suppression of cortisol secretion.

Risk Factors: No specific risk factors known.

Related Drugs: Ketoconazole has been reported to inhibit the metabolism of *prednisolone (Prelone)*.

Management Options:

- *Monitor.* Patients receiving methylprednisolone may require dosage adjustments when ketoconazole is added to or removed from their drug regimens.

References:

1. Glynn AM et al. Effects of ketoconazole on methylprednisolone pharmacokinetics and cortisol secretion. Clin Pharmacol Ther. 1986;39:654.
2. Kandrotas RJ et al. Ketoconazole effects on methylprednisolone disposition and their joint suppression of endogenous cortisol. Clin Pharmacol Ther. 1987;42:465.

## Ketoconazole (Nizoral)

### Midazolam (Versed)

Summary: Oral midazolam concentrations were markedly increased following ketoconazole administration; increased sedation and psychomotor impairment should be expected.

Risk Factors:

- *Route of Administration.* Plasma midazolam concentrations will increase to a greater extent following oral administration than after IV midazolam dosing.

Related Drugs: *Itraconazole (Sporanox)*, *fluconazole (Diflucan)*, and *miconazole (Monistat)* are likely to reduce midazolam's metabolism. Ketoconazole is likely to inhibit other benzodiazepines that are metabolized by CYP3A4 such as *alprazolam (Xanax)* and *triazolam (Halcion)*. Benzodiazepines not metabolized via the CYP3A4 enzyme [e.g., *lorazepam (Ativan)*, *oxazepam (Serax)*, *temazepam (Restoril)*] are less likely to be affected.

Management Options:

- *Consider Alternative.* Patients maintained on ketoconazole should be prescribed a benzodiazepine that is not metabolized via the CYP3A4 enzyme. (See Related Drugs.) Patients stabilized on midazolam requiring antifungal therapy should be considered for terbinafine.
- *Monitor.* Patients receiving both midazolam and ketoconazole should be carefully monitored for increased sedation and reduced psychomotor performance.

References:

1. Olkkola KT et al. Midazolam should be avoided in patients receiving the systemic antimycotics ketoconazole and itraconazole. Clin Pharmacol Ther. 1994;55:481.

### Ketoconazole (Nizoral)

### Omeprazole (Prilosec)

Summary: An increase in gastric pH will reduce the absorption of keto-conazole (Nizoral).

Risk Factors: No specific risk factors known.

Related Drugs: Any agent that increases the pH of the stomach will reduce the absorption of ketoconazole. Thus, antacids, $H_2$-antagonist drugs [e.g., *cimetidine (Tagamet)*, *ranitidine (Zantac)*], and *lansoprazole (Prevacid)* would reduce ketoconazole absorption. *Fluconazole (Diflucan)* absorption is not affected by the pH of the stomach.[2]

Management Options:

- *Circumvent/Minimize.* The administration of an acidic drink such as Coca-Cola will help to minimize this interaction. The dose of keto-conazole may need to be increased when used with drugs that increase gastric pH. With long duration of acid suppression caused by the proton pump inhibitors, it would be difficult to separate doses to minimize the effects on ketoconazole absorption.
- *Consider Alternative.* Consider using fluconazole in patients with a gastric pH that is higher than usual as a result of other medications.
- *Monitor* for therapeutic failure when ketoconazole is administered to patients with elevated gastric pH.

References:

1. Chin TWF et al. Effects of an acidic beverage (Coca-Cola) on absorption of keto-conazole. Antimicrob Agents Chemother. 1995;39:1671.
2. Blum RA et al. Increased gastric pH and the bioavailability of fluconazole and keto-conazole. Ann Intern Med. 1991;114:755.

### Ketoconazole (Nizoral)

### Quinidine

Summary: In a patient stabilized on quinidine, ketoconazole was associated with a marked increase in quinidine plasma concentrations.

Risk Factors: No specific risk factors known.

Related Drugs: Other azole CYP3A4-inhibiting antifungals [e.g., *fluconazole (Diflucan)*, *miconazole (Monistat)*, *itraconazole (Sporanox)*] would be expected to have similar effects on quinidine metabolism.

## Significance Classification

 - *Avoid Combination.* Risk always outweighs benefit.

 - *Usually Avoid Combination.* Use combination only under special circumstances.

 - *Minimize Risk.* Take action as necessary to reduce risk.

Management Options:

- *Monitor.* Until more definitive studies are available, patients stabilized on quinidine should be observed for increased plasma concentrations and electrocardiographic changes (prolonged QRS) when ketoconazole is added to their regimen.

References:

1. McNulty RM et al. Transient increase in plasma quinidine concentrations during ketoconazole-quinidine therapy. Clin Pharm. 1989;8:222.

## Ketoconazole (Nizoral)

### Ranitidine (Zantac)

Summary: Ranitidine administration reduces the plasma concentrations of ketoconazole, potentially resulting in loss of antifungal effect.

Risk Factors: No specific risk factors known.

Related Drugs: Other oral antifungal agents may be similarly affected by ranitidine administration. Other $H_2$-receptor antagonists [e.g., *cimetidine (Tagamet), nizatidine (Axid), famotidine (Pepcid)*] and proton pump inhibitors [e.g., *omeprazole (Prilosec), lansoprazole (Prevacid)*] would be expected to produce similar reactions with ketoconazole.

Management Options:

- *Circumvent/Minimize.* Several recommendations have been made to avoid this interaction in patients with elevated gastric pH. The product information for ketoconazole suggests that each ketoconazole tablet should be dissolved in 4 mL of an aqueous solution of 0.2 N hydrochloric acid with the resulting mixture ingested with a straw (to avoid contact with teeth) and followed by a glass of water.[2] Others suggest that an easier and equally effective method is to give 2 capsules of glutamic acid hydrochloride (Acidulin) 15 minutes before the ketoconazole.[3]

- *Monitor.* Until more is known about this interaction, be alert for evidence of reduced ketoconazole effect when ranitidine or other agents that increase gastric pH are coadministered.

References:

1. Piscitelli SC et al. Effects of ranitidine and sucralfate on ketoconazole bioavailability. Antimicrob Agents Chemother. 1991;35:1795.
2. Nizoral. Physician's Desk Reference. 47th ed. Oradell: Medical Economics Data; 1993:1172.
3. Lelawongs P et al. Effect of food and gastric acidity on absorption of orally administered ketoconazole. Clin Pharm. 1988;7:228.

## Ketoconazole (Nizoral)

### Rifampin (Rifadin)

Summary: Rifampin and isoniazid (INH) decrease the plasma concentration of ketoconazole, and ketoconazole appears to decrease the peak plasma concentration of rifampin.

Risk Factors: No specific risk factors known.

Related Drugs: Rifampin reduces the concentration of *fluconazole (Diflucan)* and *itraconazole (Sporanox)*.

Management Options:
- *Circumvent/Minimize.* Separation of the rifampin and ketoconazole doses by 12 hours may prevent depression of rifampin concentrations.
- *Monitor.* Patients should be observed for therapeutic failure when rifampin or INH are administered with ketoconazole. Likewise, the response to rifampin should be checked when ketoconazole is coadministered.

References:
1. Engelhard D et al. Interaction of ketoconazole with rifampin and isoniazid. N Engl J Med. 1984;311:1681.
2. Meunier F. Serum fungistatic and fungicidal activity in volunteers receiving antifungal agents. Eur J Clin Microbiol. 1986;5:103.
3. Doble N et al. Pharmacokinetic study of the interaction between rifampicin and ketoconazole. J Antimicrob Chemother. 1988;21:633.

### Ketoconazole (Nizoral)
### Saquinavir (Invirase)

Summary: Ketoconazole administration can result in a large increase in saquinavir serum concentrations; toxicity may result in some patients.

Risk Factors: No specific risk factors known.

Related Drugs: Ketoconazole is known to increase the serum concentration of *indinavir (Crixivan)*. The effects of other azole antifungal agents [e.g., itraconazole (Sporanox), fluconazole (Diflucan)] that inhibit CYP3A4 metabolism on saquinavir is unknown, but some increase in saquinavir serum concentration would be expected. *Terbinafine (Lamisil)* does not appear to inhibit CYP3A4 activity and may not increase saquinavir concentrations.

Management Options:
- *Consider Alternative.* Although no specific data are available, terbinafine does not appear to inhibit CYP3A4 activity and might provide an alternative antifungal agent that may not increase saquinavir concentrations.
- *Circumvent/Minimize.* It may be necessary to reduce the dose of saquinavir when ketoconazole is coadministered.
- *Monitor.* Pending further information on this interaction, monitor patients for increased saquinavir serum concentrations and abdominal discomfort or diarrhea.

References:
1. Hoffman-La Roche, Inc. Saquinavir (Invirase) package insert. 1995.

### Ketoconazole (Nizoral)

### Sucralfate (Carafate)

Summary: The concomitant administration of sucralfate and ketoconazole reduces the plasma concentration of the antifungal agent; the clinical importance of the reduction is unknown.

Risk Factors: No specific risk factors known.

Related Drugs: No information available.

Management Options:

• *Circumvent/Minimize.* Ketoconazole should be administered at least 2 hours before sucralfate to minimize any interaction.

• *Monitor.* If ketoconazole and sucralfate are coadministered, monitor for reduced antifungal effects.

References:

1. Piscitelli SC et al. Effects of ranitidine and sucralfate on ketoconazole bioavailability. Antimicrob Agents Chemother. 1991;35:1765.
2. Carver PL et al. In vivo interaction of ketoconazole and sucralfate in healthy volunteers. Antimicrob Agents Chemother. 1994;38:326.

### Ketoconazole (Nizoral)

### Tacrolimus (Prograf)

Summary: Ketoconazole increases the concentration of orally administered tacrolimus; toxicity may result.

Risk Factors:

• *Route of Administration.* The oral administration of tacrolimus will produce an interaction of greater magnitude with ketoconazole than that following the intravenous (IV) administration of tacrolimus.

Related Drugs: *Cyclosporine (Sandimmune)* is similarly affected by ketoconazole administration. Other azole antifungal agents [e.g., *itraconazole (Sporanox)* and *fluconazole (Diflucan)*] are likely to affect orally administered tacrolimus in a similar manner.

Management Options:

• *Consider Alternative.* Patients stabilized on tacrolimus who require antifungal therapy should be considered for an alternative antifungal agent. Since itraconazole and fluconazole may produce similar effects on the bioavailability of tacrolimus, terbinafine (Lamisil), which does not appear to reduce CYP3A4 or P-glycoprotein activity, should be considered.

• *Circumvent/Minimize.* The dose of tacrolimus should be reduced, based upon blood concentrations, if it is administered with ketoconazole.

• *Monitor.* Tacrolimus blood concentrations should be checked during coadministration with ketoconazole.

References:

1. Floren LC et al. Tacrolimus oral bioavailability doubles with coadministration of ketoconazole. Clin Pharmacol Ther. 1997;62:41.

## Ketoconazole (Nizoral)

### Terfenadine (Seldane)

**Summary:** Excessive terfenadine concentrations following concomitant ketoconazole administration may increase the risk of cardiac arrhythmias.

**Risk Factors:**
- *Concurrent Diseases.* Pre-existing cardiac conduction problems increase the risk for the interaction.

**Related Drugs:** Other oral antifungal agents [e.g., *itraconazole (Sporanox)*, *fluconazole (Diflucan)*] have been reported to inhibit the metabolism of terfenadine. *Astemizole (Hismanal)* metabolism also has been noted to be reduced during oral antifungal therapy.

**Management Options:**
- *Avoid Combination.* Until more information on the interaction between ketoconazole and terfenadine is available, it would be prudent to avoid giving the 2 drugs together. The use of sedating antihistamines or perhaps cetirizine (Zyrtec) or loratadine (Claritin) instead of terfenadine would seem to be preferred in patients taking ketoconazole or other oral antifungal agents.

**References:**
1. Zimmermann M et al. Torsades de pointes after treatment with terfenadine and ketoconazole. Eur Heart J. 1992;13:1002.
2. Eller MG et al. Pharmacokinetic interaction between terfenadine and ketoconazole. Clin Pharmacol Ther. 1991;49:130. Abstract.
3. Honig P et al. The pharmacokinetics and cardiac consequences of the terfenadine-ketoconazole interaction. Clin Pharmacol Ther. 1993;53:206. Abstract.

## Ketoconazole (Nizoral)

### Triazolam (Halcion)

**Summary:** Triazolam plasma concentrations are markedly elevated by the coadministration of ketoconazole; increased toxicity is likely to result.

**Risk Factors:** No specific risk factors known.

**Related Drugs:** *Itraconazole (Sporanox)*, *fluconazole (Diflucan)*, and *miconazole (Monistat)* are likely to reduce triazolam's metabolism. Ketoconazole is likely to inhibit other benzodiazepines that are metabolized by CYP3A4 such as *alprazolam (Xanax)* and oral *midazolam (Versed)*. Benzodiazepines not metabolized via the CYP3A4 enzyme [e.g., *lorazepam (Ativan)*, *oxazepam (Serax)*] are less likely to be affected.

**Management Options:**
- *Consider Alternative.* Patients maintained on ketoconazole should be prescribed a benzodiazepine that is not metabolized via the CYP3A4 enzyme. (See Related Drugs.) Patients stabilized on triazolam requiring antifungal therapy should be considered for terbinafine.
- *Monitor.* Patients receiving both triazolam and ketoconazole should be carefully monitored for increased sedation and reduced psychomotor performance.

References:
1. von Moltke LL et al. Triazolam biotransformation by human liver microsomes *in vitro*: effects of metabolic inhibitors and clinical confirmation of a predicted interaction with ketoconazole. J Pharmacol Exper Ther. 1996;276:370.
2. Wright CE et al. Ketoconazole inhibition of triazolam and alprazolam clearance: differential kinetic and dynamic consequences. Clin Pharmacol Ther. 1997;61:183. Abstract.

## Ketoconazole (Nizoral)

### Warfarin (Coumadin)

Summary: Isolated case reports, as well as the known interactive properties of the 2 drugs, suggest that ketoconazole increases the hypoprothrombinemic response of warfarin.

Risk Factors: No specific risk factors known.

Related Drugs: Other azole antifungal agents such as *fluconazole (Diflucan)*, *itraconazole (Sporanox)*, and *miconazole (Monistat)* also have been reported to increase the hypoprothrombinemic response to warfarin. The effect of ketoconazole on oral anticoagulants other than warfarin is not established, but an interaction may occur (with the possible exception of *phenprocoumon*, which is metabolized primarily by glucuronidation).

Management Options:
• *Monitor* for altered oral anticoagulant effect if ketoconazole is initiated, discontinued, or changed in dosage. Adjust the anticoagulant dose as needed.

References:
1. Smith AG. Potentiation of oral anticoagulants by ketoconazole. Br Med J. 1984; 288:188.

## Ketoprofen (Orudis)

### Methotrexate (Mexate)

Summary: Isolated cases indicate that ketoprofen may increase the toxicity of antineoplastic doses of methotrexate.

Risk Factors:
• *Dosage Regimen.* The risk of adverse effects from this interaction is primarily in patients receiving antineoplastic doses of methotrexate, rather than the lower doses used to treat rheumatoid arthritis, psoriasis, and related diseases.

## Significance Classification

 - *Avoid Combination.* Risk always outweighs benefit.

 - *Usually Avoid Combination.* Use combination only under special circumstances.

 - *Minimize Risk.* Take action as necessary to reduce risk.

- *Concurrent Diseases.* Particular caution is suggested in patients with pre-existing renal impairment [who may be more susceptible to non-steroidal anti-inflammatory drug (NSAID)-induced renal failure].

Related Drugs: Other NSAIDs may interact similarly, however, more information is needed.

Management Options:

- *Avoid Unless Benefit Outweighs Risk.* Until more information is available on this interaction, it would be prudent to avoid ketoprofen (as well as other NSAIDs) in patients receiving antineoplastic doses of methotrexate. Particular caution is suggested in patients with pre-existing renal impairment, who may be more susceptible to NSAID-induced renal failure.

- *Monitor.* If the combination is used, monitor for methotrexate toxicity. Findings in methotrexate toxicity can include stomatitis, severe gastrointestinal symptom (nausea, diarrhea, vomiting), bone marrow suppression, fever, bleeding, skin rashes, nephrotoxicity, and hepatotoxicity. Although decreasing the methotrexate dosage would be expected to reduce the likelihood of toxicity, the magnitude of the required reduction in methotrexate dosage has not been established.

References:

1. Furst DE et al. Effect of aspirin and sulindac on methotrexate clearance. J Pharm Sci. 1990;79:782.
2. Dupuis LL et al. Methotrexate-nonsteroidal antiinflammatory drug interaction in children with arthritis. J Rheumatol. 1990;17:1469.
3. Skeith KJ et al. Lack of significant interaction between low dose methotrexate and ibuprofen or flurbiprofen in patients with arthritis. J Rheumatol. 1990;17:1008.

### Ketoprofen (Orudis)

### Warfarin (Coumadin)

**2**

Summary: A patient well controlled on chronic warfarin therapy developed excessive hypoprothrombinemia and bleeding after starting ketoprofen therapy. However, this patient may have been particularly predisposed to the interaction, and more study will be needed to determine the incidence and magnitude of the effect.

Risk Factors:

- *Concurrent Diseases.* Patients with peptic ulcer disease or a history of gastrointestinal (GI) bleeding are probably at greater risk for the interaction.

Related Drugs: All NSAIDs inhibit platelet function, cause gastric erosions, and probably increase the risk of GI bleeding. Some NSAIDs, however, such as *ibuprofen (Advil)*, *naproxen (Naprosyn)*, or *diclofenac (Voltaren)*, may be less likely to increase oral anticoagulant-induced hypoprothrombinemia than other NSAIDs.

Management Options:

- *Avoid Unless Benefit Outweighs Risk.* Since all NSAIDs probably increase the risk of GI bleeding in patients on oral anticoagulants,

use the combination only after careful consideration of the benefit versus risk. If an NSAID must be used with an oral anticoagulant, it would be prudent to use NSAIDs that are unlikely to affect the hypoprothrombinemic response to oral anticoagulants. If the NSAID is being used as an analgesic or antipyretic, acetaminophen (Tylenol) probably is safer to use with oral anticoagulants. Nonacetylated salicylates (e.g., choline salicylate, magnesium salicylate, salsalate, sodium salicylate) also probably are safer with oral anticoagulants than NSAIDs, since such salicylates have minimal effects on platelet function and the gastric mucosa.

- *Monitor.* If any NSAID is used with an oral anticoagulant, one should carefully monitor the prothrombin time and watch for evidence of bleeding, especially from the GI tract.

References:
1. Flessner MF et al. Prolongation of prothrombin time and severe gastrointestinal bleeding associated with combined use of warfarin and ketoprofen. JAMA. 1988; 259:353.
2. Shorr RI et al. Concurrent use of nonsteroidal anti-inflammatory drugs and oral anticoagulants places elderly persons at high risk for hemorrhagic peptic ulcer disease. Arch Intern Med. 1993;153:1665.
3. Mieszczak C et al. Lack of interaction of ketoprofen with warfarin. Eur J Clin Pharmacol. 1993;44:205.

## Ketorolac (Toradol)

### Lithium (Eskalith)

Summary: A patient receiving lithium developed about a doubling of his lithium serum concentrations after starting ketorolac, but the incidence and magnitude of this interaction is not established.

Risk Factors: No specific risk factors known.

Related Drugs: Most NSAIDs increase lithium serum concentrations, but *sulindac (Clinoril)* and *aspirin* appear to have minimal effects.

Management Options:

- *Consider Alternative.* If appropriate for the patient, consider using an anti-inflammatory agent that is less likely to affect lithium, such as sulindac or aspirin.

- *Monitor.* If ketorolac therapy is initiated in a patient taking lithium, monitor serum lithium concentrations and look for evidence of lithium toxicity (e.g., nausea, vomiting, diarrhea, anorexia, coarse tremor, slurred speech, vertigo, confusion, and lethargy; in severe cases, seizures, stupor, coma, and cardiovascular collapse). In a patient stabilized on lithium and an NSAID, discontinuation of the NSAID may result in inadequate lithium serum concentrations.

References:
1. Langlois R et al. Increased serum lithium levels due to ketorolac therapy. Can Med Assoc J. 1994;150:1455.

### Lamotrigine (Lamictal)

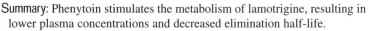

### Phenytoin (Dilantin)

Summary: Phenytoin stimulates the metabolism of lamotrigine, resulting in lower plasma concentrations and decreased elimination half-life.

Risk Factors: No specific risk factors known.

Related Drugs: The effect of **phenobarbital** on lamotrigine has not been studied directly. However, the known inducing properties of phenobarbital and carbamazepine would be consistent with decreasing lamotrigine concentrations.

Management Options:

- *Monitor.* In patients stabilized on enzyme inducing drugs, monitor for the need to use larger than expected doses of lamotrigine. Also be aware that discontinuing phenytoin may affect lamotrigine dosage requirements.

References:

1. Jawad S et al. Lamotrigine: single dose pharmacokinetics and initial 1 week experience in refractory epilepsy. Epilepsy Res. 1987;1:194.
2. Cohen AF et al. Lamotrigine, a new anticonvulsant: pharmacokinetics in normal humans. Clin Pharmacol Ther. 1987;41:535.
3. Wolf P et al. Lamotrigine: preliminary clinical observations on pharmacokinetics and interactions with traditional antiepileptic drugs. J Epilepsy. 1992;5:73.

### Lamotrigine (Lamictal)

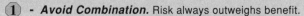

### Valproic Acid (Depakene)

Summary: Valproic acid inhibits the metabolism of lamotrigine, resulting in higher plasma concentrations and increased elimination half-life. Lamotrigine stimulates the metabolism of valproic acid, resulting in lower plasma concentrations.

Risk Factors: No specific risk factors known.

Related Drugs: No information available.

Management Options:

- *Monitor.* In patients stabilized on valproic acid, lower doses of lamotrigine are necessary, initially. Starting with low doses of lamotrigine and a slow rate of therapy escalation, appears to decrease the incidence of rash. One also should be aware that discontinuation of valproic acid may affect lamotrigine dosage requirements. The clin-

## Significance Classification

(1) - *Avoid Combination.* Risk always outweighs benefit.

(2) - *Usually Avoid Combination.* Use combination only under special circumstances.

(3) - *Minimize Risk.* Take action as necessary to reduce risk.

ical significance of the effect of lamotrigine on valproic acid is unclear; however, increasing doses of valproic acid on initiation of lamotrigine is probably not necessary.

References:
1. Cohen AF et al. Lamotrigine, a new anticonvulsant: pharmacokinetics in normal humans. Clin Pharmacol Ther. 1987;41:535.
2. Anderson GD et al. Effect of lamotrigine on the pharmacokinetics and biotransformation of valproate. Epilepsia. 1992;33:82. Abstract.
3. Smith D et al. Outcomes of add-on treatment of lamotrigine in partial epilepsy. Epilepsia. 1993;34:312.

## Levodopa (Larodopa)

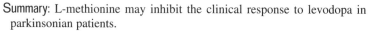

### Methionine

Summary: L-methionine may inhibit the clinical response to levodopa in parkinsonian patients.

Risk Factors: No specific risk factors known.

Related Drugs: No information available.

Management Options:
- *Circumvent/Minimize.* Large doses of methionine probably should be avoided in parkinsonian patients receiving levodopa.
- *Monitor* for reduced levodopa effect if the combination is used.

References:
1. Pearce LA et al. L-methionine: a possible levodopa antagonist. Neurology. 1974; 24:640.

## Levodopa (Larodopa)

### Moclobemide

Summary: Moclobemide appeared to increase the risk of adverse effects (e.g., headache, nausea) in healthy subjects receiving levodopa; but more study is needed.

Risk Factors: No specific risk factors known.

Related Drugs: The effect of other MAO-A inhibitors on levodopa is not established.

Management Options:
- *Monitor.* If moclobemide is used in a patient receiving levodopa, one should monitor for the need to adjust the levodopa dosage.

References:
1. Dingemanse J. An update of recent moclobemide interaction data. Int Clin Psychopharmacol. 1993;7:167.

## Levodopa (Larodopa)

### Phenelzine (Nardil)

Summary: The administration of levodopa with nonselective monoamine oxidase inhibitors (MAOIs) may result in a hypertensive response.

Risk Factors:
- *Dosage Regimen.* One patient receiving phenelzine became hypertensive with a 50 mg dose of levodopa but not with a 25 mg dose.[1]
- *Other Drugs.* Concurrent use of carbidopa with levodopa appears to minimize the interaction with nonselective MAOIs.

Related Drugs: All nonselective MAOIs including **isocarboxazid (Marplan)** and tranylcypromine would be expected to interact with levodopa in the absence of a decarboxylase inhibitor. **Nialamide** and **tranylcypromine (Parnate)** interact similarly with levodapa.

Management Options:
- *Circumvent/Minimize.* The use of a decarboxylase inhibitor (e.g., carbidopa) with levodopa apparently prevents the hypertensive reactions.
- *Monitor.* The use of nonselective MAOIs with levodopa (in the absence of a decarboxylase inhibitor) generally should be avoided. Remember that the effects of nonselective MAOIs should be assumed to persist for 2 weeks after they are discontinued. If they are given concomitantly, blood pressure must be monitored very carefully. If hypertension ensues, the results of 1 case indicate that phentolamine (Regitine) may reverse the hypertension.[1]

References:
1. Hunter KR et al. Monoamine oxidase inhibitors and L-dopa. Br Med J. 1970;3:388.
2. Corder CN et al. Postural hypotension: adrenergic responsivity and levodopa therapy. Neurology. 1977;27:921.
3. Collier DS et al. Parkinsonism treatment: Part III—update. Ann Pharmacother. 1992;26:227.

## Levodopa (Larodopa)

## Phenytoin (Dilantin)

Summary: Preliminary patient data indicate that phenytoin may inhibit the antiparkinsonian effect of levodopa.

Risk Factors: No specific risk factors known.

Related Drugs: No information available.

Management Options:
- *Consider Alternative.* Although this interaction is based on limited evidence, consider alternatives to phenytoin in parkinsonian patients receiving levodopa.
- *Circumvent/Minimize.* If the combination is used, a larger dose of levodopa may be required.
- *Monitor.* Be alert for evidence of levodopa's reduced antiparkinson effect if phenytoin is taken concurrently.

References:
1. Mendez JS et al. Diphenylhydantoin blocking of levodopa effects. Arch Neurol. 1975;32:44.

## Levodopa (Larodopa)

## Pyridoxine (Vitamin B₆)

Summary: Pyridoxine inhibits the antiparkinsonian effect of levodopa, but few patients are affected since concurrent use of carbidopa negates the interaction.

Risk Factors:
- *Other Drugs.* The interaction occurs only in the absence of concurrent therapy with a peripheral decarboxylase inhibitor (e.g., carbidopa).

Related Drugs: No information available.

Management Options:
- *Circumvent/Minimize.* Pyridoxine and vitamin preparations containing pyridoxine should be avoided in patients receiving levodopa unless a peripheral decarboxylase inhibitor (e.g., carbidopa) is also being given.
- *Monitor* for reduced levodopa response if pyridoxine is used in the absence of a decarboxylase inhibitor.

References:
1. Fahn S. "On-off" phenomenon with levodopa therapy in parkinsonism. Neurology. 1974;24:431.
2. Mars H. Levodopa, carbidopa, and pyridoxine in Parkinson disease. Metabolic interactions. Arch Neurol. 1974;30:444.
3. Mims RB et al. Inhibition of L-dopa-induced growth hormone stimulation of pyridoxine and chlorpromazine. J Clin Endocrinol Metab. 1975;40:256.

## Levodopa (Larodopa)

## Spiramycin (Rovamycine)

Summary: Spiramycin reduces the plasma concentration of levodopa; antiparkinson efficacy may be reduced.

Risk Factors: No specific risk factors known.

Related Drugs: It is not known whether other macrolide antibiotics (e.g., erythromycin) that stimulate gastric motility would produce a similar effect. **Carbidopa** interacts similarly with spiramycin.

Management Options:
- *Monitor.* Until studies in patients with Parkinson's disease are available, spiramycin and other macrolide antibiotics that increase gastrointestinal transit should be administered to patients taking levodopa-carbidopa combinations only with close observation for increased symptoms of Parkinson's disease.

References:
1. Brion N et al. Effect of a macrolide (spiramycin) on the pharmacokinetics of l-dopa and carbidopa in healthy volunteers. Clin Neuropharmacol. 1992;15:229.

## Levodopa (Larodopa)

### Tacrine (Cognex)

Summary: Tacrine may inhibit the effect of levodopa in patients with parkinsonism; dosage adjustments of one or both drugs may be required.

Risk Factors: No specific risk factors known.

Related Drugs: No information available.

Management Options:

- *Consider Alternative.* Before giving tacrine to a patient with parkinsonism (whether on levodopa or not) one should consider the risk of worsening the parkinsonism.
- *Monitor.* If tacrine is used in a patient with parkinsonism, the doses of the tacrine and/or the antiparkinson drugs may need to be adjusted.

References:

1. Ott BR, Lannon MC. Exacerbation of parkinsonism by tacrine. Clin Neuropharmacol. 1992;15:322.

## Lidocaine (Xylocaine)

### Propranolol (Inderal)

Summary: Lidocaine concentrations may become excessive during concomitant propranolol administration.

Risk Factors: No specific risk factors known.

Related Drugs: **Metoprolol (Lopressor)** and **nadolol (Corgard)** interact similarly with lidocaine. Other beta blockers also may enhance the negative inotropic effects of lidocaine. **Pindolol (Visken)** reportedly has no effect on lidocaine clearance.[2]

Management Options:

- *Monitor.* Patients who receive concurrent therapy with beta blockers and lidocaine should be monitored carefully for increased lidocaine effects. The magnitude of the reduction in lidocaine clearance probably varies with different beta blockers, but no generalizations are possible at this time.

References:

1. Bax NDS et al. The impairment of lidocaine clearance by propranolol—major contribution from enzyme inhibition. Br J Clin Pharmacol. 1985;19:597.
2. Svendsen TL et al. Effects of propranolol and pindolol on plasma lignocaine clearance in man. Br J Clin Pharmacol. 1982;13:223S.
3. Schneck DW et al. Effects of nadolol and propranolol on plasma lidocaine clearance. Clin Pharmacol Ther. 1984;36:584.

## Lisinopril (Prinivil)

### Lithium (Eskalith)

Summary: Several case reports suggest that lisinopril and other angiotensin-converting enzyme (ACE) inhibitors may increase the risk of serious lithium toxicity, but the incidence of this effect is unknown.

Risk Factors: No specific risk factors known.

Related Drugs: Given the proposed mechanism, it appears likely that all ACE inhibitors [e.g., *enalapril (Vasotec)*] have the potential to produce lithium toxicity.

Management Options:

- *Consider Alternative.* If possible, avoid the concurrent use of ACE inhibitors and lithium. Although it appears that patients can be stabilized on the two drugs, it is possible that other factors (e.g., diarrhea) may unmask the interaction, resulting in lithium toxicity. If an alternative to an ACE inhibitor is used, remember that other antihypertensives, such as thiazides, calcium channel blockers, methyldopa (Aldomet), and possibly propranolol (Inderal) and spironolactone (Aldactone), may affect lithium response as well.

- *Monitor.* If the combination of an ACE inhibitor and lithium is used, monitor the serum lithium concentration if ACE inhibitors are initiated, discontinued, or changed in dosage. Monitor the patient for clinical evidence of lithium toxicity (e.g., nausea, vomiting, diarrhea, anorexia, coarse tremor, slurred speech, vertigo, confusion, lethargy; in severe cases, seizures, stupor, coma, and cardiovascular collapse). Adjust lithium dose as needed.

References:

1. Navis GJ et al. Volume homeostasis, angiotensin converting enzyme inhibition, and lithium therapy. Am J Med. 1989;86:621.
2. Baldwin CM et al. A case of lisinopril-induced lithium toxicity. DICP, Ann Pharmacother. 1990;24:946.
3. Correa FJ et al. Angiotensin-converting enzyme inhibitors and lithium toxicity. Am J Med. 1992;93:108.

## Lithium (Eskalith)

## Losartan (Cozaar)

Summary: An elderly patient developed lithium toxicity after starting losartan, but more study is needed to establish the clinical importance of this effect.

Risk Factors: No specific risk factors known.

Related Drugs: The effect of angiotensin-2 receptor antagonists other than losartan on lithium is not established; theoretically they should interact similarly.

## Significance Classification

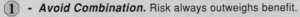

① - *Avoid Combination.* Risk always outweighs benefit.

② - *Usually Avoid Combination.* Use combination only under special circumstances.

③ - *Minimize Risk.* Take action as necessary to reduce risk.

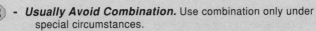

Management Options:
- *Monitor.* Be alert for evidence of lithium toxicity (nausea, vomiting, diarrhea, anorexia, coarse tremor, slurred speech, vertigo, confusion, lethargy; in severe cases, seizures, stupor, coma, and cardiovascular collapse). Adjust lithium dose as needed.

References:
1. Blanche P et al. Lithium intoxication in an elderly patient after combined treatment with losartan. Eur J Clin Pharmacol. 1997;52:501.

### Lithium (Eskalith)

### Mefenamic Acid (Ponstel)

Summary: Isolated cases of lithium toxicity have been associated with mefenamic acid therapy.

Risk Factors: No specific risk factors known.

Related Drugs: Most NSAIDs increase lithium serum concentrations, but **sulindac (Clinoril)** and **aspirin** appear to have minimal effects.

Management Options:
- *Consider Alternative.* If appropriate for the patient, consider using an anti-inflammatory agent that is less likely to affect lithium, such as sulindac or aspirin.
- *Monitor.* If mefenamic acid therapy is initiated in the presence of lithium therapy, monitor serum lithium concentrations and for symptoms consistent with lithium toxicity (e.g., nausea, vomiting, diarrhea, anorexia, coarse tremor, slurred speech, vertigo, confusion, lethargy; in severe cases, seizures, stupor, coma, and cardiovascular collapse). In a patient stabilized on lithium and an NSAID, discontinuation of the NSAID may result in inadequate serum lithium concentrations.

References:
1. MacDonald J et al. Toxic interaction of lithium carbonate and mefenamic acid. Br Med J. 1988;297:1339.
2. Shelly RK. Lithium toxicity and mefenamic acid: a possible interaction and the role of prostaglandin inhibition. Br J Psychiatry. 1987;151:847.

### Lithium (Eskalith)

### Methyldopa (Aldomet)

Summary: Methyldopa was associated with evidence of lithium toxicity in several patients, but a causal relationship was not firmly established.

Risk Factors: No specific risk factors known.

Related Drugs: No information available.

Management Options:
- *Consider Alternative.* In patients who need lithium therapy, consider using antihypertensive therapy other than methyldopa.
- *Monitor.* If the combination is used, monitor for evidence of lithium intoxication (e.g., nausea, vomiting, tremor, confusion, weakness,

dizziness, slurred speech). Plasma lithium concentrations may not be useful in detecting this interaction since they may be in the therapeutic range.

References:
1. Yassa R. Lithium-methyldopa interaction. Can Med Assoc J. 1986;134:141.
2. Osanloo E et al. Interaction of lithium and methyldopa. Ann Intern Med. 1980; 92:433.
3. Walker N et al. Lithium-methyldopa interactions in normal subjects. Drug Intell Clin Pharm. 1980;14:638.

## Lithium (Eskalith)
## Naproxen (Naprosyn)

Summary: Naproxen increases lithium serum concentrations and may increase the risk of lithium toxicity; the magnitude of the effect appears to vary considerably from patient to patient.

Risk Factors: No specific risk factors known.

Related Drugs: Most NSAIDs increase lithium serum concentrations, but *sulindac (Clinoril)* and *aspirin* appear to have minimal effects.

Management Options:
- *Consider Alternative.* If appropriate for the patient, consider using an anti-inflammatory agent that is less likely to affect lithium, such as sulindac or aspirin.
- *Monitor.* If naproxen therapy is initiated in the presence of lithium therapy, monitor serum lithium concentrations and for symptoms consistent with lithium toxicity (e.g., nausea, vomiting, diarrhea, anorexia, coarse tremor, slurred speech, vertigo, confusion, lethargy; in severe cases, seizures, stupor, coma, and cardiovascular collapse). In a patient stabilized on lithium and an NSAID, discontinuation of the NSAID may result in inadequate serum lithium concentrations.

References:
1. Ragheb M et al. Lithium interaction with sulindac and naproxen. J Clin Psychopharmacol. 1986;6:150.

## Lithium (Eskalith)
## Phenelzine (Nardil)

Summary: Two fatal cases of malignant hyperpyrexia have been reported in patients taking lithium and phenelzine, but a causal relationship was not established.

Risk Factors: No specific risk factors known.

Related Drugs: Until more information is available, one should assume that other nonselective monoamine oxidase inhibitors (MAOIs) such as *isocarboxazid (Marplan)* and *tranylcypromine (Parnate)* also can interact with lithium.

Management Options:
- *Avoid Unless Benefit Outweighs Risk.* Given the severity of the reported interactions, it would be prudent to avoid concurrent use of lithium with nonselective MAOIs until additional information is available. The effects of nonselective MAOIs should be assumed to persist for 2 weeks after they are discontinued.
- *Monitor.* Patients treated with nonselective MAOIs and lithium should be observed closely for evidence of neuroleptic malignant-like syndrome.

References:
1. Brennan D et al. Neuroleptic malignant syndrome without neuroleptics. Br J Psychiatry. 1988;152:578.
2. Staufenberg EF et al. Malignant hyperpyrexia syndrome in combined treatment. Br J Psychiatry. 1989;154:577.

### Lithium (Eskalith)

### Phenylbutazone (Butazolidin)

Summary: Phenylbutazone appears to increase lithium serum concentrations, but the magnitude of the effect appears to vary considerably from patient to patient. Limited evidence suggests that phenylbutazone may result in adverse psychiatric symptoms in patients receiving lithium.

Risk Factors: No specific risk factors known.

Related Drugs: Most NSAIDs increase lithium serum concentrations, but **sulindac (Clinoril)** and **aspirin** appear to have minimal effects.

Management Options:
- *Consider Alternative.* If appropriate for the patient, consider using an anti-inflammatory agent that is less likely to affect lithium, such as sulindac or aspirin.
- *Monitor* serum lithium concentrations and for symptoms consistent with lithium toxicity (e.g., nausea, vomiting, diarrhea, anorexia, coarse tremor, slurred speech, vertigo, confusion, lethargy; in severe cases, seizures, stupor, coma, and cardiovascular collapse) when phenylbutazone therapy is initiated. In a patient stabilized on lithium and an NSAID, discontinuation of the NSAID may result in inadequate serum lithium concentrations.

References:
1. Ragheb M. The interaction of lithium with phenylbutazone in bipolar affective patients. J Clin Psychopharmacol. 1990;10:149. Letter.

## Significance Classification

(1) - *Avoid Combination.* Risk always outweighs benefit.

(2) - *Usually Avoid Combination.* Use combination only under special circumstances.

(3) - *Minimize Risk.* Take action as necessary to reduce risk.

## Lithium (Eskalith)

## Phenytoin (Dilantin)

Summary: Some patients have developed lithium intoxication following phenytoin use, but a causal relationship has not been established.

Risk Factors: No specific risk factors known.

Related Drugs: No information available.

Management Options:
- *Monitor.* Until more information is available, be alert for evidence of lithium toxicity when phenytoin is given concurrently.

References:
1. Salem RB et al. Ataxia as the primary symptom of lithium toxicity. Drug Intell Clin Pharm. 1980;14:621.
2. Spiers J et al. Severe lithium toxicity within normal serum concentrations. Br Med J. 1978;1:815.
3. MacCallum WAG. Interaction of lithium and phenytoin. Br Med J. 1980;280:610.

## Lithium (Eskalith)

## Piroxicam (Feldene)

Summary: Piroxicam was associated with symptoms of lithium toxicity in one well-documented case report, but the incidence of this effect in patients receiving this drug combination is not known.

Risk Factors: No specific risk factors known.

Related Drugs: Most nonsteroidal anti-inflammatory drugs increase lithium serum concentrations, but **sulindac (Clinoril)** and **aspirin** appear to have minimal effects.

Management Options:
- *Consider Alternative.* If appropriate for the patient, consider using an anti-inflammatory agent that is less likely to affect lithium, such as sulindac or aspirin.
- *Monitor.* Be alert for evidence of increased lithium effect when piroxicam is started or stopped (e.g., nausea, vomiting, diarrhea, anorexia, coarse tremor, slurred speech, vertigo, confusion, lethargy; in severe cases, seizures, stupor, coma, and cardiovascular collapse). Serum lithium determinations would be useful in monitoring this interaction.

References:
1. Kerry RJ et al. Possible toxic interaction between lithium and piroxicam. Lancet. 1983;1:418.

## Lithium (Eskalith)

## Potassium Iodide

Summary: Hypothyroidism may be more likely in patients receiving both lithium and potassium iodide than in those receiving either drug alone, but the degree of increased risk is not established.

Risk Factors: No specific risk factors known.

Related Drugs:  No information available.

Management Options:

- *Monitor.* If it is necessary to use lithium and iodide concomitantly, monitor the patient for signs of hypothyroidism.

References:

1. Shopsin B et al. Iodine and lithium-induced hypothyroidism: documentation of synergism. Am J Med. 1973;55:695.
2. Swedberg K et al. Heart failure as complication of lithium treatment. Acta Med Scand. 1974;196:279.
3. Jorgensen JV et al. Possible synergism between iodine and lithium carbonate. JAMA. 1973;223:192. Letter.

## Lithium (Eskalith)

### Sodium Bicarbonate

Summary: Sodium bicarbonate may lower plasma lithium concentrations.

Risk Factors: No specific risk factors known.

Related Drugs: No information available.

Management Options:

- *Monitor.* Patients on combined sodium bicarbonate and lithium therapy should be monitored for decreased lithium effect. Lithium blood levels may be helpful in assessing this interaction.

References:

1. Thomsen K et al. Renal lithium excretion in man. Am J Physiol. 1968;215:823.

## Lithium (Eskalith)

### Sodium Chloride

Summary: High sodium intake may reduce serum lithium concentrations, while restriction of sodium may increase serum lithium.

Risk Factors: No specific risk factors known.

Related Drugs: No information available.

Management Options:

- *Circumvent/Minimize.* Extremely large or small intakes of sodium chloride should be avoided in patients receiving lithium carbonate. Patients on severe salt-restricted diets probably should not be given lithium carbonate.
- *Monitor* for increased lithium response if sodium intake is reduced and for decreased lithium response if sodium intake is increased.

References:

1. Hurtig HI et al. Lithium toxicity enhanced by diuresis. N Engl J Med. 1974;290:748.
2. Levy ST et al. Lithium-induced diabetes insipidus: manic symptoms, brain and electrolyte correlates, and chlorothiazide treatment. Am J Psychiatry. 1973;130:1014.
3. Demers RG et al. Sodium intake and lithium treatment in mania. Am J Psychiatry. 1971;128:1.

## Lithium (Eskalith)

### Theophylline

Summary: Theophylline appears to increase renal lithium clearance in most patients; the magnitude of the effect probably is sufficient to reduce lithium efficacy in some patients.

Risk Factors: No specific risk factors known.

Related Drugs: No information available.

Management Options:

- *Circumvent/Minimize.* Intermittent use of theophylline in a patient on chronic lithium is best avoided, since the patient's response to lithium may fluctuate each time the theophylline is started or stopped.

- *Monitor.* When initiating theophylline therapy in a patient on chronic lithium, be alert for evidence of reduced lithium response. Discontinuation of theophylline therapy in a patient receiving lithium may result in excessive lithium response. When initiating lithium therapy in a patient on chronic theophylline, lithium dosage requirements may be higher than anticipated. Measurement of serum lithium concentrations would be useful in monitoring this interaction.

References:
1. Thomsen K et al. Renal lithium excretion in man. Am J Physiol. 1968;215:823.
2. Sierles FS et al. Concurrent use of theophylline and lithium in a patient with chronic obstructive lung disease and bipolar disorder. Am J Psychiatry. 1982;139:117.
3. Cook BL et al. Theophylline-lithium interaction. J Clin Psychiatry. 1985;46:278.

## Lithium (Eskalith)

### Verapamil (Calan)

Summary: The addition of verapamil or diltiazem (Cardizem) to patients stabilized on lithium therapy may result in neurotoxicity.

Risk Factors: No specific risk factors known.

Related Drugs: If this interaction is due to additive effects on cellular calcium transport, other calcium channel blockers might interact in a similar manner. Other case reports describe the development of stiffness and rigidity[2] or psychosis[3] after **diltiazem (Cardizem)** was added to lithium therapy.

Management Options:

- *Monitor.* The use of calcium blockers in the treatment of patients with bipolar disorders receiving lithium should be commenced carefully with observation for neurotoxic effects. More experience with this interaction is necessary to determine if anticholinergic agents will be useful in controlling some of the symptoms associated with the interaction.

References:
1. Price WA et al. Lithium-verapamil toxicity in the elderly. J Am Geriatr Soc. 1987;35:177.

Чад

2. Valdiserri EV. A possible interaction between lithium and diltiazem: case report. J Clin Psychiatry. 1985;46:540.
3. Binder EF et al. Diltiazem-induced psychosis and a possible diltiazem-lithium interaction. Arch Intern Med. 1991;151:373.

## Lorazepam (Ativan) / Loxapine (Loxitane)  [3]

**Summary:** Isolated cases of respiratory depression, stupor, and hypotension have been observed in patients receiving loxapine and lorazepam, but the role that a drug interaction played in these cases was not established.

**Risk Factors:** No specific risk factors known.

**Related Drugs:** Positive results of combining benzodiazepines and neuroleptics also have been reported. Diazepam increased the antipsychotic response to neuroleptic agents in schizophrenic patients,[2] and lorazepam appeared to alleviate auditory hallucinations in a schizophrenic patient receiving 1 gm/day of *chlorpromazine (Thorazine).*[3] Other combinations of neuroleptics and benzodiazepines have been used without excessive adverse effects.

**Management Options:**
- *Monitor.* Until more information is available, patients receiving loxapine and lorazepam should be monitored carefully for excessive sedation and respiratory depression. With any other combination of a neuroleptic and a benzodiazepine, consider the possibility of additive sedative effects and monitor patients accordingly.

**References:**
1. Battaglia et al. Loxapine-lorazepam-induced hypotension and stupor. J Clin Psychopharmacol. 1989;9:227. Letter.
2. Lingjaerde O et al. Antipsychotic effect of diazepam when given in addition to neuroleptics in chronic psychotic patients: a double-blind clinical trial. Curr Ther Res. 1979;26:505.
3. Yassa R et al. Lorazepam as an adjunct in the treatment of auditory hallucinations in a schizophrenic patient. J Clin Psychopharmacol. 1989;9:386. Letter.

## Lovastatin (Mevacor) / Nicotinic Acid (Niacin)  [3]

**Summary:** Isolated cases of myopathy and rhabdomyolysis have occurred in patients receiving lovastatin and niacin, but a causal relationship has not been established.

**Risk Factors:** No specific risk factors known.

**Related Drugs:** Little is known about whether niacin increases the risk of myopathy when it is combined with simvastatin (Zocor). *Fluvastatin (Lescol)* does not appear to result in myopathy when combined with niacin. Theoretically, *pravastatin (Pravachol)* also would be unlikely to interact with niacin.

**Management Options:**
- *Monitor.* Although the interaction between lovastatin and niacin is not well documented, patients receiving the combination should be

alert for muscular symptoms such as pain, tenderness, or weakness; creatine kinase should be measured in patients with such symptoms. Early recognition of this disorder is important as it may progress to acute renal failure in some patients if the drugs are not discontinued promptly.

References:

1. Reaven P et al. Lovastatin, nicotinic acid, and rhabdomyolysis. Ann Intern Med. 1988;109:597.
2. Tobert JA. Rhabdomyolysis in patients receiving lovastatin after cardiac transplantation. N Engl J Med. 1988;318:47.
3. Norman DJ et al. Myolysis and acute renal failure in a heart-transplant recipient receiving lovastatin. N Engl J Med. 1988;318:46.

### Lovastatin (Mevacor)

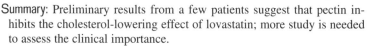

### Pectin (Kapectolin)

Summary: Preliminary results from a few patients suggest that pectin inhibits the cholesterol-lowering effect of lovastatin; more study is needed to assess the clinical importance.

Risk Factors: No specific risk factors known.

Related Drugs: The effect of pectin on HMG-CoA reductase inhibitors other than lovastatin is not established.

Management Options:

• *Circumvent/Minimize*. Although it is unknown whether separating the administration of lovastatin and pectin would avoid the interaction, it would be prudent to give lovastatin 2 hours before or 4 hours after pectin.

• *Monitor* for reduced lovastatin response if the combination is given.

References:

1. Richter WO et al. Interaction between fibre and lovastatin. Lancet. 1991;338:706.

### Lovastatin (Mevacor)

### Warfarin (Coumadin)

Summary: Lovastatin has been associated with increased hypoprothrombinemic response to warfarin in a number of patients, but the incidence with magnitude of this effect is not established.

Risk Factors: No specific risk factors known.

## Significance Classification

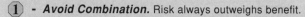
(1) - *Avoid Combination.* Risk always outweighs benefit.

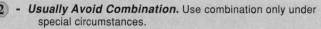
(2) - *Usually Avoid Combination.* Use combination only under special circumstances.

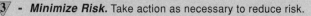
(3) - *Minimize Risk.* Take action as necessary to reduce risk.

Related Drugs: The effect of lovastatin on oral anticoagulants other than warfarin is unknown, but assume that an interaction occurs until proven otherwise. *Fluvastatin (Lescol)* appears to inhibit CYP2C9, the primary enzyme in the metabolism of S-warfarin; thus, one would expect fluvastatin to increase warfarin response.[3] *Simvastatin (Zocor)* appears to produce a small increase in warfarin effect, while available evidence suggests that *pravastatin (Pravachol)* does not affect warfarin. *Clofibrate (Atromid-S)* and *gemfibrozil (Lopid)* may enhance the hypoprothrombinemic response to warfarin, while *cholestyramine (Questran)* and *colestipol (Colestid)* may reduce its effect.

Management Options:

- *Consider Alternative.* Pravastatin appears less likely to interact with warfarin, but one still should monitor for altered hypoprothrombinemic response.
- *Monitor.* If lovastatin is used with oral anticoagulants, monitor for altered hypoprothrombinemic response if lovastatin is initiated, discontinued, or changed in dosage. Adjust the anticoagulant dose as needed.

References:

1. Ahmad S. Lovastatin warfarin interaction. Arch Intern Med. 1990;150:2407.
2. Merck Sharp & Dohme Mevacor Product Information. West Point, PA: 1993.
3. Transon C et al. In vivo inhibition profile of cyctochrome P450TB (CYP2C9) by (±) fluvastatin. Clin Pharmacol Ther. 1995;58:412.

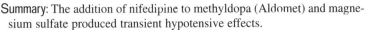

**Magnesium**

**Nifedipine (Procardia)**

Summary: The addition of nifedipine to methyldopa (Aldomet) and magnesium sulfate produced transient hypotensive effects.

Risk Factors: No specific risk factors known.

Related Drugs: Other calcium channel blockers would be expected to enhance the hypotensive actions of magnesium.

Management Options:

- *Monitor.* Patients receiving magnesium for pre-eclampsia should be carefully monitored for hypotension if calcium channel blockers are given concomitantly.

References:

1. Waisman GD et al. Magnesium plus nifedipine: potentiation of hypotensive effect in preeclampsia? Am J Obstet Gynecol. 1988;159:308.

**Mebendazole (Vermox)**

**Phenytoin (Dilantin)**

Summary: In patients receiving high oral doses of mebendazole for *Echinococcus multilocularis* or *Echinococcus granulosus* (hydatid disease), phenytoin has been shown to lower plasma mebendazole concentrations, possibly impairing its therapeutic effect.

Risk Factors:
- *Concurrent Diseases.* Patients with tissue-dwelling organisms appear to be at greater risk for the interaction than those with intestinal helminths.

Related Drugs: Other enzyme-inducing agents would be expected to produce a similar effect.

Management Options:
- *Avoid Unless Benefit Outweighs Risk.* In patients receiving mebendazole for tissue-dwelling organisms, try to avoid using enzyme-inducing drugs. No precautions appear necessary during cotherapy with phenytoin in patients receiving mebendazole to treat intestinal helminths. If possible, valproic acid (Depakene) should be used in place of phenytoin because it does not appear to reduce plasma mebendazole concentrations.
- *Monitor.* Be alert for evidence of reduced mebendazole response if phenytoin or other enzyme inducers are used with mebendazole.

References:
1. Luder PJ et al. Treatment of hydatid disease with high oral doses of mebendazole. Long-term follow-up of plasma mebendazole levels and drug interactions. Eur J Clin Pharmacol. 1986;31:443.
2. Witassek F et al. Chemotherapy of larval echinococcus with mebendazole: microsomal liver function and cholestasis as determinants of plasma drug level. Eur J Clin Pharmacol. 1983;25:85.
3. Bekhti A et al. A correlation between serum mebendazole concentrations and the aminopyrine breath test. Implications in the treatment of hydatid disease. Br J Clin Pharmacol. 1986;21:223.

### Meclofenamate (Meclomen)

### Warfarin (Coumadin)

**2**

Summary: Preliminary evidence indicates that meclofenamate may increase the hypoprothrombinemic response to warfarin; presumably, it also might effect the response to other oral anticoagulants. The possible detrimental effects of meclofenamate on the gastric mucosa and platelet function is another reason to undertake cotherapy with caution.

Risk Factors:
- *Concurrent Diseases.* Patients with peptic ulcer disease (PUD) or a history of gastrointestinal (GI) bleeding probably are at greater risk for the interaction.

Related Drugs: All NSAIDs inhibit platelet function, cause gastric erosions, and probably increase the risk of GI bleeding. Some nonsteroidal anti-inflammatory drugs, however, such as *ibuprofen (Advil), naproxen (Naprosyn),* or *diclofenac (Voltaren),* may be less likely to increase oral anticoagulant-induced hypoprothrombinemia than other NSAIDs.

Management Options:
- *Avoid Unless Benefit Outweighs Risk.* Since all NSAIDs probably increase the risk of GI bleeding in patients on oral anticoagulants,

use the combination only after careful consideration of the benefit versus risk. If an NSAID must be used with an oral anticoagulant, it would be prudent to use NSAIDs that are unlikely to affect the hypoprothrombinemic response to oral anticoagulants as mentioned in Related Drugs above. If the NSAID is being used as an analgesic or antipyretic, acetaminophen (Tylenol) probably is safer to use with oral anticoagulants. Nonacetylated salicylates (e.g., choline salicylate, magnesium salicylate, salsalate, sodium salicylate) also probably are safer with oral anticoagulants than NSAIDs, since such salicylates have minimal effects on platelet function and the gastric mucosa.

- *Monitor.* If any NSAID is used with an oral anticoagulant, one should carefully monitor the prothrombin time and watch for evidence of bleeding, especially from the GI tract.

References:
1. AMA Drug Evaluation. 6th ed. American Medical Association. Chicago; 1986:1066.
2. Park-Davis. Meclomen product information. Morris Plains, NJ; 1990.
3. Shorr RI et al. Concurrent use of nonsteroidal anti-inflammatory drugs and oral anticoagulants places elderly persons at high risk for hemorrhagic peptic ulcer disease. Arch Intern Med. 1993;153:1665.

## Mefenamic Acid (Ponstel)

## Warfarin (Coumadin)

**2**

Summary: Limited clinical evidence indicates that mefenamic acid may produce a small increase in the hypoprothrombinemic response to warfarin and, presumably, other oral anticoagulants. Another reason for caution during cotherapy with these drugs is the possible detrimental effects of mefenamic acid on the gastric mucosa and platelet function.

Risk Factors:
- *Concurrent Diseases.* Patients with peptic ulcer disease (PUD) or a history of gastrointestinal (GI) bleeding probably are at greater risk for the interaction.

Related Drugs: All NSAIDs inhibit platelet function, cause gastric erosions, and probably increase the risk of GI bleeding. Some nonsteroidal anti-inflammatory drugs, however, such as *ibuprofen (Advil)*, *naproxen (Naprosyn)*, or *diclofenac (Voltaren)*, may be less likely to increase oral anticoagulant-induced hypoprothrombinemia than other NSAIDs.

Management Options:
- *Avoid Unless Benefit Outweighs Risk.* Since all NSAIDs probably increase the risk of GI bleeding in patients on oral anticoagulants, use the combination only after careful consideration of the benefit versus risk. If an NSAID must be used with an oral anticoagulant, it would be prudent to use NSAIDs that are unlikely to affect the hypoprothrombinemic response to oral anticoagulants as mentioned

in the Related Drugs section above. If the NSAID is being used as an analgesic or antipyretic, acetaminophen (Tylenol) probably is safer to use with oral anticoagulants. Nonacetylated salicylates (e.g., choline salicylate, magnesium salicylate, salsalate, sodium salicylate) also probably are safer with oral anticoagulants than NSAIDs, since such salicylates have minimal effects on platelet function and the gastric mucosa.

- *Monitor.* If any NSAID is used with an oral anticoagulant, one should carefully monitor the prothrombin time and watch for evidence of bleeding, especially from the GI tract.

References:
1. Sellers EM et al. Displacement of warfarin from human albumin by diazoxide and ethacrynic, mefenamic and nalidixic acids. Clin Pharmacol Ther. 1970;11:524.
2. Sellers EM et al. Kinetics and clinical importance of displacement of warfarin from albumin by acidic drugs. Ann NY Acad Sci. 1971;179:213.
3. Shorr RI et al. Concurrent use of nonsteroidal anti-inflammatory drugs and oral anticoagulants places elderly persons at high risk for hemorrhagic peptic ulcer disease. Arch Intern Med. 1993;153:1665.

### Meperidine (Demerol)

### Phenelzine (Nardil)

Summary: Some patients receiving nonselective monoamine oxidase inhibitors (MAOIs) and meperidine have developed life-threatening serotonin syndrome.

Risk Factors: No specific risk factors known.

Related Drugs: Meperidine is contraindicated in patients receiving any nonselective MAOI, including *isocarboxazid (Marplan)* and *tranylcypromine (Parnate)*. *Morphine* does not appear likely to cause such severe reactions; thus, although it cannot be used with impunity with nonselective MAOIs, it is preferable to meperidine. Epidural *fentanyl (Sublimaze)* has been reported to be an acceptable analgesic for postoperative pain in a patient taking tranylcypromine.[3]

Management Options:
- *Avoid Combination.* Meperidine should be avoided in patients receiving nonselective MAOIs. Remember that the effects of nonselective MAOIs should be assumed to persist for 2 weeks after they

## Significance Classification

① - *Avoid Combination.* Risk always outweighs benefit.

② - *Usually Avoid Combination.* Use combination only under special circumstances.

③ - *Minimize Risk.* Take action as necessary to reduce risk.

are discontinued. Available evidence suggests that morphine is safer than meperidine in patients receiving nonselective MAOIs.

References:
1. Evans-Prosser CDG. The use of pethidine and morphine in the presence of monoamine oxidase inhibitors. Br J Anaesthesiol. 1968;40:279.
2. Browne B et al. Monoamine oxidase inhibitors and narcotic analgesics. A critical review of the implications for treatment. Br J Psych. 1987;151:210.
3. Youssef MS et al. Epidural fentanyl and monoamine oxidase inhibitors. Anaesthesia. 1988;43:210.

## Meperidine (Demerol)

### Phenobarbital

Summary: Phenobarbital and meperidine cotherapy can result in excessive central nervous system (CNS) depression.

Risk Factors: No specific risk factors known.

Related Drugs: Most combinations of barbiturates and narcotic analgesics would be expected to exhibit additive CNS depressant effects. Moreover, the metabolism of narcotic analgesics that are converted to inactive products might be enhanced by barbiturates thus reducing their effect.

Management Options:
- *Monitor* for excessive CNS depression when barbiturates and narcotic analgesics are given concurrently; adjust dosage of one or both drugs as needed.

References:
1. Stambaugh JE et al. A potentially toxic drug interaction between pethidine (meperidine) and phenobarbitone. Lancet. 1977;1:398.
2. Bellville JW et al. The hypnotic effects of codeine and secobarbital and their interaction in man. Clin Pharmacol Ther. 1971;12:607.
3. Stambaugh JE et al. The effect of phenobarbital on the metabolism of meperidine in normal volunteers. J Clin Pharmacol. 1978;18:482.

## Meperidine (Demerol)

### Phenytoin (Dilantin)

Summary: Phenytoin may reduce meperidine serum concentrations, but the clinical importance of this effect is not established.

Risk Factors: No specific risk factors known.

Related Drugs: No information available.

Management Options:
- *Monitor.* Until more information is available, be alert for evidence of reduced analgesic efficacy and/or increased toxicity when meperidine is used in patients receiving phenytoin.

References:
1. Pond SM et al. Effect of phenytoin on meperidine clearance and normeperidine formation. Clin Pharmacol Ther. 1981;30:680.

## Meperidine (Demerol)

## Selegiline (Eldepryl)

Summary: A patient on selegiline developed agitation, delirium, rigidity, sweating, and hyperpyrexia after starting meperidine, but it was not established that it resulted from an interaction between selegiline and meperidine.

Risk Factors:
- *Other Drugs.* The concurrent use of other drugs that inhibit serotonin reuptake may increase the risk.

Related Drugs: Theoretically, **morphine** would be less likely to interact than meperidine, but little is known about other opiates.

Management Options:
- *Use Alternative.* Although it is not clear that the reported reaction resulted from a selegiline-meperidine interaction, the potential severity of the reaction dictates caution. Until more data are available, it would be prudent to use analgesics other than meperidine in patients on selegiline. Nonetheless, the manufacturer recommends caution.

References:
1. Zornberg GL et al. Severe adverse interaction between pethidine and selegiline. Lancet. 1991;337:246. Letter.
2. Eldepryl product information. Physician's Desk Reference. 50th ed. Oradell: Medical Economics Data; 1996:2550.

## Mercaptopurine (6-MP)

## Warfarin (Coumadin)

Summary: Mercaptopurine appeared to inhibit the hypoprothrombinemic response to warfarin in 1 patient, a finding consistent with animal studies. More study is needed to evaluate the incidence and significance of this interaction.

Risk Factors: No specific risk factor known.

Related Drugs: **Azathioprine (Imuran)** is metabolized to mercaptopurine and also has been reported to inhibit the hypoprothrombinemic response to warfarin. The effect of mercaptopurine on oral anticoagulants other than warfarin is unknown, but be alert for a similar effect with all oral anticoagulants until information to the contrary is available.

Management Options:
- *Monitor* for altered oral anticoagulant effect if mercaptopurine is initiated, discontinued, or changed in dosage. Adjust the anticoagulant dose as needed.

References:
1. Martini A et al. Studies in rats on the mechanisms by which 6-mercaptopurine inhibits the anticoagulant effect of warfarin. J Pharmacol Exp Ther. 1977;210:547.
2. Spiers ASD et al. Increased warfarin requirement during mercaptopurine therapy: a new drug interaction. Lancet. 1974;2:221. Letter.

### Metaraminol (Aramine)

### Pargyline

Summary: Metaraminol administration to patients taking a monoamine oxidase inhibitor (MAOI) such as pargyline may result in a severe hypertensive response.

Risk Factors: No specific risk factors known.

Related Drugs: Metaraminol is contraindicated in patients receiving any nonselective MAOI, including *isocarboxazid (Marplan)*, *phenelzine (Nardil)*, and *tranylcypromine (Parnate)*. *Norepinephrine (Levarterenol)* is likely to be a safer pressor agent than metaraminol in such patients.

Management Options:
- *Avoid Combination*. Metaraminol should be avoided in patients taking an MAOI. Remember that the effects of nonselective MAOIs should be assumed to persist for 2 weeks after they are discontinued.

References:
1. Sjoqvist F. Psychotropic drugs (2). Interaction between monoamine oxidase (MAO) inhibitors and other substances. Proc R Soc Med. 1965;58:967.
2. Horler AR et al. Hyperstensive crisis due to pargyline and metaraminol. Br Med J. 1965;3:460.

### Methadone (Dolophine)

### Phenobarbital

Summary: Phenobarbital may enhance methadone metabolism, resulting in methadone withdrawal.

Risk Factors: No specific risk factors known.

Related Drugs: All barbiturates would be expected to enhance methadone metabolism.

Management Options:
- *Monitor* for methadone withdrawal if barbiturates are given concurrently.

References:
1. Liu S-J et al. Case report of barbiturate-induced enhancement of methadone metabolism and withdrawal syndrome. Am J Psychiatry. 1984;141:1287.

### Methadone (Dolophine)

### Phenytoin (Dilantin)

Summary: Phenytoin may reduce serum methadone concentrations, resulting in symptoms of methadone withdrawal.

Risk Factors: No specific risk factors known.

Related Drugs: Other enzyme inducers such as barbiturates, *carbamazepine (Tegretol)*, *primidone (Mysoline)*, and *rifampin (Rifadin)* probably also enhance methadone metabolism.

Management Options:
- *Avoid Unless Benefit Outweighs Risk*. If possible, avoid using methadone with enzyme inducers such as phenytoin.

- *Monitor.* If the combination is necessary, monitor for the need to adjust the methadone dose if phenytoin therapy is initiated, discontinued, or changed in dosage.

References:
1. Finelli PF. Phenytoin and methadone tolerance. N Engl J Med. 1976;294:227. Letter.
2. Tong TG et al. Phenytoin-induced methadone withdrawal. Ann Intern Med. 1981; 94:349.

## Methadone (Dolophine)

### Rifampin (Rifadin)

Summary: Rifampin can decrease methadone serum concentrations resulting in withdrawal symptoms.

Risk Factors: No specific risk factors known.

Related Drugs: No information available.

Management Options:

- *Monitor.* Methadone-treated patients should be observed for evidence of methadone withdrawal when they are started on rifampin. If the methadone dose is increased to offset the effect of rifampin, be alert for excessive methadone effect when the rifampin is discontinued.

References:
1. Kreek MJ et al. Rifampin-induced methadone withdrawal. N Engl J Med. 1976; 294:1104.
2. Bending MR et al. Rifampicin and methadone withdrawal. Lancet. 1977;1:1211. Letter.
3. Holmes VE. Rifampin-induced methadone withdrawal in AIDS. J Clin Psychopharmacol. 1990;10:443. Letter.

## Methandrostenolone (Dianabol)

### Tolbutamide (Orinase)

Summary: Anabolic steroids may enhance the hypoglycemic effect of tolbutamide and possibly other antidiabetic agents.

Risk Factors: No specific risk factors known.

Related Drugs: Although some anabolic steroids would be expected to enhance the hypoglycemic response to other antidiabetic drugs (e.g., *insulin*), specific data demonstrating this effect on hypoglycemic agents other than tolbutamide are lacking.

## Significance Classification

 - *Avoid Combination.* Risk always outweighs benefit.

 - *Usually Avoid Combination.* Use combination only under special circumstances.

 - *Minimize Risk.* Take action as necessary to reduce risk.

Management Options:
- *Consider Alternative.* Nandrolone (Durabolin) and methenolone acetate did not appear to affect tolbutamide's hypoglycemic effects.[3]
- *Monitor.* If anabolic steroids are added to antidiabetic drug therapy, the patient should be monitored more closely for evidence of hypoglycemia.

References:
1. Sotaniemi EA et al. Drug metabolism and androgen control therapy in prostatic cancer. Clin Pharmacol Ther. 1973;14:413.
2. Kontturi M et al. Estrogen-induced metabolic changes during treatment of prostatic cancer. Scan J Lab Clin Invest. 1970;25(Suppl. 113):45.
3. Landon J et al. The effect of anabolic steroids on blood sugar and plasma insulin levels in man. Metabolism. 1963;12:924.

## Methenamine

### Sodium Bicarbonate

Summary: Sodium bicarbonate administration interferes with the antibacterial activity of methenamine compounds.

Risk Factors: No specific risk factors known.

Related Drugs: Certain antacids (e.g., **magnesium, aluminum** hydroxides) and **acetazolamide (Diamox)** also may alkalinize the urine somewhat, but it is unknown whether this effect would be sufficient to affect methenamine.

Management Options:
- *Monitor.* If the urine cannot be kept at about pH 5.5 or lower during the use of sodium bicarbonate, methenamine compounds should not be used.

References:
1. Mandelamine. Physician's Desk Reference. 44th ed. Oradell: Medical Economics Data; 1990:1628.
2. Kevorkian CG et al. Methenamine mandelate with acidification: an effective urinary antiseptic in patients with neurogenic bladder. Mayo Clin Proc. 1984;59:523.
3. Pearman JW et al. The antimicrobial activity of urine of paraplegic patients receiving methenamine mandelate. Invest Urol. 1978;16:91.2.

## Methenamine

### Sulfadiazine

Summary: The combination of methenamine and sulfadiazine may result in crystalluria.

Risk Factors: No specific risk factors known.

Related Drugs: **Sulfamethizole (Thiosulfil)** and **sulfathiazole** interact similarly with methenamine. However, more soluble agents, such as sulfisoxazole, rarely interact.

Management Options:
- *Consider Alternative.* Methenamine compounds should not be used with sulfonamides that may precipitate in an acid urine. The use of sulfathiazole or sulfamethizole with methenamine compounds

should be avoided. If a methenamine product and a sulfonamide are to be used together, it would be preferable to use the more soluble sulfonamides, such as sulfisoxazole.

- *Monitor.* Patients receiving methenamine and sulfadiazine should be monitored for crystalluria.

References:

1. Mandelamine. Physician's Desk Reference. 47th ed. Oradell: Medical Economics Data; 1993:1780.

## Methotrexate (Mexate)

## Naproxen (Naprosyn)

Summary: A patient on chronic methotrexate for arthritis developed evidence of methotrexate toxicity and died after receiving naproxen.

Risk Factors:

- *Dosage Regimen.* The risk of adverse effects from this interaction is primarily in patients receiving antineoplastic doses of methotrexate, rather than the lower doses used to treat rheumatoid arthritis, psoriasis, and related diseases.

- *Concurrent Diseases.* Particular caution is suggested in patients with pre-existing renal impairment [who may be more susceptible to nonsteroidal anti-inflammatory drug (NSAID)-induced renal failure].

Related Drugs: Patients on low-dose methotrexate for rheumatoid arthritis frequently receive concurrent NSAIDs, and severe methotrexate toxicity in such patients is unusual.[2-4] Although these patients would appear to be at low risk, caution is warranted since NSAID use in patients on low-dose methotrexate occasionally is associated with severe methotrexate toxicity.[1,5]

Management Options:

- *Avoid Unless Benefit Outweighs Risk.* Until more information is available on this interaction, it would be prudent to avoid naproxen (as well as other NSAIDs) in patients receiving antineoplastic doses of methotrexate. Particular caution is suggested in patients with pre-existing renal impairment, who may be more susceptible to NSAID-induced renal failure.

- *Monitor.* If the combination is used, monitor for methotrexate toxicity. Findings in methotrexate toxicity can include stomatitis, severe gastrointestinal symptoms (nausea, diarrhea, vomiting), bone marrow suppression, fever, bleeding, skin rashes, nephrotoxicity, and hepatotoxicity. Although decreasing the methotrexate dosage would be expected to reduce the likelihood of toxicity, the magnitude of the required reduction in methotrexate dosage has not been established.

References:

1. Daly HM et al. Methotrexate toxicity precipitated by azapropazone. Br J Dermatol. 1986;114:733.
2. Boh LE et al. Low-dose weekly oral methotrexate therapy for inflammatory arthritis. Clin Pharm. 1986;5:503.

3. Anderson PA et al. Weekly pulse methotrexate in rheumatoid arthritis: clinical and immunologic effects in a randomized, double-blind study. Ann Intern Med. 1985; 103:489.

4. Tugwell P et al. Methotrexate in rheumatoid arthritis: indications, contraindications, efficacy, and safety. Ann Intern Med. 1987;107:358.

5. Adams JD et al. Drug interactions in psoriasis. Aust J Dermatol. 1976;17:39.

## Methotrexate (Mexate)

## Neomycin

Summary: Oral absorption of methotrexate is decreased by 30% to 50% in patients receiving oral antibiotic mixtures including paromomycin (Humatin), neomycin, nystatin (Mycostatin), and vancomycin (Vancocin).

Risk Factors: No specific risk factors known.

Related Drugs: No information available.

Management Options:

- **Avoid Combination.** Patients receiving oral methotrexate should not receive oral nonabsorbable antibiotics. It is not known whether this interaction occurs with parenteral methotrexate; however, the possibility cannot be excluded.

References:

1. Cohen MH et al. Effect of oral prophylactic broad spectrum nonabsorbable antibiotics on the gastrointestinal absorption of nutrients and methotrexate in small cell bronchogenic carcinoma patients. Cancer. 1976;38:1556–559.

## Methotrexate (Mexate)

## Omeprazole (Prilosec)

Summary: A patient with osteosarcoma developed elevated methotrexate serum concentrations while receiving concurrent omeprazole; more study is needed to establish the clinical importance of this purported interaction.

Risk Factors: No specific risk factors known.

Related Drugs: Theoretically, $H_2$-receptor antagonists, such as **ranitidine (Zantac)**, **cimetidine (Tagamet)**, **famotidine (Pepcid)**, and **nizatidine (Axid)**,

## Significance Classification

**①** - **Avoid Combination.** Risk always outweighs benefit.

**②** - **Usually Avoid Combination.** Use combination only under special circumstances.

**③** - **Minimize Risk.** Take action as necessary to reduce risk.

would be less likely than omeprazole to interact with methotrexate, but little clinical information is available.

Management Options:

- *Monitor.* Until more data are available, monitor for excessive methotrexate effect if omeprazole is given concurrently.

References:

1. Reid T et al. Impact of omeprazole on the plasma clearance of methotrexate. Cancer Chemother Pharmacol. 1993;33:82.

## Methotrexate (Mexate)

## Phenylbutazone (Butazolidin)

Summary: Two patients on methotrexate developed evidence of severe methotrexate toxicity after starting phenylbutazone; one patient died.

Risk Factors:

- *Dosage Regimen.* The risk of adverse effects from this interaction is primarily in patients receiving antineoplastic doses of methotrexate, rather than the lower doses used to treat rheumatoid arthritis, psoriasis, and related diseases.

- *Concurrent Diseases.* Particular caution is suggested in patients with pre-existing renal impairment [who may be more susceptible to nonsteroidal anti-inflammatory drug (NSAID)-induced renal failure].

Related Drugs: *Oxyphenbutazone* also would be expected to enhance methotrexate toxicity, but clinical data are lacking.

Management Options:

- *Avoid Unless Benefit Outweighs Risk.* Although only limited clinical evidence exists, it would be prudent to avoid phenylbutazone (as well as other NSAIDs) in patients receiving antineoplastic doses of methotrexate. Particular caution is suggested in patients with pre-existing renal impairment, who may be more susceptible to NSAID-induced renal failure.

- *Monitor.* If the combination is used, monitor for methotrexate toxicity. Findings in methotrexate toxicity can include stomatitis, severe gastrointestinal symptoms (nausea, diarrhea, vomiting), bone marrow suppression, fever, bleeding, skin rashes, nephrotoxicity, and hepatotoxicity. Although decreasing the methotrexate dosage would be expected to reduce the likelihood of toxicity, the magnitude of the required reduction in methotrexate dosage has not been established.

References:

1. Furst DE et al. Effect of aspirin and sulindac on methotrexate clearance. J Pharm Sci. 1990;79:782.
2. Dupuis LL et al. Methotrexate-nonsteroidal antiiflammatory drug interaction in children with arthritis. J Rheumatol. 1990;17:469.
3. Skeith KJ et al. Lack of significant interaction between low dose methotrexate and ibuprofen or flurbiprofen in patients with arthritis. J Rheumatol. 1990;17:1008.

### Methotrexate (Mexate)

### Polio Vaccine

Summary: Administration of live-virus vaccines such as oral polio vaccine (OPV) to immunosuppressed patients, including those undergoing cytotoxic chemotherapy, may result in infection by the live virus.

Risk Factors: No specific risk factors known.

Related Drugs: Other vaccines that may result in infections in immunocompromised patients include *BCG vaccine, typhoid vaccine, measles vaccine, mumps vaccine, rubella vaccine, smallpox vaccine,* or *yellow fever vaccine.*

Management Options:

- *Avoid Combination.* Current recommendations state that patients with leukemia in remission should not receive live vaccines until at least 3 months have passed since the completion of all chemotherapy.[2,3] Similar guidelines should be followed for patients receiving chemotherapy for other malignancies.

References:

1. Mitus A et al. Attenuated measles vaccine in children with acute leukemia. Am J Dis Child. 1962;103:243.
2. Pizzo PA et al. Infections in the cancer patient. In: DeVita VT et al., eds. Cancer: principles and practice of oncology. 4th ed. Philadelphia: J.B. Lippincott; 1993: 2292.
3. Immunization Practices Advisory Committee. Update on adult immunization. Recommendations of the Immunization practices advisory committee (ACIP). MMWR. 1991;40(RR-12):1.

### Methotrexate (Mexate)

### Probenecid (Benemid)

Summary: Probenecid markedly increases serum methotrexate concentrations and would be expected to increase both the therapeutic effect and toxicity of methotrexate.

Risk Factors: No specific risk factors known.

Related Drugs: *Sulfinpyrazone (Anturane)* would be expected to produce a similar effect on methotrexate.

Management Options:

- *Avoid Unless Benefit Outweighs Risk.* Probenecid and sulfinpyrazone generally should be avoided in patients receiving methotrexate.
- *Monitor.* If the combination is used, one should anticipate that a reduction in methotrexate dosage may be required. Serum methotrexate determinations would be helpful, and one also should monitor for excessive methotrexate effect (e.g., gastrointestinal toxicity, stomatitis, bone marrow suppression, hepatotoxicity, infection).

References:

1. Aherne GW et al. Prolongation and enhancement of serum methotrexate concentrations by probenecid. Br Med J. 1978;1:1097.

2. Lilly MB et al. Clinical pharmacology of oral intermediate-dose methotrexate with or without probenecid. Cancer Chemother Pharmacol. 1985;15:220.
3. Howell SB et al. Effect of probenecid on cerebrospinal fluid methotrexate kinetics. Clin Pharmacol Ther. 1979;26:641.

## Methotrexate (Mexate)

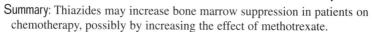

### Thiazides

Summary: Thiazides may increase bone marrow suppression in patients on chemotherapy, possibly by increasing the effect of methotrexate.

Risk Factors: No specific risk factors known.

Related Drugs: No information available.

Management Options:

- *Monitor.* Patients should be monitored for enhanced bone marrow suppression when thiazides are used with methotrexate (or other cytotoxic agents). Adjust cytotoxic drug dosage as needed.

References:

1. Orr LE. Potentiation of myelosuppression from cancer chemotherapy and thiazide diuretics. Drug Intell Clin Pharm. 1981;15:967.

## Methotrexate (Mexate)

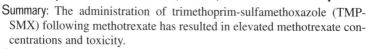

### Trimethoprim-Sulfamethoxazole (Bactrim)

Summary: The administration of trimethoprim-sulfamethoxazole (TMP-SMX) following methotrexate has resulted in elevated methotrexate concentrations and toxicity.

Risk Factors: No specific risk factors known.

Related Drugs: No information available.

Management Options:

- *Circumvent/Minimize.* Trimethoprim-sulfamethoxazole generally should be avoided in patients who are receiving methotrexate. Folinic acid may be required to treat megaloblastic changes.
- *Monitor.* If these 2 drugs are coadministered, watch for evidence of methotrexate toxicity (stomatitis, leukopenia, nausea).

References:

1. Ferrazzini G et al. Interaction between trimethoprim-sulfamethoxazole and methotrexate in children with leukemia. J Ped. 1990;117:823.
2. Groenendal H et al. Methotrexate and trimethoprim-sulphamethoxazole—a potentially hazardous combination. Clin Exper Derm. 1990;15:358.
3. Thomas MH et al. Methotrexate toxicity in a patient receiving trimethoprim-sulfamethoxazole. J Rheum. 1986;13:40.

## Methotrimeprazine (Levoprome)

### Pargyline

Summary: Coadministration of pargyline and methotrimeprazine was associated with fatality in 1 reported case.

Risk Factors: No specific risk factors known.

Related Drugs: All nonselective monoamine oxidase inhibitors (MAOIs) including *isocarboxazid (Marplan)*, *phenelzine (Nardil)*, and *tranylcypromine (Parnate)* should be considered contraindicated with methotrimeprazine.

Management Options:

- *Avoid Combination.* Although the interaction between methotrimeprazine and MAOIs is not well documented, the possibility of a fatal reaction contraindicates concomitant use of these drugs. Remember that the effects of nonselective MAOIs should be assumed to persist for 2 weeks after they are discontinued.

References:

1. Sjoqvist F. Psychotropic drugs (2). Interaction between monoamine oxidase (MAO) inhibitors and other substances. Proc R Soc Med. 1965;58:967.
2. Barsa JA et al. A comparative study of tranylcypromine and pargyline. Psychopharmacologia. 1964;6:295.

## Methoxyflurane (Penthrane)

### Secobarbital

Summary: Barbiturates like secobarbital may enhance the nephrotoxic effect of methoxyflurane.

Risk Factors: No specific risk factors known.

Related Drugs: Based upon the mechanism, one would expect all barbiturates to interact similarly with methoxyflurane.

Management Options:

- *Consider Alternative.* Consider anesthetics other than methoxyflurane in patients who are receiving enzyme inducers such as barbiturates. It should be remembered that enzyme induction dissipates slowly following discontinuation of the inducing agent, so the enhanced metabolic activity usually returns to normal within 2–3 weeks.

- *Monitor* for nephrotoxicity if the combination is given.

References:

1. Churchill D et al. Toxic nephropathy after low-dose methoxyflurane anesthesia: drug interaction with secobarbital? Can Med Assoc J. 1976;114:326.
2. Cousins MJ et al. Methoxyflurane nephrotoxicity: a study of dose response in man. JAMA. 1973;225:1611.

## Methoxyflurane (Penthrane)

### Tetracycline

Summary: Patients receiving methoxyflurane anesthesia appear to be at increased risk of developing renal toxicity if they are treated with tetracycline.

Risk Factors: No specific risk factors known.

Related Drugs: Other antibiotics, including *kanamycin (Kantrex)* and *gentamicin (Garamycin)*, have been implicated in similar nephrotoxic effects in patients who receive methoxyflurane.[2]

Management Options:
- *Use Alternative.* The severe consequences of this possible interaction warrant great caution in administering tetracycline (and perhaps other nephrotoxic antibiotics) to patients who will soon undergo or have recently undergone methoxyflurane anesthesia. Avoid the use of tetracycline with methoxyflurane.

References:
1. Churchill D. Persisting renal insufficiency after methoxyflurane anesthesia. Report of two cases and review of literature. Am J Med. 1974;56:575.
2. Cousins MJ. Tetracycline, methoxyflurane anesthesia, and renal dysfunction. Lancet. 1972;1:751. Letter.
3. Dryden GE. Incidence of tubular degeneration with microlithiasis following methoxyflurane compared with other anesthetic agents. Anesth Analg. 1974;53:383.

### Methyldopa (Aldomet)

### Norepinephrine (Levarterenol)

Summary: Methyldopa therapy may prolong the pressor response to norepinephrine.

Risk Factors: No specific risk factors known.

Related Drugs: No information available.

Management Options:
- *Monitor* for increased blood pressure response to norepinephrine in patients receiving methyldopa.

References:
1. Dollery CT. Physiological and pharmacological interactions of antihypertensive drugs. Proc R Soc Med. 1965;58:983.
2. Dollery CT et al. Haemodynamic studies with methyldopa: effect on cardiac output and response to pressor amines. Br Heart J. 1963;25:670.

### Methylprednisolone (Medrol)

### Troleandomycin (TAO)

Summary: TAO markedly enhances methylprednisolone effects and may enhance prednisolone effect in some patients.

Risk Factors: No specific risk factors known.

Related Drugs: Although **prednisolone (Prelone)** disposition was not affected by TAO in 3 steroid-dependent asthmatics, TAO did reduce prednisolone elimination somewhat in the presence of phenobarbital.[2] Little is known

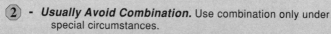

## Significance Classification

 - *Avoid Combination.* Risk always outweighs benefit.

② - *Usually Avoid Combination.* Use combination only under special circumstances.

 - *Minimize Risk.* Take action as necessary to reduce risk.

regarding the effect of TAO on other corticosteroids in humans. *Erythromycin* and *clarithromycin (Biaxin)* are likely to produce a similar effect on methylprednisolone. *Azithromycin (Zithromax)* and *dirithromycin (Dynabac)* would be unlikely to enhance the effects of methylprednisolone.

Management Options:

• *Monitor.* A considerable reduction in methylprednisolone dosage requirement is likely in the presence of TAO. Patients on other corticosteroids also should be monitored for the need to adjust corticosteroid doses when TAO is started or stopped.

References:

1. Szefler SJ et al. The effect of troleandomycin on methylprednisolone elimination. J Allergy Clin Immunol. 1980;66:447.
2. Szefler SJ et al. Steroid-specific and anticonvulsant interaction aspects of troleandomycin-steroid therapy. J Allergy Clin Immunol. 1982;69:455.
3. Nelson HS et al. A double-blind study of troleandomycin and methylprednisolone in asthmatic subjects who require daily corticosteroids. Am Rev Respir Dis. 1993; 147:398.

## Metoprolol (Lopressor)

### Propafenone (Rythmol)

Summary: Metoprolol or propranolol concentrations may significantly increase after administration of propafenone.

Risk Factors: No specific risk factors known.

Related Drugs: Propafenone 225 mg Q 8 hr for 7 days in healthy subjects resulted in an 83% and 213% increase in *propranolol (Inderal)* peak and steady-state serum concentrations, respectively.[2] Beta blocking effects were minimally enhanced during combination therapy. Beta blockers that are renally eliminated such as *atenolol (Tenormin)* or *nadolol (Corgard)* would be unlikely to be affected by propafenone.

Management Options:

• *Monitor.* Patients receiving metoprolol or propranolol should be monitored for increased beta blockade (bradycardia, hypotension, heart failure) when propafenone is added to their therapy and for a reduced effect when it is withdrawn.

References:

1. Wegner F et al. Drug interaction between propafenone and metoprolol. Br J Clin Pharmacol. 1987;24:213.
2. Kowey PR et al. Interaction between propranolol and propafenone in healthy volunteers. J Clin Pharmacol. 1989;29:512.

## Metoprolol (Lopressor)

### Propoxyphene (Darvon)

Summary: Propoxyphene may increase the plasma concentration of highly metabolized beta blockers such as metoprolol; increased beta blocker effects may occur.

Risk Factors: No specific risk factors known.

Related Drugs: *Propranolol (Inderal)* interacts similarly with propoxyphene. It is unlikely that beta blockers excreted primarily by the kidneys [e.g., *atenolol (Tenormin)*, *nadolol (Corgard)*, and *sotalol (Betapace)*] would be affected by propoxyphene.

Management Options:
- *Monitor.* Until more information is available, be aware of increased response to metoprolol and propranolol when propoxyphene is initiated and a decreased response when it is discontinued.

References:
1. Lundborg P et al. The effect of propoxyphene pretreatment on the disposition of metoprolol and propranolol. Clin Pharmacol Ther. 1981;29:263.

## Metoprolol (Lopressor)

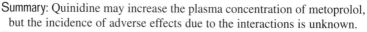

### Quinidine

Summary: Quinidine may increase the plasma concentration of metoprolol, but the incidence of adverse effects due to the interactions is unknown.

Risk Factors:
- *Pharmacogenetics.* Patients who are rapid metabolizers of metoprolol are at increased risk for the interaction.

Related Drugs: Quinidine also decreases the metabolism of *propranolol (Inderal)*, and *timolol (Blocadren)*. Preliminary evidence suggests that quinidine has no effect on *labetalol (Normodyne)* pharmacokinetics or pharmacodynamics.[3] *Atenolol (Tenormin)* and other renally excreted beta blockers are less likely to interact.

Management Options:
- *Consider Alternative.* Renally excreted beta blockers (e.g., atenolol) should be less likely to interact with quinidine, since their clearance is unlikely to be affected by quinidine. Nevertheless, additive cardiac depressant effects cannot be overlooked.
- *Monitor.* Concomitant use of quinidine and metoprolol should be undertaken with careful monitoring. Watch for bradycardia, heart failure, and arrhythmias.

References:
1. Leeman NT et al. Single dose quinidine treatment inhibits metoprolol oxidation in extensive metabolizers. Eur J Clin Pharmacol. 1986;29:739.
2. Schlanz KD et al. Loss of stereoselective metoprolol metabolism following quinidine inhibition of P450IID6. Pharmacotherapy. 1991;11:271. Abstract.
3. Gearhart MO et al. Lack of effects on labetalol pharmacodynamics with quinidine inhibition of P450IID6. Pharmacotherapy. 1991;11:P-36. Abstract.

## Metoprolol (Lopressor)

### Rifampin (Rifadin)

Summary: Plasma concentrations of beta blockers that are metabolized in the liver, such as metoprolol, may decline with concomitant rifampin therapy.

Risk Factors: No specific risk factors known.

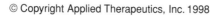

Related Drugs: Rifampin is likely to increase the clearance of all beta blockers that are oxidatively metabolized by the liver, such as **propranolol (Inderal)** and **bisprolol (Zebeta)**. **Atenolol (Tenormin)** and other renally excreted beta blockers are less likely to interact.

Management Options:
- *Consider Alternative.* Beta-adrenergic blockers that are primarily eliminated by the kidneys, such as atenolol, could be used.
- *Circumvent/Minimize.* Beta blocker dosages may need to be increased when rifampin therapy is initiated and decreased when rifampin is discontinued.
- *Monitor.* Watch for reduced beta-adrenergic effects if rifampin is administered with beta-adrenergic blockers that are eliminated by hepatic metabolism.

References:
1. Shaheen O et al. Effect of debrisoquine phenotype on the inducibility of propranolol metabolism. Clin Pharmacol Ther. 1989;45:439.
2. Bennett PN et al. Effects of rifampin on metoprolol and antipyrine kinetics. Br J Clin Pharmacol. 1982;13:387.
3. Kirch W et al. Interaction of bisoprolol with cimetidine and rifampicin. Eur J Clin Pharmacol. 1986;31:59.

### Metoprolol (Lopressor)
### Terbutaline (Brethaire)

Summary: Beta blocker-induced bronchoconstriction may antagonize the bronchodilating effect of beta-agonists; metoprolol increases terbutaline serum concentrations. The use of $\beta_1$-selective beta blockers is preferable in asthmatics receiving beta-agonists.

Risk Factors:
- *Pharmacogenetics.* Patients who are slow metoprolol metabolizers are at increased risk for the interaction.

Related Drugs: Nonspecific beta blockers, such as **propranolol (Inderal)**, would appear more likely to antagonize bronchodilators, such as terbutaline. **Practolol** does not appear to impair the bronchodilator activity of terbutaline.

Management Options:
- *Use Alternative.* If possible, beta blockers should be avoided in patients receiving beta-agonists or theophylline for bronchospastic pulmonary disease. If beta blockers are required, cardioselective

**Significance Classification**
1 - *Avoid Combination.* Risk always outweighs benefit.
2 - *Usually Avoid Combination.* Use combination only under special circumstances.
3 - *Minimize Risk.* Take action as necessary to reduce risk.

agents are preferable. If a cardioselective beta blocker is administered to a patient with asthma taking a beta agonist, observe the patient for worsening asthma.

References:
1. Formgren H et al. Effects of practolol in combination with terbutaline in the treatment of hypertension and arrhythmics in asthmatic patients. Scand J Respir Dis. 1975;56:217.
2. Jonkers RE et al. Debrisoquine phenotype and the pharmacokinetics and beta-2 receptor pharmacodynamics of metoprolol and its enantiomers. J Pharmacol Exp Ther. 1991;256:959.

## Metronidazole (Flagyl)
## Phenytoin (Dilantin)

Summary: Metronidazole may moderately increase phenytoin serum concentrations.

Risk Factors: No specific risk factors known.

Related Drugs: No information available.

Management Options:
- *Monitor.* Patients who have serum phenytoin concentrations near the upper limit of the therapeutic range should be monitored more carefully for increased phenytoin effect when metronidazole is added to their therapy.

References:
1. Blyden GT et al. Metronidazole impairs clearance of phenytoin but not alprazolam or lorazepam. J Clin Pharmacol. 1988;28:240.

## Metronidazole (Flagyl)
## Trimethoprim-Sulfamethoxazole (Bactrim)

Summary: Metronidazole may produce a disulfiram-like reaction when administered with intravenous (IV) trimethoprim-sulfamethoxazole (TMP-SMX).

Risk Factors:
- *Route of Administration.* Administration of *intravenous* TMP-SMX increases the risk for the interaction.

Related Drugs: The coadministration of metronidazole and IV drugs containing ethanol [e.g., *phenytoin (Dilantin)*, *phenobarbital*, *diazepam (Valium)*, and *nitroglycerin*] may result in flushing and vomiting. *Disulfiram (Antabuse)* may react with IV TMP-SMX.

Management Options:
- *Circumvent/Minimize.* The use of oral dosage forms of these agents will prevent this interaction.
- *Monitor.* Watch for signs of disulfiram-like reaction when metronidazole is administered with IV drugs containing ethanol.

References:
1. Edwards DL et al. Disulfiram-like reaction associated with intravenous trimethoprim-sulfamethoxazole and metronidazole. Clin Pharm. 1986;5:999.

## Metronidazole (Flagyl)

## Warfarin (Coumadin)

Summary: Metronidazole increases the hypoprothrombinemic response to warfarin, and bleeding has occurred in some patients receiving both drugs. Adjustments in warfarin dosage may be needed during cotherapy.

Risk Factors: No specific risk factors known.

Related Drugs: No information available.

Management Options:

- *Avoid Unless Benefit Outweighs Risk.* Concomitant use of metronidazole and oral anticoagulants should be avoided if possible.

- *Monitor.* Patients receiving oral anticoagulants should be monitored for an increased anticoagulant effect when metronidazole is started and the converse when it is stopped. If oral anticoagulant therapy is begun in a patient receiving metronidazole, use conservative doses until the maintenance dose is established.

References:

1. O'Reilly RA. The stereoselective interaction of warfarin and metronidazole in man. N Engl J Med. 1976;295:354.
2. Kazmier FJ. A significant interaction between metronidazole and warfarin. Mayo Clin Proc. 1976;51:782.
3. Dean RP et al. Bleeding associated with concurrent warfarin and metronidazole therapy. Drug Intell Clin Pharm. 1980;14:864.

## Mexiletine (Mexitil)

## Phenytoin (Dilantin)

Summary: A study in healthy subjects suggests that phenytoin substantially reduces mexiletine concentrations.

Risk Factors: No specific risk factors known.

Related Drugs: No information available.

Management Options:

- *Circumvent/Minimize.* Mexiletine dosage requirements are likely to increase when phenytoin is administered and decrease when it is discontinued.

- *Monitor.* Measurement of mexiletine concentrations would be helpful to assure that dosage adjustments are adequate. Monitor patients for a decreased therapeutic response when phenytoin is used concurrently and an increased response if phenytoin is discontinued.

References:

1. Begg EJ et al. Enhanced metabolism of mexiletine after phenytoin administration. Br J Clin Pharmacol. 1982;14:219.

## Mexiletine (Mexitil)

## Quinidine

Summary: Quinidine administration increases mexiletine concentrations and increases its antiarrhythmic effects.

Risk Factors:
- *Pharmacogenetics.* Patients who are extensive mexiletine metabolizers are at increased risk for the interaction.

Related Drugs: No information available.

Management Options:
- *Monitor.* Patients stabilized on mexiletine should be monitored for increased serum concentrations and electrophysiologic effects of mexiletine when quinidine is administered.

References:
1. Turgeon J et al. Influence of debrisoquine phenotype and of quinidine on mexiletine disposition in man. J Pharmacol Exper Ther. 1991;259:789.
2. Duff HJ et al. Role of quinidine in the mexiletine-quinidine interaction: electrophysiologic correlates of enhanced antiarrhythmic efficacy. J Cardiovasc Pharmacol. 1990;16:685.
3. Duff HJ et al. Electropharmacologic synergism with mexiletine and quinidine. J Cardiovasc Pharmacol. 1986;8:840.
4. Duff HJ et al. Mexiletine/quinidine combination therapy: electrophysiology correlates of anti-arrhythmic efficacy. Clin Invest Med. 1991;14:476.

**Mexiletine (Mexitil)**

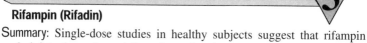

**Rifampin (Rifadin)**

Summary: Single-dose studies in healthy subjects suggest that rifampin administration substantially reduces the plasma concentration of mexiletine.

Risk Factors: No specific risk factors known.

Related Drugs: No information available.

Management Options:
- *Circumvent/Minimize.* Mexiletine dosage may need to be increased when rifampin is added to a patient's regimen and reduced when rifampin is discontinued. Based upon the reported changes in the mexiletine clearance, doses should be adjusted by 25% to 50% to maintain the plasma concentration of mexiletine in the therapeutic range (0.5–2 µg/mL).
- *Monitor.* Patients taking both agents should be monitored for reduced mexiletine concentrations and lowered efficacy.

References:
1. Pentikainen PJ et al. Effect of rifampicin treatment on the kinetics of mexiletine. Eur J Clin Pharmacol. 1982;23:261.

**Mexiletine (Mexitil)**

**Sodium Bicarbonate**

Summary: An increase in urine pH could result in clinically significant increases in mexiletine concentrations.

Risk Factors: No specific risk factors known.

Related Drugs: Other agents that alkalinize the urine [e.g., **acetazolamide (Diamox)**] would be expected to produce a similar interaction with mexiletine.

Management Options:
- *Monitor.* Patients receiving mexiletine who have large changes in their urine pH as a result of concurrent drug therapy should be monitored for changes in mexiletine plasma concentration.

References:
1. Begg EJ et al. Enhanced metabolism of mexiletine after phenytoin administration. Br J Clin Pharmacol. 1982;14:219.
2. Pentikainen PJ et al. Effect of rifampicin treatment on the kinetics of mexiletine. Eur J Clin Pharmacol. 1982;23:261.
3. Kiddie MA et al. The influence of urinary pH on the elimination of mexiletine. Br J Clin Pharmacol. 1974;1:229.

### Mexiletine (Mexitil)

### Theophylline

Summary: Patients maintained on theophylline may develop elevated theophylline serum concentrations and toxicity after initiating concomitant mexiletine therapy.

Risk Factors: No specific risk factors known.

Related Drugs: No information available.

Management Options:
- *Use Alternative.* Patients taking mexiletine should avoid receiving theophylline. The use of a beta-agonist or steroid should be considered. An alternative to mexiletine should be considered in patients receiving theophylline. Patients stabilized on theophylline who receive mexiletine should be carefully monitored for increased theophylline concentrations and potentially toxic symptoms, including tachycardia, arrhythmias, gastrointestinal upset, and seizures.

References:
1. Kendall JD et al. Theophylline-mexiletine interaction: a case report. Pharmacotherapy. 1992;12:416.
2. Hurwitz A et al. Mexiletine effects on theophylline disposition. Clin Pharmacol Ther. 1991;50:299.
3. Stoysich AM et al. Influence of mexiletine on the pharmacokinetics of theophylline in healthy volunteers. J Clin Pharmacol. 1991:31:354.

### Mibefradil (Posicor)

### Simvastatin (Zocor)

Summary: Mibefradil coadministration with simvastatin or lovastatin may increase the risk of rhabdomyolysis. Pending further data, the combination should be avoided.

Risk Factors: No specific risk factors known.

Related Drugs: Since *lovastatin (Mevacor)* is metabolized similarly to simvastatin, mibefradil would be expected to reduce lovastatin's clearance and potentially induce muscle toxicity. While no data are currently available, *atorvastatin (Lipitor)* and *cerivastatin (Baycol)* metabolism also may be reduced by mibefradil administration. Mibefradil is unlikely to reduce the clearance of *fluvastatin (Lescol)* or *pravastatin (Pravachol)*. *Verapamil (Isoptin)* and *diltiazem (Cardizem)* are also likely to reduce lovastatin, simvastatin, atorvastatin, and cerivastatin clearance.

Management Options:
- *Use Alternative.* Patients taking mibefradil who require a HMG-CoA reductase inhibitor should receive fluvastatin or pravastatin.

References:
1. Roche Laboratories, Inc.. Mibefradil (Posicor) package insert. 1997.

### Mibefradil (Posicor)
### Terfenadine (Seldane)

Summary: Terfenadine concentrations can increase during mibefradil coadministration; cardiac arrhythmias may result. Avoid concurrent use of terfenadine and mibefradil.

Risk Factors: No specific risk factors known.

Related Drugs: It is likely that mibefradil administration would cause an accumulation of *astemizole (Hismanal)* and potentially produce cardiac toxicity. Other calcium channel blockers [e.g., *amlodipine (Norvasc)*, *nifedipine (Procardia)*, *nicardipine (Cardene)*] would not be expected to change terfenadine plasma concentrations. The metabolism of *fexofenadine (Allegra)*, *cetirizine (Zyrtec)*, and *loratadine (Claritin)* would be unlikely to be affected by concomitant mibefradil administration.

Management Options:
- *Use Alternative.* Due to the risk of a possibly serious arrhythmia, the combination of mibefradil and terfenadine (or astemizole) should be avoided. Noninteracting antihistamines are available and should be used in patients receiving mibefradil.

References:
1. Roche Laboratories, Inc. Mibefradil (Posicor) package insert. 1997.

### Miconazole (Monistat)
### Warfarin (Coumadin)

Summary: Miconazole given systemically and as an oral gel has been associated with enhanced hypoprothrombinemia and bleeding in some patients receiving oral anticoagulants.

## Significance Classification

① - *Avoid Combination.* Risk always outweighs benefit.

② - *Usually Avoid Combination.* Use combination only under special circumstances.

③ - *Minimize Risk.* Take action as necessary to reduce risk.

Risk Factors: No specific risk factors known.

Related Drugs: The effect of miconazole on oral anticoagulants other than warfarin is not known, but be alert for a similar effect with all oral anticoagulants until information to the contrary is available.

Management Options:
- *Monitor* for altered oral anticoagulant effect if miconazole is initiated, discontinued, or changed in dosage. Adjust the anticoagulant dose as needed.

References:
1. Watson PG et al. Drug interaction with coumarin derivative anticoagulants. Br Med J. 1982;285:1045.
2. Goenen M et al. A case of *Candida albicans* endocarditis 3 years after an aortic valve replacement: successful combined medical and surgical therapy. J Cardiovasc Surg. 1977;18:391.
3. Coloquhorn MC et al. Interaction between warfarin and miconazole oral gel. Lancet. 1987;1:695.

## Midazolam (Versed)

### Phenytoin (Dilantin)

Summary: Phenytoin markedly reduces the effect of oral midazolam, but parenteral midazolam is likely to be less affected.

Risk Factors:
- *Route of Administration.* Since the majority of the interaction is likely due to increased presystemic metabolism of oral midazolam by the gut wall and liver, parenteral midazolam is likely to be much less affected.

Related Drugs: **Carbamazepine (Tegretol)** interacts similarly with midazolam. **Triazolam (Halcion)**, **alprazolam (Xanax)**, and to some extent **diazepam (Valium)** also are metabolized by CYP3A4 and would be expected to interact with enzyme inducers in a manner similar to midazolam.

Management Options:
- *Consider Alternative.* When midazolam is used orally as a sedative-hypnotic (as it is in several countries), patients receiving enzyme inducers such as phenytoin are unlikely to respond unless very large doses of midazolam are used. Thus, it may be preferable to use alternative sedative-hypnotics in such patients.
- *Monitor.* Although parenteral midazolam is likely to be much less affected, monitor for inadequate midazolam effect and increase its dose if needed.

References:
1. Backman JT et al. Concentrations and effects of oral midazolam are greatly reduced in patients treated with carbamazepine or phenytoin. Epilepsia. 1996;37:253.

## Misoprostol (Cytotec)

### Phenylbutazone

Summary: The combined use of phenylbutazone and misoprostol has been associated with adverse effects (e.g., tingling, headache, hot flushes, dizziness, nausea) in some patients, but a causal relationship is not established.

Risk Factors: No specific risk factors known.

Related Drugs: **Naproxen (Naprosyn)** and **etodolac (Lodine)** do not appear to affect misoprostol. The effect of other nonsteroidal anti-inflammatory drugs on misoprostol is not established.

Management Options:
- *Monitor.* Until more information is available, be alert for adverse effects such as tingling, headache, hot flushes, dizziness, and nausea when misoprostol is used in patients receiving phenylbutazone.

References:
1. Chassagne P et al. Neurosensory adverse effects after combined phenylbutazone and misoprostol. Br J Rheumatol. 1991;30:392. Letter.
2. Jacquemier JM et al. Neurosensory adverse effects after phenylbutazone and misoprostol combined treatment. Lancet. 1989;2:1283. Letter.

## Mitomycin (Mutamycin)

### Vinblastine (Velban)

Summary: Administration of vinblastine following treatment with mitomycin has been associated with acute bronchospasm and dyspnea.

Risk Factors: No specific risk factors known.

Related Drugs: No information available.

Management Options:
- *Avoid Unless Benefit Outweighs Risk.* Although most patients do not appear to develop pulmonary toxicity, the severity of the reaction dictates that the combination generally should be avoided.
- *Monitor.* In instances where the combination is felt to be necessary, patients should be advised to contact their physician or go to the emergency room immediately if they develop difficulty in breathing. Both drugs should be discontinued immediately at the first sign of respiratory compromise. Further therapy with this combination should be avoided in patients who experience dyspnea, as it appears to recur upon repeated administration.

References:
1. Kris MG et al. Dyspnea following vinblastine or vindesine administration in patients receiving mitomycin plus vinca alkaloid combination therapy. Cancer Treat Rep. 1984;68:1029.

2. Rao SX et al. Fatal acute respiratory failure after vinblastine-mitomycin therapy in lung carcinoma. Arch Intern Med. 1985;145:1905.
3. Hoelzer KL. Vinblastine-associated pulmonary toxicity in patients receiving combination therapy with mitomycin and cisplatin. Drug Intell Clin Pharm. 1986; 20:287.

## Mitotane (Lysodren)

## Spironolactone (Aldactone)

Summary: Spironolactone may antagonize the activity of mitotane.

Risk Factors: No specific risk factors known.

Related Drugs: No information available.

Management Options:
- *Avoid Combination.* Patients on mitotane should not receive concurrent spironolactone.

References:
1. Wortsman J et al. Mitotane. Spironolactone antagonism in Cushing's syndrome. JAMA. 1977;238:2527.

## Mitotane (Lysodren)

## Warfarin (Coumadin)

Summary: Mitotane appears to inhibit the hypoprothrombinemic response to warfarin and probably other oral anticoagulants as well. Oral anticoagulant dose requirements may be increased in patients taking both drugs.

Risk Factors: No specific risk factors known.

Related Drugs: The effect of mitotane on oral anticoagulants other than warfarin is not known, but be alert for a similar effect with all oral anticoagulants until information to the contrary is available.

Management Options:
- *Monitor* for altered oral anticoagulant effect if mitotane is initiated, discontinued, or changed in dosage. Adjust the anticoagulant dose as needed.

References:
1. Cuddy PG et al. Influence of mitotane on the hypoprothrombinemic effect of warfarin. South Med J. 1986;79:387.

## Significance Classification

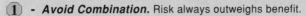

(1) - *Avoid Combination.* Risk always outweighs benefit.

(2) - *Usually Avoid Combination.* Use combination only under special circumstances.

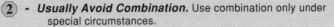

(3) - *Minimize Risk.* Take action as necessary to reduce risk.

## Moclobemide

### Selegiline (Eldepryl)

Summary: Combined use of selegiline and moclobemide substantially increases the pressor effect of tyramine over either drug used alone.

Risk Factors: No specific risk factors known.

Related Drugs: This interaction is likely to occur with any combination of an MAO-B and MAO-A inhibitor.

Management Options:

- *Consider Alternative.* Given the likely increase in risk of adverse drug or food interactions, one should consider using an antidepressant other than moclobemide in patients receiving MAO-B inhibitors such as selegiline.

- *Circumvent/Minimize.* Until more data are available, patients receiving combined therapy with moclobemide and selegiline (or any other combination of an MAO-A and MAO-B inhibitor) should be given the same dietary and drug interaction instructions as patients receiving nonselective MAOI such as phenelzine or tranylcypromine.

- *Monitor* for evidence of tyramine-induced hypertension if the combination is used.

References:

1. Dingemanse J. An update of recent moclobemide interaction data. Int Clin Psychopharmacol. 1993;7:167.

## Moclobemide

### Tyramine

Summary: Moclobemide may increase the pressor response to large amounts of tyramine; high-tyramine foods (e.g., aged cheese) should be avoided.

Risk Factors: No specific risk factors known.

Related Drugs: Other MAO-A inhibitors may interact similarly with tyramine.

Management Options:

- *Circumvent/Minimize.* Although moclobemide appears much less likely to interact with dietary tyramine than nonselective MAOIs, it would be prudent to avoid foods with high tyramine content. It also has been suggested that moclobemide be taken after meals to minimize the interaction,[3] but more study is needed to assess the value of this precaution.

- *Monitor* blood pressure if the interaction is suspected.

References:

1. Dingemanse J. An update of recent moclobemide interaction data. Int Clin Psychopharmacol. 1993;7:167.

2. Simpson GM et al. Comparison of the pressor effect of tyramine after treatment with phenelzine and moclobemide in healthy male volunteers. Clin Pharmacol Ther. 1992;52:286.

3. Freeman H. Moclobemide. Lancet. 1993;342:1528.

## Moricizine (Ethmozine)

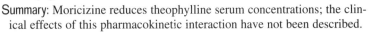

### Theophylline

Summary: Moricizine reduces theophylline serum concentrations; the clinical effects of this pharmacokinetic interaction have not been described.

Risk Factors: No specific risk factors known.

Related Drugs: No information available.

Management Options:

• *Monitor.* Patients taking theophylline should be monitored for reduced theophylline concentrations and potential loss of effect when moricizine is added to their therapy.

References:

1. Pieniaszek HJ et al. Effect of moricizine on the pharmacokinetics of single-dose theophylline in healthy subjects. Ther Drug Monit. 1993;15:199.

## Moxalactam (Moxam)

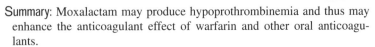

### Warfarin (Coumadin)

Summary: Moxalactam may produce hypoprothrombinemia and thus may enhance the anticoagulant effect of warfarin and other oral anticoagulants.

Risk Factors:

• *Concurrent Diseases.* Renal dysfunction, hepatic dysfunction, and reduced dietary vitamin K can place one at risk.

Related Drugs: Cephalosporins with a methylthiotetrazole (MTT) ring [e.g., *cefoperazone (Cefobid)*, *cefamandole (Mandol)*, *cefotetan (Cefotan)*, and *cefmetazole (Zefazone)*] have been associated with prolonged prothrombin times and bleeding. *Cefoxitin (Mefoxin)*, *cefazolin (Ancef)*, and *ceftriaxone (Rocephin)* also interact with warfarin. IV *cefonicid (Monocid)* 2 mg/day for 7 days did not affect the hypoprothrombinemic response.[3]

Management Options:

• *Use Alternative.* Moxalactam, cefoperazone, cefamandole, cefotetan, and cefmetazole probably should be avoided in patients taking warfarin. Intravenous cefonicid may be an alternative.

References:

1. Conjura A et al. Cefotetan and hypoprothrombinemia. Ann Intern Med. 1988; 108: 644.

2. Angaran DM et al. The comparative influence of prophylactic antibiotics on the prothrombin response to warfarin in the postoperative prosthetic cardiac valve patient: cefamandole, cefazolin, vancomycin. Ann Surg. 1987;206:155.

3. Anagaran DM et al. Effect of cefonicid (CN) on prothrombin time (PT) in outpatients (OP) receiving warfarin (W) therapy. Pharmacotherapy. 1988;8:120. Abstract.

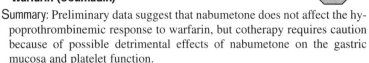

## Nabumetone (Relafen)

## Warfarin (Coumadin)

Summary: Preliminary data suggest that nabumetone does not affect the hypoprothrombinemic response to warfarin, but cotherapy requires caution because of possible detrimental effects of nabumetone on the gastric mucosa and platelet function.

Risk Factors:
- *Concurrent Diseases.* Patients with peptic ulcer disease (PUD) or a history of gastrointestinal (GI) bleeding are probably at greater risk.

Related Drugs: All NSAIDs inhibit platelet function, cause gastric erosions, and probably increase the risk of GI bleeding.

Management Options:
- *Avoid Unless Benefit Outweighs Risk.* Since all NSAIDs probably increase the risk of GI bleeding in patients on oral anticoagulants, use the combination only after careful consideration of the benefit versus risk. If the NSAID is being used as an analgesic or antipyretic, acetaminophen probably is safer to use with oral anticoagulants. Nonacetylated salicylates (e.g., choline salicylate, magnesium salicylate, salsalate, sodium salicylate) probably also are safer with oral anticoagulants than NSAIDs since they have minimal effects on platelet function and the gastric mucosa.
- *Monitor.* If any NSAID is used with an oral anticoagulant, one should monitor carefully the prothrombin time and watch for evidence of bleeding, especially from the GI tract.

References:
1. Hilleman DE et al. Hypoprothrombinemic effect of nabumetone in warfarin-treated patients. Pharmacotherapy. 1993;13:270. Abstract.
2. Shorr RI et al. Concurrent use of nonsteroidal anti-inflammatory drugs and oral anticoagulants places elderly persons at high risk for hemorrhagic peptic ulcer disease. Arch Intern Med. 1993;153:1665.

## Nafcillin

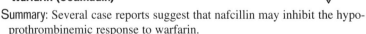

## Warfarin (Coumadin)

Summary: Several case reports suggest that nafcillin may inhibit the hypoprothrombinemic response to warfarin.

Risk Factors: No specific risk factors known.

Related Drugs: **Dicloxacillin (Dynapen)** also may inhibit the hypoprothrombinemic response to warfarin, but data are limited.

Management Options:
- *Monitor.* In patients receiving warfarin or other oral anticoagulants, monitor for a decreased hypoprothrombinemic response whenever nafcillin or other penicillinase-resistant penicillins are given. Available evidence suggests that the onset of the interaction is delayed for several days after starting the penicillin, and the effect may persist for weeks after the penicillin is discontinued.

References:
1. Fraser GL et al. Warfarin resistance associated with nafcillin therapy. Am J Med. 1989;87:237.
2. Davis RL et al. Warfarin-nafcillin interaction. J Pediatr. 1991;118:300.
3. Shovick VA et al. Decreased hypoprothrombinemic response to warfarin secondary to the warfarin-nafcillin interaction. DICP, Ann Pharmacother. 1991;25:598.

## Nalidixic Acid (NegGram)

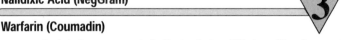

## Warfarin (Coumadin)

Summary: Isolated case reports indicate that nalidixic acid enhances the hypoprothrombinemic response to warfarin and acenocoumarol, but the incidence of this interaction in patients receiving the combination is unknown.

Risk Factors:
- *Concurrent Diseases.* Patients with fever or low albumin concentrations are at risk.

Related Drugs: Acenocoumarol interacts similarly with nalidixic acid. Little is known regarding the effect of nalidixic acid on other anticoagulants, but assume that an interaction may occur with all oral anticoagulants until evidence to the contrary is available.

Management Options:
- *Monitor* patients for an altered hypoprothrombinemic response when nalidixic acid therapy is started or stopped in patients receiving oral anticoagulants.

References:
1. Sellers EM et al. Displacement of warfarin from human albumin by diazoxide and ethacrynic, mefenamic and nalidixic acids. Clin Pharmacol Ther. 1970;11:524.
2. Potasman I et al. Nicoumalone and nalidixic acid interaction. Ann Intern Med. 1980;92:572.
3. Leor J et al. Interaction between nalidixic acid and warfarin. Ann Intern Med. 1987;107:601.

## Naproxen (Naprosyn)

## Warfarin (Coumadin)

Summary: Naproxen does not appear to affect the hypoprothrombinemic response to warfarin in most patients; however, naproxen should be used cautiously because of its possible detrimental effects on gastric mucosa and platelet function.

Risk Factors:
- *Concurrent Diseases.* Patients with peptic ulcer disease (PUD) or a history of gastrointestinal (GI) bleeding are probably at greater risk.

Related Drugs: All NSAIDs inhibit platelet function, cause gastric erosions, and probably increase the risk of GI bleeding.

Management Options:
- *Avoid Unless Benefit Outweighs Risk.* Since all NSAIDs probably increase the risk of GI bleeding in patients on oral anticoagulants,

use the combination only after careful consideration of the benefit versus risk. If the NSAID is being used as an analgesic or antipyretic, acetaminophen probably is safer to use with oral anticoagulants. Nonacetylated salicylates (e.g., choline salicylate, magnesium salicylate, salsalate, sodium salicylate) probably also are safer with oral anticoagulants than NSAIDs since they have minimal effects on platelet function and the gastric mucosa.

- *Monitor.* If any NSAID is used with an oral anticoagulant, one should monitor carefully the prothrombin time and watch for evidence of bleeding, especially from the GI tract.

References:

1. Jain A et al. Effect of naproxen on the steady-state serum concentration and anticoagulant activity of warfarin. Clin Pharmacol Ther. 1979;25:61.
2. Slattery JT et al. Effect of naproxen on the kinetics of elimination and anticoagulant activity of single dose warfarin. Clin Pharmacol Ther. 1979;25:51.
3. Shorr RI et al. Concurrent use of nonsteroidal anti-inflammatory drugs and oral anticoagulants places elderly persons at high risk for hemorrhagic peptic ulcer disease. Arch Intern Med. 1993;153:1665.

### Nefazodone (Serzone)

### Simvastatin (Zocor)

**2**

Summary: A patient on simvastatin developed muscle damage (myositis and rhabdomyolysis) after starting nefazodone therapy.

Risk Factors:

- *Dosage Regimen.* The ability of simvastatin to produce damage to skeletal muscle appears to be dose related. Thus, the risk of combined therapy with nefazodone is probably higher in patients on larger doses of simvastatin.

Related Drugs: **Lovastatin (Mevacor)** also is known to result in muscle damage when given with CYP3A4 inhibitors, while **pravastatin (Pravachol)**, **fluvastatin (Lescol)**, and **atorvastatin (Lipitor)** may be less likely to do so. **Fluoxetine (Prozac)** may inhibit CYP3A4 to a lesser extent than nefazodone (see Management Options below).

Management Options:

- *Use Alternative.* The use of an HMG-CoA reductase inhibitor other than simvastatin or lovastatin probably reduces the risk. Nefazodone

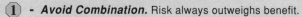
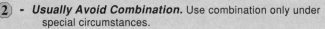

## Significance Classification

1. - *Avoid Combination.* Risk always outweighs benefit.

2. - *Usually Avoid Combination.* Use combination only under special circumstances.

3. - *Minimize Risk.* Take action as necessary to reduce risk.

is probably one of the most potent CYP3A4 inhibitors among anti-depressants, so using an alternative antidepressant may reduce the interaction. Fluoxetine also may inhibit CYP3A4, but probably to a lesser extent than nefazodone. If the combination is used, be alert for evidence of muscle damage (e.g., muscle pain, weakness, dark-ened urine, elevated muscle enzymes such as creatine kinase). It also would be prudent to use conservative doses of simvastatin or lovastatin when they are used with a CYP3A4 inhibitor such as nefazodone.

References:
1. Jacobson RH et al. Myositis and rhabdomyolysis associated with concurrent use of simvastatin and nefazodone. JAMA. 1997;277:296. Letter.

## Nelfinavir (Viracept)

## Rifampin (Rifadin)

**2**

Summary: Rifampin increases nelfinavir clearance; loss of efficacy is like-ly to result.

Risk Factors: No specific risk factors known.

Related Drugs: Rifampin increases the clearance of *ritonavir (Norvir)*, *indin-avir (Crixivan)*, and *saquinavir (Invirase)*. *Rifabutin (Mycobutin)* would be expected to have a similar affect on nelfinavir clearance.

Management Options:
- *Use Alternative.* Based on the magnitude of this interaction, it would be difficult to administer an effective dose of nelfinavir. Since other protease inhibitors are also likely to be affected, an alternative to rifampin should be considered.

References:
1. Yuen GJ et al. The pharmacokinetics of nelfinavir administration alone and with rifampin in healthy volunteers. Clin Pharmacol Ther. 1997;61:147. Abstract.

## Neomycin

## Warfarin (Coumadin)

**3**

Summary: Oral administration of aminoglycosides like neomycin appears to enhance the hypoprothrombinemic response to oral anticoagulants like warfarin in certain predisposed patients.

Risk Factors:
- *Dosage Regimen.* Large oral aminoglycoside doses produce a greater risk.
- *Concurrent Diseases.* Deficiency of dietary vitamin K and impaired liver function place a patient at greater risk.

Related Drugs: Other orally administered aminoglycosides may increase hypoprothrombinemic response to warfarin.

Management Options:
- *Monitor.* Careful monitoring of hypoprothrombinemia appears warranted when an oral aminoglycoside is coadministered for more than 1 to 2 days, particularly when a patient is predisposed to a dietary vitamin K deficiency.

References:
1. Remmel RP et al. The effect of broad-spectrum antibiotics on warfarin excretion and metabolism in the rat. Res Commun Chem Pathol Pharmacol. 1981;34:503.
2. Rodriguez-Erdmann F et al. Interaction of antibiotics with vitamin K. JAMA. 1981;246:937.
3. Schade RWB et al. A comparative study of the effects of cholestyramine and neomycin in the treatment of type II hyperlipoproteinaemia. Acta Med Scand. 1976;199:175.

## Neostigmine (Prostigmin)

### Procainamide (Procan SR)

Summary: In patients receiving cholinergic agents for myasthenia gravis, symptoms may be exacerbated by procainamide administration.

Risk Factors: No specific risk factors known.

Related Drugs: Although lidocaine (Xylocaine) and propranolol also might be expected to worsen myasthenia,[1] limited use of lidocaine in 2 myasthenic patients did not result in aggravation of symptoms.[2] *Edrophonium (Tensilon)* tests may be unreliable in procainamide-treated patients.[2]

Management Options:
- *Monitor.* Watch for increased weakness in patients with myasthenia gravis if procainamide is coadministered.

References:
1. Flacke W. Treatment of myasthenia gravis. N Engl J Med. 1973;288:27.
2. Kornfeld P et al. Myasthenia gravis unmasked by antiarrhythmic agents. Mt Sinai J Med. 1976;43:10.

## Neostigmine (Prostigmin)

### Propranolol (Inderal)

Summary: Both neostigmine and beta-adrenergic blockers, such as propranolol, can slow the heart rate; additive bradycardia would be expected, but the risk of adverse consequences from the combination is not known.

Risk Factors: No specific risk factors known.

Related Drugs: Other beta blockers [e.g., *atenolol (Tenormin)*, *nadolol (Corgard)*] may produce similar effects. *Physostigmine* affects propranolol similarly.

Management Options:
- *Monitor* for excessive bradycardia in patients receiving beta-adrenergic blockers concurrently with neostigmine or other cholinergic agents.

References:
1. Seidl DC, Martin DE. Prolonged bradycardia after neostigmine administration in a patient taking nadolol. Anesth Analg. 1984;63:365.
2. Baraka A, Dajani A. Severe bradycardia following physostigmine in the presence of beta-adrenergic blockade. Middle East J Anesthesiol. 1984;7:291.
3. Eldor J et al. Prolonged bradycardia and hypotension after neostigmine administration in a patient receiving atenolol. Anesthesia. 1987;42:1294.

## Nicardipine (Cardene)

## Propranolol (Inderal)

Summary: Nicardipine administration increases propranolol concentrations; an increase in beta blocker effect may occur in some patients.

Risk Factors: No specific risk factors known.

Related Drugs: A single dose of nicardipine 30 mg had no effect on the pharmacokinetics of *atenolol (Tenormin)*.[4] Nicardipine increased *metoprolol (Lopressor)* concentration by about 25%.[5] *Nimodipine (Nimotop)* and propranolol had minimal effect on each other's plasma concentrations.[6] *Nisoldipine (Sular)* and *nifedipine (Procardia)* increased the AUC of propranolol.[1,2] Conversely, nisoldipine AUC and peak serum concentrations were increased 30% and 57%, respectively, by propranolol. Others found no change in drug concentrations during chronic nisoldipine and propranolol dosing.[7] Propranolol also blunted the increase in cardiac output observed following nisoldipine alone. *Isradipine (DynaCirc)* 10 mg increased the AUC of propranolol 28% and its peak concentration 60%.[3]

Management Options:

• *Monitor.* Patients receiving combined therapy with propranolol and nicardipine should be monitored for enhanced effects resulting from pharmacokinetic or pharmacodynamic interactions.

References:
1. Levine MAH et al. Pharmacokinetic and pharmacodynamic interactions between nisoldipine and propranolol. Clin Pharmacol Ther. 1988;43:39.
2. Vinceneux PH et al. Pharmacokinetic and pharmacodynamic interactions between nifedipine and propranolol or betaxolol. Int J Clin Pharmacol Ther Toxicol. 1986; 24:153.
3. Rosenkranz B et al. Interaction between nifedipine and atenolol: pharmacokinetics and pharmacodynamics in normotensive volunteers. J Cardiovasc Pharmacol. 1986; 8:943.
4. Vercruysse I et al. Nicardipine does not influence the pharmacokinetics and pharmacodynamics of atenolol. Br J Clin Pharmacol. 1990;30:499. Letter.
5. Funck-Brentano C et al. Influence of CYP2D6-dependent metabolism on the steady-state pharmacokinetics and pharmacodynamics of metoprolol and nicardipine, alone and in combination. Br J Clin Pharmacol. 1993;36:531.
6. Breuel HP et al. Chronic administration of nimodipine and propranolol in elderly normotensive subjects—an interaction study. Int J Clin Pharmacol Ther. 1995; 33:103.
7. Shaw-Stiffel TA et al. Pharmacokinetic and pharmacodynamic interactions during multiple-dose administration of nisoldipine and propranolol. Clin Pharmacol Ther. 1994;55:661.

### Nifedipine (Procardia)

### Phenobarbital

Summary: Phenobarbital substantially reduces the plasma concentrations of nifedipine.

Risk Factors: No specific risk factors known.

Related Drugs: Phenobarbital also increases the metabolism of **verapamil (Calan)**. Other calcium channel blockers may be affected similarly by phenobarbital.

Management Options:
- *Circumvent/Minimize.* Patients receiving phenobarbital may require higher than usual doses of nifedipine.
- *Monitor.* Patients stabilized on nifedipine should be monitored for the possibility of decreased effectiveness when phenobarbital is administered concomitantly.

References:
1. Schellens JHM et al. Influence of enzyme induction and inhibition on the oxidation of nifedipine, sparteine, mephenytoin and antipyrine in humans as assessed by a cocktail study design. J Pharmacol Exp Ther. 1989;249:638.

### Nifedipine (Procardia)

### Phenytoin (Dilantin)

Summary: Nifedipine was associated with increased plasma phenytoin concentration in one case; more study is needed.

Risk Factors: No specific risk factors known.

Related Drugs: The bioavailability of most calcium channel blockers appears to be reduced by enzyme inducers such as phenytoin.

Management Options:
- *Monitor.* Until more information regarding this potential interaction is available, patients receiving phenytoin should be monitored carefully when nifedipine or diltiazem is added to or removed from their regimen.

References:
1. Ahmad S. Nifedipine-phenytoin interaction. J Am Coll Cardiol. 1984;3:1581.

## Significance Classification

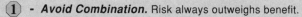
① - *Avoid Combination.* Risk always outweighs benefit.

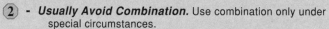
② - *Usually Avoid Combination.* Use combination only under special circumstances.

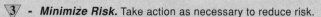
③ - *Minimize Risk.* Take action as necessary to reduce risk.

## Nifedipine (Procardia)

## Propranolol (Inderal)

Summary: The combination of nifedipine and propranolol may result in hypotension; nifedipine can increase propranalol concentrations.

Risk Factors: No specific risk factors known.

Related Drugs: *Atenolol (Tenormin)* and *metoprolol (Lopressor)* may interact similarly with nifedipine. *Felodipine (Plendil)* 10 mg BID increased the AUC of metoprolol by 31%,[2] but the AUC of felodipine was not altered by chronic metoprolol or atenolol therapy.[4] *Nisoldipine (Sular)* 20 mg increased the propranolol AUC by about 50%.[1,5] Conversely, nisoldipine AUC and peak serum concentrations were increased 30% and 57%, respectively, by propranolol. Propranolol also blunted the increase in cardiac output observed following nisoldipine alone. *Isradipine (DynaCirc)* 10 mg increased the AUC of propranolol 28% and its peak concentration 60%.[3]

Management Options:

- *Monitor.* Patients receiving combined therapy with propranolol and nifedipine should be monitored for enhanced effects resulting from pharmacokinetic or pharmacodynamic interactions.

References:

1. Levine MAH et al. Pharmacokinetic and pharmacodynamic interactions between nisoldipine and propranolol. Clin Pharmacol Ther. 1988;43:39.
2. Smith SR et al. Pharmacokinetic interactions between felodipine and metoprolol. Eur J Clin Pharmacol. 1987;31:575.
3. Shepherd AMM et al. Pharmacokinetic interaction between isradipine and propranolol. Clin Pharmacol Ther. 1988;43:194. Abstract.
4. Bengtsson-Hasselgren B et al. Haemodynamic effects and pharmacokinetics of felodipine at rest and during exercise in hypertensive patients treated with metoprolol. Eur J Clin Pharmacol. 1989;37:459.
5. Elliott HL et al. The interactions between nisoldipine and two beta-adrenoceptor antagonists-atenolol and propranolol. Br J Clin Pharmacol. 1991;32:379.

## Nifedipine (Procardia)

## Quinidine

Summary: Nifedipine appears to reduce the serum concentrations of quinidine, and quinidine appears to increase the serum concentration of nifedipine.

Risk Factors: No specific risk factors known.

Related Drugs: *Verapamil (Calan)* increases quinidine concentrations. *Diltiazem (Cardizem)* 120 mg/day had no effect on quinidine concentrations.[3]

Management Options:

- *Circumvent/Minimize.* Quinidine doses may require upward adjustment when nifedipine is added or downward adjustment if quinidine is discontinued.

• *Monitor.* Nifedipine and quinidine coadministration may reduce quinidine concentration and increase nifedipine concentration; patients should be monitored carefully.

References:

1. Matera MG et al. Quinidine-diltiazem: pharmacokinetic interaction in humans. Curr Ther Res. 1986;40:653.
2. Bowles SK et al. Evaluation of the pharmacokinetic and pharmacodynamic interaction between quinidine and nifedipine. J Clin Pharmacol. 1993;33:727.
3. Bailey DG et al. Quinidine interaction with nifedipine and felodipine: pharmacokinetic and pharmacodynamic evaluation. Clin Pharmacol Ther. 1993;53:354.

### Nifedipine (Procardia)

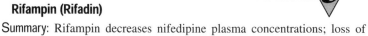

### Rifampin (Rifadin)

Summary: Rifampin decreases nifedipine plasma concentrations; loss of therapeutic effect may result.

Risk Factors: No specific risk factors known.

Related Drugs: Rifampin probably affects other calcium channel blockers in a similar manner. *Rifabutin (Mycobutin)* would be expected to affect nifedipine in a similar manner.

Management Options:

• *Consider Alternative.* Because this interaction is likely to reduce the efficacy of nifedipine, one should consider an alternative agent for nifedipine. Other calcium channel blockers also may be affected; a therapeutic substitution to a different class of agent may be required.

• *Circumvent/Minimize.* Larger doses of calcium channel blockers (particularly those administered orally) may be required when rifampin is coadministered.

• *Monitor.* Patients taking calcium channel blockers should be monitored for a reduction in efficacy when rifampin is given.

References:

1. Tsuchihashi K et al. A case of variant angina exacerbated by administration of rifampicin. Heart Vessels. 1987;3:214.
2. Tada Y et al. Case report: nifedipine-rifampicin interaction attenuates the effect on blood pressure in a patient with essential hypertension. Am J Med Sci. 1992;303:25.

### Nifedipine (Procardia)

### Vincristine (Oncovin)

Summary: Nifedipine appeared to increase markedly the half-life of vincristine; the clinical significance is unknown.

Risk Factors: No specific risk factors known.

Related Drugs: Little is known regarding the effect of other calcium channel blockers on vincristine, but consider the possibility that they also interact.

Management Options:
- *Monitor.* Until further information is available, monitor patients receiving vincristine and nifedipine concomitantly for enhanced pharmacodynamic effects of vincristine. It may be necessary to adjust vincristine dose.

References:
1. Tsuruo T et al. Potentiation of vincristine and adriamycin effects in human hemopoietic tumor cell lines by calcium antagonists and calmodulin inhibitors. Cancer Res. 1983;43:2267.
2. Fedeli L et al. Pharmacokinetics of vincristine in cancer patients treated with nifedipine. Cancer. 1989;64:1805.

### Nimodipine (Nimotop)

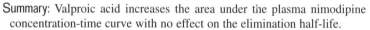

### Valproic Acid (Depakene)

Summary: Valproic acid increases the area under the plasma nimodipine concentration-time curve with no effect on the elimination half-life.

Risk Factors: No specific risk factors known.

Related Drugs: No information available.

Management Options:
- *Monitor.* Patients receiving both nimodipine and valproic acid should be monitored for altered nimodipine effect if valproic acid is initiated, discontinued, or changed in dosage.

References:
1. Tartara A et al. Differential effects of valproic acid and enzyme-inducing anticonvulsants on nimodipine pharmacokinetics in epileptic patients. Br J Clin Pharmacol. 1991;32:335.

### Norepinephrine (Levarterenol)

### Phenelzine (Nardil)

Summary: Monoamine oxidase inhibitors (MAOIs) may slightly increase the pressor response to norepinephrine.

Risk Factors: No specific risk factors known.

Related Drugs: Theoretically other nonselective MAOIs, including *isocarboxazid (Marplan)* and *tranylcypromine (Parnate)*, would interact with norepinephrine in a similar manner.

## Significance Classification

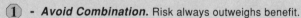
- **Avoid Combination.** Risk always outweighs benefit.

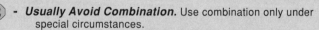
- **Usually Avoid Combination.** Use combination only under special circumstances.

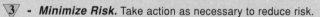
- **Minimize Risk.** Take action as necessary to reduce risk.

Management Options:

- *Monitor* blood pressure carefully if patients on nonselective MAOIs receive norepinephrine. Remember that the effects of nonselective MAOIs should be assumed to persist for 2 weeks after they are discontinued.

References:

1. Boakes AJ et al. Interactions between sympathomimetic amines and antidepressant agents in man. Br Med J. 1973;1:311.
2. Sjoqvist F. Psychotropic drugs (2). Interaction between monoamine oxidase (MAO) inhibitors and other substances. Proc R Soc Med. 1965;58:967.
3. Ellis J et al. Modification by monoamine oxidase inhibitors of the effect of some sympathomimetics on blood pressure. Br Med J. 1967;2:75.

## Norfloxacin (Noroxin)

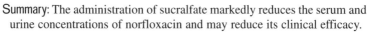

## Sucralfate (Carafate)

Summary: The administration of sucralfate markedly reduces the serum and urine concentrations of norfloxacin and may reduce its clinical efficacy.

Risk Factors: No specific risk factors known.

Related Drugs: **Aluminum**-containing antacids also reduce the absorption of norfloxacin. Sucralfate inhibits the absorption of **ciprofloxacin (Cipro)**, **fleroxacin**, and **ofloxacin (Floxin)**.

Management Options:

- *Consider Alternative.* If dosage separation is not possible, an alternative to sucralfate [e.g., $H_2$-receptor antagonist, omeprazole (Prilosec), but *not* an antacid] should be considered.
- *Circumvent/Minimize.* Until further information is available, the co-administration of norfloxacin and sucralfate should be avoided. Norfloxacin should be administered several hours before sucralfate.
- *Monitor.* If sucralfate and a quinolone are coadministered, monitor the patient for reduced antibiotic efficacy.

References:

1. Parpia SH et al. Sucralfate reduces the gastrointestinal absorption of norfloxacin. Antimicrob Agents Chemother. 1989;33:99.
2. Lehto P et al. Effect of sucralfate on absorption of norfloxacin and ofloxacin. Antimicrob Agents Chemother. 1994;38:248.

## Norfloxacin (Noroxin)

## Theophylline

Summary: Norfloxacin may increase the serum concentration of theophylline; however, the increase is unlikely to result in the development of theophylline toxicity in most patients.

Risk Factors: No specific risk factors known.

Related Drugs: Quinolones reported to inhibit the metabolism of drugs include **ciprofloxacin (Cipro)**, **enoxacin (Penetrex)**, **pipemidic acid**, and **pefloxacin**.

Management Options:
- *Consider Alternative.* Quinolones reported to produce no or minor changes in theophylline pharmacokinetics include fleroxacin, flosequinan, lomefloxacin (Maxaquin), ofloxacin (Floxin), rufloxacin, sparfloxacin, and temafloxacin.
- *Monitor.* Patients maintained on theophylline are at limited risk to develop theophylline toxicity (palpitations, tachycardia, nausea, tremor) during concomitant administrations of norfloxacin.

References:
1. Ho G et al. Evaluation of the effect of norfloxacin on the pharmacokinetics of theophylline. Clin Pharmacol Ther. 1989;44:35.
2. Prince RA et al. The effect of quinolone antibiotics on theophylline pharmacokinetics. J Clin Pharmacol. 1989;20:650.
3. Davis RL et al. The effect of norfloxacin on theophylline metabolism. Antimicrob Agents Chemother. 1989;33:212.

### Norfloxacin (Noroxin)

### Warfarin (Coumadin)

Summary: A patient on chronic warfarin therapy developed excessive hypoprothrombinemia and fatal hemorrhage during therapy with norfloxacin, but a study in healthy subjects suggests that norfloxacin does not affect warfarin response.

Risk Factors:
- *Concurrent Diseases.* Fever may place a patient at increased risk.

Related Drugs: **Ciprofloxacin (Cipro)** and **ofloxacin (Floxin)** have been noted to increase INRs in a few case reports.

Management Options:
- *Monitor.* Until additional information is available, monitor the prothrombin time carefully if norfloxacin therapy is initiated or discontinued in a patient receiving warfarin or other anticoagulants.

References:
1. Linville T et al. Norfloxacin and warfarin. Ann Intern Med. 1989;110:751. Letter.
2. Vlasses PH et al. Warfarin in healthy men. Pharmacotherapy. 1988;8:120. Abstract.

### Nortriptyline (Pamelor)

### Rifampin (Rifadin)

Summary: Rifampin and isoniazid administration appeared to decrease nortriptyline concentrations in one patient; the significance of this interaction is not known.

Risk Factors: No specific risk factors known.

Related Drugs: If this interaction is confirmed, other cyclic antidepressants also may be affected by rifampin administration.

Management Options:
- *Circumvent/Minimize.* The dose of nortriptyline may have to be adjusted when rifampin is started or discontinued.
- *Monitor.* Until information is available, patients taking both nortriptyline and rifampin should be monitored for reduced nortriptyline concentration and effect. Discontinuation of rifampin may result in toxic antidepressant concentrations.

References:
1. Bebchuk JM et al. Drug interaction between rifampin and nortriptyline: a case report. Int J Psychiatry Med. 1991;21:183.

## Ofloxacin (Floxin)

## Procainamide (Procan)

Summary: Ofloxacin administration increases procainamide concentrations; it is possible that some patients may experience clinically significant increases in procainamide effects.

Risk Factors: No specific risk factors known.

Related Drugs: *Lomefloxacin (Maxaquin)* is also partially eliminated by the organic cationic transport system and may affect procainamide renal clearance to some degree.[2] The effects of other quinolone antibiotics on procainamide renal clearance are unknown.

Management Options:
- *Monitor.* Patients stabilized on procainamide therapy should have procainamide plasma concentrations monitored during concomitant administration of ofloxacin. Electrocardiogram monitoring for widened QRS and QTc intervals would be warranted.

References:
1. Martin DE et al. Effects of ofloxacin on the pharmacokinetics and pharmacodynamics of procainamide. J Clin Pharmacol. 1996;36:85.
2. Hoffler D et al. Pharmacokinetics of lomefloxacin in normal and impaired renal function. Acta Ther. 1989;15:321.

## Ofloxacin (Floxin)

## Sucralfate (Carafate)

Summary: The concomitant administration of sucralfate with ofloxacin results in a marked reduction in ofloxacin serum concentrations and potentially reduced clinical efficacy.

Risk Factors: No specific risk factors known.

Related Drugs: Sucralfate also inhibits the absorption of *ciprofloxacin (Cipro)*, *fleroxacin*, and *norfloxacin (Noroxin)*. *Aluminum*-containing antacids also reduce ofloxacin absorption.

Management Options:
- *Consider Alternative.* If dosage separation is not possible, an alternative to sucralfate [e.g., $H_2$-receptor antagonist, omeprazole (Prilosec), but *not* an antacid] should be considered.
- *Circumvent/Minimize.* Patients prescribed sucralfate and ofloxacin should avoid concomitant administration of the two agents. To avoid the interaction the ofloxacin should be taken 2 hours before the sucralfate dose.
- *Monitor.* If sucralfate and a quinolone are coadministered, monitor the patient for reduced antibiotic efficacy.

References:
1. Lehto P et al. Effect of sucralfate on absorption of norfloxacin and ofloxacin. Antimicrob Agents Chemother. 1994;38:248.
2. Kawakami J et al. The effect of food on the interaction of ofloxacin with sucralfate in healthy volunteers. Cur J Clin Pharmacol. 1994;47:67.

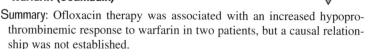

**Ofloxacin (Floxin)**

**Warfarin (Coumadin)**

Summary: Ofloxacin therapy was associated with an increased hypoprothrombinemic response to warfarin in two patients, but a causal relationship was not established.

Risk Factors:
- *Concurrent Diseases.* Fever may place a patient at increased risk.

Related Drugs: *Ciprofloxacin (Cipro)* and *norfloxacin (Noroxin)* have been noted to increase INRs in a few case reports.

Management Options:
- *Monitor.* Until more information is available, monitor patients for an altered hypoprothrombinemic response to warfarin if ofloxacin is initiated, discontinued, or changed in dosage.

References:
1. Leor J et al. Ofloxacin and warfarin. Ann Intern Med. 1988;109:761. Letter.
2. Baciewicz AM et al. Interaction of ofloxacin and warfarin. Ann Intern Med. 1993; 119:1223. Letter.

**Omeprazole (Prilosec)**

**Phenytoin (Dilantin)**

Summary: Omeprazole increases plasma phenytoin concentrations modestly in healthy subjects given single oral or IV doses of phenytoin, but the importance of the interaction in patients on chronic phenytoin therapy is not established.

Risk Factors:
- *Dosage Regimen.* Omeprazole doses $\geq 40$ mg/day may inhibit phenytoin metabolism.

Related Drugs: The effect of *lansoprazole (Prevacid)* on phenytoin is not established, but lansoprazole generally is less likely to inhibit drug metabolism than omeprazole.

Management Options:

- *Monitor.* Until data from patients on chronic phenytoin therapy are available, monitor for an excessive phenytoin response when omeprazole is started and for a reduced phenytoin response when omeprazole is stopped. It may be necessary to adjust the phenytoin dose in some cases.

References:

1. Andersson T et al. Identification of human liver cytochrome P450 isoforms medicating secondary omeprazole metabolism. Br J Clin Pharmacol. 1994;37:597.
2. Andersson T. Omeprazole drug interaction studies. Clin Pharmacokinet. 1991; 21:195.
3. Prichard PJ et al. Oral phenytoin pharmacokinetics during omeprazole therapy. Br J Clin Pharmacol. 1987;24:543.

## Oral Contraceptives

## Phenobarbital

Summary: Phenobarbital may reduce the efficacy of oral contraceptives; menstrual irregularities and unintended pregnancies may occur.

Risk Factors:

- *Dosage Regimen.* It is likely that patients taking low-dose oral contraceptives that contain the lowest doses of steroids are most susceptible to this interaction.

Related Drugs: All barbiturates are likely to enhance *estrogen* metabolism.

Management Options:

- *Circumvent/Minimize.* Patients receiving chronic barbiturate therapy may require oral contraceptives with a higher estrogen content. If barbiturate use is short-term, alternative methods of contraception should be used (in addition to the oral contraceptives) during, and for at least several weeks after, barbiturate therapy has been discontinued.

## Significance Classification

(1) - *Avoid Combination.* Risk always outweighs benefit.

(2) - *Usually Avoid Combination.* Use combination only under special circumstances.

(3) - *Minimize Risk.* Take action as necessary to reduce risk.

- *Monitor.* Spotting or breakthrough bleeding may be an indication that significant enzyme induction is occurring, but a lack of menstrual irregularities does not ensure that the interaction has not occurred.

References:
1. Conney AH. Pharmacological implications of microsomal enzyme induction. Pharmacol Rev. 1967;19:317.
2. Robertson YR et al. Interactions between oral contraceptives and other drugs: a review. Curr Med Res Opin. 1976;3:647.
3. Hempel E et al. Drug stimulated biotransformation of hormonal steroid contraceptives: clinical implications. Drugs. 1976;12:442.

## Oral Contraceptives

### Phenytoin (Dilantin)

Summary: Phenytoin and other enzyme-inducing anticonvulsants, such as barbiturates, carbamazepine, and primidone, may inhibit the effect of oral contraceptives resulting in menstrual irregularities and unplanned pregnancies.

Risk Factors: No specific risk factors known.

Related Drugs: *Valproic acid (Depakene)* does not appear to affect the pharmacokinetics of oral contraceptives;[1] both clinical evidence and theoretical considerations suggest that benzodiazepine anticonvulsants are unlikely to affect oral contraceptive efficacy. *Carbamazepine (Tegretol)* and *primidone (Mysoline)* may inhibit the effect of oral contraceptives resulting in menstrual irregularities and unplanned pregnancies.

Management Options:
- *Consider Alternative.* When pregnancy is to be avoided in women receiving enzyme-inducing anticonvulsants such as carbamazepine, phenobarbital, phenytoin, and primidone, some recommend the use of a means of contraception other than oral contraceptives. Others prefer to use an oral contraceptive with a higher estrogen content for women who are being treated with an enzyme-inducing anticonvulsant. This method would work best for women on a relatively stable anticonvulsant regimen.
- *Monitor.* This method also should be individualized based on patient response (e.g., lack of breakthrough bleeding). Spotting or breakthrough bleeding in patients who are taking oral contraceptives and enzyme-inducing anticonvulsants could indicate that the drugs are interacting, although lack of breakthrough bleeding does not ensure contraceptive protection.[3] Also be alert for evidence of increased phenytoin effect in patients taking oral contraceptives.

References:
1. Crawford P et al. The lack of effect of sodium valproate on the pharmacokinetics or oral contraceptive steroids. Contraception. 1986;33:23.
2. Haukkamaa M. Contraception by Norplant subdermal capsules is not reliable in epileptic patients on anticonvulsant treatment. Contraception. 1986;33:559.
3. Mattson RH et al. Use of oral contraceptives by women with epilepsy. JAMA. 1986;256:238.

## Oral Contraceptives

### Prednisolone (Prelone)

Summary: Oral contraceptives and estrogens may enhance the effect of hydrocortisone, prednisolone, and possibly other corticosteroids; adjustments in corticosteroid dosage may be required.

Risk Factors: No specific risk factors known.

Related Drugs: **Estrogen** enhances the anti-inflammatory effect of **hydrocortisone** in patients with chronic inflammatory skin diseases.[2] The glucosuric effect of **prednisone (Deltasone)**, **dexamethasone (Decadron)**, and **methylprednisolone (Medrol)** was not consistently affected by estrogen in one study.[1] Most combinations of oral contraceptives and corticosteroids probably interact.

Management Options:
- *Monitor.* In patients receiving both corticosteroids and oral contraceptives estrogen, watch for evidence of excessive corticosteroid effects. It may be necessary to reduce the dose of the corticosteroid.

References:
1. Nelson DH et al. Potentiation of the biologic effect of administered cortisol by estrogen treatment. J Clin Endocrinol Metab. 1963;23:261.
2. Spangler AS et al. Enhancement of the anti-inflammatory action of hydrocortisone by estrogen. J Clin Endocrinol. 1969;29:650.
3. Boekenoogen SJ et al. Prednisolone disposition and protein binding in oral contraceptive users. J Clin Endocrinol Metab. 1983;56:702.

## Oral Contraceptives

### Rifampin (Rifadin)

Summary: Rifampin therapy can induce menstrual irregularities, ovulation, and occasionally contraceptive failure in women taking birth control pills.

Risk Factors:
- *Dosage Regimen.* Patients receiving oral contraceptives with low estrogen content may be especially susceptible to a reduction in effectiveness by rifampin.

Related Drugs: **Rifabutin (Mycobutin)** might affect oral contraceptives in a similar manner.

Management Options:
- *Consider Alternative.* Patients receiving rifampin should use contraceptive methods other than oral contraceptives or use additional contraceptive methods during and for at least 1 cycle after rifampin administration is completed.
- *Monitor.* Watch for evidence of reduced estrogen effect, including menstrual irregularities, as evidence of rifampin-induced estrogen metabolism. Patients taking oral contraceptives should be counseled on the risk of potential pregnancy during rifampin administration.

References:
1. Joshi JV et al. A study of interaction of a low-dose combination oral contraceptive with anti-tubercular drugs. Contraception. 1980;21:617.

2. Meyer B et al. A model to detect interactions between roxithromycin and oral contraceptives. Clin Pharmacol Ther. 1990;47:671.
3. Back DJ et al. The effect of rifampin on the pharmacokinetics of ethynyl estradiol in women. Contraception. 1980;21:135.

## Oral Contraceptives

### Ritonavir (Norvir)

Summary: Ritonavir is reported to reduce ethinyl estradiol concentrations. Loss of contraceptive activity could occur.

Risk Factors: No specific risk factors known.

Related Drugs: *Indinavir (Crixivan)* has been noted to *increase* ethinyl estradiol concentrations by 24%.[3] The effect of ritonavir on other estrogens is unknown. While no data are available, *saquinavir (Invirase)* and *nelfinavir (Viracept)* would be less likely to interact with ethinyl estradiol.

Management Options:

- *Consider Alternative.* Patients receiving ritonavir and oral contraceptives should utilize an alternative method of birth control during ritonavir administration and for at least one cycle following its discontinuation. Indinavir does not appear to reduce oral contraceptive concentrations and could be considered as an alternative antiviral agent.

- *Monitor* for signs that may indicate insufficient estrogen concentrations such as breakthrough bleeding.

References:
1. Abbott Laboratories. Ritonavir (Norvir) package insert. 1996.
2. Shenfield GM. Oral Contraceptives. Drug Safety. 1993;9:21.
3. Merck and Company, Inc. Indinavir (Crixivan) package insert. 1996.

## Oral Contraceptives

### Tetracycline

Summary: Case reports suggest that tetracycline can reduce the effectiveness of oral contraceptives; a prospective study failed to demonstrate an effect in a small number of women.

## Significance Classification

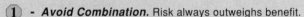

(1) - *Avoid Combination.* Risk always outweighs benefit.

(2) - *Usually Avoid Combination.* Use combination only under special circumstances.

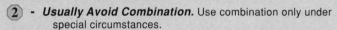 - *Minimize Risk.* Take action as necessary to reduce risk.

Risk Factors: No specific risk factors known.

Related Drugs: Other oral antibiotics [e.g., *doxycycline (Vibramycin)*] have been associated with oral contraceptive failure.

Management Options:

- *Monitor.* Although evidence of interaction between tetracyclines and oral contraceptives is scanty, women on oral contraceptives should be counseled to use additional forms of contraception during tetracycline therapy.

References:

1. Back DJ et al. Evaluation of committee on safety of medicines yellow card reports on oral contraceptive-drug interactions with anticonvulsants and antibiotics. Br J Clin Pharmacol. 1988;25:527.
2. Murphy AA et al. The effect of tetracycline on levels of oral contraceptives. Am J Obstet Gynecol. 1991;164:28.
3. Neely JL et al. The effect of doxycycline on serum levels of ethinyl estradiol, norethindrone, and endogenous progesterone. Obstet Gynecol. 1991;77:416.

## Oral Contraceptives

## Warfarin (Coumadin)

Summary: Oral contraceptives have been reported to both increase and decrease the anticoagulant response, depending upon the oral anticoagulant. Most patients requiring oral anticoagulants probably should avoid oral contraceptives since they may increase the risk of thromboembolic disorders.

Risk Factors: No specific risk factors known.

Related Drugs: Seven women on various oral contraceptives (containing 30 to 50 μ estrogen) were given a single oral dose of *phenprocoumon* (0.22 mg/kg).[3] The clearance of phenprocoumon was 25% higher in these women than in 7 matched controls not receiving oral contraceptives. Similarly, oral contraceptives have been shown clinically to decrease the anticoagulant response to *dicumarol*.[1]

Management Options:

- *Avoid Unless Benefit Outweighs Risk.* Patients on oral anticoagulants generally should avoid oral contraceptives because the contraceptives may increase the risk of thromboembolic disorders.

- *Monitor.* If an oral contraceptive must be used in a patient receiving an oral anticoagulant, monitor for altered hypoprothrombinemic response when the oral contraceptive is initiated, discontinued, or if the hormone content of the oral contraceptive is changed.

References:

1. Schrogie JJ et al. Effect of oral contraceptives on vitamin K-dependent clotting activity. Clin Pharmacol Ther. 1967;8:670.

2. de Teresa E et al. Interaction between anticoagulants and contraceptives: an unexpected finding. Br Med J. 1979;2:1260.
3. Monig H et al. Effect of oral contraceptive steroids on the pharmacokinetics of phenprocoumon. Br J Clin Pharmacol. 1990;30:115.

## Oxymetholone (Anadrol)

## Warfarin (Coumadin)

**2**

Summary: Several anabolic steroids have been shown to enhance the hypoprothrombinemic response to oral anticoagulants; bleeding episodes have been reported in some cases.

Risk Factors: No specific risk factors known.

Related Drugs: Some evidence indicates that 17-alpha-alkylated anabolic steroids such as *methandrostenolone (Dianabol)*, *norethandrolone*, *methyltestosterone (Metandren)*, and *stanozolol (Winstrol)* are more likely to potentiate oral anticoagulants than anabolic steroids that are not so substituted. *Testosterone* also interacts with warfarin.

Management Options:

- *Avoid Unless Risk Outweighs Benefit.* Concomitant use of oral anticoagulants and anabolic steroids should be avoided if possible.
- *Monitor.* If the combination is necessary, patients should be monitored carefully for altered anticoagulant response when the anabolic steroid is initiated, discontinued, or changed in dosage.

References:

1. Lorentz SM et al. Potentiation of warfarin anticoagulation by topical testosterone ointment. Clin Pharm. 1985;4:333.
2. Acomb C et al. A significant interaction between warfarin and stanozolol. Pharmaceutical J. 1985;234;73.
3. Shaw PW et al. Possible interaction of warfarin and stanozolol. Clin Pharm. 1987; 6:500.

## Pancuronium (Pavulon)

## Polymyxin

**2**

Summary: Polymyxin may prolong apnea following the use of muscle relaxants such as pancuronium.

Risk Factors: No specific risk factors known.

Related Drugs: Other neuromuscular blockers may interact with polymyxin.

Management Options:

- *Avoid Unless Benefit Outweighs Risk.* Polymyxin only should be given with caution during surgery or in the postoperative period.
- *Monitor.* If the polymyxin and neuromuscular blocking drugs are used together, monitor the patient carefully for enhanced neuromuscular blockade.

References:

1. Levine RA et al. Polymyxin B-induced respiratory paralysis reversed by intravenous calcium chloride. J Mt Sinai Hosp. 1969;36:380.

2. Pittinger CB et al. Antibiotic-induced paralysis. Anesth Analg. 1970;49:487.
3. Fogdall RP et al. Prolongation of a pancuronium-induced neuromuscular blockage by polymyxin B. Anesthesiology. 1974;40:84.

### Para-Aminobenzoic Acid (Potaba)

### Sulfamethoxazole (Gantanol)

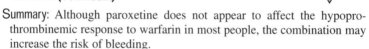

**Summary:** Para-aminobenzoic acid (PABA) may interfere with the antibacterial activity of sulfonamides.

**Risk Factors:** No specific risk factors known.

**Related Drugs:** PABA may be found in some vitamin supplements.

**Management Options:**

- *Use Alternative.* PABA should not be administered to patients receiving antibacterial sulfonamides.

**References:**

1. Mandell GL et al. Antimicrobial agents. Sulfonamides, trimethoprim-sulfamethoxazole, quinolones, and agents for urinary tract infections. In: Gilman AG et al., eds. The Pharmacological Basis of Therapeutics. 8th ed. New York: Pergamon; 1990: 1048.

### Paroxetine (Paxil)

### Warfarin (Coumadin)

**Summary:** Although paroxetine does not appear to affect the hypoprothrombinemic response to warfarin in most people, the combination may increase the risk of bleeding.

**Risk Factors:** No specific risk factors known.

**Related Drugs:** The effect of paroxetine on the response to other oral anticoagulants is not established, but the same precautions would apply until data are available. Data are insufficient to determine the relative risk of paroxetine versus other selective serotonin reuptake inhibitors (SSRIs) in anticoagulated patients.

**Management Options:**

- *Consider Alternative.* Although the ability of paroxetine to increase the risk of bleeding in patients on warfarin is not well established, it would be prudent to avoid the combination when possible. The use of an SSRI other than paroxetine may or may not reduce the risk.

- *Monitor.* If the combination is used, monitor for altered hypoprothrombinemic response to warfarin if paroxetine is initiated, discontinued, or changed in dosage. Note an increased bleeding risk may occur in the absence of excessive hypoprothrombinemia.

**References:**

1. Bannister SJ et al. Evaluation of the potential for interactions of paroxetine with diazepam, cimetidine, warfarin, and digoxin. Acta Psychiatr Scand. 1989;80(Suppl. 350):102.

## Pentoxifylline (Trental)

### Theophylline

Summary: Pentoxifylline increased plasma theophylline concentrations in healthy subjects; theophylline toxicity may be increased in patients receiving the combination, but more study is needed.

Risk Factors: No specific risk factors known.

Related Drugs: Whether other forms of theophylline would be affected similarly by pentoxifylline is unknown. If the mechanism of the interaction is inhibition of theophylline elimination, the interaction is likely to be similar with all forms of theophylline. If another mechanism is involved (e.g., increased theophylline absorption), the interaction may or may not be similar for other theophylline dosage forms.

Management Options:

- *Monitor* for evidence of altered theophylline effect if pentoxifylline therapy is initiated and for decreased theophylline effect if it is discontinued. Alteration of theophylline dose may be needed.

References:

1. Ellison MJ et al. Influence of pentoxifylline on steady-state theophylline serum concentrations from sustained-release formulation. Pharmacotherapy. 1990;10:383.
2. Cummings DM et al. Interference potential of pentoxifylline and its major metabolite with theophylline assays. Am J Hosp Pharm. 1985;42:2717.
3. Cohen IA et al. Effect of pentoxifylline and its metabolites on three theophylline assays. Clin Pharm. 1988;7:457.

## Phenelzine (Nardil)

### Phenylephrine (Neo-Synephrine)

Summary: Monoamine oxidase inhibitors (MAOIs) like phenelzine enhance the effects of phenylephrine, especially when it is administered orally. Concomitant use of these drugs may result in hypertensive reactions.

Risk Factors:

- *Route of Administration.* The interaction is likely to be much greater with oral than with parenteral phenylephrine.

Related Drugs: All nonselective MAOIs including *isocarboxazid (Marplan)* and *tranylcypromine (Parnate)* would be expected to interact with phenylephrine.

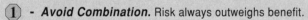
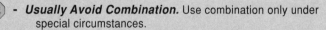

## Significance Classification

1. - **Avoid Combination.** Risk always outweighs benefit.

2. - **Usually Avoid Combination.** Use combination only under special circumstances.

3. - **Minimize Risk.** Take action as necessary to reduce risk.

Management Options:
- *Avoid Combination.* Oral phenylephrine should be avoided in patients taking an MAOI. It should be noted that phenylephrine is found in many nonprescription cold remedies. Parenteral phenylephrine should be used with great care in patients on an MAOI. The effect of phenylephrine-containing nose sprays in those taking an MAOI has not been studied, but they should probably be avoided until information on their safety is available. Remember that effects of nonselective MAOIs should be assumed to persist for 2 weeks after they are discontinued.

References:
1. Boakes AJ et al. Interactions between sympathomimetic amines and antidepressant agents in man. Br Med J. 1973;1:311.
2. Davies B et al. Pressor amines and monoamine-oxidase inhibitors for treatment of postural hypotension in autonomic failure. Limitations and hazards. Lancet. 1978; 1:172.
3. Harrison W et al. MAOIs and hypertensive crises: the role of OTC drugs. J Clin Psychiatry. 1989;50:64.

### Phenelzine (Nardil)

### Phenylpropanolamine

Summary: Phenylpropanolamine administration can result in severe hypertensive reactions in patients on monoamine oxidase inhibitors (MAOIs) like phenelzine.

Risk Factors: No specific risk factors known.

Related Drugs: All nonselective MAOIs including *isocarboxazid (Marplan)* and *tranylcypromine (Parnate)* would be expected to interact with phenylpropanolamine.

Management Options:
- *Avoid Combination.* Phenylpropanolamine should not be given to patients receiving nonselective MAOIs. Remember that the effects of nonselective MAOIs should be assumed to persist for 2 weeks after they are discontinued.

References:
1. Cuthbert MF et al. Cough and cold remedies: potential danger to patients on monoamine oxidase inhibitors. Br Med J. 1969;1:404.
2. Terry R et al. Sinutab. Med J Aust. 1975;2:763. Letter.
3. Harrison W et al. MAOIs and hypertensive crises: the role of OTC drugs. J Clin Psychiatry. 1989;50:64.

### Phenelzine (Nardil)

### Pseudoephedrine (Sudafed)

Summary: Indirect-acting sympathomimetics like pseudoephedrine may produce severe hypertension when administered to patients receiving a monoamine oxidase inhibitor (MAOI) like phenelzine.

Risk Factors: No specific risk factors known.

Related Drugs: All nonselective MAOIs including *isocarboxazid (Marplan)* and *tranylcypromine (Parnate)* would be expected to interact with pseudoephedrine [as well as other indirect-acting sympathomimetics and *phenylephrine (Neo-Synephrine)*].

Management Options:

- *Avoid Combination.* Pseudoephedrine should not be given to patients receiving nonselective MAOIs. Remember that the effects of nonselective MAOIs should be assumed to persist for 2 weeks after they are discontinued.

References:

1. Wright SP. Hazards with monoamine-oxide inhibitors: a persistent problem. Lancet. 1978;1:284. Letter.
2. Harrison W et al. MAOIs and hypertensive crises: the role of OTC drugs. J Clin Psychiatry. 1989;50:64.

### Phenelzine (Nardil)

### Reserpine (Serpalan)

Summary: Reserpine reportedly may cause a hypertensive reaction in patients receiving a monoamine oxidase inhibitor (MAOI) like phenelzine, but supporting clinical evidence is scanty.

Risk Factors:

- *Order of Administration.* Theoretically, this interaction is most likely to occur in a patient who has been taking nonselective MAOIs who then is started on reserpine (rather than the reverse order of administration).

Related Drugs: Theoretically, all nonselective MAOIs including *isocarboxazid (Marplan)* and *tranylcypromine (Parnate)* would be expected to interact with reserpine.

Management Options:

- *Consider Alternative.* Although more clinical information is needed to clarify this interaction, it would be prudent to consider antihypertensive therapy other than reserpine in patients on nonselective MAOIs. Remember that the effects of nonselective MAOIs should be assumed to persist for 2 weeks after they are discontinued.
- *Monitor* for evidence of hypertensive reaction if the combination is given.

References:

1. Goldberg LI. Monoamine oxidase inhibitors. Adverse reactions and possible mechanisms. JAMA. 1964;190:456.

### Phenobarbital

### Phenytoin (Dilantin)

Summary: Phenobarbital tends to decrease serum phenytoin concentrations; it occasionally does not change and sometimes even increases the serum phenytoin concentration. Combined use of barbiturates and phenytoin can be beneficial in many patients; however, the phenytoin serum concentration can be affected when phenobarbital is started or stopped.

Risk Factors: No specific risk factors known.

Related Drugs: Little is known regarding the effect of barbiturates other than phenobarbital on phenytoin, but they probably will reduce phenytoin serum concentrations.

Management Options:

- *Circumvent/Minimize.* Large doses of phenobarbital probably should be avoided in patients with high blood levels of phenytoin because of the potential for competitive inhibition of phenytoin metabolism.

- *Monitor.* Patients maintained on phenytoin and a barbiturate should be observed for signs of phenytoin intoxication if the barbiturate therapy is stopped. Epileptic patients who manifest decreases in phenytoin blood concentrations due to phenobarbital administration do not appear to be adversely affected clinically, and no action is required.

References:

1. Callaghan N et al. The effect of anticonvulsant drugs which induce liver enzymes on derived and ingested phenobarbitone levels. Acta Neurol Scand. 1977;56:1.

2. Lambie DG et al. Therapeutic and pharmacokinetic effects of increasing phenytoin in chronic epileptics on multiple drug therapy. Lancet. 1976;2:386.

3. Cuzzolin L et al. Phenytoin-phenobarbital interaction: importance of free plasma phenytoin monitoring. Pharmacol Res Commun. 1988;20: 627.

## Phenobarbital

## Prednisone

Summary: Barbiturates may reduce serum concentrations of prednisone and other corticosteroids sufficiently to impair their therapeutic effect.

Risk Factors: No specific risk factors known.

Related Drugs: **Dexamethasone (Decadron), prednisolone (Prelone)**, and **methylprednisolone (Medrol)** interact similarly with phenobarbital. Assume that all combinations of barbiturates and corticosteroids interact until proven otherwise.

Management Options:

- *Consider Alternative.* If appropriate, consider possible alternatives to barbiturates (e.g., benzodiazepines).

- *Monitor* for altered corticosteroid effect if a barbiturate is initiated, discontinued, or changed in dosage; substantial adjustments in corticosteroid dosage may be needed.

References:

1. Wassner SJ et al. The adverse effect of anticonvulsant therapy on renal allograft survival. J Pediatr. 1976;88:134.

2. Brooks PM et al. Effects of enzyme induction on metabolism of prednisolone. Clinical and laboratory study. Ann Rheum Dis. 1976;35:339.

3. Gambertoglio J et al. Enhancement of prednisolone elimination by anticonvulsants in renal transplant recipients. Clin Pharmacol Ther. 1982;31:228.

### Phenobarbital

### Primidone (Mysoline)

Summary: The combination of primidone and phenobarbital may result in excessive serum phenobarbital concentrations.

Risk Factors: No specific risk factors known.

Related Drugs: No information available.

Management Options:
- *Consider Alternative.* For most patients, it is illogical to use primidone and phenobarbital concomitantly.
- *Monitor.* If the combination is used, the patient should be monitored for excessive phenobarbital serum concentrations.

References:
1. Gallagher BB et al. Primidone, diphenylhydantoin and phenobarbital. Aspects of acute and chronic toxicity. Neurology. 1973;23:145.
2. Fincham FW et al. The influence of diphenylhydantoin on primidone metabolism. Arch Neurol. 1974;30:259.
3. Griffin GD et al. Primidone-phenobarbital intoxication. Drug Ther. 1976;60:76.

### Phenobarbital

### Propafenone (Rythmol)

Summary: Phenobarbital increases the metabolism of propafenone and reduces its plasma concentrations in healthy subjects; the clinical importance of this interaction is not established.

Risk Factors: No specific risk factors known.

Related Drugs: No information available.

Management Options:
- *Monitor.* Until this interaction is studied in patients receiving chronic propafenone and phenobarbital, patients should be monitored for diminished propafenone efficacy and toxicity when phenobarbital is added to or removed from the drug regimen.

References:
1. Chan GL-Y et al. The effect of phenobarbital on the pharmacokinetics of propafenone in man. Pharmaceut Res. 1988;5:S-153. Abstract.

### Phenobarbital

### Protriptyline (Vivactil)

Summary: Phenobarbital and other barbiturates may reduce serum concentrations of protriptyline and other tricyclic antidepressants (TCAs); the therapeutic response to the antidepressants probably is reduced in some patients.

Risk Factors:
- *Dosage Regimen.* Barbiturate-induced enzyme induction is known to be dose related; small and/or occasional doses are unlikely to sig-

nificantly affect drug metabolism. Depending upon the barbiturate, it may take 1–2 weeks or more for the maximal reduction in serum concentrations of the affected drug.

Related Drugs: Other barbiturates also may reduce serum concentrations of protriptyline and other TCAs. Unlike barbiturates, benzodiazepines do not appear likely to affect TCA serum concentrations.

Management Options:

- *Consider Alternative.* Patients on TCAs probably respond better without barbiturates, and it has been recommended that barbiturates be avoided in such patients.[2]
- *Monitor* for altered TCA effect if barbiturate therapy is initiated, discontinued, or changed in dosage; adjust tricyclic antidepressant dose as needed.

References:
1. Moody JP et al. Pharmacokinetic aspects of protriptyline plasma levels. Eur J Clin Pharmacol. 1977;11:51.
2. Burrows GD et al. Antidepressants and barbiturates. Br Med J. 1971;4:113. Letter.
3. Royds R et al. Tricyclic antidepressant poisoning. Practitioner. 1970; 204:282.

### Phenobarbital

### Quinidine

Summary: Barbiturates can reduce quinidine plasma concentrations; loss of efficacy could result.

Risk Factors: No specific risk factors known.

Related Drugs: Other barbiturates would be expected to produce a similar response. **Phenytoin (Dilantin)** appears to affect quinidine similarly.

Management Options:

- *Circumvent/Minimize.* Initiation or discontinuation of phenobarbital therapy in patients taking quinidine may necessitate a change in quinidine dosage.
- *Monitor.* Quinidine response and plasma concentrations may be reduced when barbiturates are added or increased when phenobarbital is discontinued.

References:
1. Data JL et al. Interaction of quinidine with anticonvulsant drugs. N Engl J Med. 1976;294:699.

## Significance Classification

1 - *Avoid Combination.* Risk always outweighs benefit.

2 - *Usually Avoid Combination.* Use combination only under special circumstances.

3 - *Minimize Risk.* Take action as necessary to reduce risk.

2. Chapron DJ et al. Apparent quinidine-induced digoxin toxicity after withdrawal of pentobarbital. A case of sequential drug interactions. Arch Intern Med. 1979; 139:363.

3. Kroboth FJ et al. Phenytoin-theophylline-quinidine interaction. N Engl J Med. 1983;308:725. Letter.

## Phenobarbital

### Theophylline

Summary: Barbiturates like phenobarbital may reduce serum theophylline concentrations; in some patients, the effect may be large enough to reduce the therapeutic response to theophylline.

Risk Factors: No specific risk factors known.

Related Drugs: **Pentobarbital (Nembutal)** and **secobarbital (Seconal)** interact similarly with theophylline. All barbiturates probably have a similar effect on theophylline.

Management Options:
- *Monitor.* Patients receiving chronic theophylline therapy should be monitored for altered theophylline effect when barbiturate therapy is started or stopped.

References:
1. Gibson GA et al. Influence of high-dose pentobarbital theophylline pharmacokinetics: a case study. Ther Drug Monit. 1985;7:181.
2. Paladino JA et al. Effect of secobarbital on theophylline clearance. Ther Drug Monit. 1983;5:135.
3. Landay RA et al. Effect of phenobarbital on theophylline disposition. J Allergy Clin Immunol. 1978;62:27.

## Phenobarbital

### Valproic Acid (Depakene)

Summary: Valproic acid increases serum phenobarbital concentrations; phenobarbital intoxication may occur in some patients.

Risk Factors: No specific risk factors known.

Related Drugs: No information available.

Management Options:
- *Monitor* for excessive phenobarbital effect when valproic acid is given concurrently; reductions in the phenobarbital dose may be necessary for many patients.

References:
1. Wilder BJ et al. Valproic acid: interaction with other anticonvulsant drugs. Neurology. 1978;28:892.
2. Patel IH et al. Phenobarbital-valproic acid interaction. Clin Pharmacol Ther. 1980; 27:515.
3. Bruni J et al. Valproic acid and plasma levels of phenobarbital. Neurology. 1980; 30:94.

## Phenobarbital

### Verapamil (Calan)

Summary: Phenobarbital substantially reduces the plasma concentrations of verapamil, especially when verapamil is given orally.

Risk Factors:
- *Route of Administration.* Oral verapamil dosing can increase the risk of interaction.

Related Drugs: Phenobarbital also increases the metabolism of *nifedipine (Procardia)*. Other calcium channel blockers may be similarly affected by phenobarbital and other barbiturates.

Management Options:
- *Circumvent/Minimize.* Patients receiving phenobarbital may require higher than usual doses of verapamil, especially if the verapamil is administered orally.
- *Monitor.* Patients stabilized on verapamil (especially if taken orally) should be monitored for the possibility of decreased effectiveness when phenobarbital is administered concomitantly.

References:
1. Rutledge DR et al. Effects of chronic phenobarbital on verapamil disposition in humans. J Pharmacol Exp Ther. 1988;246:7.

## Phenobarbital

### Warfarin (Coumadin)

Summary: Barbiturates inhibit the hypoprothrombinemic response to oral anticoagulants like warfarin. Fatal bleeding episodes have occurred when barbiturates were discontinued in patients stabilized on an anticoagulant.

Risk Factors:
- *Dosage Regimen.* The effect of barbiturates on anticoagulants may be dose related. For example, plasma warfarin did not change in one patient when 100 mg/day of secobarbital was given, but it decreased considerably when the dosage was increased to 200 mg/day.[1] However, in 6 healthy subjects, 100 mg/day of secobarbital was sufficient to enhance warfarin metabolism.[2] A decrease in the anticoagulant response usually develops gradually after a barbiturate is initiated, with maximal effects occurring at about 2 weeks. The time course following discontinuation of the barbiturate is similar; the results of enzyme induction usually begin to diminish within a week, with little induction remaining by 2 to 3 weeks. Note that the onset and offset of enzyme induction by barbiturates will vary depending upon the half-life of the specific barbiturate.

Related Drugs: *Phenobarbital (Solfoton)*, *butabarbital (Butisol)*, *heptabarbital*, *pentobarbital (Nembutal)*, *secobarbital (Seconal)*, and *amobarbital (Amytal)* have all been shown to decrease the response to coumarin anticoagulants. Most barbiturates [including **primidone (Mysoline)**, which is metabolized to phenobarbital] probably have this ability. Most of the interaction studies have involved warfarin or **dicumarol**, but barbiturates also appear to increase the metabolism of other anticoagulants such as **phenprocoumon**,[4] **acenocoumarol**,[5,6] and **ethyl biscoumacetate**.[5]

Management Options:

- *Avoid Unless Benefit Outweighs Risk.* If the barbiturate is being used as a sedative/hypnotic, its use with an oral anticoagulant generally should be avoided. Alternative sedative/hypnotic drugs unlikely to interact with oral anticoagulants include flurazepam (Dalmane), chlordiazepoxide (Librium), diazepam (Valium), or diphenhydramine (Benadryl). Nonetheless, the consistent use of stable doses of barbiturates, as in epileptic patients, does not appear to interfere significantly with anticoagulant control.[3]

- *Monitor.* If a barbiturate is used in a patient receiving an oral anticoagulant, monitor for altered hypoprothrombinemic response if the barbiturate is initiated, discontinued, or changed in dosage. Moreover, patients stabilized on a barbiturate and an oral anticoagulant should be advised not to stop taking the barbiturate or change its dosage without consulting with their physician for careful monitoring of their anticoagulant response.

References:

1. Whitfield JB et al. Changes in plasma gamma-glutamyl transpeptidase activity associated with alterations in drug metabolism in man. Br Med J. 1973;1:316.
2. O'Reilly RA et al. Interaction of secobarbital with warfarin pseudoracemates. Clin Pharmacol Ther. 1980;28:187.
3. Williams JRB et al. Effect of concomitantly administered drugs on the control of long term anticoagulant therapy. Q J Med. 1976;45:63.
4. Antlitz AM et al. Effect of butabarbital on orally administered anticoagulants. Curr Ther Res. 1968;10:70.
5. Dayton PG et al. The influence of barbiturates on coumarin plasma levels and prothrombin response. J Clin Invest. 1961;40:1797.
6. Kroon C et al. Interaction between single dose acenocoumarol and cimetidine or pentobarbitone: validation of a single dose model to predict interactions in steady state. Br J Clin Pharmacol. 1990;29:643P.

### Phenylbutazone (Butazolidin)
### Tolbutamide (Orinase)

**2**

Summary: Phenylbutazone increases the serum concentrations of tolbutamide and several other oral hypoglycemic drugs and may increase their hypoglycemic action.

Risk Factors: No specific risk factors known.

Related Drugs: It is not known whether other oral hypoglycemics are affected by phenylbutazone. Other nonsteroidal anti-inflammatory drugs appear to be safer than phenylbutazone to use with hypoglycemic drugs.

Management Options:
- *Use Alternative.* Do not administer phenylbutazone to patients taking oral hypoglycemic agents. **Oxyphenbutazone** appears to affect tolbutamide in a similar manner.[1] Other nonsteroidal anti-inflammatory drugs [e.g., **piroxicam (Feldene), pirprofen, tolmetin (Tolectin), tenoxicam**, and **naproxen (Naprosyn)**] appear to be acceptable alternatives though **acetohexamide (Dymelor)** appears to be affected similarly and phenylbutazone potentiates the action of **insulin** and **chlorpropamide (Diabinase)**.

References:
1. Pond SM et al. Mechanisms of inhibition of tolbutamide metabolism: phenylbutazone, oxyphenbutazone, sulfaphenazole. Clin Pharmacol Ther. 1977;22:573.
2. Day RO et al. The effect of tenoxicam on tolbutamide pharmacokinetics and glucose concentrations in healthy volunteers. Internat J Clin Pharmacol Ther. 1995; 33:308.
3. Diwan PV et al. Potentiation of hypoglycemic response of glibenclamide by piroxicam in rats and humans. Indian J Exp Biol. 1992;30:317.

### Phenylbutazone (Butazolidin)

### Warfarin (Coumadin)

Summary: Phenylbutazone dramatically enhances the hypoprothrombinemic response to warfarin, leading to severe bleeding in some patients. This combination should be avoided.

Risk Factors:
- *Concurrent Diseases.* Patients with peptic ulcer disease (PUD) or a history of gastrointestinal (GI) bleeding are probably at greater risk.

Related Drugs: All NSAIDs inhibit platelet function, cause gastric erosions, and probably increase the risk of GI bleeding. Some NSAIDs, however, such as **ibuprofen (Motrin), naproxen (Naprosyn)**, or **diclofenac (Voltaren)** may be less likely to increase oral anticoagulant-induced hypoprothrombinemia than other NSAIDs. **Oxyphenbutazone** appears to interact similarly.

Management Options:
- *Avoid Combination.* Phenylbutazone should be avoided in patients receiving oral anticoagulants. Probably no condition exists in which the benefit of phenylbutazone therapy outweighs the serious risk of concomitant therapy with oral anticoagulants. It would be prudent to

## Significance Classification

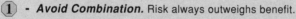

(1) - ***Avoid Combination.*** Risk always outweighs benefit.

(2) - ***Usually Avoid Combination.*** Use combination only under special circumstances.

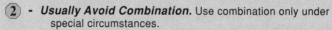

(3) - ***Minimize Risk.*** Take action as necessary to reduce risk.

use NSAIDs that are unlikely to affect the hypoprothrombinemic response to oral anticoagulants. If the NSAID is being used as an analgesic or antipyretic, acetaminophen is probably safer to use with oral anticoagulants. Nonacetylated salicylates (e.g., choline salicylate, magnesium salicylate, salsalate, sodium salicylate) probably also are safer with oral anticoagulants than NSAIDs, since such salicylates have minimal effects on platelet function and the gastric mucosa. If any NSAID is used with an oral anticoagulant, one should carefully monitor the prothrombin time and watch for evidence of bleeding, especially from the GI tract.

References:
1. O'Reilly RA. Phenylbutazone and sulfinpyrazone interaction with oral anticoagulant phenprocoumon. Arch Int Med. 1982;142:1634.
2. O'Reilly RA et al. Comparative interaction of sulfinpyrazone and phenylbutazone with racemic warfarin: alteration *in vivo* of free fraction of plasma warfarin. J Pharmacol Exp Ther. 1981;219:691.
3. Shorr RI et al. Concurrent use of nonsteroidal anti-inflammatory drugs and oral anticoagulants places elderly persons at high risk for hemorrhagic peptic ulcer disease. Arch Intern Med. 1993;153:1665.

### Phenylpropanolamine (Propadrine)

### Thioridazine (Mellaril)

Summary: A patient on thioridazine died after taking a single dose of phenylpropanolamine, but a causal relationship was not established.

Risk Factors: No specific risk factors known.

Related Drugs: The effect of other combinations of phenothiazines and sympathomimetics is not established, but consider the possibility that they also interact.

Management Options:
• *Consider Alternative.* In patients on thioridazine (and possibly other neuroleptics) consider using alternatives to systemic phenylpropanolamine (or other sympathomimetics). Although there is very little evidence to support the existence of this interaction, the severity of the reported reaction (death) dictates caution.
• *Monitor.* If the combination is used, monitor for evidence of ventricular arrhythmias (e.g., palpitations, fainting).

References:
1. Chouinard G et al. Death attributed to ventricular arrhythmia induced by thioridazine in combination with a single Contac-C capsule. Can Med Assoc J. 1978;119:729.
2. Giles TD et al. Death associated with ventricular arrhythmia and thioridazine. JAMA. 1968;205:98.

### Phenytoin (Dilantin)

### Primidone (Mysoline)

Summary: Phenytoin appears to enhance the conversion of primidone to phenobarbital. Excessive phenobarbital serum concentrations may occur in some patients.

Risk Factors:
- *Other Drugs.* Concurrent therapy with phenobarbital or carbamazepine can increase the magnitude of this interaction.

Related Drugs: No information available.

Management Options:
- *Monitor.* No special precautions are necessary with the concomitant use of phenytoin and primidone, although relatively high concentrations of phenobarbital can be generated. The finding of supratherapeutic concentrations of phenobarbital in patients receiving phenytoin, primidone, and phenobarbital[2] sheds doubt on the advantage of adding phenobarbital to a regimen of phenytoin and primidone.

References:
1. Gallagher BB et al. Primidone, diphenylhydantoin and phenobarbital. Aspects of acute and chronic toxicity. Neurology. 1973;23:145.
2. Fincham RW et al. The influence of diphenylhydantoin on primidone metabolism. Arch Neurol. 1974;30:259.
3. Callaghan N et al. The effect of anticonvulsant drugs which induce liver enzymes on derived and ingested phenobarbitone levels. Acta Neurol Scand. 1977;56:1.

### Phenytoin (Dilantin)

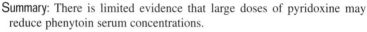

### Pyridoxine (Vitamin B<sub>6</sub>)

Summary: There is limited evidence that large doses of pyridoxine may reduce phenytoin serum concentrations.

Risk Factors:
- *Dosage Regimen.* The potential effect was seen with very large doses of pyridoxine; smaller doses, such as in multivitamins, probably have a minimal effect.

Related Drugs: No information available.

Management Options:
- *Monitor.* No special precautions appear necessary when small doses of pyridoxine (as in multivitamins) are given to patients receiving phenytoin. Monitoring for reduced serum phenytoin concentrations is probably warranted if large doses of pyridoxine are used.

References:
1. Hansson O et al. Pyridoxine and serum concentrations of phenytoin and phenobarbitone. Lancet. 1976;1:256. Letter.

### Phenytoin (Dilantin)

### Quinidine

Summary: Phenytoin may substantially decrease quinidine serum concentrations.

Risk Factors: No specific risk factors known.

Related Drugs: No information available.

Management Options:
- *Monitor.* Starting or stopping phenytoin therapy in patients receiving quinidine may necessitate a change in quinidine dosage.

References:
1. Data JL et al. Interaction of quinidine with anticonvulsant drugs. N Engl J Med. 1976;294:699.
2. Kroboth FJ et al. Phenytoin-theophylline-quinidine interaction. N Engl J Med. 1983;308:725. Letter.
3. Urbano AM. Phenytoin-quinidine interaction in a patient with recurrent ventricular tachyarrhythmias. N Engl J Med. 1982;308:225. Letter.

### Phenytoin (Dilantin)

### Rifampin (Rifadin)

**Summary:** Pharmacokinetic data and a case report indicate that rifampin decreases serum phenytoin concentrations; adjustments in the phenytoin dose may be needed.

**Risk Factors:** No specific risk factors known.

**Related Drugs:** No information available.

**Management Options:**
- *Circumvent/Minimize.* The phenytoin dose may require adjustment if rifampin is added or removed from a patient's regimen.
- *Monitor.* Patients on phenytoin therapy who receive rifampin should be monitored carefully for reduced serum phenytoin concentrations.

References:
1. Kay L et al. Influence of rifampicin and isoniazid on the kinetics of phenytoin. Br J Clin Pharmacol. 1985;20:323.
2. Wagner JC. Rifampin-phenytoin drug interaction. Drug Intell Clin Pharm. 1984; 18:497. Abstract.

### Phenytoin (Dilantin)

### Sucralfate (Carafate)

**Summary:** Sucralfate modestly reduces the gastrointestinal absorption of phenytoin, but the clinical importance of this effect is not established.

**Risk Factors:** No specific risk factors known.

**Related Drugs:** No information available.

**Management Options:**
- *Circumvent/Minimize.* Although any reduction in phenytoin absorption is likely to be modest, it would be prudent to give phenytoin 2 hours before or 6 hours after the sucralfate and keep the interval between the drugs as constant as possible.

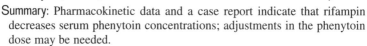

## Significance Classification

① - **Avoid Combination.** Risk always outweighs benefit.

② - **Usually Avoid Combination.** Use combination only under special circumstances.

③ - **Minimize Risk.** Take action as necessary to reduce risk.

- *Monitor* for altered phenytoin response if sucralfate is initiated, discontinued, or if the interval between the drugs is changed.

References:
1. Smart HL et al. The effects of sucralfate upon phenytoin absorption in man. Br J Clin Pharmacol. 1985;20:238.
2. Hall TG et al. Effect of sucralfate on phenytoin bioavailability. Drug Intell Clin Pharm. 1986;20:607.

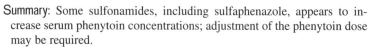

## Phenytoin (Dilantin)

### Sulfaphenazole

Summary: Some sulfonamides, including sulfaphenazole, appears to increase serum phenytoin concentrations; adjustment of the phenytoin dose may be required.

Risk Factors: No specific risk factors known.

Related Drugs: **Sulfamethoxazole (Gantanol)** appears to increase phenytoin half-life only modestly.[3] Phenytoin half-life increased from an average of 11.3 hours before, to 20.5 hours after, **sulfamethizole (Thiosulfil)** administration (4 gm/day for 7 days). Sulfamethizole also inhibits phenytoin metabolism. Sulfisoxazole, sulfadimethoxine, and sulfamethoxypyridazine do not appear to inhibit phenytoin metabolism.[1]

Management Options:
- *Consider Alternative.* Consider using a sulfonamide that does not inhibit phenytoin metabolism.
- *Monitor* patients for increased phenytoin serum concentrations and signs of phenytoin toxicity (e.g., ataxia, nystagmus, mental impairment) when sulfamethizole or sulfaphenazole is started. Stopping these sulfonamides may cause a fall in serum phenytoin concentrations.

References:
1. Siersbaek-Nielsen K et al. Sulfamethizole-induced inhibition of diphenylhydantoin and tolbutamide metabolism in man. Clin Pharmacol Ther. 1973;14:148. Abstract.
2. Lumholtz B et al. Sulfamethizole-induced inhibition of diphenylhydantoin, tolbutamide, and warfarin metabolism. Clin Pharmacol Ther. 1975;17:731.
3. Hansen JM et al. The effect of different sulfonamides on phenytoin metabolism in man. Acta Med Scand (Suppl.). 1979;624:106.

## Phenytoin (Dilantin)

### Tacrolimus (Prograf)

Summary: Phenytoin probably reduces tacrolimus blood concentrations; increased tacrolimus dosage may be needed.

Risk Factors: No specific risk factors known.

Related Drugs: Other enzyme inducers such as **aminoglutethimide (Cytadren)**, barbiturates, **carbamazepine (Tegretol)**, **glutethimide (Doriden)**, **primidone (Mysoline)**, **rifabutin (Mycobutin)**, and **rifampin (Rifadin)** also may reduce tacrolimus blood concentrations.

Management Options:
   • *Monitor* for subtherapeutic tacrolimus blood concentrations if phenytoin or other enzyme inducers are used concurrently.

References:
   1. Thompson PA et al. Tacrolimus-phenytoin interaction. Ann Pharmacother. 1996; 30:544. Letter.

### Phenytoin (Dilantin)

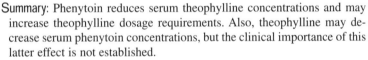

### Teniposide (Vumen)

Summary: Phenytoin substantially increased the systemic clearance of teniposide and may reduce teniposide's efficacy.

Risk Factors: No specific risk factors known.

Related Drugs: No information available.

Management Options:
   • *Monitor* for altered teniposide effect if phenytoin is initiated, discontinued, or changed in dosage; adjust teniposide dose as needed.

References:
   1. Baker et al. Increased teniposide clearance with concomitant anticonvulsant therapy. J Clin Oncol. 1992;10:311.

### Phenytoin (Dilantin)

### Theophylline

Summary: Phenytoin reduces serum theophylline concentrations and may increase theophylline dosage requirements. Also, theophylline may decrease serum phenytoin concentrations, but the clinical importance of this latter effect is not established.

Risk Factors: No specific risk factors known.

Related Drugs: Other enzyme inducers also are likely to enhance theophylline metabolism.

Management Options:
   • *Monitor.* Be alert for the need to increase the theophylline dose when phenytoin is started and decrease the dose when phenytoin is stopped. Patients on chronic phenytoin therapy may require larger-than-expected theophylline doses. Also monitor for a reduced phenytoin response in patients receiving theophylline.

References:
   1. Miller M et al. Influence of phenytoin on theophylline clearance. Clin Pharmacol Ther. 1984;35:666.
   2. Reed RC et al. Phenytoin-theophylline-quinidine interaction. N Engl J Med. 1983; 308:724.
   3. Sklar SJ èt al. Enhanced theophylline clearance secondary to phenytoin therapy. Drug Intell Clin Pharm. 1985;19:34.

## Phenytoin (Dilantin)

### Thyroid

Summary: Limited evidence indicates phenytoin may increase thyroid replacement dose requirements in some patients.

Risk Factors: No specific risk factors known.

Related Drugs: No information available.

Management Options:
- *Monitor.* In patients on thyroid replacement, starting or stopping phenytoin therapy may increase or decrease thyroid dose requirements, respectively. Also, patients requiring thyroid replacement therapy should be given IV phenytoin with caution, especially if they also have a cardiac disease.

References:
1. Fulop M et al. Possible diphenylhydantoin-induced arrhythmia in hypothyroidism. JAMA. 1966;196:454.
2. Blackshear JL et al. Thyroxine replacement requirements in hypothyroid patients receiving phenytoin. Ann Intern Med. 1983;99:341.

## Phenytoin (Dilantin)

### Ticlopidine (Ticlid)

Summary: Patients have developed phenytoin toxicity after ticlopidine was added to their therapy; it may be necessary to reduce phenytoin dose in the presence of ticlopidine.

Risk Factors: No specific risk factors known.

Related Drugs: No information available.

Management Options:
- *Monitor* for altered phenytoin effect if ticlopidine is initiated, discontinued, or changed in dosage; adjust phenytoin dose as needed. If phenytoin is initiated in the presence of ticlopidine therapy, it would be prudent to begin with conservative doses of phenytoin.

References:
1. Rindone JP et al. Phenytoin toxicity associated with ticlopidine administration. Arch Intern Med. 1996;156:1113. Letter.
2. Privitera M et al. Acute phenytoin toxicity followed by seizure breakthrough from a ticlopidine-phenytoin interaction. Arch Neurol. 1996;53:1191–192.
3. Riva R et al. Ticlopidine impairs phenytoin clearance: a case report. Neurology. 1996;46:1172–173.

## Phenytoin (Dilantin)

### Tolbutamide (Orinase)

Summary: Although excessive phenytoin doses may result in hyperglycemia, alteration in glucose tolerance appears unlikely in patients with free serum phenytoin concentrations within the usual therapeutic range. Tolbutamide may transiently increase free serum phenytoin concentrations, but the incidence of toxicity from this effect is unknown.

Risk Factors: No specific risk factors known.

Related Drugs: The effect of other sulfonylureas on phenytoin is not well established, although one possible case of *tolazamide (Tolinase)*-induced phenytoin toxicity has been reported.[3]

Management Options:

- *Monitor* for alterations in antidiabetic drug requirements if phenytoin therapy is started, stopped, or changed in dosage. Patients stabilized on phenytoin should be warned of the possibility of transient phenytoin toxicity (e.g., ataxia, dizziness, nausea, headache) when tolbutamide therapy is begun.

References:

1. Saudek CD et al. Phenytoin in the treatment of diabetic symmetrical polyneuropathy. Clin Pharmacol Ther. 1977;22:196.
2. Wesseling H et al. Diphenylhydantoin (DPH) and tolbutamide in man. Eur J Clin Pharmacol. 1975;8:75.
3. Beech E et al. Phenytoin toxicity produced by tolbutamide. Br Med J. 1988;297:1613.

**Phenytoin (Dilantin)** ⟶ ▽3

**Trimethoprim (Proloprim)**

Summary: Trimethoprim may increase serum phenytoin concentrations; phenytoin toxicity may occur in some patients.

Risk Factors: No specific risk factors known.

Related Drugs: Phenytoin half-life was similarly prolonged by *trimethoprim-sulfamethoxazole (Bactrim)*, but *sulfamethoxazole (Gantanol)* alone produced only a small increase in phenytoin half-life.

Management Options:

- *Monitor* for signs of phenytoin toxicity (e.g., nystagmus, ataxia, mental impairment) when trimethoprim is given concurrently with phenytoin. Serum phenytoin determinations would be useful if the interaction is suspected.

References:

1. Hansen JM et al. The effect of different sulfonamides on phenytoin metabolism in man. Acta Med Scand. 1979;624(Suppl.):106.

## Significance Classification

① - *Avoid Combination.* Risk always outweighs benefit.

② - *Usually Avoid Combination.* Use combination only under special circumstances.

③ - *Minimize Risk.* Take action as necessary to reduce risk.

## Phenytoin (Dilantin)

### Valproic Acid (Depakene)

Summary: Valproic acid can increase, decrease, or have no effect on total phenytoin plasma concentrations. Phenytoin may decrease serum valproic acid concentrations.

Risk Factors: No specific risk factors known.

Related Drugs: No information available.

Management Options:

- *Monitor.* Patients receiving phenytoin may not require an alteration in the dose of phenytoin when valproic acid therapy is initiated since the free serum concentration of phenytoin may not change. Nevertheless, watch for signs of phenytoin toxicity (e.g., ataxia, nystagmus, mental impairment, involuntary muscular movements, seizures) when valproic acid is used concurrently. The decreased total serum phenytoin concentrations seen during the first few weeks of valproic acid therapy should not prompt an increase in phenytoin dose unless poor seizure control occurs concurrently. Free phenytoin in plasma concentrations should be followed whenever possible since total phenytoin concentrations may be altered without a change in the free phenytoin plasma concentration.

References:

1. Monks A et al. Effect of single doses of sodium valproate on serum phenytoin levels and protein binding in epileptic patients. Clin Pharmacol Ther. 1980;27:89.
2. Bruni J et al. Interactions of valproic acid with phenytoin. Neurology. 1980;30:1233.
3. Miles MV et al. Predictability of unbound antiepileptic drug concentrations in children treated with valproic acid and phenytoin. Clin Pharm. 1988;7:688.

## Phenytoin (Dilantin)

### Vigabatrin (Sabril)

Summary: Vigabatrin has been found to decrease the serum concentrations of phenytoin by 20% to 30%.

Risk Factors: No specific risk factors known.

Related Drugs: No information available.

Management Options:

- *Monitor.* Phenytoin plasma concentrations should be monitored for 1 month after initiation/or removal of vigabatrin therapy. Patients receiving phenytoin may require an increase in the dose of phenytoin when vigabatrin therapy is initiated.

References:

1. Tartara A et al. Vigabatrin in the treatment of epilepsy: a long-term follow-up study. J Neurol Neurosurg Psych. 1989;52:467.
2. Rimmer EM et al. Interaction between vigabatrin and phenytoin. Br J Clin Pharmacol. 1989;27(Suppl. 1):S27.
3. Gatti G et al. Vigabatrin induced decrease in serum phenytoin concentration does not involve a change in phenytoin bioavailability. Br J Clin Pharmacol. 1993;35:603.

### Phenytoin (Dilantin)

### Warfarin (Coumadin)

**Summary:** Initiation of phenytoin therapy may transiently increase the hypoprothrombinemic response to warfarin (and probably other oral anticoagulants). This is followed within 1 to 2 weeks by an inhibition of the hypoprothrombinemic response. Patients on chronic phenytoin therapy may require larger-than-expected doses of oral anticoagulants. Dicumarol and phenprocoumon may increase serum phenytoin concentrations, whereas warfarin does not appear to do so.

**Risk Factors:** No specific risk factors known.

**Related Drugs:** Interactions of phenytoin with oral anticoagulants other than warfarin, *dicumarol* and *phenprocoumon* are not established.

**Management Options:**
- *Consider Alternative.* Warfarin is preferable to dicumarol in patients receiving phenytoin, since warfarin does not appear to affect phenytoin serum concentrations.
- *Monitor* for altered oral anticoagulant effect if phenytoin is initiated, discontinued, or changed in dosage. Adjust the anticoagulant dose as needed. If an oral anticoagulant is started in the presence of phenytoin therapy, remember that the anticoagulant dosage requirements may be greater than usual.

**References:**
1. Skovsted L et al. The effect of different oral anticoagulants on diphenylhydantoin (DPH) and tolbutamide metabolism. Acta Med Scand. 1976;199:513.
2. Nappi JM. Warfarin and phenytoin interaction. Ann Intern Med. 1979;90:852.
3. Taylor JW et al. Oral anticoagulant-phenytoin interactions. Drug Intell Clin Pharm. 1980;14:669.

### Piroxicam (Feldene)

### Warfarin (Coumadin)

**Summary:** Preliminary clinical evidence indicates that piroxicam may increase the hypoprothrombinemic response to warfarin, acenocoumarol, and possibly other oral anticoagulants.

**Risk Factors:**
- *Concurrent Diseases.* Patients with peptic ulcer disease (PUD) or a history of gastrointestinal (GI) bleeding are probably at greater risk.

**Related Drugs:** All NSAIDs inhibit platelet function, cause gastric erosions, and probably increase the risk of gastrointestinal bleeding. Some NSAIDs, however, such as *ibuprofen (Advil), naproxen (Naprosyn),* or *diclofenac (Voltaren)* may be less likely to increase oral anticoagulant-induced hypoprothrombinemia than other NSAIDs. *Acenocoumarol* appears to interact similarly.

**Management Options:**
- *Avoid Unless Benefit Outweighs Risk.* Since all NSAIDs probably increase the risk of gastrointestinal bleeding in patients on oral anti-

coagulants, use the combination only after careful consideration of the benefit versus risk. If an NSAID must be used with an oral anti-coagulant, it would be prudent to use NSAIDs that are unlikely to affect the hypoprothrombinemic response to oral anticoagulants. (See Related Drugs above.) If the NSAID is being used as an analgesic or antipyretic, acetaminophen is probably safer to use with oral anticoagulants. Non-acetylated salicylates (e.g., choline salicylate, magnesium salicylate, salsalate, sodium salicylate) are probably also safer with oral anticoagulants than NSAIDs, since such salicylates have minimal effects on platelet function and the gastric mucosa.

- *Monitor.* If any NSAID is used with an oral anticoagulant, one should monitor carefully the prothrombin time and watch for evidence of bleeding, especially from the GI tract.

References:

1. Rhodes RS et al. A warfarin-piroxicam drug interaction. Drug Intell Clin Pharm. 1985;19:556.
2. Emergy P. Gastrointestinal blood loss and piroxicam. Lancet. 1982;1:1302.
3. Shorr RI et al. Concurrent use of nonsteroidal anti-inflammatory drugs and oral anticoagulants places elderly persons at high risk for hemorrhagic peptic ulcer disease. Arch Intern Med. 1993;153:1665.

## Potassium

### Spironolactone (Aldactone)

Summary: Coadministration of potassium supplements and spironolactone may result in severe hyperkalemia.

Risk Factors:

- *Age.* The elderly may be at greater risk.
- *Concurrent Diseases.* Patients with impaired renal function and/or severe diabetes may be at greater risk. Patients with diet-controlled diabetes do not appear to be predisposed particularly to potassium-sparing diuretic-induced hyperkalemia if no other predisposing factors are present.[3]
- *Diet/Food.* A high potassium diet (including salt substitutes) may enhance the risk of hyperkalemia.
- *Other Drugs.* Concurrent administration of ACE inhibitors may enhance the risk.

Related Drugs: ***Amiloride (Midamor)*** and ***triamterene (Dyrenium)*** also can result in hyperkalemia when combined with potassium supplements.

Management Options:

- *Avoid Unless Benefit Outweighs Risk.* The combination of potassium-sparing diuretics and potassium supplementation should be used only for severe and/or refractory hypokalemia. Particular caution is needed in predisposed patients (e.g., an elderly diabetic with impaired renal function).
- *Monitor.* If the combination is used, serum potassium concentrations should be monitored carefully.

References:

1. Kalbian VV. Iatrogenic hyperkalemic paralysis with electrocardiographic changes. South Med J. 1974;67:342.
2. Simborg DN. Medication prescribing on a university medical service—the incidence of drug combinations with potential adverse interactions. Johns Hopkins Med J. 1976;139:23.
3. Lowenthal DT et al. Effects of amiloride on oral glucose loading, serum potassium, renin, and aldosterone in diet-controlled diabetes. Clin Pharmacol Ther. 1980; 27:671.

## Potassium

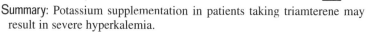

### Triamterene (Dyrenium)

Summary: Potassium supplementation in patients taking triamterene may result in severe hyperkalemia.

Risk Factors:

- *Age.* Elderly patients may be at greater risk.
- *Concurrent Diseases.* Patients with impaired renal function and/or severe diabetes may be at greater risk. Patients with diet-controlled diabetes do not appear to be particularly predisposed to potassium-sparing diuretic-induced hyperkalemia if no other predisposing factors are present.[2]
- *Diet/Food.* A high potassium diet (including salt substitutes) may place a patient at greater risk.
- *Other Drugs.* Concurrent administration of angiotensin-converting enzyme inhibitors may increase the risk.

Related Drugs: **Amiloride (Midamor)** and **spironolactone (Aldactone)** also can result in hyperkalemia when combined with potassium supplements.

Management Options:

- *Avoid Unless Benefit Outweighs Risk.* The combination of potassium-sparing diuretics and potassium supplementation should be used only for severe and/or refractory hypokalemia. Particular caution is needed in predisposed patients (e.g., an elderly diabetic with impaired renal function).
- *Monitor.* If the combination is used, serum potassium concentrations should be monitored carefully.

References:

1. O'Reilly MV et al. Transvenous pacemaker failure induced by hyperkalemia. JAMA. 1974;228:336.
2. Lowenthal DT et al. Effects of amiloride on oral glucose loading, serum potassium, renin, and aldosterone in diet-controlled diabetes. Clin Pharmacol Ther. 1980; 27:671.

### Prazosin (Minipress)

### Propranolol (Inderal)

Summary: The first-dose syncopal response to prazosin may be enhanced by beta blockade.

Risk Factors: No specific risk factors known.

Related Drugs: A similar increase in the incidence of first-dose hypotensive reaction was observed with combined use of prazosin and **alprenolol** in hypertensive patients.[2] The combination of other beta blockers and alpha blockers [e.g., **terazosin (Hytrin)**] may produce acute postural hypotension.

Management Options:

- *Circumvent/Minimize.* The addition of propranolol to patients stabilized on prazosin will lessen the likelihood of a syncopal episode. However, monitor for orthostatic blood pressure changes.

- *Monitor.* In patients receiving beta blockers, initiation of prazosin therapy should be undertaken with caution and with conservative (e.g., 50% of normal) doses. Taking the initial prazosin dose at bedtime would be prudent.

References:

1. Elliott HL et al. Immediate cardiovascular responses to oral prazosin—effects of concurrent beta blockers. Clin Pharmacol Ther. 1981;29:303.
2. Seideman P et al. Prazosin first dose phenomenon during combined treatment with a beta-adrenoceptor in hypertensive patients. Br J Clin Pharmacol. 1982;13:865.
3. Rubin P et al. Studies on the clinical pharmacology of prazosin. II: The influence of indomethacin and of propranolol on the action and disposition of prazosin. Br J Clin Pharmacol. 1980;10:33.

### Prazosin (Minipress)

### Verapamil (Calan)

Summary: The combination of verapamil with prazosin can enhance hypotensive effects.

Risk Factors: No specific risk factors known.

Related Drugs: The combination of verapamil and **terazosin (Hytrin)** also has been noted to produce increased pharmacodynamic effect. Verapamil apparently reduces the first-pass metabolism of terazosin.[1,2] Other calcium channel blockers may have additive hypotensive effects when administered with prazosin, terazosin, or **doxazosin (Cardura)**.

Management Options:

- *Circumvent/Minimize.* Smaller doses of prazosin may be indicated when verapamil is coadministered.

## Significance Classification

 - **Avoid Combination.** Risk always outweighs benefit.

 - **Usually Avoid Combination.** Use combination only under special circumstances.

 - **Minimize Risk.** Take action as necessary to reduce risk.

• *Monitor.* The combination of verapamil and prazosin appears to produce a potent antihypertensive effect. Patients stabilized on one of these drugs should be monitored carefully for hypotension during the institution of the second drug.

References:

1. Lenz M et al. Combined terazosin and verapamil therapy in essential hypertension; haemodynamic interactions. Clin Pharmacol Ther. 1991;49:146. Abstract.
2. Varghese A et al. Combined terazosin and verapamil therapy in essential hypertension; pharmacokinetic interactions. Clin Pharmacol Ther. 1991;49:130. Abstract.
3. Meredith PA et al. An additive or synergistic drug interaction: application of concentration-effect modeling. Clin Pharmacol Ther. 1992;51:708.

## Prednisolone

### Rifampin (Rifadin)

Summary: Rifampin appears to reduce the effect of corticosteroids like prednisolone significantly in some patients.

Risk Factors: No specific risk factors known.

Related Drugs: It is likely that most corticosteroids (e.g., *cortisone*) would be affected similarly by rifampin.

Management Options:

• *Circumvent/Minimize.* The dose of corticosteroid may require an increase.

• *Monitor.* It does not seem necessary to avoid concomitant use of corticosteroids and rifampin, but be alert for evidence of reduced corticosteroid effect.

References:

1. Yamada S et al. Induction of hepatic cortisol-6-hydroxylase by rifampicin. Lancet. 1976;2:366.
2. van Marle W et al. Concurrent steroid and rifampicin therapy. Br Med J. 1979; 1:1029.
3. Carrie F et al. Rifampin-induced nonresponsiveness of giant cell arteritis to prednisone treatment. Arch Intern Med. 1994;154:1521.

## Primidone (Mysoline)

### Valproic Acid (Depakene)

Summary: Valproic acid may increase serum concentrations of the phenobarbital that is produced from primidone; excessive phenobarbital response may occur.

Risk Factors: No specific risk factors known.

Related Drugs: No information available.

Management Options:

• *Monitor.* Patients receiving primidone should be monitored for signs of phenobarbital toxicity when valproate is given concomitantly.

References:

1. Windorfer A et al. Elevation of diphenylhydantoin and primidone serum concentration by addition of dipropylacetate, a new anticonvulsant drug. Acta Paediatr Scand. 1975;64:771.

## Probenecid (Benemid)

### Thiopental (Pentothal)

Summary: Probenecid may prolong thiopental anesthesia.

Risk Factors: No specific risk factors known.

Related Drugs: No information available.

Management Options:
- *Monitor* for prolonged anesthesia in patients receiving probenecid.

References:
1. Kaukinen S et al. Prolongation of thiopentone anaesthesia by probenecid. Br J Anæsth. 1980;52:603.

## Probenecid (Benemid)

### Zidovudine (Retrovir)

Summary: Probenecid increases the plasma concentration of zidovudine and may allow zidovudine to be administered less frequently and in lower doses.

Risk Factors: No specific risk factors known.

Related Drugs: No information available.

Management Options:
- *Circumvent/Minimize.* The dose of zidovudine should be reduced when probenecid is administered concomitantly. The concurrent administration of probenecid with zidovudine may enable Q 8 hr dosing of zidovudine that would be more convenient than taking zidovudine Q 4 hr. The decreased total daily dose of zidovudine also would decrease the financial expenditure for this costly medication.
- *Monitor.* Patients should be observed for rash and other side effects when both agents are administered.

References:
1. Hedaya MA et al. Probenecid inhibits the metabolic and renal clearances of zidovudine (AZT) in human volunteers. Pharm Res. 1990;7:411.
2. Kornhauser DM et al. Probenecid and zidovudine metabolism. Lancet. 1989;2:473.
3. Petty BG et al. Zidovudine with probenecid: a warning. Lancet. 1990;335:1044.

## Procainamide (Procan SR)

### Quinidine

Summary: Quinidine markedly increased procainamide serum concentrations in 1 patient; more study is needed.

Risk Factors: No specific risk factors known.

Related Drugs: No information available.

Management Options:
- *Circumvent/Minimize.* Until further data are available, the concomitant use of procainamide and quinidine should be avoided.
- *Monitor.* Patients receiving procainamide for antiarrhythmic therapy should be monitored for an increased response, increased serum

concentrations, and toxicity (wide QRS, QT interval) when quinidine is added to their drug regimens. Discontinuing quinidine may reduce the serum concentration and efficacy of concurrently administered procainamide.

References:
1. Hughes B et al. Increased procainamide plasma concentrations caused by quinidine: a new drug interaction. Am Heart J. 1987;114:908.

## Procainamide (Procan SR)

## Trimethoprim (Proloprim)

Summary: Trimethoprim significantly increases serum concentrations of procainamide and N-acetylprocainamide (NAPA); cardiac toxicity may result.

Risk Factors: No specific risk factors known.

Related Drugs: No information available.

Management Options:
- *Monitor.* Serum procainamide and NAPA concentrations should be monitored and patients should be observed for procainamide toxicity (wide QRS, QT interval) when trimethoprim is coadministered.

References:
1. Kosoglou T et al. Trimethoprim alters the disposition of procainamide and N-acetylprocainamide. Clin Pharmacol Ther. 1988;44:467.
2. Vlasses PH et al. Trimethoprim inhibition of the renal clearance of procainamide and N-acetylprocainamide. Arch Intern Med. 1989;149:1350.

## Procarbazine (Matulane)

## Prochlorperazine (Compazine)

Summary: Use of phenothiazines in patients receiving procarbazine has been associated with increased sedation and possibly with increased severity of extrapyramidal symptoms.

Risk Factors: No specific risk factors known.

Related Drugs: Procarbazine purportedly can increase sedation from opiates and barbiturates, but cases in humans are lacking.[2]

Management Options:
- *Monitor.* Patients and families should be instructed to watch for increased sedation and changes in extrapyramidal symptoms if phenothiazines are used with procarbazine.

References:
1. Todd IDH. Natulan in management of late Hodgkin's disease, other lymphoreticular neoplasms, and malignant melanoma. Br Med J. 1965;1:628.
2. Weiss HD et al. Neurotoxicity of commonly used antineoplastic agents. N Engl J Med. 1974;291:127.
3. Poster DS. Procarbazine-prochlorperazine interaction: an underreported phenomenon. J Med. 1978;9:519.

## Propafenone (Rythmol)

### Quinidine

Summary: Quinidine increases propafenone serum concentrations and reduces the serum concentrations of its active metabolite. The result may be no net change in response.

Risk Factors:
- *Pharmacogenetics.* Rapid propafenone metabolizers may be at increased risk for the interaction.

Related Drugs: No information available.

Management Options:
- *Circumvent/Minimize.* It should be noted that in this group of patients doses of propafenone were reduced an average of 45% before quinidine was initiated. In all likelihood this attenuated the increase in propafenone concentration and the potential for toxicity to occur. Prophylactic reduction of the propafenone dose may be the most judicious approach.
- *Monitor.* Until more data are available, patients stabilized on propafenone should be monitored carefully for toxicity when quinidine is added.

References:
1. Funck-Brentano C et al. Genetically-determined interaction between propafenone and low dose quinidine: role of active metabolites in modulating net drug effect. Br J Clin Pharmacol. 1989;27:435.
2. Siddoway LA et al. Polymorphism of propafenone metabolism and disposition in man: clinical and pharmacokinetic consequences. Circulation. 1987;75:785.
3. Morike KE et al. Quinidine-enhanced beta-blockade during treatment with propafenone in extensive metabolizer human subjects. Clin Pharmacol Ther. 1994;55:28.

## Propafenone (Rythmol)

### Rifampin (Rifadin)

Summary: Rifampin lowers propafenone plasma concentrations and may cause loss of antiarrhythmic efficacy.

Risk Factors: No specific risk factors known.

Related Drugs: *Rifabutin (Mycobutin)* would, theoretically, produce a similar reduction in propafenone concentration.

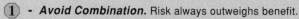
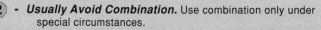

## Significance Classification

(1) - *Avoid Combination.* Risk always outweighs benefit.

(2) - *Usually Avoid Combination.* Use combination only under special circumstances.

(3) - *Minimize Risk.* Take action as necessary to reduce risk.

Management Options:
- *Monitor.* Patients receiving propafenone should be monitored for falling plasma concentrations and loss of antiarrhythmic efficacy after the addition of rifampin. One to two weeks may be required to observe the maximum effect of rifampin on propafenone concentrations.

References:
1. Castel JM et al. Rifampicin lowers plasma concentrations of propafenone and its antiarrhythmic effect. Br J Clin Pharmacol. 1990;30:155.

### Propafenone (Rythmol)

### Theophylline

Summary: Case reports suggest that propafenone elevates theophylline plasma concentrations and may produce symptoms of theophylline toxicity.

Risk Factors: No specific risk factors known.

Related Drugs: No information available.

Management Options:
- *Circumvent/Minimize.* Theophylline doses may require reduction following the addition of propafenone.
- *Monitor.* Patients stabilized on theophylline should be monitored for elevated theophylline concentrations and signs of theophylline toxicity (e.g., nausea, anorexia, tremor, tachycardia) if propafenone therapy is added. Discontinuing propafenone may result in subtherapeutic theophylline concentrations.

References:
1. Lee BL et al. Theophylline toxicity after propafenone treatment: evidence for drug interaction. Clin Pharmacol Ther. 1992;51:353.
2. Spinler SA et al. Propafenone-theophylline interaction. Pharmacotherapy. 1993; 13:68.

### Propafenone (Rythmol)

### Warfarin (Coumadin)

Summary: Propafenone increases warfarin serum concentrations and prolongs the prothrombin time in subjects taking low doses of both drugs.

Risk Factors: No specific risk factors known.

Related Drugs: In a case report, a similar enhancement of anticoagulant effect in a patient taking **phenprocoumon** and propafenone was noted.[2]

Management Options:
- *Monitor.* Although data from therapeutically anticoagulated patients are limited, the administration of propafenone in antiarrhythmic doses could enhance the anticoagulation effect of warfarin significantly. Patients stabilized on warfarin should be monitored if propafenone is added or withdrawn from therapy.

References:
1. Kates RE et al. Interaction between warfarin and propafenone in healthy volunteer subjects. Clin Pharmacol Ther. 1987;42:305.
2. Korst HA et al. Warning: propafenone potentiates the effect of oral anticoagulants. Med Klin. 1981;72:349.

## Propoxyphene (Darvocet-N)
## Warfarin (Coumadin)

Summary: Several cases of enhanced hypoprothrombinemic response to warfarin have been reported during the use of a propoxyphene-acetaminophen preparation, but an effect of propoxyphene alone on oral anticoagulant response has not been documented.

Risk Factors: No specific risk factors known.

Related Drugs: No information available.

Management Options:
- *Monitor.* Although this interaction is not well established, monitor for altered oral anticoagulant effect if propoxyphene is initiated, discontinued or changed in dosage. Adjust the anticoagulant dose as needed.

References:
1. Jones RV. Warfarin and distalgesic interaction. Br Med J. 1976;1:460.
2. Smith R et al. Propoxyphene and warfarin interaction. Drug Intell Clin Pharm. 1984;18:822.
3. Justice JL et al. Analgesic and warfarin; a case that brings up the questions and cautions. Postgrad Med J. 1988;83:217.

## Propranolol (Inderal)
## Quinidine

Summary: Quinidine may increase the plasma concentration of propranolol, but the incidence of adverse effects due to these interactions is unknown. Propranolol does not affect quinidine kinetics.

Risk Factors:
- *Pharmacogenetics.* Rapid metabolizers of propranolol may be at increased risk to develop the interaction.

Related Drugs: Quinidine decreases the metabolism of **metoprolol (Lopressor)**, and **timolol (Blocadren)**.

Management Options:
- *Consider Alternative.* Preliminary evidence suggests no effect of quinidine on labetalol pharmacokinetics or pharmacodynamics.[3] Renally excreted beta blockers [e.g., atenolol (Tenormin)] should be less likely to interact with quinidine since their metabolism is unlikely to be affected by quinidine. Nevertheless, additive cardiac depressant effects cannot be overlooked.

• *Monitor.* Concomitant use of quinidine and propranolol should be undertaken with careful monitoring. Watch for bradycardia, heart failure, and arrhythmias.

References:

1. Yasuhara M et al. Alteration of propranolol pharmacokinetics and pharmacodynamics by quinidine in man. J Pharmacobiodyn. 1990;13:681.
2. Zhou H-H et al. Quinidine reduces clearance of (+)-propranolol more than (–)-propranolol through marked reduction in 4-hydroxylation. Clin Pharmacol Ther. 1990;47:686.
3. Gearhart MO et al. Lack of effects on labetalol pharmacodynamics with quinidine inhibition of P450IID6. Pharmacotherapy. 1991;11:P-36. Abstract.

## Propranolol (Inderal)

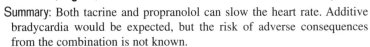

### Tacrine (Cognex)

Summary: Both tacrine and propranolol can slow the heart rate. Additive bradycardia would be expected, but the risk of adverse consequences from the combination is not known.

Risk Factors: No specific risk factors known.

Related Drugs: Other beta blockers [e.g., *atenolol (Tenormin)*, *nadolol (Corgard)*] may produce similar additive bradycardia.

Management Options:

• *Monitor* for excessive bradycardia in patients receiving beta-adrenergic blockers concurrently with tacrine or other cholinergic agents.

References:

1. Eldor J et al. Prolonged bradycardia and hypotension after neostigmine administration in a patient receiving atenolol. Anaesthesia. 1987;42:1294.
2. Taylor P. Agents acting at the neuromuscular junction and autonomic ganglia. In: Gilman AG et al., eds. The Pharmacological Basis of Therapeutics, 8th ed. New York: Pergamon Press; 1990:166–186.
3. Hartvig P et al. Pharmacokinetics and effects of 9-amino-1,2,3,4-tetrahydroacridine in the immediate postoperative period in neurosurgical patients. J Clin Anesth. 1991;3:137.

## Propranolol (Inderal)

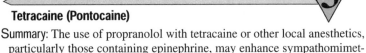

### Tetracaine (Pontocaine)

Summary: The use of propranolol with tetracaine or other local anesthetics, particularly those containing epinephrine, may enhance sympathomimetic side effects resulting in hypertensive reactions. Acute discontinuation of beta blockers before local anesthesia may increase the risk of side effects due to the anesthetic.

Risk Factors:

• *Anesthetic Combinations.* Local anesthetics containing epinephrine may be at risk for hypertensive reactions.

Related Drugs: *Bupivacaine (Marcaine)* and *lidocaine (Xylocaine)* appear to interact similarly with propranolol. Cardioselective beta blocker [e.g., *metoprolol (Lopressor)*, *acebutolol (Sectral)*, *atenolol (Tenormin)*] are probably less likely to predispose patients to epinephrine-induced hypertension. In 10 patients on propranolol who received small doses of *local anesthetic* plus *epinephrine (Adrenalin)* (mean epinephrine dose ≈50.03 mg), no hypertensive reactions were noted.[3]

Management Options:

- *Consider Alternative.* If possible, local anesthetics containing epinephrine should be avoided in patients receiving propranolol or other nonselective beta blockers, such as nadolol, pindolol or timolol.

- *Circumvent/Minimize.* These studies indicate that chronic beta blocker therapy should *not* be discontinued before the use of local anesthetics such as tetracaine or bupivacaine although one should be alert for evidence of cardiodepression.

- *Monitor.* If local anesthetics and beta blockers are coadministered, monitor for hypertensive or cardiotoxic reactions.

References:

1. Roitman K et al. Enhancement of bupivacaine cardiotoxicity with cardiac glycosides and beta-adrenergic blockers: a case report. Anesth Analg. 1993;76:658.
2. Foster CA et al. Propranolol-epinephrine interaction: a potential disaster. Plast Reconstr Surg. 1983;72:74.
3. Dzubow LM. The interaction between propranolol and epinephrine as observed in patients undergoing Mohs' surgery. J Am Acad Dermatol. 1986;15:71.

## Propranolol (Inderal)

## Theophylline

Summary: Propranolol increases theophylline serum concentrations in a dose-dependent manner. Theophylline and beta blockers have antagonistic pharmacodynamic effects.

Risk Factors:

- *Dosage Regimen.* Higher doses of propranolol may reduce theophylline clearance.

Related Drugs: *Metoprolol (Lopressor)* appears to interact similarly with theophylline. *Atenolol (Tenormin)* and *nadolol (Corgard)* do not appear to alter the theophylline pharmacokinetics but may interact pharmacodynamically.[2,3] Other beta blockers may produce similar antagonistic effects with theophylline.

## Significance Classification

 - *Avoid Combination.* Risk always outweighs benefit.

 - *Usually Avoid Combination.* Use combination only under special circumstances.

 - *Minimize Risk.* Take action as necessary to reduce risk.

Management Options:
- *Use Alternative.* If possible, beta blockers should be avoided in patients receiving theophylline for bronchospastic pulmonary disease. If beta blockers are required, cardioselective agents are preferable.
- *Monitor.* If cardioselective beta blockers are administered to asthmatics, monitor carefully for reduced bronchodilator response.

References:
1. Lombardi TP et al. The effects of a beta$_2$ agonist and a nonselective beta antagonist on theophylline clearance. Drug Intell Clin Pharm. 1986;20:455.
2. Cerasa LA et al. Lack of effect of atenolol on the pharmacokinetics of theophylline. Br J Clin Pharmacol. 1988;26:800.
3. Corsi CM et al. Lack of effect of atenolol and nadolol on the metabolism of theophylline. Br J Clin Pharmacol. 1990;29:265.

## Propranolol (Inderal)

## Verapamil (Calan)

Summary: Propranolol serum concentrations may be increased by verapamil; beta blocker and verapamil combinations may result in a greater risk of bradycardia or hypotension than when either is used alone.

Risk Factors: No specific risk factors known.

Related Drugs: **Atenolol (Tenormin), metoprolol (Lopressor)**, and **timolol (Timoptic)** appear to interact similarly with verapamil. **Diltiazem (Cardizem)** reduces the metabolism of several beta blockers.

Management Options:
- *Circumvent/Minimize.* The use of beta blockers that are not metabolized (e.g., atenolol) should minimize pharmacokinetic (but not pharmacodynamic) interactions with verapamil.
- *Monitor.* Patients receiving therapy with beta blockers and verapamil should be monitored for enhanced effects, particularly atrioventricular conduction slowing, resulting from pharmacokinetic or pharmacodynamic interactions.

References:
1. Murdoch DL et al. Evaluation of potential pharmacodynamic and pharmacokinetic interactions between verapamil and propranolol in normal subjects. Br J Clin Pharmacol. 1991;31:323.
2. Hunt BA et al. Effects of calcium channel blockers on the pharmacokinetics of propranolol stereoisomers. Clin Pharmacol Ther. 1990;47:584.
3. Bailey DG et al. Interaction between oral verapamil and beta-blockers during submaximal exercise: relevance of ancillary properties. Clin Pharmacol Ther. 1991: 49:370.

## Quinidine

## Rifampin (Rifadin)

Summary: Rifampin markedly reduces quinidine plasma concentrations.

Risk Factors: No specific risk factors known.

Related Drugs: Theoretically **rifabutin (Mycobutin)** would affect quinidine in a similar manner.

Management Options:

- *Circumvent/Minimize.* In patients receiving rifampin, the quinidine dose may have to be increased substantially to maintain therapeutic efficacy. Discontinuation of rifampin will result in increased quinidine concentrations.

- *Monitor.* Plasma quinidine determinations can be used to achieve the optimal dose of quinidine in the presence of rifampin. Patients should be observed carefully for changes in quinidine response for several days to two weeks following the addition or removal of rifampin therapy.

References:
1. Schwartz A et al. Quinidine-rifampin interaction. Am Heart J. 1984;107:789.
2. Twum-Barima Y et al. Quinidine-rifampin interaction. N Engl J Med. 1981;304:1466.
3. Bussey HI et al. Influence of rifampin on quinidine and digoxin. Arch Intern Med. 1984;144:1021.

## Quinidine

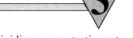

### Sodium Bicarbonate

Summary: Sodium bicarbonate can increase quinidine concentrations; toxicity could result.

Risk Factors: No specific risk factors known.

Related Drugs: Other agents that alkalinize the urine [e.g., **antacids**, **acetazolamide (Diamox)**] would be expected to produce similar results.

Management Options:

- *Monitor.* When a urinary alkalizer such as sodium bicarbonate is initiated, the quinidine dose may have to be reduced to avoid toxicity.

References:
1. Knouss RF et al. Variation in quinidine excretion with changing urine pH. Ann Intern Med. 1968;68:1157. Abstract.
2. Milne MD. Influence of acid-base balance on the efficacy and toxicity of drugs. Proc R Soc Med. 1965;58:961.

## Quinidine

### Timolol (Blocadren)

Summary: Quinidine may increase the plasma concentration of timolol, but the incidence of adverse effects due to these interactions is unknown.

Risk Factors:

- *Pharmacogenetics.* Patients who are rapid metabolizers of timolol are at increased risk for the interaction.

Related Drugs: Quinidine also decreases the metabolism of **metoprolol (Lopressor)** and **propranolol (Inderal)**. It would not likely affect renally eliminated beta blockers such as *atenolol (Tenormin)*. Preliminary evidence suggests no effect of quinidine on *labetalol (Normodyne)* pharmacokinetics or pharmacodynamics.[3]

Management Options:
- *Consider Alternative.* Renally excreted beta blockers (e.g., atenolol) should be less likely to interact with quinidine, since their metabolism is unlikely to be affected by quinidine. Nevertheless, additive cardiac depressant effects cannot be overlooked.
- *Monitor.* Concomitant use of quinidine and timolol should be undertaken with careful monitoring. Watch for bradycardia, heart failure, and arrhythmias.

References:
1. Dinai Y et al. Bradycardia induced by interaction between quinidine and ophthalmic timolol. Ann Intern Med. 1985;103:890.
2. Kaila T et al. Beta blocking effects of timolol at low plasma concentrations. Clin Pharmacol Ther. 1991;49:53.
3. Gearhart MO et al. Lack of effects on labetalol pharmacodynamics with quinidine inhibition of P450IID6. Pharmacotherapy. 1991;11:P-36. Abstract.

### Quinidine

### Tubocurarine

Summary: Quinidine administration may enhance the effects of tubocurarine and other neuromuscular blockers.

Risk Factors: No specific risk factors known.

Related Drugs: A similar effect might be seen with other neuromuscular blockers [e.g., *succinylcholine (Anectine)*].[1,2]

Management Options:
- *Monitor.* If possible, quinidine should be avoided in the immediate postoperative period when the effects of muscle relaxants still may be present. If quinidine must be used, the need for respiratory support should be anticipated.

References:
1. Schmidt JL et al. The effect of quinidine on the action of muscle relaxants. JAMA. 1963;183:669.

## Significance Classification

1 - *Avoid Combination.* Risk always outweighs benefit.

2 - *Usually Avoid Combination.* Use combination only under special circumstances.

3 - *Minimize Risk.* Take action as necessary to reduce risk.

2. Cuthbert MF. The effect of quinidine and procainamide on the neuromuscular blocking action of suxamethonium. Br J Anaesth. 1966;38:775.
3. Kambam JR et al. Effect of quinidine on plasma cholinesterase activity and succinylcholine neuromuscular blockade. Anesthesiology. 1987;67:858.

## Quinidine

### Verapamil (Calan)

Summary: Verapamil administration with quinidine increases quinidine concentrations and may result in quinidine toxicity.

Risk Factors: No specific risk factors known.

Related Drugs: **Nifedipine (Procardia)** reduces quinidine concentrations. **Diltiazem (Cardizem)** 120 mg/day had no effect on quinidine concentrations.[3] The effects of combining other calcium channel blockers and quinidine are unknown, but are likely to be limited.

Management Options:
- *Circumvent/Minimize.* The addition of verapamil to quinidine therapy may necessitate a reduction in the dose of quinidine.
- *Monitor.* If quinidine and verapamil are coadministered, monitor for quinidine toxicity including hypotension and heart block.

References:
1. Trohman RG et al. Increased quinidine plasma concentrations during administration of verapamil; a new quinidine-verapamil interaction. Am J Cardiol. 1986; 57:706.
2. Edwards DJ et al. The effect of co-administration of verapamil on the pharmacokinetics and metabolism of quinidine. Clin Pharmacol Ther. 1987;41:68.
3. Matera MG et al. Quinidine-diltiazem: pharmacokinetic interaction in humans. Curr Ther Res. 1986;40:653.

## Quinidine

### Warfarin (Coumadin)

Summary: A few patients experienced enhanced anticoagulation after quinidine was added to warfarin therapy. Prospective studies do not indicate that the interaction is widespread or of substantial magnitude.

Risk Factors: No specific risk factors known.

Related Drugs: Theoretically, the same effect could be seen with other oral anticoagulants.

Management Options:
- *Monitor.* Patients on oral anticoagulants who subsequently receive quinidine should be observed closely for prolonged prothrombin times and signs of bleeding.

References:
1. Gazzaniga AB et al. Possible quinidine-induced hemorrhage in a patient on warfarin sodium. N Engl J Med. 1969;280:711.

2. Sopher IM et al. Fatal corpus luteum hemorrhage during anti-coagulant therapy. Obstet Gynecol. 1971;37:695.

3. Udall JA. Drug interference with warfarin therapy. Clin Med. 1970;77:20.

## Radioactive Iodine ($I^{131}$)

### Theophylline

Summary: A patient developed theophylline toxicity following $I^{131}$ therapy for thyrotoxicosis; this response is consistent with known effect of thyroid function on theophylline elimination.

Risk Factors:
- *Concurrent Diseases.* Patients who develop hypothyroidism following $I^{131}$ are at increased risk for the interaction.

Related Drugs: Theoretically, antithyroid drugs such as **methimazole (Tapazole)** and **propylthiouracil** would produce an effect similar to that of $I^{131}$ (i.e., an increase in serum theophylline concentrations).

Management Options:
- *Monitor* for theophylline toxicity in patients who receive $I^{131}$ therapy for hyperthyroidism. Although hypothyroidism following $I^{131}$ therapy is not unusual, it may take months or years to occur; thus, the time course of any increase in serum theophylline concentrations would be highly variable.

References:
1. Johnson CE et al. Theophylline toxicity after iodine 131 treatment for hyperthyroidism. Clin Pharm. 1988;7:620.

## Rifabutin (Mycobutin)

### Ritonavir (Norvir)

Summary: Ritonavir administration produces marked increases in rifabutin concentrations; rifabutin toxicity may result.

Risk Factors: No specific risk factors known.

Related Drugs: **Indinavir (Crixivan)** also inhibits the metabolism of rifabutin. Rifabutin decreases the area under the concentration-time curve of **saquinavir (Invirase)**. The effects of saquinavir and nelfinavir (Viracept) on rifabutin are unknown.

Management Options:
- *Consider Alternative.* If monotherapy for *Mycobacterium avium* complex (MAC) is required, azithromycin or clarithromycin should be considered. Note that ritonavir inhibits the metabolism of clarithromycin and lower doses of clarithromycin may be required.
- *Circumvent/Minimize.* Pending further information on this interaction, the use of ritonavir and rifabutin should be avoided if possible. Rifabutin dose and frequency may require reduction during coadministration with ritonavir.

- *Monitor.* If the ritonavir and rifabutin are coadministered, watch for signs of rifabutin toxicity including arthralgia, dyspepsia, anemia, or skin discoloration. Be alert for subtherapeutic rifabutin concentrations when ritonavir is discontinued.

References:
1. Abbott Laboratories. Ritonavir (Norvir) package insert. 1996.

## Rifabutin (Mycobutin)
## Saquinavir (Invirase)

Summary: Rifabutin markedly reduces the serum concentration of saquinavir; loss of efficacy or development of resistant organisms may result.

Risk Factors: No specific risk factors known.

Related Drugs: Rifabutin reduces the concentrations of other protease inhibitors including *ritonavir (Norvir)*, *indinavir (Crixivan)*, and probably *nelfinavir (Viracept)*. *Rifampin (Rifadin)* also reduces saquinavir serum concentrations.

Management Options:
- *Circumvent/Minimize.* The dose of saquinavir may require substantial increase to produce therapeutic serum concentrations. If possible, saquinavir serum concentrations should be monitored if dosage adjustments are attempted.
- *Monitor.* Watch for loss of saquinavir efficacy during rifabutin coadministration.

References:
1. Hoffman-La Roche, Inc. Saquinavir (Invirase) package insert. 1995.

## Rifampin (Rifadin)

## Ritonavir (Norvir)

Summary: Rifampin appears to reduce ritonavir plasma concentrations; loss of antiviral efficacy may result.

Risk Factors: No specific risk factors known.

Related Drugs: *Rifabutin (Mycobutin)* also may reduce the concentrations of ritonavir. Other protease inhibitors such as *indinavir (Crixivan)*, *saquinavir (Invirase)*, and *nelfinavir (Viracept)* may be affected by rifampin in a similar manner.

Management Options:
- *Circumvent/Minimize.* Pending further clinical data, one should consider increasing the dosage of ritonavir during coadministration of rifampin.
- *Monitor* for reduced ritonavir efficacy.

References:
1. Abbott Laboratories. Ritonavir (Norvir) package insert. 1996.

### Rifampin (Rifadin)

### Saquinavir (Invirase)

**Summary:** Rifampin markedly reduces the serum concentration of saquinavir; loss of efficacy or development of resistant organisms may result.

**Risk Factors:** No specific risk factors known.

**Related Drugs:** Rifampin reduces the concentrations of other protease inhibitors including *ritonavir (Norvir)*, *indinavir (Crixivan)*, and *nelfinavir (Viracept)*. *Rifabutin (Mycobutin)* also reduces saquinavir serum concentrations.

**Management Options:**

- *Use Alternative.* Based on the magnitude of this interaction, it would be difficult to administer an effective dose of saquinavir. Since other protease inhibitors are also likely to be affected, an alternative to rifampin should be considered.

**References:**

1. Hoffman-La Roche, Inc. Saquinavir (Invirase) package insert. 1995.

### Rifampin (Rifadin)

### Theophylline

**Summary:** Rifampin lowers the plasma concentration of theophylline; a reduction of theophylline efficacy may result.

**Risk Factors:** No specific risk factors known.

**Related Drugs:** No information available.

**Management Options:**

- *Monitor.* Be alert for the need to adjust the theophylline dose when rifampin therapy is started or stopped. Theophylline dose requirement may be higher in patients receiving rifampin.

**References:**

1. Straughn AB et al. Effect of rifampin on theophylline disposition. Ther Drug Monit. 1984;6:153.
2. Boyce EG et al. The effect of rifampin on theophylline kinetics. Clin Pharmacol Ther. 1985;37:183.
3. Brocks DR et al. Theophylline-rifampin interaction in a pediatric patient. Clin Pharm. 1986;5:602.

### Rifampin (Rifadin)

### Tocainide (Tonocard)

**Summary:** Rifampin administration to healthy subjects reduces tocainide serum concentrations considerably. There appears to be a potential for a loss of efficacy resulting from diminished tocainide concentrations.

**Risk Factors:** No specific risk factors known.

**Related Drugs:** No information available.

**Management Options:**

- *Monitor.* Patients stabilized on tocainide should be monitored for a decreased response and serum concentrations if rifampin is instituted. Discontinuing concomitant rifampin therapy could result in an increased tocainide concentration and effect.

References:
1. Rice TL et al. Influence of rifampin on tocainide pharmacokinetics in humans. Clin Pharm. 1989;8:200.
2. Edgar B et al. The pharmacokinetics of r- and s-tocainide in healthy subjects. Br J Clin Pharmacol. 1984;17:216P.
3. Hoffmann K-J et al. Stereoselective disposition of rs-tocainide in man. Eur J Drug Metab and Pharmacokinet. 1984;9:215.

## Rifampin (Rifadin)

## Tolbutamide (Orinase)

Summary: Rifampin reduces tolbutamide and glyburide serum concentrations and may reduce hypoglycemic activity.

Risk Factors: No specific risk factors known.

Related Drugs: A 67-year-old patient taking rifampin 600 mg/day and *glyburide (DiaBeta)* 15 mg/day had glyburide concentrations between 30 and 40 ng/mL.[3] After cessation of the rifampin therapy, the glyburide concentrations increased to >160 ng/mL. Blood glucose concentrations did not appear to be altered by the change in glyburide concentrations. Little is known concerning the effect of rifampin on other oral antidiabetic drugs, but their metabolism also might be enhanced by rifampin. *Rifabutin (Mycobutin)* might affect tolbutamide in a similar manner.

Management Options:
 • *Monitor.* When rifampin is administered concomitantly with tolbutamide or glyburide and possibly other sulfonylureas, be alert for the potential for diminished hypoglycemic activity. Discontinuation of rifampin could result in hypoglycemia.

References:
1. Syvalahti E et al. Effect of tuberculostatic agents on the response of serum growth hormone and immunoreactive insulin to intravenous tolbutamide, and on the half-life of tolbutamide. Int J Clin Pharmacol. 1976;13:83.
2. Zilly W et al. Stimulation of drug metabolism by rifampicin in patients with cirrhosis or cholestasis measured by increased hexobarbital and tolbutamide clearance. Eur J Clin Pharmacol. 1977;11:287.
3. Self TH et al. Interaction of rifampin and glyburide. Chest. 1989;96:1443.

## Significance Classification

① - *Avoid Combination.* Risk always outweighs benefit.

② - *Usually Avoid Combination.* Use combination only under special circumstances.

③ - *Minimize Risk.* Take action as necessary to reduce risk.

**Rifampin (Rifadin)**

**Triazolam (Halcion)**

Summary: Rifampin markedly reduces the plasma concentrations of triazolam; loss of triazolam effect is likely to occur during coadministration.

Risk Factors: No specific risk factors known.

Related Drugs: **Rifabutin (Mycobutin)** is likely to produce a similar effect on triazolam pharmacokinetics. Rifampin is known to increase the elimination of other benzodiazepines including **midazolam (Versed)** and **diazepam (Valium)**. Benzodiazepines that do not interact with rifampin include **temazepam (Restoril)** and **oxazepam (Serax)**.

Management Options:
- *Consider Alternative.* Selection of a benzodiazepine that does not interact with rifampin (see Related Drugs) would avoid the interaction.
- *Monitor.* Patients receiving rifampin should be monitored for reduced triazolam efficacy. If rifampin is discontinued in a patient receiving both agents, the dose of triazolam may require reduction during the next week or two to avoid excess sedation.

References:
1. Villikka K et al. Triazolam is ineffective in patients taking rifampin. Clin Pharmacol Ther. 1997;61:8.

**Rifampin (Rifadin)**

**Verapamil (Calan)**

Summary: Rifampin decreases verapamil plasma concentrations; loss of therapeutic effect may result.

Risk Factors:
- *Route of Administration.* Administration of verapamil orally increases the magnitude of this interaction.

Related Drugs: Rifampin is likely to affect other calcium channel blockers in a similar manner. **Rifabutin (Mycobutin)** might affect verapamil similarly.

Management Options:
- *Consider Alternative.* Because this interaction is likely to reduce the efficacy of verapamil, one should consider an alternative agent for verapamil. Other calcium channel blockers also may be affected; a therapeutic substitution to a different class of agent may be required.
- *Circumvent/Minimize:* Larger doses of calcium channel blockers (particularly those administered orally) may be required when rifampin is coadministered.
- *Monitor.* Patients taking calcium channel blockers should be monitored for a reduction in efficacy when rifampin is given.

References:
1. Rahn KH et al. Reduction of bioavailability of verapamil by rifampin. N Engl J Med. 1985;312:920.
2. Barbarash RA et al. Near-total reduction in verapamil bioavailability by rifampin. Chest. 1988;94:954.
3. Mooy J et al. The influence of antituberculosis drugs on the plasma level of verapamil. Eur J Clin Pharmacol. 1987;32:107.

## Rifampin (Rifadin)

### Warfarin (Coumadin)

Summary: Rifampin reduces the hypoprothrombinemic effect of warfarin and other oral anticoagulants in most patients to a clinically significant extent; anticoagulant dosage adjustments are likely to be necessary during cotherapy with these drugs.

Risk Factors: No specific risk factors known.

Related Drugs: **Phenprocoumon** and **acenocoumarol (Sintrom)** interact similarly with rifampin.

Management Options:
- *Avoid Unless Benefit Outweighs Risk.* Rifampin and oral anticoagulants should not be coadministered unless no alternative is available.
- *Monitor.* If rifampin is administered to patients requiring warfarin, clinicians should evaluate the patient's anticoagulant response carefully and readjust the anticoagulant dose as needed when rifampin is started, stopped, or changed in dosage.

References:
1. Self TH et al. Interaction of rifampin and warfarin. Chest. 1975;67:490.
2. Ranankiewicz JA et al. Rifampin and warfarin: a drug interaction. Ann Intern Med. 1975;82:224.
3. Heimark LD et al. The mechanism of the warfarin-rifampin drug interaction in humans. Clin Pharmacol Ther. 1987;42:388.

## Rifampin (Rifadin)

### Zidovudine (Retrovir)

Summary: Zidovudine plasma concentrations are reduced by the concomitant administration of rifampin; loss of efficacy could result.

Risk Factors: No specific risk factors known.

Related Drugs: No information available.

Management Options:
- *Monitor.* Patients taking zidovudine should have their zidovudine plasma concentrations monitored and be watched for a change in zidovudine response if rifampin therapy is added or discontinued. Zidovudine dose adjustments are likely to be necessary.

References:
1. Burger DM et al. Pharmacokinetic interaction between rifampin and zidovudine. Antimicrob Agents Chemother. 1993;37:1426.

## Ritonavir (Norvir)

### Saquinavir (Invirase)

Summary: Ritonavir increases saquinavir plasma concentrations; saquinavir toxicity may result.

Risk Factors: No specific risk factors known.

Related Drugs: Other protease inhibitors such as *indinavir (Crixivan)* and *nelfinavir (Viracept)* may affect saquinavir metabolism in a similar manner although the magnitude of the inhibition may be less than that observed with ritonavir. Ritonavir may inhibit the metabolism of other protease inhibitors such as *indinavir (Crixivan)* and *nelfinavir (Viracept)*.

Management Options:

- *Consider Alternative*. Using another protease inhibitor instead of ritonavir may reduce but not eliminate the interaction. Be alert for evidence of increased saquinavir plasma concentrations.
- *Circumvent/Minimize*. Reduction of the saquinavir dose may be necessary to avoid toxicity such as gastrointestinal upset and increased liver function tests.
- *Monitor* for gastrointestinal upset and elevated liver function tests when saquinavir is administered with ritonavir.

References:

1. Abbott Laboratories. Ritonavir (Norvir) package insert. 1996.
2. Hoffman-La Roche Inc. Saquinavir (Invirase) package insert. 1996.

## Ritonavir (Norvir)

### Theophylline

Summary: Ritonavir reduces theophylline plasma concentrations; a reduction in theophylline efficacy may result.

Risk Factors: No specific risk factors known.

Related Drugs: The effect of other protease inhibitors such as indinavir (Crixivan), saquinavir (Invirase), and nelfinavir (Viracept) on theophylline metabolism is unknown.

Management Options:

- *Consider Alternative*. While specific information is not available, other protease inhibitors may avoid the interaction with theophylline.

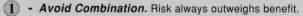
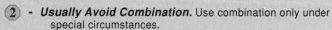

## Significance Classification

①  - *Avoid Combination*. Risk always outweighs benefit.

②  - *Usually Avoid Combination*. Use combination only under special circumstances.

③  - *Minimize Risk*. Take action as necessary to reduce risk.

- *Circumvent/Minimize.* The coadministration of theophylline and ritonavir may require increasing the dose of theophylline to maintain therapeutic concentrations.
- *Monitor* theophylline concentrations to ensure adequate plasma levels are maintained during ritonavir administration. Watch for inadequate theophylline response such as bronchospasm or wheezing.

References:
1. Abbot Laboratories. Ritonavir (Norvir) package insert. 1996.

## Selegiline (Eldepryl)

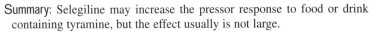

## Tyramine

Summary: Selegiline may increase the pressor response to food or drink containing tyramine, but the effect usually is not large.

Risk Factors:
- *Dosage Regimen.* Selegiline doses of up to 10 mg/day usually have only a small inhibitory effect on monoamine oxidase (MAO)-A, but larger doses can have a clinically important effect.

Related Drugs: **Mofegiline**, another MAO-B inhibitor, does not appear to lose its MAO-B selectivity when large doses are used.

Management Options:
- *Circumvent/Minimize.* Although strict avoidance of tyramine-containing foods is not necessary, it would be prudent to avoid high-tyramine foods, especially if the patient is taking >10 mg/day of selegiline.
- *Monitor* for evidence of tyramine-induced hypertension.

References:
1. Elsworth JD et al. Deprenyl administration in man: a selective monoamine oxidase B inhibitor without the "cheese effect." Psychopharmacology. 1978;57:33.
2. Schulz R et al. Tyramine kinetics and pressor sensitivity during monoamine oxidase inhibition by selegiline. Clin Pharmacol Ther. 1989; 46:528.

## Sertraline (Zoloft)

## Warfarin (Coumadin)

Summary: A preliminary report suggests that sertraline may slightly increase the hypoprothrombinemic response to warfarin.

Risk Factors: No specific risk factors known.

Related Drugs: Some selective serotonin reuptake inhibitors [e.g., **fluoxetine (Prozac)**, **paroxetine (Paxil)**] have been reported to have an intrinsic inhibitory effect on hemostasis, but it is not known if sertraline has a similar effect. The effect of sertraline on oral anticoagulants other than warfarin is not established.

Management Options:
- *Monitor.* Although data are scanty, be alert for evidence of an altered hypoprothrombinemic response to warfarin (or other anticoagu-

lants) if sertraline is initiated, discontinued, or changed in dosage. Although not reported for sertraline, some SSRIs may impair hemostasis; thus, be alert for evidence of bleeding even if the hypoprothrombinemic response is in the desired range.

References:
1. Wilner KD et al. The effects of sertraline on the pharmacodynamics of warfarin in healthy volunteers. Biol Psychiatry. 1991;29:333S.

## Sucralfate (Carafate)

### Warfarin (Coumadin)

Summary: In isolated cases sucralfate appeared to inhibit the effect of warfarin, but subsequent studies have failed to demonstrate an interaction.

Risk Factors: No specific risk factors known.

Related Drugs: The effect of sucralfate on oral anticoagulants other than warfarin is not established. *Ranitidine (Zantac)* and *famotidine (Pepcid)* do not interact.

Management Options:
- *Consider Alternative.* Consider using a noninteracting H$_2$-receptor antagonist, such as ranitidine (Zantac) or famotidine (Pepcid).
- *Circumvent/Minimize.* Take oral anticoagulants at least 2 hours before or 6 hours after sucralfate and try to maintain a relatively constant interval and sequence of administration of the 2 drugs.
- *Monitor.* Although this interaction is not well established, monitor for altered oral anticoagulant effect if sucralfate is initiated, discontinued, or changed in dosage. Adjust the anticoagulant dose as needed.

References:
1. Talbert RL et al. Effect of sucralfate on plasma warfarin concentration in patients requiring chronic warfarin therapy. Drug Intell Clin Pharm. 1985;19:456.
2. Neuvonen PJ et al. Clinically significant sucralfate-warfarin interaction is not likely. Br J Clin Pharmacol. 1985;20:178.
3. Rey AM et al. Altered absorption of digoxin, sustained-release quinidine, and warfarin with sucralfate administration. DICP Ann Pharmacother. 1991;25:745.

## Sulfinpyrazone (Anturane)

### Tolbutamide (Orinase)

Summary: Sulfinpyrazone may increase the hypoglycemic effects of tolbutamide.

Risk Factors: No specific risk factors known.

Related Drugs: Sulfinpyrazone could potentially affect other sulfonylureas.

Management Options:
- *Monitor.* Diabetic patients receiving tolbutamide may require dosage adjustments when therapy with sulfinpyrazone is initiated or with-

drawn. Monitor blood glucose and watch for symptoms of hypoglycemia if sulfinpyrazone is initiated or hyperglycemia if it is withdrawn.

References:
1. Miners JO. The effect of sulfinpyrazone on oxidative drug metabolism in man: inhibition of tolbutamide elimination. Eur J Clin Pharmacol. 1982;22:321.

## Sulfinpyrazone (Anturane)

## Warfarin (Coumadin)

Summary: Sulfinpyrazone markedly increases the hypoprothrombinemic response to warfarin, acenocoumarol, and possibly other oral anticoagulants. If the combination must be used, monitor carefully for excessive hypoprothrombinemia and clinical evidence of bleeding.

Risk Factors: No specific risk factors known.

Related Drugs: *Acenocoumarol (Sintrom)* is affected similarly by sulfinpyrazone. *Phenprocoumon* does not appear to interact with sulfinpyrazone.[3] The effect of sulfinpyrazone on other oral anticoagulants is unknown, but assume that they interact until proven otherwise.

Management Options:

- *Avoid Unless Benefit Outweighs Risk.* Sulfinpyrazone should not be used in anticoagulated patients unless the potential benefit clearly outweighs the substantial risk.

- *Monitor.* If sulfinpyrazone is used, the hypoprothrombinemic response should be monitored very closely. When warfarin therapy is initiated in patients receiving sulfinpyrazone, increased sensitivity to warfarin's hypoprothrombinemic effect may occur.

References:
1. O'Reilly RA. Stereoselective interaction of sulfinpyrazone with racemic warfarin and its separated enantiomorphs in man. Circulation. 1982;65:202.
2. Girolami A et al. Potentiation of anticoagulated response to warfarin by sulfinpyrazone: a double-blind study in patients with prosthetic heart values. Clin Lab Haematol. 1982;4:23.
3. O'Reilly RA. Phenylbutazone and sulfinpyrazone interaction with oral anticoagulant phenprocoumon. Arch Intern Med. 1982;142:1634.

## Sulindac (Clinoril)

## Warfarin (Coumadin)

Summary: Although sulindac did not affect the response to warfarin in healthy subjects, several patients receiving warfarin have developed excessive hypoprothrombinemia following sulindac therapy.

Risk Factors:

- *Concurrent Diseases.* Patients with peptic ulcer disease (PUD) or a history of gastrointestinal bleeding probably are at greater risk.

Related Drugs: All NSAIDs inhibit platelet function, cause gastric erosions, and probably increase the risk of GI bleeding. Some NSAIDs, however, such as **ibuprofen (Advil)**, **naproxen (Naprosyn)**, or **diclofenac (Voltaren)** may be less likely to increase oral anticoagulant-induced hypoprothrombinemia than other NSAIDs.

Management Options:
- *Avoid Unless Benefit Outweighs Risk.* Since all NSAIDs probably increase the risk of GI bleeding in patients on oral anticoagulants, use the combination only after careful consideration of the benefit versus risk. If an NSAID must be used with an oral anticoagulant, it would be prudent to use NSAIDs that are unlikely to affect the hypoprothrombinemic response to oral anticoagulants. If the NSAID is being used as an analgesic or antipyretic, acetaminophen (Tylenol) is probably safer to use with oral anticoagulants. Nonacetylated salicylates (e.g., choline salicylate, magnesium salicylate, salsalate, sodium salicylate) probably also are safer with oral anticoagulants than NSAIDs, since such salicylates have minimal effects on platelet function and the gastric mucosa.
- *Monitor.* If any NSAID is used with an oral anticoagulant, one should carefully monitor the prothrombin time and watch for evidence of bleeding, especially from the GI tract.

References:
1. Ross JRY et al. Sulindac, prothrombin time, and anticoagulants. Lancet. 1979; 2:1075.
2. Carter SA. Potential effect of sulindac on response of prothrombin time to oral anticoagulants. Lancet. 1979;2:698.
3. Shorr RI et al. Concurrent use of nonsteroidal anti-inflammatory drugs and oral anticoagulants places elderly persons at high risk for hemorrhagic peptic ulcer disease. Arch Intern Med. 1993;153:1665.

## Tacrine (Cognex)

## Theophylline

Summary: Tacrine can substantially increase theophylline plasma concentrations; reductions in theophylline dosage are likely to be necessary.

Risk Factors: No specific risk factors known.

Related Drugs: No information available.

Management Options:
- *Consider Alternative.* In patients already receiving tacrine who are being started on theophylline, consider using alternatives to theophylline. If theophylline is used, it would be prudent to begin with smaller than usual doses until the response is determined.
- *Circumvent/Minimize.* Given the potential magnitude of the interaction, it may be prudent to adjust theophylline dosage prophylactically in patients at higher risk (e.g., those with high pre-existing theophylline plasma concentrations).

- *Monitor.* In patients receiving theophylline monitor clinical status and theophylline plasma concentrations if tacrine is initiated, discontinued, or changed in dosage.

References:
1. Madden S et al. An investigation into the formation of stable, protein-reactive and cytotoxic metabolites from tacrine *in vitro*: studies with human and rat liver microsomes. Biochem Pharmacol. 1993;46:13.
2. de Vries TM et al. Effect of multiple-dose tacrine administration on single-dose pharmacokinetics of digoxin, diazepam, and theophylline. Pharm Res. 1993;10: S333. Abstract.
3. Parke-Davis. Cognex Product Information. Morris Plains, NJ: 1993.

## Tacrine (Cognex)

### Trihexyphenidyl (Artane)

Summary: Tacrine may inhibit the therapeutic effect of anticholinergic agents such as trihexyphenidyl, and centrally acting anticholinergics may inhibit the therapeutic effect of tacrine.

Risk Factors: No specific risk factors known.

Related Drugs: Although more study is needed, one would expect all centrally acting anticholinergic agents to inhibit tacrine response. Peripherally acting anti-cholinergics [e.g., ***glycopyrrolate (Robinul)***] would be expected to inhibit the adverse cholinergic effects of tacrine without affecting the therapeutic effect. Tacrine may inhibit the therapeutic effect of anticholinergics.

Management Options:
- *Consider Alternative.* It would be prudent to avoid centrally acting anticholinergic agents in patients receiving tacrine, since they would be expected to antagonize the favorable effects of tacrine in Alzheimer's disease.
- *Monitor.* If the combination is used, monitor for reduced tacrine response.

References:
1. Ott BR, Lannon MC. Exacerbation of parkinsonism by tacrine. Clin Neuropharmacol. 1992;15:322.
2. Summers WK et al. Use of THA in treatment of Alzheimer-like dementia: pilot study in twelve patients. Biol Psychiatry. 1981;16:145.

## Significance Classification

- (1) - ***Avoid Combination.*** Risk always outweighs benefit.
- (2) - ***Usually Avoid Combination.*** Use combination only under special circumstances.
- (3) - ***Minimize Risk.*** Take action as necessary to reduce risk.

**Terfenadine (Seldane)**

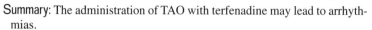

**Troleandomycin (TAO)**

Summary: The administration of TAO with terfenadine may lead to arrhythmias.

Risk Factors: No specific risk factors known.

Related Drugs: ***Erythromycin*** and ***clarithromycin (Biaxin)*** inhibit terfenadine metabolism. ***Astemizole (Hismanal)*** metabolism would be inhibited by TAO. ***Azithromycin (Zithromax)*** and ***dirithromycin (Dynabac)*** do not alter terfenadine concentrations.

Management Options:
- *Use Alternative.* Patients should avoid taking terfenadine and TAO due to the risk of arrhythmias. Astemizole may not be a safe alternative to terfenadine since it has been associated with arrhythmias when administered with drugs that inhibit its metabolism. The use of sedating antihistamines, cetirizine (Zyrtec) or loratadine (Claritin) may be preferable in patients who require antihistamine therapy during TAO treatment.

References:
1. Fournier P et al. Une nouvelle cause de torsades de pointes: association terfenadine et troleandomycine. Ann Cardiol Angeiol. 1993;42:249.

**Terfenadine (Seldane)**

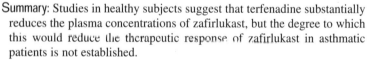

**Zafirlukast (Accolate)**

Summary: Studies in healthy subjects suggest that terfenadine substantially reduces the plasma concentrations of zafirlukast, but the degree to which this would reduce the therapeutic response of zafirlukast in asthmatic patients is not established.

Risk Factors: No specific risk factors known.

Related Drugs: The effect of other antihistamines on zafirlukast pharmacokinetics is not established. Since ***astemizole (Hismanal)*** has interactive properties similar to terfenadine, it might be expected to interact with zafirlukast in a similar manner. However, no information is available.

Management Options:
- *Consider Alternative.* In patients on zafirlukast, consider using antihistamines with fewer interactive properties than terfenadine or astemizole.
- *Monitor.* If the combination is used, monitor for reduced zafirlukast response (i.e., uncontrolled asthma).

References:
1. Zeneca Pharmaceuticals. Accolate Product Information. Wilmington, DE: 1996.

## Tetracycline

### Zinc

Summary: Zinc may reduce the serum concentration of tetracycline enough to reduce its antibacterial efficacy.

Risk Factors: No specific risk factors known.

Related Drugs: ***Doxycycline (Vibramycin)*** absorption was not significantly affected by concomitant zinc administration.[1]

Management Options:

- *Consider Alternative.* Doxycycline might be considered as an alternative.

- *Circumvent/Minimize.* When patients are receiving both tetracycline and zinc sulfate, the drugs should be taken as far apart as possible to minimize mixing in the GI tract. Take the tetracycline 2 to 3 hours before the zinc.

- *Monitor.* If tetracycline and foods or dairy products containing large amounts of cations are coadministered, be alert for reduced antibiotic effects.

References:

1. Penttila O et al. Effect of zinc sulphate on the absorption of tetracycline and doxycycline in man. Eur J Clin Pharmacol. 1975;9:131.

2. Mapp RK et al. The effect of zinc sulphate and of bicitropeptide on tetracycline absorption. S Afr Med J. 1976;50:1829.

3. Andersson KE et al. Inhibition of tetracycline absorption by zinc. Eur J Clin Pharmacol. 1976;10:59.

## Theophylline

### Thiabendazole (Mintezol)

Summary: Case reports suggest that thiabendazole can substantially increase serum theophylline concentrations; theophylline toxicity may result.

Risk Factors: No specific risk factors known.

Related Drugs: ***Mebendazole (Vermox)*** does not interact.

Management Options:

- *Circumvent/Minimize.* Theophylline dosages should be reduced in patients who must take thiabendazole with theophylline. Alternative drugs for theophylline (e.g., beta-agonists, steroids) should be considered during thiabendazole treatment.

- *Monitor.* Patients taking theophylline should be monitored carefully for increased theophylline concentrations and manifestations of theophylline toxicity (tachycardia, nervousness, nausea) if they require a course of thiabendazole therapy.

References:
1. Sugar AM et al. Possible thiabendazole-induced theophylline toxicity. Am Rev Respir Dis. 1980;122:501.
2. Lew G et al. Theophylline-thiabendazole drug interaction. Clin Pharm. 1989;8:225.
3. Schneider D et al. Theophylline and antiparasitic drug interactions. A case report and study of the influence of thiabendazole and mebendazole on theophylline pharmacokinetics in adults. Chest. 1990;97:84.

## Theophylline
## Thyroid

**Summary:** Initiation of thyroid replacement therapy in patients receiving theophylline may reduce serum theophylline concentrations.

**Risk Factors:**
* *Order of Administration.* Patients on theophylline therapy who are started on thyroid replacement are at increased risk for the interaction. (Patients stabilized on thyroid replacement before theophylline therapy is started probably are at minimal risk for the interaction.)

**Related Drugs:** No information available.

**Management Options:**
* *Monitor* patients for a reduced theophylline response when thyroid replacement therapy is initiated for hypothyroidism.

References:
1. Johnson CE et al. Theophylline toxicity after iodine 131 treatment for hyperthyroidism. Clin Pharm. 1988;7:620.

## Theophylline
## Ticlopidine (Ticlid)

**Summary:** Ticlopidine substantially increased plasma theophylline concentrations in healthy subjects and may increase the risk of theophylline toxicity in patients.

**Risk Factors:** No specific risk factors known.

**Related Drugs:** No information available.

**Management Options:**
* *Monitor* for altered theophylline effect if ticlopidine therapy is initiated, discontinued, or changed in dosage; adjustments in theophylline dosage may be needed.

References:
1. Colli A et al. Ticlopidine-theophylline interaction. Clin Pharmacol Ther. 1987;41:358.

## Theophylline
## Troleandomycin (TAO)

**Summary:** TAO may increase theophylline serum concentrations and the potential for theophylline toxicity.

Risk Factors:
- *Dosage Regimen.* TAO doses above 250 mg/day increases the risk for the interaction.

Related Drugs: **Erythromycin** and **clarithromycin (Biaxin)** will inhibit theophylline metabolism. **Azithromycin (Zithromax)** has been shown to have no effect on theophylline metabolism.

Management Options:
- *Use Alternative.* Patients should avoid theophylline and TAO administration. Azithromycin may be an alternative.

References:
1. Weinberger M et al. Inhibition of theophylline clearance by troleandomycin. J Allergy Clin Immunol. 1977;59:228.
2. Kamada AK et al. Effect of low-dose troleandomycin on theophylline clearance: implications for therapeutic drug monitoring. Pharmacotherapy. 1992;12:98.

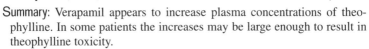

### Theophylline

### Verapamil (Calan)

Summary: Verapamil appears to increase plasma concentrations of theophylline. In some patients the increases may be large enough to result in theophylline toxicity.

Risk Factors:
- *Pharmacogenetics.* Children and cigarette smokers are at increased risk for the interaction.

Related Drugs: The clearance of theophylline was decreased ($\approx$20%)[4,13] or not affected by **diltiazem (Cardizem)**.[3,5–8,11,12] Diltiazem attenuated rifampin (Rifadin)-induced theophylline clearance,[9] but not smoking-induced clearance.[4] Theophylline absorption was noted to be moderately reduced following **felodipine (Plendil)** administration.[10] Additional study is needed to substantiate these findings and establish clinical significance. **Isradipine (DynaCirc)**[13] and **nifedipine (Procardia)** appear to have no[3,5–8,11,12] or minimal[1,2] effect on theophylline pharmacokinetics.

Management Options:
- *Consider Alternative.* Isradipine and nifedipine may be alternatives to verapamil.

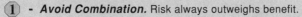
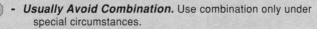

## Significance Classification

(1) - *Avoid Combination.* Risk always outweighs benefit.

(2) - *Usually Avoid Combination.* Use combination only under special circumstances.

(3) - *Minimize Risk.* Take action as necessary to reduce risk.

• *Monitor.* Patients receiving verapamil and perhaps diltiazem should be monitored carefully for evidence of theophylline toxicity (e.g., tachycardia, tremor, GI upset). Theophylline plasma concentration determinations may be helpful.

References:

1. Parrillo SJ et al. Elevated theophylline blood levels from institution of nifedipine therapy. Ann Emerg Med. 1984;13:216.
2. Harrod CS. Theophylline toxicity and nifedipine. Ann Intern Med. 1987;106:480.
3. Sirmans S et al. Effect of calcium channel blockers on theophylline disposition. Clin Pharmacol Ther. 1988;44:29.
4. Nafziger AN et al. Inhibition of theophylline elimination by diltiazem therapy. J Clin Pharmacol. 1987;27:862.
5. Jackson SHD et al. The interaction between IV theophylline and chronic oral dosing with slow-release nifedipine in volunteers. Br J Clin Pharmacol. 1986;21:389.
6. Christopher MA et al. Clinical relevance of the interaction of theophylline with diltiazem or nifedipine. Chest. 1989;95:309.
7. Garty M et al. Effect of nifedipine and theophylline in asthma. Clin Pharmacol Ther. 1986;40:195.
8. Robson RA et al. Selective inhibitory effects of nifedipine and verapamil on oxidative metabolism: effects of theophylline. Br J Clin Pharmacol. 1988;25:397.
9. Adebayo GI et al. Attenuation of rifampicin-induced theophylline metabolism by dilitiazem/rifampicin coadministration in healthy volunteers. Eur J Clin Pharmacol. 1989;37:127.
10. Bratel T et al. Felodipine reduces the absorption of theophylline in man. Eur J Clin Pharmacol. 1989;36:481.
11. Abernethy DR et al. Substrate-selective inhibition by verapamil and diltiazem: differential disposition of antipyrine and theophylline in humans. J Pharmacol Exp Ther. 1989;244:994.
12. Yilmaz E et al. Nifedipine alters serum theophylline levels in asthmatic patients with hypertension. Fundam Clin Pharmacol. 1991;5:341.
13. Perreault M et al. The effect of isradipine on theophylline pharmacokinetics in healthy volunteers. Pharmacotherapy. 1993;13:149.

## Theophylline

### Zafirlukast (Accolate)

Summary: The manufacturer reports that theophylline can decrease plasma concentrations of zafirlukast; adjustments in zafirlukast dose may be needed.

Risk Factors: No specific risk factors known.

Related Drugs: No information available.

Management Options:

• *Monitor* for altered zafirlukast effect if theophylline is initiated, discontinued, or changed in dosage.

References:

1. Zeneca Pharmaceuticals. Accolate manufacturer's product information. 1997.

## Thyroid

### Warfarin (Coumadin)

Summary: The hypoprothrombinemic response to oral anticoagulants is altered by changes in clinical thyroid status; adjustments in anticoagulant dosage are likely to be required if the thyrometabolic status changes.

Risk Factors:
- *Order of Administration.* The primary risk is in starting thyroid replacement therapy in the presence of chronic oral anticoagulants, while the risk appears small if the oral anticoagulant is started in the presence of chronic thyroid therapy.

Related Drugs: Given the mechanism, it is likely that all oral anticoagulants are affected by all types of thyroid replacement.

Management Options:
- *Monitor* for altered oral anticoagulant effect if thyroid replacement therapy is initiated, discontinued, or changed in dosage. Adjust the anticoagulant dose as needed. No special precautions appear necessary when oral anticoagulant therapy is begun in a patient already stabilized on maintenance thyroid replacement therapy.

References:
1. Hansten PD. Oral anticoagulants and drugs which alter thyroid function. Drug Intell Clin Pharm. 1980;14:331.
2. Van Dosterom AT et al. The influence of the thyroid function on the metabolic rate of prothrombin, factor VII, and factor X in the rat. Thromb Haemost. 1976;3:607.
3. Costigan DC et al. Potentiation of oral anticoagulant effect by 1-thyroxine. Clin Pediatr. 1984;23:172.

### Tolbutamide (Orinase)

### Trimethoprim-Sulfamethoxazole (Bactrim)

Summary: Several sulfonamides like trimethoprim-sulfamethoxazole (TMP-SMX) can increase plasma concentration of oral antidiabetic agents like tolbutamide and enhance their hypoglycemic effects.

Risk Factors: No specific risk factors known.

Related Drugs: *Glipizide (Glucotrol)*, *glyburide (DiaBeta)*, and *chlorpropamide (Diabenese)* are affected similarly by sulfonamides such as TMP-SMX, *sulfamethizole (Thiosulfil)*, *sulfaphenazole*, and *sulfisoxazole (Gantrisin)*. Sulfonamides have not been reported to affect the response to insulin.

Management Options:
- *Monitor.* Concomitant TMP-SMX and tolbutamide administration should be undertaken with the realization that enhanced hypoglycemic effects may occur. Sulfadiazine and sulfadimethoxine do not appear to have this effect.

References:
1. Wing LMH et al. Cotrimoxazole as an inhibitor of oxidative drug metabolism: effects of trimethoprim and sulphamethoxazole separately and combined on tolbutamide disposition. Br J Clin Pharmacol. 1985;20:482.
2. Johnson JF et al. Symptomatic hypoglycemia secondary to a glipizide-trimethoprim/sulfamethoxazole drug interaction. DICP, Ann Pharmacother. 1990;24:250.
3. Baciewicz AM et al. Hypoglycemia induced by the interaction of chlorpropamide and co-trimoxazole. Drug Intell Clin Pharm. 1984;18:309.

## Tolmetin (Tolectin)

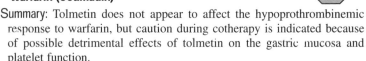

## Warfarin (Coumadin)

Summary: Tolmetin does not appear to affect the hypoprothrombinemic response to warfarin, but caution during cotherapy is indicated because of possible detrimental effects of tolmetin on the gastric mucosa and platelet function.

Risk Factors:
- *Concurrent Diseases.* Patients with peptic ulcer disease (PUD) or a history of gastrointestinal bleeding probably are at greater risk for the interaction.

Related Drugs: All NSAIDs inhibit platelet function, cause gastric erosions, and probably increase the risk of GI bleeding.

Management Options:
- *Avoid Unless Benefit Outweighs Risk.* Since all NSAIDs probably increase the risk of GI bleeding in patients on oral anticoagulants, use the combination only after careful consideration of the benefit versus risk. If the NSAID is being used as an analgesic or antipyretic, acetaminophen (Tylenol) probably is safer to use with oral anticoagulants. Nonacetylated salicylates (e.g., choline salicylate, magnesium salicylate, salsalate, sodium salicylate) probably also are safer with oral anticoagulants than NSAIDs since they have minimal effects on platelet function and the gastric mucosa.
- *Monitor.* If any NSAID is used with an oral anticoagulant, one should carefully monitor the prothrombin time and watch for evidence of bleeding, especially from the GI tract.

References:
1. Pullar T. Interaction between oral anti-coagulant drugs and nonsteroidal anti-inflammatory agents: a review. Scott Med J. 1983;28:42.
2. Shorr RI et al. Concurrent use of nonsteroidal anti-inflammatory drugs and oral anticoagulants places elderly persons at high risk for hemorrhagic peptic ulcer disease. Arch Intern Med. 1993;153:1665.

## Toloxatone

## Tyramine

Summary: Large doses of toloxatone [a selective monoamine oxidase (MAO)-A inhibitor] may increase the pressor response to large amounts of tyramine; high tyramine foods (e.g., aged cheese) should be avoided.

Risk Factors: No specific risk factors known.

Related Drugs: Other MAO-A inhibitors, such as *moclobemide*, may interact similarly with tyramine.

Management Options:

- *Circumvent/Minimize.* Although toloxatone appears less likely to interact with dietary tyramine than nonselective MAOIs, it would be prudent to avoid foods with a high tyramine content.
- *Monitor* blood pressure if the interaction is suspected.

References:

1. Provost JC et al. Pharmacokinetic and pharmacodynamic interaction between to-loxatone, a new reversible monoamine oxidase-A inhibitor, and oral tyramine in healthy subjects. Clin Pharmacol Ther. 1992; 52:384.
2. Freeman H Moclobemide. Lancet. 1993;342:1528.
3. Simpson GM et al. Comparison of the pressor effect of tyramine after treatment with phenelzine and moclobemide in healthy male volunteers. Clin Pharmacol Ther. 1992;52:286.

## Tramadol (Ultram)

## Tranylcypromine (Parnate)

**2**

Summary: Tramadol theoretically increases the risk of seizures and serotonin syndrome in patients taking monoamine oxidase inhibitors (MAOIs).

Risk Factors: No specific risk factors known.

Related Drugs: Until clinical data are available, all MAOIs, including *phenelzine (Nardil)* and *isocarboxazid (Marplan)*, should be considered equally likely to interact with tramadol.

Management Options:

- *Avoid Unless Benefit Outweighs Risk.* Although published clinical information appears lacking, theoretical and medicolegal considerations suggest that the combination should generally be avoided.
- *Monitor.* If the combination is used, monitor for seizures and for early evidence of serotonin syndrome. Serotonin syndrome can result in neurotoxicity (myoclonus, tremors, rigidity, incoordination, restlessness, hyperreflexia, seizures, coma), psychiatric symptoms (agitation, confusion, hypomania), and temperature regulation abnormalities (fever, sweating).

References:

1. McNeil Pharmaceutical. Ultram manufacturer's product information. 1997.

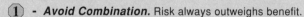
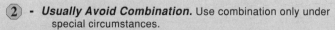

## Significance Classification

1. - **Avoid Combination.** Risk always outweighs benefit.

2. - **Usually Avoid Combination.** Use combination only under special circumstances.

3. - **Minimize Risk.** Take action as necessary to reduce risk.

### Tranylcypromine (Parnate)

### Tyramine

Summary: The consumption of foods containing large amounts of tyramine can result in hypertensive reactions in patients taking monoamine oxidase inhibitors (MAOIs).

Risk Factors: No specific risk factors known.

Related Drugs: One patient receiving *phenelzine (Nardil)* developed a hypertensive reaction and headache following ingestion of a cup of miso soup.[4] All nonselective MAOIs including *isocarboxazid (Marplan)* interact with tyramine-containing *foods*.

Management Options:

- *Avoid Combination.* Patients taking MAOIs should be instructed to avoid foods that may have a high tyramine content. Remember that the effects of nonselective MAOIs should be assumed to persist for 2 weeks after they are discontinued. Estimates of the tyramine content of various foods and beverages have been published.[1–3] Foods to be avoided include cheeses (especially aged), red wines, caviar, herring (dried or pickled), canned figs, fermented or spoiled meat (including salami, pepperoni, summer sausage), fava beans, yeast extracts, miso soup, and avocados (especially if overripe).

References:
1. Shullman KI et al. Dietary restriction, tyramine, and the use of monoamine oxidase inhibitors. J Clin Psychopharmacol. 1989;9:397.
2. Sen NP. Analysis and significance of tyramine in foods. J Food Sci. 1969;34:22.
3. Anon. Monoamine oxidase inhibitors for depression. Med Lett. 1980;22:58.
4. Mesmer RE et al. Don't mix miso with MAOIs. JAMA. 1987;258:3515.

### Triazolam (Halcion)

### Troleandomycin (TAO)

Summary: Troleandomycin causes considerable increase in triazolam serum concentrations and increased sedation may result.

Risk Factors: No specific risk factors known.

Related Drugs: *Erythromycin* and *clarithromycin (Biaxin)* may inhibit the metabolism of triazolam. *Azithromycin (Zithromax)* would not be expected to affect triazolam. Other benzodiazepines metabolized by CYP3A4 [e.g., *alprazolam (Xanax)*, *midazolam (Versed)*, and *diazepam (Valium)*] may be inhibited similarly by TAO.

Management Options:

- *Monitor.* Patients receiving triazolam who are prescribed TAO should be observed carefully for enhanced triazolam effects. Several days may be required for the maximum effect of TAO to become evident, and triazolam dosages may require adjustment after addition of the antibiotic and again when it is discontinued.

References:
1. Warot D et al. Troleandomycin-induced interaction in healthy volunteers: pharmacokinetic and psychometric evaluation. Eur J Clin Pharmacol. 1987;32:389.

## Triclofos

### Warfarin (Coumadin)

Summary: Because triclofos transiently increases the hypoprothrombinemic response to warfarin, alternative hypnotics are preferable in patients on oral anticoagulants.

Risk Factors: No specific risk factors known.

Related Drugs: Alternative sedative/hypnotic drugs unlikely to interact with oral anticoagulants include **flurazepam (Dalmane), chlordiazepoxide (Librium), diazepam (Valium),** or **diphenhydramine (Benadryl).**

Management Options:
- *Consider Alternative.* Consider an alternative sedative/hypnotic which is unlikely to interact, such as flurazepam, chlordiazepoxide, diazepam, or diphenhydramine.
- *Monitor.* If triclofos is used, monitor for altered oral anticoagulant effect when triclofos is initiated, discontinued, or changed in dosage. Adjust the anticoagulant dose as needed.

References:
1. Sellers EM et al. Enhancement of warfarin-induced hypoprothrombinemia by triclofos. Clin Pharmacol Ther. 1972;13:911.
2. Beliles RP et al. Interaction of bishydroxycoumarin with chloral hydrate and trichloroethyl phosphate. Toxicol Appl Pharmacol. 1974; 27:225.

## Trimethoprim-Sulfamethoxazole (Bactrim)

### Warfarin (Coumadin)

Summary: Trimethoprim-sulfamethoxazole (TMP-SMX) increases the hypoprothrombinemic response to warfarin; adjustments in warfarin dose may be required during cotherapy. Oral anticoagulants and other sulfonamides may also interact, but supporting evidence is limited.

Risk Factors:
- *Concurrent Diseases.* Fever may enhance the catabolism of clotting factors, thus increasing the interaction.

Related Drugs: Preliminary clinical evidence indicates that **sulfamethizole (Thiosulfil)** inhibits warfarin metabolism[2] and that **sulfaphenazole (Thiosulf)** enhances the hypoprothrombinemic response to **phenindione.**[3] The effect on phenindione appeared to be more pronounced in patients with hypoalbuminemia.

Management Options:
- *Consider Alternative.* If possible, TMP-SMX should not be used in patients anticoagulated with oral agents. A non-interacting antibiotic or heparin anticoagulation could be considered.
- *Monitor.* If the combination is used, monitor the patient carefully for an increased hypoprothrombinemic response and risk of bleeding during initiation and decreased effects upon discontinuation of TMP-SMX.

References:
1. O'Reilly RA. Stereoselective interaction of trimethoprim-sulfamethoxazole with the separated enantiomorphs of racemic warfarin in man. N Engl J Med. 1980; 302:33.
2. Lumholtz B et al. Sulfamethizole-induced inhibition of diphenylhydantoin, tolbutamide, and warfarin metabolism. Clin Pharmacol Ther. 1975;17:731.
3. Varma DL et al. Prothrombin response to phenindione during hypoalbuminaemia. Br J Clin Pharmacol. 1975;2:467. Letter.

## Vecuronium (Norcuron)

## Verapamil (Calan)

**Summary:** Verapamil (and perhaps other calcium channel blocking drugs) appears to prolong the neuromuscular blockade of nondepolarizing neuromuscular blockers such as vecuronium and pancuronium (Pavulon).

**Risk Factors:** No specific risk factors known.

**Related Drugs:** Other calcium channel blockers [e.g., *nicardipine (Cardene)*, *diltiazem (Cardizem)*] may produce similar interactions with vercuronium and other neuromuscular blockers [e.g., *pancuronium (Pavulon)*].

**Management Options:**
- *Circumvent/Minimize.* Reduction in the dose of muscle relaxant may be needed. Edrophonium may be required to reverse the muscle blockade.
- *Monitor.* Until additional information is available, patients receiving verapamil or other calcium channel blockers should be observed carefully for prolongation of neuromuscular blockade.

References:
1. Van Poorten JF et al. Verapamil and reversal of vecuronium neuromuscular blockade. Anesth Analg. 1984;63:155.
2. Jones RM et al. Verapamil potentiation of neuromuscular blockade: failure of reversal with neostigmine but prompt reversal with edrophonium. Anesth Analg. 1985; 64:1021.
3. Kazunaga K et al. Decrease in vecuronium infusion dose requirements by nicardipine in humans. Anesth Analg. 1994;79:1159.

## Vitamin E

## Warfarin (Coumadin)

**Summary:** Vitamin E may increase the hypoprothrombinemic response to warfarin and other oral anticoagulants. Although the incidence of this interaction in patients receiving the combination is not known, vitamin E should be avoided in anticoagulated patients.

**Risk Factors:**
- *Dosage Regimen.* The risk is probably greater with large doses of vitamin E than the small amounts normally present in multivitamin preparations.

**Related Drugs:** Three healthy subjects showed a mild increase in hypoprothrombinemic response to *dicumarol* 150 mg when they were given vitamin E 42 IU/day for 30 days.[3]

Management Options:
- *Monitor* for altered oral anticoagulant effect if vitamin E is initiated, discontinued, or changed in dosage. Adjust the anticoagulant dose as needed.

References:
1. Corrigan JJ et al. Coagulopathy associated with vitamin E ingestion. JAMA. 1974;230:1300.
2. Anon. Vitamin K, vitamin E and the coumarin drugs. Nutr Rev. 1982;40:180.
3. Schrogie JJ et al. Coagulopathy and fat-soluble vitamins. JAMA. 1975;232:19. Letter.

## Vitamin K

## Warfarin (Coumadin)

Summary: Ingestion of large amounts of foods high in vitamin K may antagonize the hypoprothrombinemic effect of oral anticoagulants.

Risk Factors: No specific risk factors known.

Related Drugs: All oral anticoagulants would be similarly affected by vitamin K.

Management Options:
- *Circumvent/Minimize.* Patients on oral anticoagulants should avoid sudden increases in their intake of leafy vegetables or other foods high in vitamin K content. However, warfarin requirements should not change if patients are consistent in their intake of these foods.
- *Monitor* for altered hypoprothrombinemic response if vitamin K intake changes substantially.

References:
1. Karlson B et al. On the influence of vitamin K-rich vegetables and wine on the effectiveness of warfarin treatment. Acta Med Scand. 1986;220:347.
2. Quick A. Leafy vegetables in diet alter prothrombin time in patients taking anticoagulant drugs. JAMA. 1987;187:27.
3. Chow WH et al. Anticoagulation instability with life-threatening complication after dietary modification. Postgrad. Med J. 1990;66:855.

## Warfarin (Coumadin)

## Zafirlukast (Accolate)

Summary: Zafirlukast appears to increase the hypoprothrombinemic response to warfarin; adjustments in warfarin dosage may be necessary.

## Significance Classification

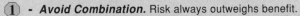 - *Avoid Combination.* Risk always outweighs benefit.

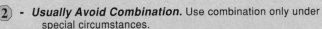 - *Usually Avoid Combination.* Use combination only under special circumstances.

- *Minimize Risk.* Take action as necessary to reduce risk.

Risk Factors: No specific risk factors known.

Related Drugs: The effect of zafirlukast on oral anticoagulants other than warfarin is not established. If the mechanism of the interaction is inhibition of CYP2C9, *phenprocoumon* (which is metabolized primarily by glucuronide conjugation) theoretically would be less likely to interact with zafirlukast than warfarin.

Management Options:

- *Consider Alternative.* Given the substantial effect of zafirlukast on warfarin response, consider using alternative antiasthmatic medications. In countries where phenprocoumon is available, consider it as an alternative to warfarin which (theoretically) would be less likely to interact.

- *Monitor* for altered hypoprothrombincmic response to warfarin if zafirlukast is initiated, discontinued, or changed in dosage; adjust warfarin dose as needed.

References:

1. Zeneca Pharmaceuticals. Accolate Product Information. Wilmington, DE: 1996.

# Index

The key to the effective use of **Hansten and Horn's Managing Clinically Important Drug Interactions** is the Index. The drug interaction monographs are listed in alphabetical order beginning on page 1.

All drug interaction monographs are listed by generic name except for combination products (e.g., antacids, oral contraceptives) and drugs that interact equally within the class (e.g., thyroid hormones, thiazide diuretics). The term "homogeneous interactions" is used within the text to refer to drug interactions that apply to all drugs equally within a pharmacological class.

The manufacturer's data for many drugs newly approved for use in the United States have included cautions on possible drug interactions. Although the potential for a drug interaction exists with some of these drugs, the scientific literature may, in the opinion of Drs. Hansten and Horn, be insufficient at the time of publication to warrant an in-depth drug-drug interaction monograph. The available information for these drugs will be found in the Related Drugs section of another related drug monograph. To find this information, use the Index to locate the drug and then look in the Related Drugs section of the indicated monograph.

The asterisks (*) next to a page number in the Index refer to specific drug interaction monographs. Page numbers without an asterisk indicate the location where the drug interaction is merely mentioned (e.g., in the Related Drugs section).

Drug interactions that warrant special attention (i.e., those classified as Category 1 or Category 2) are listed in bold print. Descriptions of intervention categories can be found on each monograph page and are provided below as well.

## Significance Classification

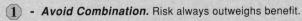 - *Avoid Combination.* Risk always outweighs benefit.

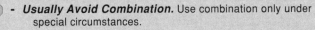 - *Usually Avoid Combination.* Use combination only under special circumstances.

- *Minimize Risk.* Take action as necessary to reduce risk.

Adenocard
  Also see Antiarrhythmics
  *3* atenolol 50
  *3* dipyridamole 6*
  *3* theophylline 7*
Adenosine
  Also see Antiarrhythmics
  *3* atenolol 50
  *3* dipyridamole 6*
  *3* theophylline 7*
Adrenalin
  Also see
    Sympathomimetics
  *3* alprenolol 240
  *3* chlorpromazine 93*
  *3* clozapine 93
  *2* imipramine 240*
  *3* labetalol 240
  *3* nadolol 240
  *3* pindolol 240
  *3* propranolol 240*, 429
  *2* protriptyline 240
  *3* thioridazine 93
  *3* timolol 240
Adriamycin
  Also see Antineoplastics
  *3* cyclosporine 167*
  *3* tacrolimus 168
  *3* verapamil 231*
Adrucil
  Also see Antineoplastics
  *2* metronidazole 268*
  *3* warfarin 269*
Advil
  Also see Nonsteroidal anti-
    inflammatory drugs
  *3* digoxin 212
  *3* furosemide 281
  *3* lithium 298*
  *3* methotrexate 299*
  *2* phenprocoumon 276,
    299
  *3* prazosin 306
  *3* triamterene 308
  *2* warfarin 53, 208, 262,
    299*, 309, 335, 352, 353,
    409, 418, 444
Aerosporin
  *2* pancuronium 398*
Alconefrin
  *3* guanethidine 295*
  *3* imipramine 302*

*1* isocarboxazid 400
*1* phenelzine 400*
*1* tranylcypromine 400
Aldactone
  Also see Diuretics;
    Potassium-sparing diuret-
    ics
  *3* digoxin 218*
  *1* mitotane 377*
  *2* potassium 419*, 420
Aldomet
  *3* iron 314*
  *3* lithium 343*
  *3* norepinephrine 366*
Aleve
  Also see Nonsteroidal anti-
    inflammatory drugs
  *3* cyclosporine 178*, 183
  *3* furosemide 281
  *3* lithium 343*
  *2* methotrexate 359*
  *3* propranolol 307
  *2* warfarin 53, 208, 262,
    309, 335, 352, 353, 381*,
    409, 418, 444
Alfenta
  *3* cimetidine 7*
  *3* clarithromycin 8
  *3* diltiazem 8*
  *3* erythromycin 8*
  *3* mibefradil 8
  *3* troleandomycin 8
  *3* verapamil 8
Alfentanil
  *3* cimetidine 7*
  *3* clarithromycin 8
  *3* diltiazem 8*
  *3* erythromycin 8*
  *3* mibefradil 8
  *3* troleandomycin 8
  *3* verapamil 8
Alka-Mints
  Also see Antacids
  *3* allopurinol 9
  *3* amphetamines 37
  *3* aspirin 29*
  *3* cefpodoxime 29*
  *3* cefuroxime 85
  *3* ciprofloxacin 30*, 35, 36,
    130, 134
  *3* doxycycline 39
  *3* Ecotrin 29
  *3* enoxacin 31*

*3* ephedrine 31*, 37
*3* glipizide 32*
*3* glyburide 32*
*3* iron 33*
*3* isoniazid 34*
*3* itraconazole 34
*3* ketoconazole 34
*3* lithium 346*
*3* lomefloxacin 30, 34*,
  35*, 36
*3* methenamine 358*
*3* mexiletine 372*
*3* nifedipine 351
*3* norfloxacin 35*, 36, 390
*3* ofloxacin 30, 35, 36*,
  392
*3* penicillamine 37*
*3* phenylpropanolamine 37
*3* pseudoephedrine 37*
*3* quinidine 6, 38*, 431*
*3* sodium polystyrene sulfonate resin 38*
*3* tetracycline 39*
*3* thiazides 64*
*3* tocainide 40*
Alkeran
  Also see Antineoplastics
  *3* cimetidine 117*
  *3* cyclosporine 175*
Allermed
  Also see
    Sympathomimetics
  *3* aluminum 37*
  *3* antacids 37*
  *1* isocarboxazid 402
  *3* magnesium 37*
  *2* moclobemide 239
  *1* phenelzine 402*
  *3* sodium bicarbonate 37*
  *1* tranylcypromine 402
Allopurinol
  *3* aluminum 9*
  *3* antacids 9*
  *2* azathioprine 9*, 12
  *3* calcium 9
  *2* captopril 10*
  *3* cyclophosphamide 11*
  *3* cyclosporine 11*
  *2* enalapril 10
  *3* magnesium 9
  *3* mercaptopurine 10, 11*
  *3* tacrolimus 11

Allopurinol *(Continued)*
  *3* theophylline 12*
  *3* vidarabine 13*
  *3* warfarin 13*
Alpha agonists
  Also see Clonidine; Guanabenz; Guanfacine
  *2* **amitriptyline 25, 152**
  *3* amitriptyline 25*
  *3* chlorpromazine 93*
  *3* cyclosporine 151*
  *2* **desipramine 152***
  *3* fluphenazine 93
  *3* haloperidol 93
  *2* **imipramine 152**
  *3* imipramine 25
  *3* insulin 153*
  *3* nitroprusside 153*
  *3* propranolol 154*
  *3* sotalol 154
  *3* tacrolimus 151
  *3* trazodone 152
Alpha blockers
  Also see Doxazosin; Labetalol; Prazosin; Terazosin; Trimazosin
  *3* cimetidine 125
  *3* diazepam 202
  *3* enalapril 62
  *3* epinephrine 240
  *3* ibuprofen 306
  *3* indomethacin 306*, 307
  *3* nifedipine 253*
  *3* propranolol 420*, 421
  *3* verapamil 421*
Alprazolam
  Also see Benzodiazepines
  *3* carbamazepine 76
  *3* cimetidine 111
  *3* clarithromycin 13
  *3* erythromycin 13*, 62
  *3* fluoxetine 14*, 200
  *3* fluvoxamine 14
  *3* grapefruit juice 291
  *3* itraconazole 322
  *3* ketoconazole 90, 327
  *3* phenytoin 375
  *3* troleandomycin 13, 454
Alprenolol
  Also see Beta-adrenergic blockers
  *3* epinephrine 240
  *3* insulin 311

AlternaGEL
  Also see Antacids
  *3* allopurinol 9*
  *3* aspirin 29*
  *3* cefpodoxime 29*
  *3* cefuroxime 85
  *3* ciprofloxacin 30*, 130, 134
  *3* glipizide 32*
  *3* glyburide 32*
  *3* iron 33*
  *3* isoniazid 34*
  *3* ketoconazole 34
  *3* lomefloxacin 35*
  *3* methenamine 358
  *3* norfloxacin 35*, 36, 390
  *3* ofloxacin 35, 36*, 392
  *3* penicillamine 37*
  *3* pseudoephedrine 37
  *3* tetracycline 39*
Altretamine
  Also see Antineoplastics
  *3* imipramine 14*
Alu-Cap
  Also see Antacids
  *3* allopurinol 9*
  *3* aspirin 29*
  *3* cefpodoxime 29*
  *3* cefuroxime 85
  *3* ciprofloxacin 30*, 130, 134
  *3* glipizide 32*
  *3* glyburide 32*
  *3* iron 33*
  *3* isoniazid 34*
  *3* ketoconazole 34
  *3* lomefloxacin 35*
  *3* methenamine 358
  *3* norfloxacin 35*, 36, 390
  *3* ofloxacin 35, 36*, 392
  *3* penicillamine 37*
  *3* pseudoephedrine 37
  *3* tetracycline 39*
Aludrox
  Also see Antacids
  *3* allopurinol 9*
  *3* aspirin 29*
  *3* cefpodoxime 29*
  *3* cefuroxime 85
  *3* ciprofloxacin 30*, 130, 134
  *3* glipizide 32*

  *3* glyburide 32*
  *3* iron 33*
  *3* isoniazid 34*
  *3* ketoconazole 34
  *3* lomefloxacin 35*
  *3* methenamine 358
  *3* nifedipine 351
  *3* norfloxacin 35*, 36, 390
  *3* ofloxacin 35, 36*, 392
  *3* penicillamine 37*
  *3* quinidine 38*
  *3* sodium polystyrene sulfonate resin 38*
  *3* pseudoephedrine 37
  *3* tetracycline 39*
Aluminum
  Also see Antacids
  *3* allopurinol 9*
  *3* aspirin 29*
  *3* cefpodoxime 29*
  *3* cefuroxime 85
  *3* ciprofloxacin 30*, 130, 134
  *3* glipizide 32*
  *3* glyburide 32*
  *3* iron 33*
  *3* isoniazid 34*
  *3* ketoconazole 34
  *3* lomefloxacin 35*
  *3* methenamine 358
  *3* norfloxacin 35*, 36, 390
  *3* ofloxacin 35, 36*, 392
  *3* penicillamine 37*
  *3* pseudoephedrine 37
  *3* tetracycline 39*
Alu-Tab
  Also see Antacids
  *3* allopurinol 9*
  *3* aspirin 29*
  *3* cefpodoxime 29*
  *3* cefuroxime 85
  *3* ciprofloxacin 30*, 130, 134
  *3* glipizide 32*
  *3* glyburide 32*
  *3* iron 33*
  *3* isoniazid 34*
  *3* ketoconazole 34
  *3* lomefloxacin 35*
  *3* methenamine 358
  *3* norfloxacin 35*, 36, 390
  *3* ofloxacin 35, 36*, 392

*3* penicillamine 37*
*3* pseudoephedrine 37
*3* tetracycline 39*
Ambenonium
 *3* tacrine 56
Amikacin
 Also see Aminoglycosides
 *3* carboplatin 82
 *3* indomethacin 286
Amikin
 Also see Aminoglycosides
 *3* carboplatin 82
 *3* indomethacin 286
Amiloride
 Also see Diuretics; Potassium-sparing diuretics
 *2* **potassium 419, 420**
Aminoglutethimide
 *3* acenocoumarol 17
 *3* cortisone 15
 *3* dexamethasone 15*
 *3* hydrocortisone 15
 *3* medroxyprogesterone 15*
 *3* methylprednisolone 15
 *3* prednisolone 15
 *3* prednisone 15
 *3* tacrolimus 413
 *2* **tamoxifen 16***
 *3* theophylline 16*
 *3* warfarin 17*
Aminoglycosides
 Also see Amikacin; Gentamicin; Kanamycin;
  Neomycin; Netilmicin;
  Streptomycin; Tobra-
  mycin
 *3* amphotericin B 27*
 *2* **atracurium 51***
 *3* carboplatin 82*, 141
 *3* cisplatin 141*
 *3* cyclosporine 170*
 *2* **ethacrynic acid 248***
 *3* indomethacin 286*
 *1* **methotrexate 360***
 *3* methoxyflurane 365
 *2* **succinylcholine 51**
 *3* vancomycin 286*
 *2* **vecuronium 51**
 *3* warfarin 383*
Aminophylline
 *3* adenosine 7*
 *3* allopurinol 12*

*3* aminoglutethimide 16*
*3* amiodarone 23*
*3* atenolol 429
*3* carbamazepine 78*
*3* cigarette smoking 108*
*3* cimetidine 127*
*3* ciprofloxacin 134*, 238,
  390
*3* disulfiram 228*
*2* **enoxacin 134, 238*, 390**
*3* erythromycin 245*, 449
*2* **fluvoxamine 278***
*3* imipenem 300*
*3* interferon 313*
*3* isoniazid 319*
*3* lithium 347*
*3* methimazole 434
*3* metoprolol 429
*2* **mexiletine 373***
*3* moricizine 378*
*3* nadolol 429
*3* norfloxacin 134, 238,
  390*
*3* pefloxacin 134, 238, 390,
*3* pentobarbital 406
*3* pentoxifylline 400*
*3* phenobarbital 406*
*3* phenytoin 414*
*3* pipemidic acid 134, 238,
  390
*3* propafenone 426*
*2* **propranolol 429***
*3* propylthiouracil 434
*3* radioactive iodine 434*
*3* rifampin 436*
*3* ritonavir 440*
*3* secobarbital 406
*3* tacrine 444*
*3* thiabendazole 447*
*3* thyroid 448*
*3* ticlopidine 448*
*2* **troleandomycin 246,
  448***
*3* verapamil 449*
*3* zafirlukast 450*
Amiodarone
 Also see Antiarrythmics
 *3* acenocoumarol 23
 *3* cholestyramine 17*
 *3* cimetidine 18*
 *3* colestipol 18
 *3* cyclosporine 18*
 *3* digitoxin 19

*3* digoxin 19*
*3* diltiazem 19*
*3* encainide 20
*3* flecainide 20*
*3* metoprolol 20*, 23
*3* phenytoin 21*
*3* procainamide 22*
*3* propranolol 21, 23
*3* quinidine 22*
*3* sotalol 22*
*3* tacrolimus 18
*3* theophylline 23*
*3* verapamil 19
*3* warfarin 23*
Amitriptyline
 Also see Cyclic antidepressants; Tricyclic antidepressants
 *3* carbamazepine 71
 *3* cimetidine 111, 113
 *2* **clonidine 25, 152**
 *3* fluoxetine 24*
 *3* guanabenz 25
 *3* guanfacine 25*
 *3* isoproterenol 25*
 *3* lithium 26*
 *2* **norepinephrine 301**
 *3* paroxetine 24
 *2* **phenelzine 150, 301**
 *3* tolazamide 231
Amobarbital
 Also see Barbiturates
 *2* **warfarin 408**
Amodiaquine
 *3* chlorpromazine 91
Amodopa
 *3* iron 314*
 *3* lithium 343*
 *3* norepinephrine 366*
Amoxapine
 Also see Cyclic antidepressants
 *3* cimetidine 111, 113
Amphetamines
 Also see
  Dextroamphetamine
 *3* furazolidone 192*, 193
 *3* guanadrel 192
 *3* guanethidine 192*
 *3* imipramine 193*
 *1* **isocarboxazid 193**
 *1* **phenelzine 193**

Amphetamines *(Continued)*
**2 selegiline 193**
**1 tranylcypromine 193***
Amphojel
Also see Antacids
3 allopurinol 9*
3 aspirin 29*
3 cefpodoxime 29*
3 cefuroxime 85
3 ciprofloxacin 30*, 130, 134
3 glipizide 32*
3 glyburide 32*
3 iron 33*
3 isoniazid 34*
3 ketoconazole 34
3 lomefloxacin 35*
3 methenamine 358
3 norfloxacin 35*, 36, 390
3 ofloxacin 35, 36*, 392
3 penicillamine 37*
3 pseudoephedrine 37
3 tetracycline 39*
Amphotericin B
Also see Antifungals
3 atracurium 27
3 cyclosporine 26*
3 gentamicin 27*
3 succinylcholine 27*
3 vecuronium 27
Ampicillin
Also see Penicillins
3 atenolol 28*
3 oral contraceptives 28*
Amytal
Also see Barbiturates
**2 warfarin 408**
Anabolic steroids
Also see Danazol;
Methandrostenolone;
Stanozolol
**2 carbamazepine 66***
**2 cyclosporine 165***
3 insulin 358
3 lovastatin 185*
3 tacrolimus 165
3 tolbutamide 358*
**2 warfarin 186*, 398***
Anadrol
Also see Anabolic steroids
**2 warfarin 398***

Anafranil
Also see Cyclic antidepressants; Tricyclic antidepressants
3 fluvoxamine 148*
3 grapefruit juice 149*
**1 isocarboxazid 150**
**2 moclobemide 149***
**1 phenelzine 150*, 301**
**1 tranylcypromine 150**
Anaprox
Also see Nonsteroidal antiinflammatory drugs
3 cyclosporine 178*, 183
3 furosemide 281
3 lithium 343*
**2 methotrexate 359***
3 propranolol 307
**2 warfarin 53, 208, 262, 309, 335, 352, 353, 381*, 409, 418, 444**
Ancef
Also see Cephalosporins
**2 warfarin 379**
Androgens
Also see Testosterone
**2 warfarin 398**
Android
3 cyclosporine 165
**2 warfarin 398**
Anectine
Also see Neuromuscular blockers
3 amphotericin B 27*
3 cyclophosphamide 164*
**2 echothiophate iodide 234***
**2 gentamicin 51**
3 quinidine 432
Anesthetics, local
Also see Bupivacaine;
Cocaine; Lidocaine;
Tetracaine
3 acebutolol 428
3 atenolol 428
3 cimetidine 116*
3 disopyramide 224*
3 metoprolol 342, 428
3 nadolol 341
3 propranolol 158*, 341*, 428*

Angiotensin-converting enzyme inhibitors
Also see Benazepril;
Captopril; Enalapril;
Lisinopril
**2 allopurinol 10***
3 aspirin 40*
3 azathioprine 54*
3 bumetanide 235
3 bunazosin 62*
3 cyclosporine 168*
3 doxazosin 62
3 ethacrynic acid 235
3 furosemide 234*
3 insulin 64*
3 iron 235*
3 lithium 341*
3 mercaptopurine 54
3 prazosin 62
3 sulindac 41
3 terazosin 62
3 torsemide 235
3 trimazosin 62
Angiotensin receptor antagonists
Also see Losartan
3 fluconazole 263*
3 lithium 342*
3 terbinafine 263
Ansaid
Also see Nonsteroidal antiinflammatory drugs
3 furosemide 281
3 methotrexate 275*
**2 phenprocoumon 276***
**2 warfarin 276**
Antabuse
3 chlordiazepoxide 198
3 clonazepam 198
3 clorazepate 198
3 diazepam 198*
**1 ethanol 226***
**2 isoniazid 226***
3 flurazepam 198
3 halazepam 198
3 metronidazole 227*
3 phenytoin 227*
3 prazepam 198
3 theophylline 228*
3 tranylcypromine 228*
3 triazolam 198

Antivirals *(Continued)*
 **3** troleandomycin 144, 244
 **1** zidovudine 283*
Anturane
 **2** acenocoumarol 443
 **3** aspirin 46*
 **2** methotrexate 363
 **3** propranolol 307
 **3** tolbutamide 442*
 **2** warfarin 443*
Apresoline
 **3** indomethacin 298*
Ara-A
 **3** allopurinol 13*
Ara-C
 **3** chlorpromazine 91*
 **3** cyclosporine 91*
 **3** methotrexate 91*
 **3** praziquantel 92*
 **3** tacrolimus 91
Aralen
 **3** chlorpromazine 91*
 **3** cyclosporine 91*
 **3** methotrexate 91*
 **3** praziquantel 92*
 **3** tacrolimus 91
Aramine
 **1** isocarboxazid 356
 **1** pargyline 356*
 **1** phenelzine 356
 **1** tranylcypromine 356
Artane
 Also see Anticholinergics
 **3** haloperidol 55
 **3** tacrine 445*
Asendin
 Also see Cyclic antidepressants
 **3** cimetidine 111, 113
Aspirin
 Also see Salicylates
 **2** acetazolamide 5*
 **3** aluminum 29*
 **3** antacids 29*
 **3** captopril 40*
 **3** chlorpropamide 41*
 **3** diltiazem 42*
 **3** enalapril 40
 **3** ethanol 42*
 **3** glyburide 41
 **3** griseofulvin 43*

 **3** insulin 41
 **3** Maalox 29*
 **3** magnesium 29*
 **2** methotrexate 43*, 299
 **3** pentazocine 44*
 **3** prednisone 45*
 **3** probenecid 45*
 **3** sulfinpyrazone 46*
 **3** tolbutamide 41
 **2** warfarin 4, 46*
 **3** zafirlukast 47*
Astemizole
 **2** clarithromycin 48, 146
 **1** erythromycin 47*
 **1** fluconazole 49
 **2** fluoxetine 272
 **1** fluvoxamine 48*, 278
 **3** grapefruit juice 290
 **1** itraconazole 48, 49, 323
 **1** ketoconazole 48, 49*, 332
 **2** mibefradil 49, 374
 **1** miconazole 49
 **1** troleandomycin 48, 446
 **3** zafirlukast 446
Atenolol
 Also see Beta-adrenergic blockers
 **3** adenosine 50
 **3** ampicillin 28*
 **3** dipyridamole 50*
 **3** indomethacin 307
 **3** neostigmine 384
 **3** nifedipine 386
 **3** tacrine 428
 **3** tetracaine 428
 **3** theophylline 429
 **3** verapamil 430
Ativan
 Also see Benzodiazepines
 **3** clozapine 155, 157*
 **3** ethanol 199
 **2** fluconazole 267
 **3** loxapine 348*
Atorvastatin
 Also see HMG-CoA reductase inhibitors
 **3** clarithromycin 51
 **3** erythromycin 50*
 **2** itraconazole 321
 **2** ketoconazole 326
 **2** mibefradil 373

 **3** nefazodone 382
 **3** troleandomycin 51
Atracurium
 Also see Muscle relaxants; Neuromuscular blockers
 **3** amphotericin B 27
 **2** gentamicin 51*
 **3** tobramycin 51
Atromid-S
 **3** chlorpropamide 98*
 **3** furosemide 147*
 **2** lovastatin 284
 **3** pravastatin 285
 **3** rifampin 147*
 **2** warfarin 148*, 286, 350
Attenuvax
 **1** methotrexate 362
Avlosulfan
 **3** didanosine 186*
 **3** probenecid 187*
 **3** rifampin 187*
 **3** trimethoprim 188*
 **3** trimethoprim-sulfamethoxazole 188
Axid
 Also see H$_2$-receptor antagonists
 **3** cefpodoxime 29, 84
 **3** cefuroxime 85
 **3** enoxacin 31, 236
 **3** glipizide 32, 287
 **3** glyburide 32
 **3** ketoconazole 115, 329
 **3** nisoldipine 120
 **3** nitrendipine 120
 **3** tolbutamide 128
Aygestin
 **3** ampicillin 28*
 **3** carbamazepine 76*, 394
 **1** cigarette smoking 107*
 **3** cyclosporine 165, 179*
 **3** dexamethasone 395
 **2** dicumarol 397
 **3** doxycycline 397
 **3** griseofulvin 292*
 **3** hydrocortisone 395
 **3** methylprednisolone 395
 **3** phenobarbital 394*
 **2** phenprocoumon 397
 **3** phenytoin 394*
 **3** prednisolone 395*
 **3** prednisone 395

*3* primidone 394
*3* rifabutin 396
*3* rifampin 395*
*3* tetracycline 397*
*2* **warfarin 397***
Azapropazone
*2* **methotrexate 52***
*2* **warfarin 53***
Azathioprine
*2* **allopurinol 9*, 12**
*3* captopril 54*
*3* warfarin 54*, 356
Azithromycin
Also see Macrolides
*3* buspirone 62
*3* ergotamine 143
*3* indinavir 144
*3* itraconazole 144
AZT
Also see Antivirals
*1* **ganciclovir 283***
*3* interferon 313*
*3* probenecid 423*
*3* rifampin 439*
Azulfidine
Also see Sulfonamides
*3* digoxin 218*
Bactrim
*3* chlorpropamide 451
*3* dapsone 188
*3* disulfiram 370
*3* glipizide 451
*3* glyburide 451
*3* methotrexate 363*
*3* metronidazole 252, 370*
*3* phenindione 455
*3* phenytoin 416
*3* tolbutamide 451*
*3* warfarin 455*
Barbiturates
Also see Amobarbital;
   Butabarbital;
   Heptabarbital;
   Pentobarbital;
   Phenobarbital;
   Primidone; Secobarbital;
   Thiopental
*2* **acenocoumarol 408**
*3* acetaminophen 2*, 3
*3* acetazolamide 6*
*3* chloramphenicol 89*
*3* chlorpromazine 97*

*3* clozapine 65
*3* cyclosporine 66, 180*
*3* dexamethasone 403
*2* **dicumarol 408**
*3* digitoxin 209*
*3* disopyramide 225*
*3* doxycycline 232*
*3* estrogen 394
*3* ethanol 253*
*2* **ethyl biscoumacetate 408**
*3* felbamate 258*
*3* furosemide 282
*3* griseofulvin 292*
*3* haloperidol 97
*3* lamotrigine 336
*3* meperidine 354*
*3* methadone 357*
*3* methoxyflurane 365*
*3* methylprednisolone 403
*3* nifedipine 385*, 407
*3* oral contraceptives 394*
*3* phenobarbital 404*
*2* **phenprocoumon 408**
*3* phenytoin 403*, 410*
*3* prednisolone 403
*3* prednisone 403*
*3* primidone 404*
*3* probenecid 423*
*3* propafenone 404*
*3* protriptyline 405*
*3* tacrolimus 413
*3* theophylline 406*
*3* thioridazine 97
*3* valproic acid 406*, 422*
*3* verapamil 386, 407*
*2* **warfarin 407*, 408**
Basaljel
Also see Antacids
*3* allopurinol 9*
*3* aspirin 29*
*3* cefpodoxime 29*
*3* cefuroxime 85
*3* ciprofloxacin 30*, 130, 134
*3* glipizide 32*
*3* glyburide 32*
*3* iron 33*
*3* isoniazid 34*
*3* ketoconazole 34
*3* lomefloxacin 35*
*3* methenamine 358

*3* norfloxacin 35*, 36, 390
*3* ofloxacin 35, 36*, 392
*3* penicillamine 37*
*3* pseudoephedrine 37
*3* tetracycline 39*
Baycol
Also see HMG-CoA reductase inhibitors
*2* **mibefradil 373**
Bayer
Also see Salicylates
*2* **acetazolamide 5***
*3* aluminum 29*
*3* antacids 29*
*3* captopril 40*
*3* chlorpropamide 41*
*3* diltiazem 42*
*3* enalapril 40
*3* ethanol 42*
*3* glyburide 41
*3* griseofulvin 43*
*3* insulin 41
*3* Maalox 29*
*3* magnesium 29*
*2* **methotrexate 43*, 299**
*3* pentazocine 44*
*3* prednisone 45*
*3* probenecid 45*
*3* sulfinpyrazone 46*
*3* tolbutamide 41
*2* **warfarin 4, 46***
*3* zafirlukast 47*
Baypress
Also see Calcium channel blockers
*3* cimetidine 112, 119, 120*, 128
*3* cyclosporine 167, 169, 179, 184
*3* famotidine 120
*3* grapefruit juice 290
*3* nizatidine 120
*3* omeprazole 120
*3* ranitidine 120
BCG vaccine
*1* **methotrexate 362**
Benazepril
Also see Angiotensin-converting enzyme inhibitors
*3* bunazosin 62
Benemid
*3* aspirin 45*
*3* dapsone 187*

*2* **norepinephrine 300\*, 301**
*3* paroxetine 24, 189
*3* perphenazine 275
*2* **phenelzine 150\*, 301\***
*3* phenobarbital 405\*
*3* phenylephrine 302\*
*3* propoxyphene 230\*
*3* quinidine 302\*
*3* rifampin 391\*
*3* ritonavir 190\*
*3* tolazamide 231\*
*1* **tranylcypromine 150**
*3* trifluoperazine 98, 275
*3* verapamil 303\*

Calan
Also see Antiarrhythmics;
    Calcium channel blockers
*3* alfentanil 8
*3* amiodarone 19
*3* atenolol 430
*2* **carbamazepine 81\***
*3* cimetidine 112, 119, 120, 128\*
*3* cyclosporine 167, 178, 184\*
*3* diclofenac 205\*
*3* digitoxin 219
*3* digoxin 55, 210, 214, 219\*
*3* doxazosin 421
*3* doxorubicin 231\*
*3* encainide 220
*2* **ethanol 255\***
*3* imipramine 304\*
*3* lithium 348\*
*3* lovastatin 220
*3* metoprolol 430
*3* midazolam 221
*3* pancuronium 456\*
*3* phenobarbital 386, 407\*
*3* prazosin 421\*
*3* propranolol 223, 430\*
*3* quinidine 387, 433\*
*3* rifabutin 438
*3* rifampin 438\*
*3* simvastatin 374
*3* tacrolimus 184
*3* terazosin 421
*3* theophylline 449\*
*3* timolol 430
*3* vecuronium 456\*

Calcet Plus
Also see Antacids
*3* allopurinol 9
*3* amphetamines 37
*3* aspirin 29\*
*3* cefpodoxime 29\*
*3* cefuroxime 85
*3* ciprofloxacin 30\*, 35, 36, 130, 134
*3* doxycycline 39
*3* Ecotrin 29
*3* enoxacin 31\*
*3* ephedrine 31\*, 37
*3* glipizide 32\*
*3* glyburide 32\*
*3* iron 33\*
*3* isoniazid 34\*
*3* itraconazole 34
*3* ketoconazole 34
*3* lithium 346\*
*3* lomefloxacin 30, 34\*, 35\*, 36
*3* methenamine 358\*
*3* mexiletine 372\*
*3* nifedipine 351
*3* norfloxacin 35\*, 36, 390
*3* ofloxacin 30, 35, 36\*, 392
*3* penicillamine 37\*
*3* phenylpropanolamine 37
*3* pseudoephedrine 37\*
*3* quinidine 6, 38\*, 431\*
*3* sodium polystyrene sulfonate resin 38\*
*3* tetracycline 39\*
*3* thiazides 64\*
*3* tocainide 40\*

Calcilac
Also see Antacids
*3* allopurinol 9
*3* amphetamines 37
*3* aspirin 29\*
*3* cefpodoxime 29\*
*3* cefuroxime 85
*3* ciprofloxacin 30\*, 35, 36, 130, 134
*3* doxycycline 39
*3* Ecotrin 29
*3* enoxacin 31\*
*3* ephedrine 31\*, 37
*3* glipizide 32\*
*3* glyburide 32\*

*3* iron 33\*
*3* isoniazid 34\*
*3* itraconazole 34
*3* ketoconazole 34
*3* lithium 346\*
*3* lomefloxacin 30, 34\*, 35\*, 36
*3* methenamine 358\*
*3* mexiletine 372\*
*3* nifedipine 351
*3* norfloxacin 35\*, 36, 390
*3* ofloxacin 30, 35, 36\*, 392
*3* penicillamine 37\*
*3* phenylpropanolamine 37
*3* pseudoephedrine 37\*
*3* quinidine 6, 38\*, 431\*
*3* sodium polystyrene sulfonate resin 38\*
*3* tetracycline 39\*
*3* thiazides 64\*
*3* tocainide 40\*

Calcium
Also see Antacids
*3* allopurinol 9
*3* amphetamines 37
*3* aspirin 29\*
*3* cefpodoxime 29\*
*3* cefuroxime 85
*3* ciprofloxacin 30\*, 35, 36, 130, 134
*3* doxycycline 39
*3* Ecotrin 29
*3* enoxacin 31\*
*3* ephedrine 31\*, 37
*3* glipizide 32\*
*3* glyburide 32\*
*3* iron 33\*
*3* isoniazid 34\*
*3* itraconazole 34
*3* ketoconazole 34
*3* lithium 346\*
*3* lomefloxacin 30, 34\*, 35\*, 36
*3* methenamine 358\*
*3* mexiletine 372\*
*3* nifedipine 351
*3* norfloxacin 35\*, 36, 390
*3* ofloxacin 30, 35, 36\*, 392
*3* penicillamine 37\*
*3* phenylpropanolamine 37

**Catapres** *(Continued)*
**3** fluphenazine 93
**3** haloperidol 93
**2 imipramine 152**
**3** insulin 153*
**3** nitroprusside 153*
**3** propranolol 154*
**3** sotalol 154
**3** tacrolimus 151
**3** trazodone 152
**Cefamandole**
Also see Cephalosporins
**3** ethanol 83*
**2 warfarin 379**
**Cefazolin**
Also see Cephalosporins
**2 warfarin 379**
**Cefmetazole**
Also see Cephalosporins
**2 warfarin 379**
**Cefobid**
Also see Cephalosporins
**3** ethanol 84
**2 warfarin 379**
**Cefoperazone**
Also see Cephalosporins
**3** ethanol 84
**2 warfarin 379**
**Cefotan**
Also see Cephalosporins
**3** ethanol 84
**2 warfarin 379**
**Cefotetan**
Also see Cephalosporins
**3** ethanol 84
**2 warfarin 379**
**Cefoxitin**
Also see Cephalosporins
**2 warfarin 379**
**Cefpodoxime**
Also see Cephalosporins
**3** aluminum 29*
**3** antacids 29*
**3** cimetidine 29, 84
**3** famotidine 29, 84
**3** lansoprazole 29, 84
**3** Maalox 29*
**3** magnesium 29*
**3** nizatidine 29, 84
**3** omeprazole 29, 84
**3** ranitidine 29, 84, 85

**Ceftin**
Also see Cephalosporins
**3** aluminum 85
**3** Amphojel 85
**3** cimetidine 85
**3** famotidine 85
**3** lansoprazole 85
**3** nizatidine 85
**3** omeprazole 85
**3** ranitidine 84, 85*
**3** sodium bicarbonate 85
**Ceftriaxone**
Also see Cephalosporins
**2 warfarin 379**
**Cefuroxime**
Also see Cephalosporins
**3** aluminum 85
**3** Amphojel 85
**3** cimetidine 85
**3** famotidine 85
**3** lansoprazole 85
**3** nizatidine 85
**3** omeprazole 85
**3** ranitidine 84, 85*
**3** sodium bicarbonate 85
**Centrex**
Also see Benzodiazepines
**3** cimetidine 111
**3** disulfiram 198
**3** rifampin 203
**Cephaloridine**
**3** ethacrynic acid 86
**3** furosemide 85*
**Cephalosporins**
Also see Cefamandole;
Cefmetazole;
Cefoperazone; Cefotetan;
Cefoxitin; Cefpodoxime;
Ceftriaxone; Cefuroxime;
Cephalothin
**3** aluminum 29*, 85
**3** Amphojel 85
**3** antacids 29*, 85
**3** cimetidine 29, 84, 85
**3** ethanol 83*, 84
**3** famotidine 29, 84, 85
**3** furosemide 86
**3** lansoprazole 29, 84, 85
**3** Maalox 29*
**3** magnesium 29*
**3** nizatidine 29, 84, 85

**3** omeprazole 29, 84, 85
**3** ranitidine 29, 84, 85*
**3** sodium bicarbonate 85
**2 warfarin 379**
**Cephalothin**
Also see Cephalosporins
**3** furosemide 86
**Cerivastatin**
Also see HMG-CoA reductase inhibitors
**2 mibefradil 373**
**Cetirizine**
**3** ketoconazole 49
**Charcoal**
**2 digitoxin 86**
**2 digoxin 86***
**Chloral hydrate**
**3** ethanol 86*
**3** warfarin 86*
**Chloramphenicol**
**3** chlorpropamide 88*
**3** cimetidine 83
**2 dicumarol 88***
**3** phenobarbital 89*
**3** phenytoin 89*
**3** rifampin 90*
**3** tolbutamide 88
**2 warfarin 88**
**Chlordiazepoxide**
Also see Benzodiazepines
**3** cimetidine 111
**3** disulfiram 198
**3** ethanol 199
**3** fluconazole 90
**3** itraconazole 90, 201
**3** ketoconazole 90*
**3** levodopa 202
**Chloromycetin**
**3** chlorpropamide 88*
**3** cimetidine 83
**2 dicumarol 88***
**3** phenobarbital 89*
**3** phenytoin 89*
**3** rifampin 90*
**3** tolbutamide 88
**2 warfarin 88**
**Chloroptic**
**3** chlorpropamide 88*
**3** cimetidine 83
**2 dicumarol 88***
**3** phenobarbital 89*

**3** phenytoin 89*
**3** rifampin 90*
**3** tolbutamide 88
**2 warfarin 88**
Chloroquine
  **3** chlorpromazine 91*
  **3** cyclosporine 91*
  **3** methotrexate 91*
  **3** praziquantel 92*
  **3** tacrolimus 91
Chlorpromazine
  Also see Neuroleptics
  **3** amodiaquine 91
  **3** chloroquine 91*
  **3** cigarette smoking 92*
  **3** clonidine 93*
  **3** epinephrine 93*
  **3** guanadrel 94
  **3** guanethidine 94*
  **3** imipramine 275
  **2 levodopa 95***
  **3** lithium 95*
  **3** meperidine 96*
  **3** orphenadrine 96*
  **3** phenobarbital 97*
  **3** propranolol 97*
  **3** sulfadoxine pyrimethamine 91
  **3** trazodone 98*
Chlorpropamide
  Also see Antidiabetics; Sulfonylureas
  **3** chloramphenicol 88*
  **3** clofibrate 98*
  **3** doxepin 231
  **3** erythromycin 99*
  **1 ethanol 99***
  **2 phenylbutazone 409**
  **3** thiazides 312
  **3** tranylcypromine 312
  **3** trimethoprim-sulfamethoxazole 451
Chlorprothixene
  Also see Neuroleptics
  **3** bromocriptine 61
Chlorthalidone
  Also see Diuretics; Thiazides
  **3** digoxin 211
Cholestyramine
  Also see Bile acid-binding resins
  **3** acetaminophen 1*
  **3** amiodarone 17*

**3** diclofenac 100*, 160
**3** digitoxin 101
**3** digoxin 100*
**3** fluvastatin 104
**3** furosemide 101*, 161
**3** gemfibrozil 161
**3** hydrocortisone 101*
**3** imipramine 102*
**3** lovastatin 104
**3** methotrexate 103*
**3** metronidazole 103*
**3** phenprocoumon 106
**3** piroxicam 104*
**3** pravastatin 104*
**3** simvastatin 104
**3** tenoxicam 104
**3** tetracycline 162
**3** thiazides 162
**3** thyroid 105*
**3** valproic acid 106*
**3** warfarin 106*, 148, 286, 350
Cholinergics
  Also see Bethanechol; Edrophonium; Neostigmine; Pyridostigmine
  **3** atenolol 384
  **3** nadolol 384
  **3** procainamide 384*
  **3** propranolol 384*
  **3** tacrine 56*
Choloxin
  **2 warfarin 197***
Chooz
  Also see Antacids
  **3** allopurinol 9
  **3** amphetamines 37
  **3** aspirin 29*
  **3** cefpodoxime 29*
  **3** cefuroxime 85
  **3** ciprofloxacin 30*, 35, 36, 130, 134
  **3** doxycycline 39
  **3** Ecotrin 29
  **3** enoxacin 31*
  **3** ephedrine 31*, 37
  **3** glipizide 32*
  **3** glyburide 32*
  **3** iron 33*
  **3** isoniazid 34*
  **3** itraconazole 34
  **3** ketoconazole 34

**3** lithium 346*
**3** lomefloxacin 30, 34*, 35*, 36
**3** methenamine 358*
**3** mexiletine 372*
**3** nifedipine 351
**3** norfloxacin 35*, 36, 390
**3** ofloxacin 30, 35, 36*, 392
**3** penicillamine 37*
**3** phenylpropanolamine 37
**3** pseudoephedrine 37*
**3** quinidine 6, 38*, 431*
**3** sodium polystyrene sulfonate resin 38*
**3** tetracycline 39*
**3** thiazides 64*
**3** tocainide 40*
Cigarette smoking
  **3** chlorpromazine 92*
  **3** insulin 107*
  **1 oral contraceptives 107***
  **3** quinine 108*
  **3** tacrine 108*
  **3** theophylline 108*
Cimetidine
  Also see H$_2$-receptor antagonists
  **2 acenocoumarol 129**
  **3** alfentanil 7*
  **3** alprazolam 111
  **3** amiodarone 18*
  **3** amitriptyline 111, 113
  **3** amoxapine 111, 113
  **3** carmustine 83*
  **3** cefpodoxime 29, 84
  **3** cefuroxime 85
  **3** chloramphenicol 83
  **3** chlordiazepoxide 111
  **3** cisapride 109*
  **3** citalopram 109*
  **3** clorazepate 111
  **3** clozapine 110*
  **3** desipramine 110*, 113, 115, 121
  **3** desmethyldiazepam 111
  **3** diazepam 111*
  **3** dilevalol 125
  **3** diltiazem 112*, 119, 120, 128
  **3** doxepin 113*, 115, 121
  **3** femoxetine 113*
  **3** flecainide 114*

Cimetidine *(Continued)*
- *3* glipizide 32, 128, 287
- *3* glyburide 32, 128
- *3* halazepam 111
- *3* imipramine 113, 115*, 121
- *3* ketoconazole 115*, 328, 329
- *3* labetalol 125
- *3* lidocaine 116*
- *3* lomustine 83
- *3* maprotiline 111, 113
- *3* melphalan 117*
- *3* meperidine 117*
- *3* metoprolol 125
- *3* moricizine 118*
- *3* nicotine 118*
- *3* nifedipine 112, 119*, 120, 128
- *3* nimodipine 119*
- *3* nisoldipine 112, 119, 120*, 128
- *3* nitrendipine 112, 119, 120*, 128
- *3* nortriptyline 113, 115, 121*
- *3* paroxetine 122*
- *3* phenytoin 83, 122*
- *3* pindolol 125
- *3* prazepam 111
- *3* praziquantel 123*
- *3* procainamide 124*
- *3* propafenone 124*
- *3* propranolol 125*
- *3* protriptyline 111, 113, 121
- *3* quinidine 38, 126*
- *3* tacrine 126*
- *3* theophylline 127*
- *3* tolbutamide 127*
- *3* trazodone 111, 113
- *3* triazolam 111
- *3* trimipramine 111, 113
- *3* verapamil 112, 119, 120, 128*
- *2* **warfarin 129***

Cipro
Also see Quinolones
- *3* aluminum 30*, 130, 134
- *3* antacids 30*, 35, 36
- *3* diazepam 130*
- *3* didanosine 130*
- *3* food 131*
- *3* foscarnet 131*

- *3* iron 132*, 315
- *3* Maalox 30*
- *3* magnesium 30*, 130
- *3* metoprolol 132*
- *3* pentoxifylline 133*
- *3* phenytoin 133*
- *3* propranolol 132
- *3* sucralfate 30, 134*, 389, 392
- *3* theophylline 134*, 238, 390
- *3* warfarin 135*, 391, 393
- *3* zinc 135*

Ciprofloxacin
Also see Quinolones
- *3* aluminum 30*, 130, 134
- *3* antacids 30*, 35, 36
- *3* diazepam 130*
- *3* didanosine 130*
- *3* food 131*
- *3* foscarnet 131*
- *3* iron 132*, 315
- *3* Maalox 30*
- *3* magnesium 30*, 130
- *3* metoprolol 132*
- *3* pentoxifylline 133*
- *3* phenytoin 133*
- *3* propranolol 132
- *3* sucralfate 30, 134*, 389, 392
- *3* theophylline 134*, 238, 390
- *3* warfarin 135*, 391, 393
- *3* zinc 135*

Cisapride
- *3* cimetidine 109*
- *2* **clarithromycin 136*, 139**
- *3* cyclosporine 176
- *2* **erythromycin 136*, 139**
- *2* **fluconazole 137, 138, 139**
- *2* **itraconazole 137*, 138, 139**
- *2* **ketoconazole 136, 137, 138*, 139**
- *2* **mibefradil 138***
- *2* **miconazole 137, 138, 139***
- *2* **troleandomycin 136, 139***

Cisplatin
Also see Antineoplastics
- *3* bumetanide 140
- *3* diazoxide 140*

- *2* **ethacrynic acid 140***
- *3* furosemide 140
- *3* gentamicin 141*
- *3* phenytoin 141*

Citalopram
Also see Selective serotonin reuptake inhibitors
- *3* cimetidine 109*
- *2* **moclobemide 142***
- *3* omeprazole 109

Clarithromycin
Also see Macrolides
- *3* alfentanil 8
- *3* alprazolam 13
- *2* **astemizole 48, 146**
- *3* atorvastatin 51
- *3* buspirone 62
- *3* carbamazepine 65*, 68, 79
- *2* **cisapride 136*, 139**
- *3* clozapine 156
- *3* colchicine 160
- *3* cyclosporine 143*, 146, 168
- *2* **diazepam 145**
- *3* disopyramide 224
- *2* **ergotamine 143***
- *3* indinavir 144*
- *3* itraconazole 144*
- *3* lovastatin 242
- *3* methylprednisolone 366
- *2* **midazolam 145*, 243**
- *3* quinidine 243
- *3* tacrolimus 143, 145*, 244
- *2* **terfenadine 146*, 446**
- *3* triazolam 246, 454
- *3* valproic acid 247
- *3* warfarin 247

Claritin
- *3* itraconazole 323, 326
- *3* ketoconazole 49, 326*
- *3* miconazole 326

Cleocin
- *2* **kaolin-pectin 325**

Clindamycin
- *2* **kaolin-pectin 325**

Clinoril
Also see Nonsteroidal antiinflammatory drugs
- *3* bromfenac 58
- *3* captopril 41
- *3* cyclosporine 166, 173, 174, 175, 178, 183*

*3* furosemide 281
*2* **warfarin 443***
Clobazam
Also see Benzodiazepines
*3* phenytoin 146*
Clofibrate
*3* chlorpropamide 98*
*3* furosemide 147*
*2* **lovastatin 284**
*3* pravastatin 285
*3* rifampin 147*
*2* **warfarin 148*, 286, 350**
Clomipramine
Also see Cyclic antidepressants; Tricyclic antidepressants
*3* fluvoxamine 148*
*3* grapefruit juice 149*
*1* **isocarboxazid 150**
*2* **moclobemide 149***
*1* **phenelzine 150*, 301**
*1* **tranylcypromine 150**
Clonazepam
Also see Anticonvulsants; Benzodiazepines
*3* disulfiram 198
*3* valproic acid 151*
Clonidine
Also see Alpha agonists
*2* **amitriptyline 25, 152**
*3* chlorpromazine 93*
*3* cyclosporine 151*
*2* **desipramine 152***
*3* fluphenazine 93
*3* haloperidol 93
*2* **imipramine 152**
*3* insulin 153*
*3* nitroprusside 153*
*3* propranolol 154*
*3* sotalol 154
*3* tacrolimus 151
*3* trazodone 152
Clorazepate
Also see Anticonvulsants; Benzodiazepines
*3* cimetidine 111
*3* disulfiram 198
*3* rifampin 203
Clotrimazole
Also see Antifungals
*3* cyclosporine 155
*3* tacrolimus 155*

Clozapine
*3* bromocriptine 61
*3* carbamazepine 65*
*3* cimetidine 110*
*3* clarithromycin 156
*3* diazepam 155*, 157
*3* epinephrine 93
*2* **erythromycin 156***
*2* **fluvoxamine 156***
*3* lorazepam 155, 157*
*3* phenytoin 65
*3* primidone 65
*3* troleandomycin 156
*3* valproic acid 157*
Clozaril
*3* bromocriptine 61
*3* carbamazepine 65*
*3* cimetidine 110*
*3* clarithromycin 156
*3* diazepam 155*, 157
*3* epinephrine 93
*2* **erythromycin 156***
*2* **fluvoxamine 156***
*3* lorazepam 155, 157*
*3* phenytoin 65
*3* primidone 65
*3* troleandomycin 156
*3* valproic acid 157*
Cocaine
Also see Anesthetics, local
*3* propranolol 158*
Codeine
Also see Narcotic analgesics
*2* **quinidine 158***
Cogentin
Also see Anticholinergics
*3* chlorpromazine 55
*3* haloperidol 54*
Cognex
*3* ambenonium 56
*3* atenolol 428
*3* bethanechol 56*
*3* cigarette smoking 108*
*3* cimetidine 126*
*3* edrophonium 56
*3* enoxacin 237*
*3* fluoxetine 277
*2* **fluvoxamine 277***
*3* levodopa 340*
*3* nadolol 428

*3* neostigmine 56
*3* paroxetine 277
*3* propranolol 428*
*3* pyridostigmine 56
*3* sertraline 277
*3* theophylline 444*
*3* trihexyphenidyl 445*
Colchicine
*3* clarithromycin 160
*3* cyclosporine 159*
*3* erythromycin 160*
*3* tacrolimus 159
*3* troleandomycin 160
Colestid
Also see Bile-acid binding resins
*3* acetaminophen 1
*3* amiodarone 18
*3* diclofenac 100, 160*
*3* furosemide 101, 161*
*3* gemfibrozil 161*
*3* hydrocortisone 102
*3* imipramine 102
*3* methotrexate 103
*3* metronidazole 103
*3* piroxicam 104
*3* pravastatin 104
*3* tetracycline 161*
*3* thiazides 162*
*3* thyroid 105
*3* valproic acid 106
*3* warfarin 106, 148, 286, 350
Colestipol
Also see Bile-acid binding resins
*3* acetaminophen 1
*3* amiodarone 18
*3* diclofenac 100, 160*
*3* furosemide 101, 161*
*3* gemfibrozil 161*
*3* hydrocortisone 102
*3* imipramine 102
*3* methotrexate 103
*3* metronidazole 103
*3* piroxicam 104
*3* pravastatin 104
*3* tetracycline 161*
*3* thiazides 162*
*3* thyroid 105
*3* valproic acid 106
*3* warfarin 106, 148, 286, 350

Compazine
Also see Neuroleptics
*3* procarbazine 424*
Contraceptives, oral
*3* ampicillin 28*
*3* carbamazepine 76*, 394
*1* **cigarette smoking 107***
*3* cyclosporine 165, 179*
*3* dexamethasone 395
*2* **dicumarol 397**
*3* doxycycline 397
*3* griseofulvin 292*
*3* hydrocortisone 395
*3* methylprednisolone 395
*3* phenobarbital 394*
*2* **phenprocoumon 397**
*3* phenytoin 394*
*3* prednisolone 395*
*3* prednisone 395
*3* primidone 394
*3* rifabutin 396
*3* rifampin 395*
*3* tetracycline 397*
*2* **warfarin 397***
Contrast media
*3* propranolol 162*
Cordarone
Also see Antiarrythmics
*3* acenocoumarol 23
*3* cholestyramine 17*
*3* cimetidine 18*
*3* colestipol 18
*3* cyclosporine 18*
*3* digitoxin 19
*3* digoxin 19*
*3* diltiazem 19*
*3* encainide 20
*3* flecainide 20*
*3* metoprolol 20*, 23
*3* phenytoin 21*
*3* procainamide 22*
*3* propranolol 21, 23
*3* quinidine 22*
*3* sotalol 22*
*3* tacrolimus 18
*3* theophylline 23*
*3* verapamil 19
*3* warfarin 23*
Coreg
Also see Beta-adrenergic
blockers
*3* digoxin 216

Corgard
Also see Beta-adrenergic
blockers
*3* epinephrine 240
*3* insulin 311
*3* lidocaine 341
*3* neostigmine 384
*3* tacrine 428
*3* theophylline 429
Cortef
Also see Corticosteroids
*3* aminoglutethimide 15
*3* cholestyramine 101*
*3* colestipol 102
*3* oral contraceptives 395
Corticosteroids
Also see Cortisone; Dexa-
methasone; Hydrocor-
tisone; Methylprednis-
olone; Prednisolone;
Prednisone
*3* aminoglutethimide 15*
*3* aspirin 45*
*3* cholestyramine 101*
*3* clarithromycin 366
*3* colestipol 102
*3* cyclosporine 181*
*3* erythromycin 366
*3* indomethacin 307*
*3* insulin 310*
*3* isoniazid 318*
*3* ketoconazole 327*
*3* oral contraceptives 395*
*3* phenobarbital 403*
*3* rifampin 422*
*3* tacrolimus 181
*3* troleandomycin 366*
Cortisone
Also see Corticosteroids
*3* aminoglutethimide 15
*3* rifampin 422
Cotrimoxazole
*3* chlorpropamide 451
*3* dapsone 188
*3* disulfiram 370
*3* glipizide 451
*3* glyburide 451
*3* methotrexate 363*
*3* metronidazole 252, 370*
*3* phenindione 455
*3* phenytoin 416
*3* tolbutamide 451*
*3* warfarin 455*

Coumadin
Also see Anticoagulants;
Oral anticoagulants
*3* acetaminophen 4*
*3* allopurinol 13*
*3* aminoglutethimide 17*
*3* amiodarone 23*
*2* **amobarbital 408**
*2* **aspirin 4, 46***
*2* **azapropazone 53***
*3* azathioprine 54*, 356
*2* **bromfenac 58***
*2* **butabarbital 408**
*3* carbamazepine 81*
*2* **cefamandole 379**
*2* **cefazolin 379**
*2* **cefmetazole 379**
*2* **cefoperazone 379**
*2* **cefotetan 379**
*2* **cefoxitin 379**
*2* **ceftriaxone 379**
*3* chloral hydrate 87*
*2* **chloramphenicol 88**
*3* cholestyramine 106*,
148, 286, 350
*2* **cimetidine 129***
*3* ciprofloxacin 135*, 391,
393
*3* clarithromycin 247
*2* **clofibrate 148*, 286, 350**
*3* colestipol 106, 148, 286,
350
*3* cyclophosphamide 164*
*2* **danazol 186***
*2* **dextrothyroxine 197***
*2* **diclofenac 53, 206*, 208,
262, 309, 335, 352, 353,
409, 418, 444**
*2* **diflunisal 208***
*2* **disulfiram 229***
*3* doxycycline 233*
*3* erythromycin 247*
*3* ethanol 256*
*2* **etodolac 257***
*2* **fenoprofen 262***
*3* fluconazole 268*, 324,
333
*3* fluorouracil 269*
*3* fluoxetine 274*, 441
*2* **flurbiprofen 276**
*3* fluvastatin 350
*3* fluvoxamine 279*
*2* **gemfibrozil 148, 285*,
350**

Cyclic antidepressants
*(Continued)*
**2 phenelzine 150, 301***
**3** phenobarbital 405*
**3** phenylephrine 302*
**3** propoxyphene 230*
**3** quinidine 302*
**3** rifampin 391*
**3** ritonavir 190*
**3** tolazamide 231*
**1 tranylcypromine 150**
**3** trifluoperazine 275
**3** verapamil 303*
Cyclophosphamide
Also see Antineoplastics
**3** allopurinol 11*
**3** digoxin 163*
**3** succinylcholine 164*
**3** warfarin 164*
Cycloserine
**3** isoniazid 164*
Cyclosporine
**3** allopurinol 11*
**3** amiodarone 18*
**3** amphotericin B 26*
**3** carbamazepine 66*
**3** chloroquine 91*
**3** cisapride 176
**3** clarithromycin 143*, 145, 168
**3** clonidine 151*
**3** clotrimazole 155
**3** colchicine 159*
**2 danazol 165***
**3** diclofenac 166*, 173, 174, 175
**3** digoxin 166*
**3** diltiazem 167*, 178, 184
**3** doxorubicin 167*
**3** enalapril 168*
**3** erythromycin 143, 168*, 244
**3** felodipine 169*
**3** fluconazole 170*, 173, 174, 177, 265
**3** gentamicin 170*
**3** glipizide 171*
**3** grapefruit juice 171*
**3** griseofulvin 172*
**3** imipenem 172*
**3** indomethacin 166, 173*
**3** itraconazole 170, 173*, 174, 177

**3** ketoconazole 170, 172, 173, 174*, 177, 332
**3** ketoprofen 166, 174*
**3** mefenamic acid 175*
**3** melphalan 175*
**3** methotrexate 176*
**3** methylprednisolone 181
**3** methyltestosterone 165
**3** metoclopramide 176*
**3** miconazole 170, 173, 174, 177*
**3** nafcillin 177*
**3** naproxen 178*, 183
**3** nicardipine 167, 178*, 184
**3** nitrendipine 167, 169, 179, 184
**3** norethindrone 165
**3** oral contraceptives 179*
**3** phenobarbital 66, 180*
**3** phenytoin 66, 180*
**3** prednisolone 181*
**3** primidone 66
**3** probucol 182*
**2 rifampin 182***
**3** sulindac 166, 173, 174, 175, 178, 183*
**3** sulphadimidine 183*
**3** ticlopidine 184*
**3** troleandomycin 168
**3** valproic acid 66
**3** verapamil 167, 178, 184*
Cyproheptadine
**3** fluoxetine 185*
Cytadren
**3** acenocoumarol 17
**3** cortisone 15
**3** dexamethasone 15*
**3** hydrocortisone 15
**3** medroxyprogesterone 15*
**3** methylprednisolone 15
**3** prednisolone 15
**3** prednisone 15
**3** tacrolimus 413
**2 tamoxifen 16***
**3** theophylline 16*
**3** warfarin 17*
Cytotec
**3** phenylbutazone 375*
Cytovene
Also see Antivirals
**3** didanosine 206*
**1 zidovudine 283***

Cytoxan
Also see Antineoplastics
**3** allopurinol 11*
**3** digoxin 163*
**3** succinylcholine 164*
**3** warfarin 164*
Dalmane
Also see Benzodiazepines
**3** disulfiram 198
Danazol
Also see Anabolic steroids
**2 carbamazepine 66***
**2 cyclosporine 165***
**3** lovastatin 185*
**3** tacrolimus 165
**2 warfarin 186***
Danocrine
Also see Anabolic steroids
**2 carbamazepine 66***
**2 cyclosporine 165***
**3** lovastatin 185*
**3** tacrolimus 165
**2 warfarin 186***
Dapsone
**3** didanosine 186*
**3** probenecid 187*
**3** rifampin 187*
**3** trimethoprim 188*
**3** trimethoprim-sulfamethoxazole 188
Daraprim
**2 folic acid 280***
Darvocet-N
Also see Narcotic analgesics
**2 carbamazepine 78*, 231**
**3** doxepin 230*
**3** ethanol 254*
**3** metoprolol 367*
**3** propranolol 367
**3** warfarin 427*
Darvon
Also see Narcotic analgesics
**2 carbamazepine 78*, 231**
**3** doxepin 230*
**3** ethanol 254*
**3** metoprolol 367*
**3** propranolol 367
**3** warfarin 427*

Dazamide
  Also see Diuretics
  **2 aspirin 5***
  **3** methenamine 358
  **3** mexiletine 372
  **3** phenytoin 5*
  **3** primidone 6*
  **3** quinidine 6*, 431
Decadron
  Also see Corticosteroids
  **3** aminoglutethimide 15*
  **3** oral contraceptives 395
  **3** phenobarbital 403
Delavirdine
  **3** rifabutin 188
  **3** rifampin 188*
Delta-Cortef
  Also see Corticosteroids
  **3** aminoglutethimide 15
  **3** cyclosporine 181*
  **3** isoniazid 318*
  **3** oral contraceptives 395*
  **3** phenobarbital 403
  **3** rifampin 422*
  **3** tacrolimus 181
Deltasone
  Also see Corticosteroids
  **3** aminoglutethimide 15
  **3** aspirin 45*
  **3** indomethacin 307*
  **3** insulin 310*
  **3** oral contraceptives 395
  **3** phenobarbital 403*
Demadex
  Also see Diuretics; Loop
    diuretics
  **3** digoxin 211
  **3** enalapril 235
  **3** fluoxetine 269
Demerol
  Also see Narcotic
    analgesics
  **3** chlorpromazine 96*
  **3** cimetidine 117*
  **3** ethanol 250*
  **1** isocarboxazid 354
  **1** phenelzine 354*
  **3** phenobarbital 354*
  **3** phenytoin 355*
  **2** selegiline 197, 355*
  **1** tranylcypromine 354

Demulen
  Also see Estrogens
  **3** ampicillin 28*
  **3** carbamazepine 76*, 394
  **1** cigarette smoking 107*
  **3** cyclosporine 165, 179*
  **3** dexamethasone 395
  **2** dicumarol 397
  **3** doxycycline 397
  **3** griseofulvin 292*
  **3** hydrocortisone 395
  **3** methylprednisolone 395
  **3** phenobarbital 394*
  **2** phenprocoumon 397
  **3** phenytoin 394*
  **3** prednisolone 395*
  **3** prednisone 395
  **3** primidone 394
  **3** rifabutin 396
  **3** rifampin 395*
  **3** ritonavir 396*
  **3** tetracycline 397*
  **2** warfarin 397*
Depakene
  Also see Anticonvulsants
  **3** carbamazepine 80*
  **3** cholestyramine 106*
  **3** clarithromycin 247
  **3** clonazepam 151*
  **3** clozapine 157*
  **3** colestipol 106
  **3** cyclosporine 66
  **3** erythromycin 246*
  **3** felbamate 259*
  **3** isoniazid 319*
  **3** lamotrigine 337*
  **3** nimodipine 388*
  **3** phenobarbital 406*
  **3** phenytoin 417*
  **3** primidone 422*
  **3** troleandomycin 247
Depakote
  Also see Anticonvulsants
  **3** carbamazepine 80*
  **3** cholestyramine 106*
  **3** clarithromycin 247
  **3** clonazepam 151*
  **3** clozapine 157*
  **3** colestipol 106
  **3** cyclosporine 66
  **3** erythromycin 246*
  **3** felbamate 259*

**3** isoniazid 319*
**3** lamotrigine 337*
**3** nimodipine 388*
**3** phenobarbital 406*
**3** phenytoin 417*
**3** primidone 422*
**3** troleandomycin 247
Depo-Provera
  Also see Progestins
  **3** aminoglutethimide 15*
Deppen
  **3** aluminum 37*
  **3** antacids 37*
  **3** digoxin 215*
  **3** iron 316*
  **3** Maalox 37*
  **3** magnesium 37*
Desipramine
  Also see Cyclic antidepres-
    sants; Tricyclic antide-
    pressants
  **3** carbamazepine 72
  **3** cimetidine 110*, 113,
    115, 121
  **2** clonidine 152*
  **3** fluoxetine 188*
  **3** fluphenazine 275
  **2** guanabenz 152
  **3** guanadrel 190
  **3** guanethidine 190*
  **2** guanfacine 152
  **3** indinavir 190
  **2** norepinephrine 301
  **3** paroxetine 189
  **2** phenelzine 301
  **3** quinidine 302
  **3** ritonavir 190*
Desmethyldiazepam
  **3** cimetidine 111
Desogen
  Also see Estrogens
  **3** ampicillin 28*
  **3** carbamazepine 76*, 394
  **1** cigarette smoking 107*
  **3** cyclosporine 165, 179*
  **3** dexamethasone 395
  **2** dicumarol 397
  **3** doxycycline 397
  **3** griseofulvin 292*
  **3** hydrocortisone 395
  **3** methylprednisolone 395
  **3** phenobarbital 394*

Desogen *(Continued)*
  **2 phenprocoumon 397**
  *3* phenytoin 394*
  *3* prednisolone 395*
  *3* prednisone 395
  *3* primidone 394
  *3* rifabutin 396
  *3* rifampin 395*
  *3* ritonavir 396*
  *3* tetracycline 397*
  **2 warfarin 397***
Desogestrel
  *3* ampicillin 28*
  *3* carbamazepine 76*, 394
  **1 cigarette smoking 107***
  *3* cyclosporine 165, 179*
  *3* dexamethasone 395
  **2 dicumarol 397**
  *3* doxycycline 397
  *3* griseofulvin 292*
  *3* hydrocortisone 395
  *3* methylprednisolone 395
  *3* phenobarbital 394*
  **2 phenprocoumon 397**
  *3* phenytoin 394*
  *3* prednisolone 395*
  *3* prednisone 395
  *3* primidone 394
  *3* rifabutin 396
  *3* rifampin 395*
  *3* tetracycline 397*
  **2 warfarin 397***
Desyrel
  Also see Tricyclic antidepressants
  *3* chlorpromazine 98*
  *3* cimetidine 111, 113
  *3* clonidine 152
  *3* fluoxetine 189
  **2 moclobemide 149**
  **1 phenelzine 150, 301**
  *3* trifluoperazine 98
Dexamethasone
  Also see Corticosteroids
  *3* aminoglutethimide 15*
  *3* oral contraceptives 395
  *3* phenobarbital 403
Dexedrine
  Also see Amphetamines
  *3* furazolidone 192*, 193
  *3* guanadrel 192
  *3* guanethidine 192*

*3* imipramine 193*
**1 isocarboxazid 193**
**1 phenelzine 193**
**2 selegiline 193**
**1 tranylcypromine 193***
Dexfenfluramine
  **2 fluoxetine 191*, 260**
  **2 fluvoxamine 191**
  **1 isocarboxazid 191**
  **2 paroxetine 191**
  **1 phenelzine 191***
  **2 selegiline 191**
  **2 sertraline 191**
  **1 tranylcypromine 191**
Dexone
  Also see Corticosteroids
  *3* aminoglutethimide 15*
  *3* oral contraceptives 395
  *3* phenobarbital 403
Dextroamphetamine
  Also see Amphetamines
  *3* furazolidone 192*, 193
  *3* guanadrel 192
  *3* guanethidine 192*
  *3* imipramine 193*
  **1 isocarboxazid 193**
  **1 phenelzine 193**
  **2 selegiline 193**
  **1 tranylcypromine 193***
Dextromethorphan
  *3* fluoxetine 194*
  **1 isocarboxazid 196**
  **1 moclobemide 195***
  *3* paroxetine 194
  **1 phenelzine 195***
  *3* quinidine 196*
  **2 selegiline 197***
  **1 tranylcypromine 196**
Dextrothyroxine
  **2 warfarin 197***
DiaBeta
  Also see Antidiabetics;
  Sulfonylureas
  *3* aluminum 32*
  *3* antacids 32*
  *3* aspirin 41
  *3* cimetidine 32, 128
  *3* famotidine 32
  *3* gemfibrozil 283*
  *3* lansoprazole 32
  *3* Maalox 32*
  *3* magnesium 32*

*3* nizatidine 32
*3* omeprazole 32
*3* rifampin 437
*3* trimethoprim-sul-
  famethoxazole 451
*3* warfarin 289*
Diabinese
  Also see Antidiabetics;
  Sulfonylureas
  *3* chloramphenicol 88*
  *3* clofibrate 98*
  *3* doxepin 231
  *3* erythromycin 99*
  **1 ethanol 99***
  **2 phenylbutazone 409**
  *3* thiazides 312
  *3* tranylcypromine 312
  *3* trimethoprim-sul-
  famethoxazole 451
Diamox
  Also see Diuretics
  **2 aspirin 5***
  *3* methenamine 358
  *3* mexiletine 372
  *3* phenytoin 5*
  *3* primidone 6*
  *3* quinidine 6*, 431
Dianabol
  Also see Anabolic steroids
  *3* insulin 358
  *3* tolbutamide 358*
  **2 warfarin 398**
Diazepam
  Also see Anticonvulsants;
  Benzodiazepines; Muscle
  relaxants; Neuromuscular
  blockers
  *3* carbamazepine 76
  *3* cimetidine 111*
  *3* ciprofloxacin 130*
  **2 clarithromycin 145**
  *3* clozapine 155*, 157
  *3* disulfiram 198*
  *3* ethanol 199*
  *3* fluconazole 201, 264, 267
  *3* fluoxetine 200*
  *3* fluvoxamine 200
  *3* isoniazid 200*, 319
  *3* itraconazole 201*, 324
  *3* ketoconazole 201
  *3* labetalol 202
  *3* levodopa 201*
  *3* metoprolol 202*

Digitoxin *(Continued)*
- *3* furosemide 211
- *3* kaolin-pectin 213
- *3* phenobarbital 209*
- *3* propafenone 215
- *3* propranolol 216
- *3* quinine 217
- *3* rifampin 209*
- *3* verapamil 219

Digoxin
Also see Antiarrhythmics;
Digitalis glycosides
- *3* amiodarone 19*
- *3* bepridil 55*, 210, 219
- *3* bumetanide 211
- *3* carvedilol 216
- **2 charcoal 86***
- *3* chlorthalidone 211
- *3* cholestyramine 100*
- *3* cyclophosphamide 163*
- *3* cyclosporine 166*
- *3* diltiazem 55, 210*, 214, 219
- *3* erythromycin 211*
- *3* ethacrynic acid 211
- *3* furosemide 211*
- *3* hydroxychloroquine 212*
- *3* ibuprofen 212
- *3* indomethacin 212*
- *3* itraconazole 213*
- *3* kaolin-pectin 213*
- *3* lansoprazole 214
- *3* metolazone 211
- *3* mibefradil 214*
- *3* omeprazole 214*
- *3* penicillamine 215*
- *3* pentagastrin 214
- *3* phenylbutazone 213
- *3* propafenone 215*
- *3* propranolol 216*
- *3* quinidine 216*
- *3* quinine 217*
- *3* rifampin 209
- *3* spironolactone 218*
- *3* sulfasalazine 218*
- *3* tacrolimus 166
- *3* tetracycline 219*
- *3* thiazides 211
- *3* torsemide 211
- *3* verapamil 55, 210, 214, 219*

Dihydrocodeine
Also see Narcotic
analgesics
- *3* quinidine 158

Dihydropyridine calcium
channel blockers
Also see Felodipine;
Nifedipine; Nisoldipine
- *3* atenolol 386
- **2 carbamazepine 69***
- *3* cimetidine 112, 119*, 120*, 128
- *3* cyclosporine 169*
- *3* diltiazem 222*
- *3* doxazosin 230*
- *3* erythromycin 242*
- **2 ethanol 256**
- *3* famotidine 119, 120
- *3* fluconazole 260
- *3* grapefruit juice 289*, 290
- *3* itraconazole 260*
- *3* ketoconazole 260
- *3* lansoprazole 119
- *3* magnesium 351*
- *3* metoprolol 386
- *3* miconazole 260
- *3* nizatidine 120
- *3* omeprazole 120
- *3* phenobarbital 385*, 407
- *3* phenytoin 386*
- *3* propranolol 385, 386*
- *3* quinidine 387*, 433
- *3* ranitidine 119, 120
- *3* rifabutin 388
- *3* rifampin 387*
- *3* troleandomycin 242
- *3* vincristine 388*

Dilacor
Also see Calcium channel
blockers
- *3* alfentanil 8*
- *3* amiodarone 19
- *3* aspirin 42*
- **2 carbamazepine 67***
- *3* cimetidine 112*, 119, 120, 128
- *3* cyclosporine 167*, 178, 184
- *3* digitoxin 210
- *3* digoxin 55, 210*, 214, 219
- *3* encainide 220*
- *3* fentanyl 8
- *3* imipramine 303

- *3* lithium 348
- *3* lovastatin 220*
- *3* metoprolol 223
- *3* midazolam 221*
- *3* nifedipine 222*
- *3* nitroprusside 222*
- *3* propranolol 223*, 430
- *3* rifampin 223*
- *3* simvastatin 220, 374
- *3* sufentanil 8
- *3* tacrolimus 167
- *3* vecuronium 456

Dilantin
Also see Antiarrhythmics;
Anticonvulsants
- *3* acetaminophen 3*
- *3* acetazolamide 5*
- *3* alprazolam 375
- *3* amiodarone 21*
- *3* bromfenac 58*
- *3* carbamazepine 75, 77*
- *3* chloramphenicol 89*
- *3* cimetidine 83, 122*
- *3* ciprofloxacin 133*
- *3* cisplatin 141*
- *3* clobazam 146*
- *3* clozapine 65
- *3* cyclosporine 66, 180*
- *3* diazepam 375
- *3* dicumarol 418
- *3* disopyramide 225*
- *3* disulfiram 227*
- *3* dopamine 230*
- *3* doxycycline 232*
- *3* enoxacin 133
- *3* ethanol 254*
- *3* felbamate 259*
- *3* fluconazole 264*
- *3* fluoxetine 271*
- *3* folic acid 280*
- *3* furosemide 281*
- *3* gamma globulin 282*
- *3* influenza vaccine 310*
- *3* isoniazid 317*
- **2 itraconazole 322***
- *3* lamotrigine 336*
- *3* levodopa 339*
- *3* lithium 345*
- **2 mebendazole 351***
- *3* meperidine 355*
- **2 methadone 75, 357***
- *3* metronidazole 252, 369*, 370

Doan's *(Continued)*
- **3** ketoconazole 34
- **3** lomefloxacin 35*
- **3** methenamine 358
- **3** nifedipine 351
- **3** norfloxacin 35*
- **3** ofloxacin 36*
- **3** penicillamine 37*
- **3** pseudoephedrine 37
- **3** quinidine 38*
- **3** sodium polystyrene sulfonate resin 38*
- **3** tetracycline 39*

Dolobid
- Also see Salicylates
- **2 acenocoumarol 208**
- **2 warfarin 208***

Dolophine
- Also see Narcotic analgesics
- **3** carbamazepine 75*, 357
- **3** phenobarbital 356*
- **2 phenytoin 75, 357***
- **3** primidone 357
- **3** rifampin 357*

Donepezil
- **3** fluvoxamine 277

Dopamine
- **3** ergonovine 229*
- **3** phenytoin 230*

Dopar
- **3** chlordiazepoxide 202
- **2 chlorpromazine 95***
- **3** diazepam 201*
- **2 haloperidol 95**
- **3** iron 314*
- **3** isocarboxazid 338
- **3** methionine 337*
- **3** moclobemide 338*
- **3** nialamide 338
- **3** phenelzine 338*
- **3** phenytoin 339*
- **3** pyridoxine 339*
- **3** spiramycin 340*
- **3** tacrine 340*
- **3** tranylcypromine 338

Doriden
- **3** ethanol 249*
- **3** tacrolimus 413
- **2 warfarin 288***

Doryx
- Also see Tetracyclines
- **3** antacids 39

- **3** bismuth 56*, 57
- **3** carbamazepine 67*
- **3** iron 316
- **3** oral contraceptives 397
- **3** phenobarbital 232*
- **3** phenytoin 232*
- **3** warfarin 233*

Doxazosin
- Also see Alpha blockers
- **3** enalapril 62
- **3** indomethacin 306
- **3** nifedipine 253*
- **3** verapamil 421

Doxepin
- Also see Cyclic antidepressants; Tricyclic antidepressants
- **3** chlorpropamide 231
- **3** cimetidine 113*, 115, 121
- **3** fluoxetine 189
- **3** propoxyphene 230*
- **3** tolazamide 231*

Doxorubicin
- Also see Antineoplastics
- **3** cyclosporine 167*
- **3** tacrolimus 168
- **3** verapamil 231*

Doxychel Hyclate
- Also see Tetracyclines
- **3** antacids 39
- **3** bismuth 56*, 57
- **3** carbamazepine 67*
- **3** iron 316
- **3** oral contraceptives 397
- **3** phenobarbital 232*
- **3** phenytoin 232*
- **3** warfarin 233*

Doxycycline
- Also see Tetracyclines
- **3** antacids 39
- **3** bismuth 56*, 57
- **3** carbamazepine 67*
- **3** iron 316
- **3** oral contraceptives 397
- **3** phenobarbital 232*
- **3** phenytoin 232*
- **3** warfarin 233*

Duvoid
- Also see Cholinergics
- **3** tacrine 56*

Dyflex
- **3** probenecid 233*

Dymelor
- Also see Antidiabetics; Sulfonylureas
- **2 phenylbutazone 409**

Dynabac
- Also see Macrolides
- **3** buspirone 62
- **3** ergotamine 143
- **3** indinavir 144
- **3** itraconazole 144

DynaCirc
- Also see Calcium channel blockers
- **3** lovastatin 221, 321*
- **3** propranolol 385, 386

Dyphylline
- **3** probenecid 233*

Dyrenium
- Also see Diuretics; Potassium-sparing diuretics
- **3** diclofenac 308
- **3** ibuprofen 308
- **3** indomethacin 308*
- **2 potassium 420***

Echothiophate iodide
- **2 succinylcholine 234***

Ecotrin
- Also see Salicylates
- **3** antacids 44*

Edecrin
- Also see Diuretics; Loop diuretics
- **3** cephaloridine 86
- **2 cisplatin 140***
- **3** digoxin 211
- **3** enalapril 235
- **2 gentamicin 248***
- **2 kanamycin 248**
- **2 neomycin 248**
- **2 streptomycin 248**

Edrophonium
- Also see Cholinergics
- **3** procainamide 384
- **3** tacrine 56

EES
- Also see Macrolides
- **3** alfentanil 8*
- **3** alprazolam 13*, 62
- **1 astemizole 47***
- **3** atorvastatin 50*
- **3** bromocriptine 59*
- **3** buspirone 62*

*3* carbamazepine 65, 68*, 79
*3* chlorpropamide 99*
*2* cisapride 136*, 139
*2* clozapine 156*
*3* colchicine 160*
*3* cyclosporine 143, 168*, 244
*3* digoxin 211*
*3* disopyramide 224*
*2* ergotamine 143
*3* felodipine 242*
*3* indinavir 144, 244
*3* itraconazole 144
*3* lovastatin 51, 242*
*3* methylprednisolone 366
*3* midazolam 13, 62, 145, 243*
*3* nelfinavir 244
*3* quinidine 243*
*3* ritonavir 244*
*3* saquinavir 244
*3* simvastatin 51
*3* tacrolimus 145, 168, 244*
*1* terfenadine 48, 146, 245*, 446
*3* theophylline 245*, 449
*3* triazolam 13, 62, 243, 246*, 454
*3* valproic acid 246*
*3* warfarin 247*
*3* zafirlukast 247*
Elavil
  Also see Cyclic antidepressants; Tricyclic antidepressants
*3* carbamazepine 71
*3* cimetidine 111, 113
*2* clonidine 25, 152
*3* fluoxetine 24*
*3* guanabenz 25
*3* guanfacine 25*
*3* isoproterenol 25*
*3* lithium 26*
*2* norepinephrine 301
*3* paroxetine 24
*2* phenelzine 150, 301
*3* tolazamide 231
Eldepryl
  Also see Monoamine oxidase inhibitors
*2* dexfenfluramine 191
*2* dextroamphetamine 193
*2* dextromethorphan 197*

*2* fenfluramine 261
*2* fluoxetine 272*
*2* fluvoxamine 272
*2* meperidine 197, 355*
*3* moclobemide 377*
*3* morphine 355
*2* paroxetine 272
*2* sertraline 272
*3* tyramine 441*
Elixohyllin
*3* adenosine 7*
*3* allopurinol 12*
*3* aminoglutethimide 16*
*3* amiodarone 23*
*3* atenolol 429
*3* carbamazepine 78*
*3* cigarette smoking 108*
*3* cimetidine 127*
*3* ciprofloxacin 134*, 238, 390
*3* disulfiram 228*
*2* enoxacin 134, 238*, 390
*3* erythromycin 245*, 449
*2* fluvoxamine 278*
*3* imipenem 300*
*3* interferon 313*
*3* isoniazid 319*
*3* lithium 347*
*3* methimazole 434
*3* metoprolol 429
*2* mexiletine 373*
*3* moricizine 378*
*3* nadolol 429
*3* norfloxacin 134, 238, 390*
*3* pefloxacin 134, 238, 390, 
*3* pentobarbital 406
*3* pentoxifylline 400*
*3* phenobarbital 406*
*3* phenytoin 414*
*3* pipemidic acid 134, 238, 390
*3* propafenone 426*
*2* propranolol 429*
*3* propylthiouracil 434
*3* radioactive iodine 434*
*3* rifampin 436*
*3* ritonavir 440*
*3* secobarbital 406
*3* tacrine 444*
*3* thiabendazole 447*
*3* thyroid 448*
*3* ticlopidine 448*

*2* troleandomycin 246, 448*
*3* verapamil 449*
*3* zafirlukast 450*
E-Mycin
  Also see Macrolides
*3* alfentanil 8*
*3* alprazolam 13*, 62
*1* astemizole 47*
*3* atorvastatin 50*
*3* bromocriptine 59*
*3* buspirone 62*
*3* carbamazepine 65, 68*, 79
*3* chlorpropamide 99*
*2* cisapride 136*, 139
*2* clozapine 156*
*3* colchicine 160*
*3* cyclosporine 143, 168*, 244
*3* digoxin 211*
*3* disopyramide 224*
*2* ergotamine 143
*3* felodipine 242*
*3* indinavir 144, 244
*3* itraconazole 144
*3* lovastatin 51, 242*
*3* methylprednisolone 366
*3* midazolam 13, 62, 145, 243*
*3* nelfinavir 244
*3* quinidine 243*
*3* ritonavir 244*
*3* saquinavir 244
*3* simvastatin 51
*3* tacrolimus 145, 168, 244*
*1* terfenadine 48, 146, 245*, 446
*3* theophylline 245*, 449
*3* triazolam 13, 62, 243, 246*, 454
*3* valproic acid 246*
*3* warfarin 247*
*3* zafirlukast 247*
Enalapril
  Also see Angiotensin-converting enzyme inhibitors
*2* allopurinol 10
*3* aspirin 40
*3* bumetanide 235
*3* bunazosin 62*
*3* cyclosporine 168*
*3* doxazosin 62
*3* ethacrynic acid 235

Enalapril *(Continued)*
 *3* furosemide 234*
 *3* insulin 64
 *3* iron 235*
 *3* lithium 341
 *3* prazosin 62
 *3* terazosin 62
 *3* torsemide 235
 *3* trimazosin 62
Encainide
 Also see Antiarrhythmics
 *3* amiodarone 20
 *3* diltiazem 220*
 *3* quinidine 236*
 *3* verapamil 220
Endep
 Also see Cyclic antidepressants; Tricyclic antide-
 pressants
 *3* carbamazepine 71
 *3* cimetidine 111, 113
 *2* **clonidine 25, 152**
 *3* fluoxetine 24*
 *3* guanabenz 25
 *3* guanfacine 25*
 *3* isoproterenol 25*
 *3* lithium 26*
 *2* **norepinephrine 301**
 *3* paroxetine 24
 *2* **phenelzine 150, 301**
 *3* tolazamide 231
Enkaid
 Also see Antiarrhythmics
 *3* amiodarone 20
 *3* diltiazem 220*
 *3* quinidine 236*
 *3* verapamil 220
Enlon
 Also see Cholinergics
 *3* procainamide 384
 *3* tacrine 56
Enoxacin
 Also see Quinolones
 *3* antacids 31*
 *3* cimetidine 31
 *3* famotidine 236
 *3* lansoprazole 31, 236
 *3* metoprolol 132
 *3* nizatidine 31, 236
 *3* omeprazole 31, 236
 *3* pentoxifylline 133
 *3* phenytoin 133

 *3* ranitidine 31, 236*
 *3* tacrine 237*
 *2* **theophylline 134, 238*, 390**
 *3* zinc 135
Enprostil
 Also see Prostaglandins
 *3* ethanol 238*
Enteric-coated aspirin
 Also see Salicylates
 *3* antacids 44*
Ephedrine
 Also see
 Sympathomimetics
 *3* antacids 31*, 37
 *3* furazolidone 192
 *3* guanadrel 239
 *3* guanethidine 239*
 *2* **moclobemide 239***
 *3* sodium bicarbonate 31*
Epinephrine
 Also see
 Sympathomimetics
 *3* alprenolol 240
 *3* chlorpromazine 93*
 *3* clozapine 93
 *2* **imipramine 240***
 *3* labetalol 240
 *3* nadolol 240
 *3* pindolol 240
 *3* propranolol 240*, 429
 *2* **protriptyline 240**
 *3* thioridazine 93
 *3* timolol 240
Equanil
 *3* ethanol 250*
Ergonovine
 *3* dopamine 229*
Ergostat
 *3* dopamine 229*
Ergotamine
 *3* azithromycin 143
 *2* **clarithromycin 143***
 *3* dirithromycin 143
 *2* **erythromycin 143**
 *2* **nitroglycerin 241***
Ergotrate maleate
 *3* dopamine 229*
Eryc
 Also see Macrolides
 *3* alfentanil 8*
 *3* alprazolam 13*, 62

 *1* **astemizole 47***
 *3* atorvastatin 50*
 *3* bromocriptine 59*
 *3* buspirone 62*
 *3* carbamazepine 65, 68*, 79
 *3* chlorpropamide 99*
 *2* **cisapride 136*, 139**
 *2* **clozapine 156***
 *3* colchicine 160*
 *3* cyclosporine 143, 168*, 244
 *3* digoxin 211*
 *3* disopyramide 224*
 *2* **ergotamine 143**
 *3* felodipine 242*
 *3* indinavir 144, 244
 *3* itraconazole 144
 *3* lovastatin 51, 242*
 *3* methylprednisolone 366
 *3* midazolam 13, 62, 145, 243*
 *3* nelfinavir 244
 *3* quinidine 243*
 *3* ritonavir 244*
 *3* saquinavir 244
 *3* simvastatin 51
 *3* tacrolimus 145, 168, 244*
 *1* **terfenadine 48, 146, 245*, 446**
 *3* theophylline 245*, 449
 *3* triazolam 13, 62, 243, 246*, 454
 *3* valproic acid 246*
 *3* warfarin 247*
 *3* zafirlukast 247*
EryPed
 Also see Macrolides
 *3* alfentanil 8*
 *3* alprazolam 13*, 62
 *1* **astemizole 47***
 *3* atorvastatin 50*
 *3* bromocriptine 59*
 *3* buspirone 62*
 *3* carbamazepine 65, 68*, 79
 *3* chlorpropamide 99*
 *2* **cisapride 136*, 139**
 *2* **clozapine 156***
 *3* colchicine 160*
 *3* cyclosporine 143, 168*, 244
 *3* digoxin 211*
 *3* disopyramide 224*

*2* ergotamine 143
*3* felodipine 242*
*3* indinavir 144, 244
*3* itraconazole 144
*3* lovastatin 51, 242*
*3* methylprednisolone 366
*3* midazolam 13, 62, 145, 243*
*3* nelfinavir 244
*3* quinidine 243*
*3* ritonavir 244*
*3* saquinavir 244
*3* simvastatin 51
*3* tacrolimus 145, 168, 244*
*1* terfenadine 48, 146, 245*, 446
*3* theophylline 245*, 449
*3* triazolam 13, 62, 243, 246*, 454
*3* valproic acid 246*
*3* warfarin 247*
*3* zafirlukast 247*
Ery-Tab
Also see Macrolides
*3* alfentanil 8*
*3* alprazolam 13*, 62
*1* astemizole 47*
*3* atorvastatin 50*
*3* bromocriptine 59*
*3* buspirone 62*
*3* carbamazepine 65, 68*, 79
*3* chlorpropamide 99*
*2* cisapride 136*, 139
*2* clozapine 156*
*3* colchicine 160*
*3* cyclosporine 143, 168*, 244
*3* digoxin 211*
*3* disopyramide 224*
*2* ergotamine 143
*3* felodipine 242*
*3* indinavir 144, 244
*3* itraconazole 144
*3* lovastatin 51, 242*
*3* methylprednisolone 366
*3* midazolam 13, 62, 145, 243*
*3* nelfinavir 244
*3* quinidine 243*
*3* ritonavir 244*
*3* saquinavir 244
*3* simvastatin 51

*3* tacrolimus 145, 168, 244*
*1* terfenadine 48, 146, 245*, 446
*3* theophylline 245*, 449
*3* triazolam 13, 62, 243, 246*, 454
*3* valproic acid 246*
*3* warfarin 247*
*3* zafirlukast 247*
Erythrocin
Also see Macrolides
*3* alfentanil 8*
*3* alprazolam 13*, 62
*1* astemizole 47*
*3* atorvastatin 50*
*3* bromocriptine 59*
*3* buspirone 62*
*3* carbamazepine 65, 68*, 79
*3* chlorpropamide 99*
*2* cisapride 136*, 139
*2* clozapine 156*
*3* colchicine 160*
*3* cyclosporine 143, 168*, 244
*3* digoxin 211*
*3* disopyramide 224*
*2* ergotamine 143
*3* felodipine 242*
*3* indinavir 144, 244
*3* itraconazole 144
*3* lovastatin 51, 242*
*3* methylprednisolone 366
*3* midazolam 13, 62, 145, 243*
*3* nelfinavir 244
*3* quinidine 243*
*3* ritonavir 244*
*3* saquinavir 244
*3* simvastatin 51
*3* tacrolimus 145, 168, 244*
*1* terfenadine 48, 146, 245*, 446
*3* theophylline 245*, 449
*3* triazolam 13, 62, 243, 246*, 454
*3* valproic acid 246*
*3* warfarin 247*
*3* zafirlukast 247*
Erythromycin
Also see Macrolides
*3* alfentanil 8*
*3* alprazolam 13*, 62

*1* astemizole 47*
*3* atorvastatin 50*
*3* bromocriptine 59*
*3* buspirone 62*
*3* carbamazepine 65, 68*, 79
*3* chlorpropamide 99*
*2* cisapride 136*, 139
*2* clozapine 156*
*3* colchicine 160*
*3* cyclosporine 143, 168*, 244
*3* digoxin 211*
*3* disopyramide 224*
*2* ergotamine 143
*3* felodipine 242*
*3* indinavir 144, 244
*3* itraconazole 144
*3* lovastatin 51, 242*
*3* methylprednisolone 366
*3* midazolam 13, 62, 145, 243*
*3* nelfinavir 244
*3* quinidine 243*
*3* ritonavir 244*
*3* saquinavir 244
*3* simvastatin 51
*3* tacrolimus 145, 168, 244*
*1* terfenadine 48, 146, 245*, 446
*3* theophylline 245*, 449
*3* triazolam 13, 62, 243, 246*, 454
*3* valproic acid 246*
*3* warfarin 247*
*3* zafirlukast 247*
Erythromycin base
Also see Macrolides
*3* alfentanil 8*
*3* alprazolam 13*, 62
*1* astemizole 47*
*3* atorvastatin 50*
*3* bromocriptine 59*
*3* buspirone 62*
*3* carbamazepine 65, 68*, 79
*3* chlorpropamide 99*
*2* cisapride 136*, 139
*2* clozapine 156*
*3* colchicine 160*
*3* cyclosporine 143, 168*, 244
*3* digoxin 211*

Erythromycin base *(Continued)*
 *3* disopyramide 224*
 *2* **ergotamine 143**
 *3* felodipine 242*
 *3* indinavir 144, 244
 *3* itraconazole 144
 *3* lovastatin 51, 242*
 *3* methylprednisolone 366
 *3* midazolam 13, 62, 145, 243*
 *3* nelfinavir 244
 *3* quinidine 243*
 *3* ritonavir 244*
 *3* saquinavir 244
 *3* simvastatin 51
 *3* tacrolimus 145, 168, 244*
 *1* **terfenadine 48, 146, 245*, 446**
 *3* theophylline 245*, 449
 *3* triazolam 13, 62, 243, 246*, 454
 *3* valproic acid 246*
 *3* warfarin 247*
 *3* zafirlukast 247*
Erythromycin lactinobionate
 Also see Macrolides
 *3* alfentanil 8*
 *3* alprazolam 13*, 62
 *1* **astemizole 47***
 *3* atorvastatin 50*
 *3* bromocriptine 59*
 *3* buspirone 62*
 *3* carbamazepine 65, 68*, 79
 *3* chlorpropamide 99*
 *2* **cisapride 136*, 139**
 *2* **clozapine 156***
 *3* colchicine 160*
 *3* cyclosporine 143, 168*, 244
 *3* digoxin 211*
 *3* disopyramide 224*
 *2* **ergotamine 143**
 *3* felodipine 242*
 *3* indinavir 144, 244
 *3* itraconazole 144
 *3* lovastatin 51, 242*
 *3* methylprednisolone 366
 *3* midazolam 13, 62, 145, 243*
 *3* nelfinavir 244
 *3* quinidine 243*
 *3* ritonavir 244*

 *3* saquinavir 244
 *3* simvastatin 51
 *3* tacrolimus 145, 168, 244*
 *1* **terfenadine 48, 146, 245*, 446**
 *3* theophylline 245*, 449
 *3* triazolam 13, 62, 243, 246*, 454
 *3* valproic acid 246*
 *3* warfarin 247*
 *3* zafirlukast 247*
Eryzole
 Also see Macrolides
 *3* alfentanil 8*
 *3* alprazolam 13*, 62
 *1* **astemizole 47***
 *3* atorvastatin 50*
 *3* bromocriptine 59*
 *3* buspirone 62*
 *3* carbamazepine 65, 68*, 79
 *3* chlorpropamide 99*
 *2* **cisapride 136*, 139**
 *2* **clozapine 156***
 *3* colchicine 160*
 *3* cyclosporine 143, 168*, 244
 *3* digoxin 211*
 *3* disopyramide 224*
 *2* **ergotamine 143**
 *3* felodipine 242*
 *3* indinavir 144, 244
 *3* itraconazole 144
 *3* lovastatin 51, 242*
 *3* methylprednisolone 366
 *3* midazolam 13, 62, 145, 243*
 *3* nelfinavir 244
 *3* quinidine 243*
 *3* ritonavir 244*
 *3* saquinavir 244
 *3* simvastatin 51
 *3* tacrolimus 145, 168, 244*
 *1* **terfenadine 48, 146, 245*, 446**
 *3* theophylline 245*, 449
 *3* triazolam 13, 62, 243, 246*, 454
 *3* valproic acid 246*
 *3* warfarin 247*
 *3* zafirlukast 247*
Eserine
 *3* propranolol 384

Eskalith
 *3* amitriptyline 26*
 *3* bromfenac 57*
 *3* carbamazepine 74*
 *3* chlorpromazine 95*
 *3* diclofenac 204*
 *3* diltiazem 348
 *3* enalapril 341
 *3* fluoxetine 270*
 *3* fluvoxamine 277*
 *3* haloperidol 95, 296*
 *3* ibuprofen 298*
 *3* indomethacin 304*
 *2* **isocarboxazid 344**
 *3* ketorolac 336*
 *3* lisinopril 341*
 *3* losartan 342*
 *3* mefenamic acid 342*
 *3* methyldopa 343*
 *3* naproxen 343*
 *2* **phenelzine 344**
 *3* phenylbutazone 345*
 *3* phenytoin 345*
 *3* piroxicam 345*
 *3* potassium iodide 346*
 *3* sodium bicarbonate 346*
 *3* sodium chloride 347*
 *3* theophylline 347*
 *3* thioridazine 95
 *2* **tranylcypromine 344**
 *3* verapamil 348*
Estrogens
 Also see Ethinyl estradiol
 *3* ampicillin 28*
 *3* carbamazepine 76*, 394
 *1* **cigarette smoking 107***
 *3* cyclosporine 165, 179*
 *3* dexamethasone 395
 *2* **dicumarol 397**
 *3* doxycycline 397
 *3* griseofulvin 292*
 *3* hydrocortisone 395
 *3* methylprednisolone 395
 *3* phenobarbital 394*
 *2* **phenprocoumon 397**
 *3* phenytoin 394*
 *3* prednisolone 395*
 *3* prednisone 395
 *3* primidone 394
 *3* rifabutin 396
 *3* rifampin 395*

*3* ritonavir 396*
*3* tetracycline 397*
*2* **warfarin 397***
Ethacrynic acid
Also see Diuretics; Loop
diuretics
*3* cephaloridine 86
*2* **cisplatin 140***
*3* digoxin 211
*3* enalapril 235
*2* **gentamicin 248***
*2* **kanamycin 248**
*2* **neomycin 248**
*2* **streptomycin 248**
Ethanol
*3* acetaminophen 1*
*3* aspirin 42*
*3* bromazepam 199
*3* cefamandole 83*
*3* cefoperazone 84
*3* cefotetan 84
*3* chloral hydrate 86*
*3* chlordiazepoxide 199
*1* **chlorpropamide 99***
*3* diazepam 199*
*1* **disulfiram 226***
*3* enprostil 238*
*3* furazolidone 248*
*3* glutethimide 249*
*1* **insulin 99**
*1* **isocarbazid 252**
*3* isoniazid 249*
*3* ketoconazole 250*
*3* lorazepam 199
*3* meperidine 250*
*3* meprobamate 250*
*1* **methotrexate 251***
*3* metoclopramide 251*
*3* metronidazole 252*
*3* moxalactam 84
*2* **nifedipine 256**
*3* nitrazepam 199
*3* oxazepam 199
*3* pentobarbital 253
*1* **phenelzine 252***
*1* **phenformin 99**
*3* phenobarbital 253*
*3* phenprocoumon 256
*3* phenytoin 254*
*1* **procarbazine 254***
*3* propoxyphene 254*
*1* **tolbutamide 99, 255***

*1* **tranylcypromine 252**
*2* **verapamil 255***
*3* warfarin 256*
Ethinyl estradiol
Also see Estrogens
*3* ampicillin 28*
*3* carbamazepine 76*, 394
*1* **cigarette smoking 107***
*3* cyclosporine 165, 179*
*3* dexamethasone 395
*2* **dicumarol 397**
*3* doxycycline 397
*3* griseofulvin 292*
*3* hydrocortisone 395
*3* methylprednisolone 395
*3* phenobarbital 394*
*2* **phenprocoumon 397**
*3* phenytoin 394*
*3* prednisolone 395*
*3* prednisone 395
*3* primidone 394
*3* rifabutin 396
*3* rifampin 395*
*3* ritonavir 396*
*3* tetracycline 397*
*2* **warfarin 397***
Ethmozine
Also see Antiarrhythmics
*3* cimetidine 118*
*3* theophylline 378*
Ethyl alcohol
*3* acetaminophen 1*
*3* aspirin 42*
*3* bromazepam 199
*3* cefamandole 83*
*3* cefoperazone 84
*3* cefotetan 84
*3* chloral hydrate 86*
*3* chlordiazepoxide 199
*1* **chlorpropamide 99***
*3* diazepam 199*
*1* **disulfiram 226***
*3* enprostil 238*
*3* furazolidone 248*
*3* glutethimide 249*
*1* **insulin 99**
*1* **isocarbazid 252**
*3* isoniazid 249*
*3* ketoconazole 250*
*3* lorazepam 199
*3* meperidine 250*
*3* meprobamate 250*
*1* **methotrexate 251***

*3* metoclopramide 251*
*3* metronidazole 252*
*3* moxalactam 84
*2* **nifedipine 256**
*3* nitrazepam 199
*3* oxazepam 199
*3* pentobarbital 253
*1* **phenelzine 252***
*1* **phenformin 99**
*3* phenobarbital 253*
*3* phenprocoumon 256
*3* phenytoin 254*
*1* **procarbazine 254***
*3* propoxyphene 254*
*1* **tolbutamide 99, 255***
*1* **tranylcypromine 252**
*2* **verapamil 255***
*3* warfarin 256*
Ethyl biscoumacetate
Also see Anticoagulants
*2* **phenobarbital 408**
Ethynodiol diacetate
*3* ampicillin 28*
*3* carbamazepine 76*, 394
*1* **cigarette smoking 107***
*3* cyclosporine 165, 179*
*3* dexamethasone 395
*2* **dicumarol 397**
*3* doxycycline 397
*3* griseofulvin 292*
*3* hydrocortisone 395
*3* methylprednisolone 395
*3* phenobarbital 394*
*2* **phenprocoumon 397**
*3* phenytoin 394*
*3* prednisolone 395*
*3* prednisone 395
*3* primidone 394
*3* rifabutin 396
*3* rifampin 395*
*3* tetracycline 397*
*2* **warfarin 397***
Etodolac
Also see Nonsteroidal anti-
inflammatory drugs
*2* **warfarin 257***
Etretinate
*2* **methotrexate 258***
Famotidine
Also see H$_2$-receptor
antagonists
*3* cefpodoxime 29, 84

Famotidine *(Continued)*
  *3* cefuroxime 85
  *3* enoxacin 31, 236
  *3* glipizide 32, 287
  *3* glyburide 32
  *3* ketoconazole 115, 329
  *3* nifedipine 119
  *3* nisoldipine 120
  *3* nitrendipine 120
  *3* tolbutamide 128
Fansidar
  *3* chlorpromazine 91
Felbamate
  *3* carbamazepine 69*
  *3* phenobarbital 258*
  *3* phenytoin 259*
  *3* valproic acid 259*
Felbatol
  *3* carbamazepine 69*
  *3* phenobarbital 258*
  *3* phenytoin 259*
  *3* valproic acid 259*
Feldene
  Also see Nonsteroidal anti-
    inflammatory drugs
  *2* acenocoumarol 418
  *3* cholestyramine 104*
  *3* colestipol 104
  *3* furosemide 281
  *3* lithium 345*
  *3* propranolol 307
  *2* warfarin 418*
Felodipine
  Also see Calcium channel
    blockers; Dihydropyri-
    dine calcium channel
    blockers
  *2* carbamazepine 69*
  *3* cyclosporine 169*
  *3* erythromycin 242*
  *3* fluconazole 260
  *3* grapefruit juice 290
  *3* itraconazole 260*
  *3* ketoconazole 260
  *3* miconazole 260
  *3* propranolol 386
  *3* troleandomycin 242
Femoxetine
  *3* cimetidine 113*
Fenfluramine
  *2* fluoxetine 191, 260*
  *2* fluvoxamine 260

*1* isocarboxazid 261
*2* paroxetine 260
*1* phenelzine 191, 261*
*2* selegiline 261
*2* sertraline 260
*1* tranylcypromine 261
Fenoprofen
  Also see Nonsteroidal anti-
    inflammatory drugs
  *2* warfarin 262*
Fentanyl
  Also see Narcotic
    analgesics
  *3* diltiazem 8
Flagyl
  *3* carbamazepine 75*
  *3* cholestyramine 103*
  *3* colestipol 103
  *3* diazepam 252, 370
  *3* disulfiram 227*
  *3* ethanol 252*
  *2* fluorouracil 268*
  *3* nitroglycerin 252, 370
  *3* phenytoin 252, 369*, 370
  *3* trimethoprim-sul-
    famethoxazole 252, 370*
  *2* warfarin 370*
Flecainide
  Also see Antiarrhythmics
  *3* amiodarone 20*
  *3* cimetidine 114*
  *3* propranolol 262*, 263
  *3* sotalol 263*
Floxin
  Also see Quinolones
  *3* aluminum 36*, 392
  *3* antacids 30, 35, 36*
  *3* Maalox 36*
  *3* magnesium 36*
  *3* procainamide 391*
  *3* sucralfate 134, 390, 392
  *3* warfarin 135, 391, 392*
Floxyfral
  Also see Selective sero-
    tonin reuptake inhibitors
  *3* alprazolam 14
  *1* astemizole 48*, 278
  *3* carbamazepine 70*
  *3* clomipramine 148*
  *2* clozapine 156*
  *2* dexfenfluramine 191
  *3* diazepam 200

*3* donepezil 277
*2* fenfluramine 260
*3* lithium 277*
*2* selegiline 272
*2* tacrine 277*
*1* terfenadine 48, 273,
    278*
*2* theophylline 278*
*1* tranylcypromine 273
*3* warfarin 279*
Fluconazole
  Also see Antifungals;
    Imidazoles
  *1* astemizole 49
  *3* chlordiazepoxide 90
  *2* cisapride 137, 138, 139
  *3* cyclosporine 170*, 173,
    174, 177, 265
  *3* diazepam 201, 264, 267
  *3* felodipine 260
  *2* lorazepam 267
  *3* losartan 263*
  *2* lovastatin 321, 326
  *3* midazolam 264*, 267,
    322, 327
  *3* phenytoin 264*
  *3* quinidine 329
  *3* rifampin 265*, 323, 330
  *3* tacrolimus 155, 170,
    265*, 332
  *3* terfenadine 266*, 323,
    332
  *3* tolbutamide 266*
  *2* triazolam 264, 267*,
    324, 333
  *3* warfarin 268*, 324, 333
Fluogen
  *3* phenytoin 310*
Fluorouracil
  Also see Antineoplastics
  *2* metronidazole 268*
  *3* warfarin 269*
Fluoxetine
  Also see Selective sero-
    tonin reuptake inhibitors
  *3* alprazolam 14*, 200
  *3* amitriptyline 24*
  *2* astemizole 272
  *3* bumetanide 269
  *3* buspirone 63*
  *3* carbamazepine 70*
  *3* cyproheptadine 185*
  *3* desipramine 188*

Furosemide *(Continued)*
  *3* cephalothin 86
  *3* cholestyramine 101*, 161
  *3* cisplatin 140
  *3* clofibrate 147*
  *3* colestipol 101, 161*
  *3* digitoxin 211
  *3* digoxin 211*
  *3* enalapril 234*
  *3* fluoxetine 269*
  *3* flurbiprofen 281
  *3* ibuprofen 281
  *3* indomethacin 61, 281*,
    308
  *3* naproxen 281
  *3* paroxetine 269
  *3* phenobarbital 282
  *3* phenytoin 281*
  *3* piroxicam 281
  *3* sertraline 269
  *3* sulindac 281
  *3* terbutaline 282*
Furoxone
  *3* dextroamphetamine 192*,
    193
  *3* ephedrine 192
  *3* ethanol 248*
  *3* phenylpropanolamine 192
Gamma globulin
  *3* phenytoin 282*
Ganciclovir
  Also see Antivirals
  *3* didanosine 206*
  *1* zidovudine 283*
Gantanol
  Also see Sulfonamides
  *2* para-aminobenzoic acid
    399*
  *3* phenytoin 413, 416
  *3* warfarin 455
Gantrisin
  Also see Sulfonamides
  *3* tolbutamide 451
Garamycin
  Also see Aminoglycosides
  *3* amphotericin B 27*
  *2* atracurium 51*
  *3* carboplatin 82*, 141
  *3* cisplatin 141*
  *3* cyclosporine 170*
  *2* ethacrynic acid 248*

  *3* indomethacin 286*
  *3* methoxyflurane 365
  *2* succinylcholine 51
  *3* vancomycin 286*
  *2* vecuronium 51
Gaviscon
  Also see Antacids
  *3* allopurinol 9*
  *3* aspirin 29*
  *3* cefpodoxime 29*
  *3* cefuroxime 85
  *3* ciprofloxacin 30*, 130,
    134
  *3* glipizide 32*
  *3* glyburide 32*
  *3* iron 33*
  *3* isoniazid 34*
  *3* ketoconazole 34
  *3* lomefloxacin 35*
  *3* methenamine 358
  *3* nifedipine 351
  *3* norfloxacin 35*, 36, 390
  *3* ofloxacin 35, 36*, 392
  *3* penicillamine 37*
  *3* pseudoephedrine 37
  *3* quinidine 38*
  *3* sodium polystyrene sul-
    fonate resin 38*
  *3* tetracycline 39*
Gelusil
  Also see Antacids
  *3* allopurinol 9*
  *3* aspirin 29*
  *3* cefpodoxime 29*
  *3* cefuroxime 85
  *3* ciprofloxacin 30*, 130,
    134
  *3* glipizide 32*
  *3* glyburide 32*
  *3* iron 33*
  *3* isoniazid 34*
  *3* ketoconazole 34
  *3* lomefloxacin 35*
  *3* methenamine 358
  *3* nifedipine 351
  *3* norfloxacin 35*, 36, 390
  *3* ofloxacin 35, 36*, 392
  *3* penicillamine 37*
  *3* pseudoephedrine 37
  *3* quinidine 38*
  *3* sodium polystyrene sul-
    fonate resin 38*
  *3* tetracycline 39*

Gemfibrozil
  *3* cholestyramine 161
  *3* colestipol 161*
  *3* glyburide 283*
  *2* lovastatin 284*, 285
  *3* pravastatin 284, 285*
  *2* simvastatin 284, 285
  *2* warfarin 148, 285*, 350
Genora
  Also see Estrogens
  *3* ampicillin 28*
  *3* carbamazepine 76*, 394
  *1* cigarette smoking 107*
  *3* cyclosporine 165, 179*
  *3* dexamethasone 395
  *2* dicumarol 397
  *3* doxycycline 397
  *3* griseofulvin 292*
  *3* hydrocortisone 395
  *3* methylprednisolone 395
  *3* phenobarbital 394*
  *2* phenprocoumon 397
  *3* phenytoin 394*
  *3* prednisolone 395*
  *3* prednisone 395
  *3* primidone 394
  *3* rifabutin 396
  *3* rifampin 395*
  *3* ritonavir 396*
  *3* tetracycline 397*
  *2* warfarin 397*
Gentamicin
  Also see Aminoglycosides
  *3* amphotericin B 27*
  *2* atracurium 51*
  *3* carboplatin 82*, 141
  *3* cisplatin 141*
  *3* cyclosporine 170*
  *2* ethacrynic acid 248*
  *3* indomethacin 286*
  *3* methoxyflurane 365
  *2* succinylcholine 51
  *3* vancomycin 286*
  *2* vecuronium 51
Gen-Xene
  Also see Anticonvulsants;
    Benzodiazepines
  *3* cimetidine 111
  *3* disulfiram 198
  *3* rifampin 203

Geocillin
Also see Penicillins
**3** methotrexate 82*
Glipizide
Also see Antidiabetics;
Sulfonylureas
**3** aluminum 32*
**3** antacids 32*
**3** cimetidine 32, 128, 287
**3** cyclosporine 170*
**3** famotidine 32, 287
**3** lansoprazole 287
**3** magnesium 32*
**3** nizatidine 32, 287
**3** omeprazole 287
**3** ranitidine 32, 287*
**3** sodium bicarbonate 32*
**3** tacrolimus 170
**3** trimethoprim-sul-
famethoxazole 451
Glucagon
**3** acenocoumarol 288
**3** warfarin 288*
Glucotrol
Also see Antidiabetics;
Sulfonylureas
**3** aluminum 32*
**3** antacids 32*
**3** cimetidine 32, 128, 287
**3** cyclosporine 170*
**3** famotidine 32, 287
**3** lansoprazole 287
**3** magnesium 32*
**3** nizatidine 32, 287
**3** omeprazole 287
**3** ranitidine 32, 287*
**3** sodium bicarbonate 32*
**3** tacrolimus 170
**3** trimethoprim-sul-
famethoxazole 451
Glutethimide
**3** ethanol 249*
**3** tacrolimus 413
**2 warfarin 288***
Glyburide
Also see Antidiabetics;
Sulfonylureas
**3** aluminum 32*
**3** antacids 32*
**3** aspirin 41
**3** cimetidine 32, 128
**3** famotidine 32

**3** gemfibrozil 283*
**3** lansoprazole 32
**3** Maalox 32*
**3** magnesium 32*
**3** nizatidine 32
**3** omeprazole 32
**3** rifampin 437
**3** trimethoprim-sul-
famethoxazole 451
**3** warfarin 289*
Grapefruit juice
**3** alprazolam 291
**3** astemizole 290
**3** clomipramine 149*
**3** cyclosporine 171*
**3** felodipine 290
**3** midazolam 291
**3** nifedipine 289*
**3** nisoldipine 290
**3** nitrendipine 290
**3** tacrolimus 171
**3** terfenadine 290*
**3** triazolam 291*
Grifulvin
Also see Antifungals
**3** aspirin 43*
**3** cyclosporine 172*
**3** oral contraceptives 292*
**3** phenobarbital 292*
**3** tacrolimus 172
**3** warfarin 293*
Grisactin
Also see Antifungals
**3** aspirin 43*
**3** cyclosporine 172*
**3** oral contraceptives 292*
**3** phenobarbital 292*
**3** tacrolimus 172
**3** warfarin 293*
Griseofulvin
Also see Antifungals
**3** aspirin 43*
**3** cyclosporine 172*
**3** oral contraceptives 292*
**3** phenobarbital 292*
**3** tacrolimus 172
**3** warfarin 293*
Guanabenz
Also see Alpha agonists
**3** amitriptyline 25

**2 desipramine 152**
**3** insulin 153
**3** nitroprusside 153
**3** propranolol 154
Guanadrel
**3** chlorpromazine 94
**3** desipramine 190
**3** dextroamphetamine 192
**3** ephedrine 239
**3** methylphenidate 294
**3** norepinephrine 294
**3** phenelzine 295
Guanethidine
**3** chlorpromazine 94*
**3** desipramine 189*
**3** dextroamphetamine 192*
**3** ephedrine 239*
**3** haloperidol 293*
**3** imipramine 190
**3** isocarboxazid 295
**3** methylphenidate 294*
**3** norepinephrine 294*
**3** phenelzine 295*
**3** phenylephrine 295*
**3** thiothixene 295*
**3** tranylcypromine 295
Guanfacine
Also see Alpha agonists
**3** amitriptyline 25*
**2 desipramine 152**
**3** imipramine 25
**3** insulin 153
**3** nitroprusside 153
**3** propranolol 154
$H_2$-receptor antagonists
Also see Cimetidine; Fam-
otidine; Nizatidine;
Ranitidine
**2 acenocoumarol 129**
**3** alfentanil 7*
**3** alprazolam 111
**3** amiodarone 18*
**3** amitriptyline 111, 113
**3** amoxapine 111, 113
**3** carmustine 83*
**3** cefpodoxime 29, 84*, 85*
**3** cefuroxime 84, 85*
**3** chloramphenicol 83
**3** chlordiazepoxide 111
**3** cisapride 109*
**3** citalopram 109*

H₂-receptor antagonists
*(Continued)*
**3** clorazepate 111
**3** clozapine 110*
**3** desipramine 110*, 113, 115, 121
**3** desmethyldiazepam 111
**3** diazepam 111*
**3** dilevalol 125
**3** diltiazem 112*, 119, 120, 128
**3** doxepin 113*, 115, 121
**3** enoxacin 31, 236*
**3** femoxetine 113*
**3** flecainide 114*
**3** glipizide 32, 128, 287*
**3** glyburide 32, 128
**3** halazepam 111
**3** imipramine 113, 115*, 121
**3** ketoconazole 115*, 328, 329*
**3** labetalol 125
**3** lidocaine 116*
**3** lomustine 83
**3** maprotiline 111, 113
**3** melphalan 117*
**3** meperidine 117*
**3** metoprolol 125
**3** moricizine 118*
**3** nicotine 118*
**3** nifedipine 112, 119*, 120, 128
**3** nimodipine 119*
**3** nisoldipine 112, 119, 120*, 128
**3** nitrendipine 112, 119, 120*, 128
**3** nortriptyline 113, 115, 121*
**3** paroxetine 122*
**3** phenytoin 83, 122*
**3** pindolol 125
**3** prazepam 111
**3** praziquantel 123*
**3** procainamide 124*
**3** propafenone 124*
**3** propranolol 125*
**3** protriptyline 111, 113, 121
**3** quinidine 38, 126*
**3** tacrine 126*
**3** theophylline 127*

**3** tolbutamide 127*, 128
**3** trazodone 111, 113
**3** triazolam 111
**3** trimipramine 111, 113
**3** verapamil 112, 119, 120, 128*
**2 warfarin 129***
Habitrol
**3** cimetidine 118*
Halazepam
Also see Benzodiazepines
**3** cimetidine 111
**3** disulfiram 198
**3** rifampin 203
Halcion
Also see Benzodiazepines
**3** carbamazepine 76
**3** cimetidine 111
**3** clarithromycin 246, 454
**3** disulfiram 198
**3** erythromycin 13, 62, 243, 246*, 454
**2 fluconazole 264, 267*, 324, 333**
**3** grapefruit juice 291*
**3** isoniazid 201, 319*
**2 itraconazole 63, 201, 322, 324*, 333**
**3** ketoconazole 90, 324, 333*
**3** miconazole 333
**3** phenytoin 375
**3** rifabutin 438
**3** rifampin 438*
**3** troleandomycin 246, 454*
Haldol
Also see Neuroleptics
**3** benztropine 54*
**3** bromocriptine 61
**3** carbamazepine 71*
**3** clonidine 93
**3** fluoxetine 270*
**3** guanethidine 293*
**2 levodopa 95**
**3** lithium 95, 296*
**3** orphenadrine 55
**3** paroxetine 270
**3** phenobarbital 97
**3** quinidine 297*
**3** trihexyphenidyl 55

Halofed
Also see Sympatho-
mimetics
**3** aluminum 37*
**3** antacids 37*
**1 isocarboxazid 402**
**3** magnesium 37*
**2 moclobemide 239**
**1 phenelzine 402***
**3** sodium bicarbonate 37*
**1 tranylcypromine 402**
Haloperidol
Also see Neuroleptics
**3** benztropine 54*
**3** bromocriptine 61
**3** carbamazepine 71*
**3** clonidine 93
**3** fluoxetine 270*
**3** guanethidine 293*
**2 levodopa 95**
**3** lithium 95, 296*
**3** orphenadrine 55
**3** paroxetine 270
**3** phenobarbital 97
**3** quinidine 297*
**3** trihexyphenidyl 55
Heparin
Also see Anticoagulants
**3** warfarin 297*
Heptabarbital
Also see Barbiturates
**2 warfarin 408**
Hexadrol
Also see Corticosteroids
**3** aminoglutethimide 15*
**3** oral contraceptives 395
**3** phenobarbital 403
Hexalen
Also see Antineoplastics
**3** imipramine 14*
Hiprex
**3** acetazolamide 358
**3** aluminum 358
**3** magnesium 358
**3** sodium bicarbonate 358*
**3** sulfadiazine 359*
**3** sulfamethizole 359
**3** sulfathiazole 359
Hismanal
**2 clarithromycin 48, 146**
**1 erythromycin 47***

Ilotycin *(Continued)*
*3* carbamazepine 65, 68*, 79
*3* chlorpropamide 99*
*2* **cisapride 136*, 139**
*2* **clozapine 156***
*3* colchicine 160*
*3* cyclosporine 143, 168*, 244
*3* digoxin 211*
*3* disopyramide 224*
*2* **ergotamine 143**
*3* felodipine 242*
*3* indinavir 144, 244
*3* itraconazole 144
*3* lovastatin 51, 242*
*3* methylprednisolone 366
*3* midazolam 13, 62, 145, 243*
*3* nelfinavir 244
*3* quinidine 243*
*3* ritonavir 244*
*3* saquinavir 244
*3* simvastatin 51
*3* tacrolimus 145, 168, 244*
*1* **terfenadine 48, 146, 245*, 446**
*3* theophylline 245*, 449
*3* triazolam 13, 62, 243, 246*, 454
*3* valproic acid 246*
*3* warfarin 247*
*3* zafirlukast 247*

Imidazoles
Also see Fluconazole; Itraconazole; Ketoconazole; Miconazole
*3* alprazolam 90, 322, 327, 333
*3* aluminum 34
*3* antacids 34*
*1* **astemizole 48, 49*, 323**
*2* **atorvastatin 321, 326**
*3* azithromycin 144
*3* buspirone 63*
*3* calcium 34
*3* cetirizine 49
*3* chlordiazepoxide 90*, 201
*3* cimetidine 115*, 328, 329
*2* **cisapride 136, 137*, 138*, 139***
*3* clarithromycin 144*

*3* cyclosporine 170*, 172, 173*, 174*, 177*, 265, 332
*3* diazepam 201*, 264, 267, 324
*3* didanosine 207*
*3* digoxin 213*
*3* dirithromycin 144
*3* erythromycin 144
*3* ethanol 250*
*3* famotidine 115, 329
*3* felodipine 260*
*3* fluvastatin 321, 326
*3* indinavir 303*, 330
*3* lansoprazole 328, 329
*3* loratadine 49, 323, 326*
*2* **lorazepam 267**
*3* losartan 263*
*2* **lovastatin 321*, 326***
*3* magnesium 34
*3* methylprednisolone 327*
*3* midazolam 90, 201, 264*, 267, 322*, 324, 327*, 333
*3* nizatidine 115, 329
*3* omeprazole 328*, 329
*2* **phenytoin 322***
*3* phenytoin 264*
*3* pravastatin 321, 326
*3* quinidine 329*
*3* ranitidine 115, 328, 329*
*3* rifampin 265*, 323*, 330*
*3* ritonavir 303
*3* saquinavir 303, 330*
*2* **simvastatin 326**
*3* simvastatin 321
*3* sodium bicarbonate 34*
*3* tacrolimus 155, 170, 173, 174, 177, 265*, 331*, 332
*1* **terfenadine 49, 266, 323*, 332***
*3* terfenadine 266*, 323, 332
*3* tolbutamide 266*, 267
*2* **triazolam 201, 264, 267*, 322, 324*, 333**
*3* triazolam 90, 324, 327, 333*
*3* warfarin 268*, 324*, 333*, 374*

Imipenem
*3* cyclosporine 172*
*3* tacrolimus 172
*3* theophylline 300*
Imipramine
Also see Cyclic antidepressants; Tricyclic antidepressants
*3* altretamine 14*
*3* butaperazine 275
*3* carbamazepine 71*
*3* chlorpromazine 275
*3* cholestyramine 102*
*3* cimetidine 113, 115*, 121
*2* **clonidine 152**
*3* colestipol 102
*3* dextroamphetamine 193*
*3* diltiazem 303
*2* **epinephrine 240***
*3* fluoxetine 189
*3* fluphenazine 275*
*3* guanethidine 190
*3* guanfacine 25
*2* **moclobemide 149**
*2* **norepinephrine 300***
*3* perphenazine 275
*2* **phenelzine 150, 301***
*3* phenylephrine 302*
*3* quinidine 302*
*3* tolazamide 231
*3* trifluoperazine 275
*3* verapamil 303*
Imuran
*2* **allopurinol 9*, 12**
*3* captopril 54*
*3* warfarin 54*, 356
Inderal
Also see Antiarrhythmics; Beta-adrenergic blockers
*3* amiodarone 21, 23
*3* bupivacaine 428
*3* chlorpromazine 97*
*3* cimetidine 125*
*3* ciprofloxacin 133
*3* clonidine 154*
*3* cocaine 158*
*3* contrast media 162*
*3* digitoxin 216
*3* digoxin 216*
*3* diltiazem 223*, 430
*3* epinephrine 240*, 429

*3* digoxin 213*
*3* dirithromycin 144
*3* erythromycin 144
*3* felodipine 260*
*3* fluvastatin 321
*3* loratadine 323, 326
*2* **lovastatin 321\*, 326**
*3* midazolam 201, 264, 322*,324, 327
*2* **phenytoin 322\***
*3* pravastatin 321
*3* quinidine 329
*3* rifampin 265, 323*, 330
*3* simvastatin 321
*3* tacrolimus 173, 265, 332
*1* **terfenadine 266, 323\*, 332**
*3* tolbutamide 267
*2* **triazolam 201, 322, 324\*, 333**
*3* warfarin 268, 324*, 333

Janimine
Also see Cyclic antidepressants; Tricyclic antidepressants
*3* altretamine 14*
*3* butaperazine 275
*3* carbamazepine 71*
*3* chlorpromazine 275
*3* cholestyramine 102*
*3* cimetidine 113, 115*, 121
*2* **clonidine 152**
*3* colestipol 102
*3* dextroamphetamine 193*
*3* diltiazem 303
*2* **epinephrine 240\***
*3* fluoxetine 189
*3* fluphenazine 275*
*3* guanethidine 190
*3* guanfacine 25
*2* **moclobemide 149**
*2* **norepinephrine 300\***
*3* perphenazine 275
*2* **phenelzine 150, 301\***
*3* phenylephrine 302*
*3* quinidine 302*
*3* tolazamide 231
*3* trifluoperazine 275
*3* verapamil 303*

Josamycin
Also see Macrolides
*3* cyclosporine 143

Kaolin pectin
*2* **clindamycin 325**
*3* digitoxin 213
*3* digoxin 213*
*2* **lincomycin 325\***
*3* quinidine 325*

Kanamycin
Also see Aminoglycosides
*3* carboplatin 82
*2* **ethacrynic acid 248**
*3* methoxyflurane 365

Kantrex
Also see Aminoglycosides
*3* carboplatin 82
*2* **ethacrynic acid 248**
*3* methoxyflurane 365

Kayexalate
*3* antacids 38*
*3* calcium 38*
*3* Maalox 38*
*3* magnesium 38*
*3* Milk of Magnesia 38*

Keflin
Also see Cephalosporins
*3* furosemide 86

Kefto
Also see Cephalosporins
*2* **warfarin 379**

Kefurox
Also see Cephalosporins
*3* aluminum 85
*3* Amphojel 85
*3* cimetidine 85
*3* famotidine 85
*3* lansoprazole 85
*3* nizatidine 85
*3* omeprazole 85
*3* ranitidine 84, 85*
*3* sodium bicarbonate 85

Ketoconazole
Also see Antifungals; Imidazoles
*3* alprazolam 90, 327, 333
*3* aluminum 34
*3* antacids 34*
*1* **astemizole 48, 49\*, 332**
*2* **atorvastatin 326**
*3* buspirone 63
*3* calcium 34
*3* cetirizine 49

*3* chlordiazepoxide 90*
*3* cimetidine 115*, 328, 329
*2* **cisapride 136, 137, 138\*, 139**
*3* cyclosporine 170, 172, 173, 174*, 177, 332
*3* diazepam 201
*3* didanosine 207*
*3* ethanol 250*
*3* famotidine 115, 329
*3* felodipine 260
*3* fluvastatin 326
*3* indinavir 303*, 330
*3* lansoprazole 328, 329
*3* loratadine 49, 326*
*2* **lovastatin 321, 326\***
*3* magnesium 34
*3* methylprednisolone 327*
*3* midazolam 90, 264, 327*, 333
*3* nizatidine 115, 329
*3* omeprazole 328*, 329
*3* pravastatin 326
*3* quinidine 329*
*3* ranitidine 115, 328, 329*
*3* rifampin 265, 323, 330*
*3* ritonavir 303
*3* saquinavir 303, 330*
*2* **simvastatin 326**
*3* sodium bicarbonate 34*
*3* sucralfate 331*
*3* tacrolimus 174, 265, 331*
*1* **terfenadine 49, 266, 323, 332\***
*3* tolbutamide 267
*3* triazolam 90, 324, 327, 333*
*3* warfarin 268, 324, 333*

Ketoprofen
Also see Nonsteroidal antiinflammatory drugs
*3* cyclosporine 166, 174*
*2* **methotrexate 334\***
*2* **warfarin 335\***

Ketorolac
Also see Nonsteroidal antiinflammatory drugs
*3* lithium 336*

Klonopin
Also see Anticonvulsants; Benzodiazepines
*3* disulfiram 198
*3* valproic acid 151*

Lasix
Also see Diuretics; Loop
diuretics
*3* cephaloridine 85*
*3* cephalothin 86
*3* cholestyramine 101*, 161
*3* cisplatin 140
*3* clofibrate 147*
*3* colestipol 101, 161*
*3* digitoxin 211
*3* digoxin 211*
*3* enalapril 234*
*3* fluoxetine 269*
*3* flurbiprofen 281
*3* ibuprofen 281
*3* indomethacin 61, 281*,
308
*3* naproxen 281
*3* paroxetine 269
*3* phenobarbital 282
*3* phenytoin 281*
*3* piroxicam 281
*3* sertraline 269
*3* sulindac 281
*3* terbutaline 282*

Lescol
Also see HMG-CoA reduc-
tase inhibitors
*3* cholestyramine 104
*3* itraconazole 321
*3* ketoconazole 326
*3* nefazodone 382
*3* warfarin 350

Levarterenol
**2 amitriptyline 301**
**2 desipramine 301**
*3* guanadrel 294
*3* guanethidine 294*
**2 imipramine 300***
*3* isocarboxazid 389
*3* methyldopa 366*
*3* phenelzine 389*
**2 protriptyline 301**
*3* tranylcypromine 389

Levlen
Also see Estrogens
*3* ampicillin 28*
*3* carbamazepine 76*, 394
**1 cigarette smoking 107***
*3* cyclosporine 165, 179*
*3* dexamethasone 395

**2 dicumarol 397**
*3* doxycycline 397
*3* griseofulvin 292*
*3* hydrocortisone 395
*3* methylprednisolone 395
*3* phenobarbital 394*
**2 phenprocoumon 397**
*3* phenytoin 394*
*3* prednisolone 395*
*3* prednisone 395
*3* primidone 394
*3* rifabutin 396
*3* rifampin 395*
*3* ritonavir 396*
*3* tetracycline 397*
**2 warfarin 397***

Levodopa
*3* chlordiazepoxide 202
**2 chlorpromazine 95***
*3* diazepam 201*
**2 haloperidol 95**
*3* iron 314*
*3* isocarboxazid 338
*3* methionine 337*
*3* moclobemide 338*
*3* nialamide 338
*3* phenelzine 338*
*3* phenytoin 339*
*3* pyridoxine 339*
*3* spiramycin 340*
*3* tacrine 340*
*3* tranylcypromine 338

Levonorgestrel
*3* ampicillin 28*
*3* carbamazepine 76*, 394
**1 cigarette smoking 107***
*3* cyclosporine 165, 179*
*3* dexamethasone 395
**2 dicumarol 397**
*3* doxycycline 397
*3* griseofulvin 292*
*3* hydrocortisone 395
*3* methylprednisolone 395
*3* phenobarbital 394*
**2 phenprocoumon 397**
*3* phenytoin 394*
*3* prednisolone 395*
*3* prednisone 395
*3* primidone 394
*3* rifabutin 396
*3* rifampin 395*

*3* tetracycline 397*
**2 warfarin 397***

Levophed
**2 amitriptyline 301**
**2 desipramine 301**
*3* guanadrel 294
*3* guanethidine 294*
**2 imipramine 300***
*3* isocarboxazid 389
*3* methyldopa 366*
*3* phenelzine 389*
**2 protriptyline 301**
*3* tranylcypromine 389

Levoprome
**1 isocarboxazid 364**
**1 pargyline 364***
**1 phenelzine 364**
**1 tranylcypromine 364**

Levothyroxine
*3* carbamazepine 79*
*3* cholestyramine 105*
*3* colestipol 105
*3* phenytoin 79, 415*
*3* rifampin 79
*3* theophylline 448*
*3* warfarin 451

Levoxyl
*3* carbamazepine 79*
*3* cholestyramine 105*
*3* colestipol 105
*3* phenytoin 79, 415*
*3* rifampin 79
*3* theophylline 448*
*3* warfarin 451

Librium
*3* chlorpropamide 88*
*3* cimetidine 83
**2 dicumarol 88***
*3* phenobarbital 89*
*3* phenytoin 89*
*3* rifampin 90*
*3* tolbutamide 88
**2 warfarin 88**

Lidocaine
Also see Local anesthetics;
Antiarrhythmics
*3* cimetidine 116*
*3* disopyramide 224*
*3* metoprolol 342
*3* nadolol 341
*3* propranolol 341*, 428

Lincocin
  **2 kaolin-pectin 325***
Lincomycin
  **2 kaolin-pectin 325***
Lipitor
  Also see HMG-CoA reduc-
    tase inhibitors
  *3* clarithromycin 51
  *3* erythromycin 50*
  **2 itraconazole 321**
  **2 ketoconazole 326**
  **2 mibefradil 373**
  *3* nefazodone 382
  *3* troleandomycin 51
Liquaemin
  Also see Anticoagulants
  *3* warfarin 297*
Lisinopril
  Also see Angiotensin-con-
    verting enzyme inhibitors
  *3* bunazosin 62
  *3* lithium 341*
Lithane
  *3* amitriptyline 26*
  *3* bromfenac 57*
  *3* carbamazepine 74*
  *3* chlorpromazine 95*
  *3* diclofenac 204*
  *3* diltiazem 348
  *3* enalapril 341
  *3* fluoxetine 270*
  *3* fluvoxamine 277*
  *3* haloperidol 95, 296*
  *3* ibuprofen 298*
  *3* indomethacin 304*
  **2 isocarboxazid 344**
  *3* ketorolac 336*
  *3* lisinopril 341*
  *3* losartan 342*
  *3* mefenamic acid 342*
  *3* methyldopa 343*
  *3* naproxen 343*
  **2 phenelzine 344***
  *3* phenylbutazone 345*
  *3* phenytoin 345*
  *3* piroxicam 345*
  *3* potassium iodide 346*
  *3* sodium bicarbonate 346*
  *3* sodium chloride 347*
  *3* theophylline 347*

  *3* thioridazine 95
  **2 tranylcypromine 344**
  *3* verapamil 348*
Lithium
  *3* amitriptyline 26*
  *3* bromfenac 57*
  *3* carbamazepine 74*
  *3* chlorpromazine 95*
  *3* diclofenac 204*
  *3* diltiazem 348
  *3* enalapril 341
  *3* fluoxetine 270*
  *3* fluvoxamine 277*
  *3* haloperidol 95, 296*
  *3* ibuprofen 298*
  *3* indomethacin 304*
  **2 isocarboxazid 344**
  *3* ketorolac 336*
  *3* lisinopril 341*
  *3* losartan 342*
  *3* mefenamic acid 342*
  *3* methyldopa 343*
  *3* naproxen 343*
  **2 phenelzine 344***
  *3* phenylbutazone 345*
  *3* phenytoin 345*
  *3* piroxicam 345*
  *3* potassium iodide 346*
  *3* sodium bicarbonate 346*
  *3* sodium chloride 347*
  *3* theophylline 347*
  *3* thioridazine 95
  **2 tranylcypromine 344**
  *3* verapamil 348*
Lithobid
  *3* amitriptyline 26*
  3 bromfenac 57*
  *3* carbamazepine 74*
  *3* chlorpromazine 95*
  *3* diclofenac 204*
  *3* diltiazem 348
  *3* enalapril 341
  *3* fluoxetine 270*
  *3* fluvoxamine 277*
  *3* haloperidol 95, 296*
  *3* ibuprofen 298*
  *3* indomethacin 304*
  **2 isocarboxazid 344**
  *3* ketorolac 336*
  *3* lisinopril 341*

  *3* losartan 342*
  *3* mefenamic acid 342*
  *3* methyldopa 343*
  *3* naproxen 343*
  **2 phenelzine 344***
  *3* phenylbutazone 345*
  *3* phenytoin 345*
  *3* piroxicam 345*
  *3* potassium iodide 346*
  *3* sodium bicarbonate 346*
  *3* sodium chloride 347*
  *3* theophylline 347*
  *3* thioridazine 95
  **2 tranylcypromine 344**
  *3* verapamil 348*
Lithonate
  *3* amitriptyline 26*
  *3* bromfenac 57*
  *3* carbamazepine 74*
  *3* chlorpromazine 95*
  *3* diclofenac 204*
  *3* diltiazem 348
  *3* enalapril 341
  *3* fluoxetine 270*
  *3* fluvoxamine 277*
  *3* haloperidol 95, 296*
  *3* ibuprofen 298*
  *3* indomethacin 304*
  **2 isocarboxazid 344**
  *3* ketorolac 336*
  *3* lisinopril 341*
  *3* losartan 342*
  *3* mefenamic acid 342*
  *3* methyldopa 343*
  *3* naproxen 343*
  **2 phenelzine 344***
  *3* phenylbutazone 345*
  *3* phenytoin 345*
  *3* piroxicam 345*
  *3* potassium iodide 346*
  *3* sodium bicarbonate 346*
  *3* sodium chloride 347*
  *3* theophylline 347*
  *3* thioridazine 95
  **2 tranylcypromine 344**
  *3* verapamil 348*
Local anesthetics
  Also see Bupivacaine;
    Cocaine; Lidocaine;
    Tetracaine
  *3* acebutolol 428

3 atenolol 428
3 cimetidine 116*
3 disopyramide 224*
3 metoprolol 342, 428
3 nadolol 341
3 propranolol 158*, 341*, 428*

Lodine
Also see Nonsteroidal anti-inflammatory drugs
2 warfarin 257*

Loestrin
Also see Estrogens
3 ampicillin 28*
3 carbamazepine 76*, 394
1 cigarette smoking 107*
3 cyclosporine 165, 179*
3 dexamethasone 395
2 dicumarol 397
3 doxycycline 397
3 griseofulvin 292*
3 hydrocortisone 395
3 methylprednisolone 395
3 phenobarbital 394*
2 phenprocoumon 397
3 phenytoin 394*
3 prednisolone 395*
3 prednisone 395
3 primidone 394
3 rifabutin 396
3 rifampin 395*
3 ritonavir 396*
3 tetracycline 397*
2 warfarin 397*

Lomefloxacin
Also see Quinolones
3 aluminum 35*
3 antacids 30, 34*, 35, 36
3 Maalox 35*
3 magnesium 35*

Lomustine
3 cimetidine 83

Loop diuretics
Also see Bumetanide; Ethacrynic acid; Furosemide; Torsemide
3 cephaloridine 85*, 86
3 cephalothin 86
3 cholestyramine 101*, 161
2 cisplatin 140*

3 cisplatin 140
3 clofibrate 147*
3 colestipol 101, 161*
3 digitoxin 211
3 digoxin 211*
3 enalapril 234*, 235
3 fluoxetine 269*
3 flurbiprofen 281
2 gentamicin 248*
3 ibuprofen 281
3 indomethacin 61*, 281*, 308
2 kanamycin 248
3 naproxen 281
2 neomycin 248
3 paroxetine 269
3 phenobarbital 282
3 phenytoin 281*
3 piroxicam 281
3 sertraline 269
2 streptomycin 248
3 sulindac 281
3 terbutaline 282*

Lo/Ovral
Also see Estrogens
3 ampicillin 28*
3 carbamazepine 76*, 394
1 cigarette smoking 107*
3 cyclosporine 165, 179*
3 dexamethasone 395
2 dicumarol 397
3 doxycycline 397
3 griseofulvin 292*
3 hydrocortisone 395
3 methylprednisolone 395
3 phenobarbital 394*
2 phenprocoumon 397
3 phenytoin 394*
3 prednisolone 395*
3 prednisone 395
3 primidone 394
3 rifabutin 396
3 rifampin 395*
3 ritonavir 396*
3 tetracycline 397*
2 warfarin 397*

Lopid
3 cholestyramine 161
3 colestipol 161*
3 glyburide 283*
2 lovastatin 284*, 285
3 pravastatin 284, 285*

2 simvastatin 284, 285
2 warfarin 148, 285*, 350

Lopressor
Also see Beta-adrenergic blockers
3 amiodarone 20*, 23
3 bromazepam 202
3 cimetidine 125
3 ciprofloxacin 132*
3 diazepam 202*
3 diltiazem 223
3 dipyridamole 50
3 enoxacin 132
3 fluoxetine 272
3 lidocaine 341
3 nicardipine 384
3 nifedipine 386
3 norfloxacin 132
3 oxazepam 202
3 pefloxacin 132
3 pipemidic acid 132
3 propafenone 366*
3 propoxyphene 367*
3 quinidine 367*, 427, 431
3 rifampin 368*
2 terbutaline 369*
3 tetracaine 428
3 theophylline 429
3 verapamil 430

Loratadine
3 itraconazole 323, 326
3 ketoconazole 49, 326*
3 miconazole 326

Lorazepam
Also see Benzodiazepines
3 clozapine 155, 157*
3 ethanol 199
2 fluconazole 267
3 loxapine 348*

Lortab
Also see Narcotic analgesics
3 quinidine 158

Losartan
Also see Angiotensin receptor antagonists
3 fluconazole 263*
3 lithium 342*
3 terbinafine 263

Lorelco
3 cyclosporine 182*

*3* isoniazid 34*
*3* ketoconazole 34
*3* lomefloxacin 35*
*3* methenamine 358
*3* nifedipine 351
*3* norfloxacin 35*
*3* ofloxacin 36*
*3* penicillamine 37*
*3* pseudoephedrine 37
*3* quinidine 38*
*3* sodium polystyrene sulfonate resin 38*
*3* tetracycline 39*

Mag-Ox
Also see Antacids
*3* allopurinol 9
*3* aspirin 29*
*3* cefpodoxime 29*
*3* ciprofloxacin 30*, 130
*3* glipizide 32*
*3* glyburide 32*
*3* iron 33*
*3* isoniazid 34*
*3* ketoconazole 34
*3* lomefloxacin 35*
*3* methenamine 358
*3* nifedipine 351
*3* norfloxacin 35*
*3* ofloxacin 36*
*3* penicillamine 37*
*3* pseudoephedrine 37
*3* quinidine 38*
*3* sodium polystyrene sulfonate resin 38*
*3* tetracycline 39*

Mandol
Also see Cephalosporins
*3* ethanol 83*
*2* **warfarin 379**

MAOIs
Also see Isocarboxazid;
Pargyline; Phenelzine;
Selegiline; Tranylcypromine
*2* **amitriptyline 150, 301**
*3* chlorpropamide 312
*1* **clomipramine 150\*, 301**
*2* **desipramine 301**
*1* **dexfenfluramine 191\***
*2* **dexfenfluramine 191**
*1* **dextroamphetamine 193\***
*2* **dextroamphetamine 193**

*1* **dextromethorphan 195\*, 196\***
*2* **dextromethorphan 197\***
*3* disulfiram 228*
*1* **ethanol 252**
*1* **fenfluramine 191, 261\***
*2* **fenfluramine 261**
*1* **fluoxetine 273\***
*2* **fluoxetine 272\***
*1* **fluvoxamine 273**
*2* **fluvoxamine 272**
*1* **food 454**
*3* guanadrel 295
*3* guanethidine 295
*2* **imipramine 150, 301\***
*3* insulin 312*
*3* levodopa 338
*2* **lithium 344**
*1* **meperidine 354**
*2* **meperidine 197, 355\***
*1* **metaraminol 356\***
*1* **methotrimeprazine 364\***
*1* **methylphenidate 193**
*3* moclobemide 377*
*3* morphine 355
*3* norepinephrine 389
*1* **paroxetine 273**
*2* **paroxetine 272**
*1* **phenylephrine 400**
*1* **phenylpropanolamine 401**
*1* **pseudoephedrine 402**
*1* **reserpine 402**
*3* reserpine 402
*1* **sertraline 273**
*2* **sertraline 272**
*3* tolbutamide 312
*2* **tramadol 453\***
*1* **trazodone 150, 301**
*1* **tyramine 454\***
*3* tyramine 441*

Maox
Also see Antacids
*3* allopurinol 9
*3* aspirin 29*
*3* cefpodoxime 29*
*3* ciprofloxacin 30*, 130
*3* glipizide 32*
*3* glyburide 32*
*3* iron 33*
*3* isoniazid 34*

*3* ketoconazole 34
*3* lomefloxacin 35*
*3* methenamine 358
*3* nifedipine 351
*3* norfloxacin 35*
*3* ofloxacin 36*
*3* penicillamine 37*
*3* pseudoephedrine 37
*3* quinidine 38*
*3* sodium polystyrene sulfonate resin 38*
*3* tetracycline 39*

Maprotiline
Also see Cyclic antidepressants; Tricyclic antidepressants
*3* cimetidine 111, 113
*3* tolazamide 231

Marcaine
Also see Local anesthetics
*3* propranolol 428

Marplan
Also see Monoamine oxidase inhibitors
*1* **clomipramine 150**
*1* **dexfenfluramine 191**
*1* **dextroamphetamine 193**
*1* **dextromethorphan 196**
*1* **ethanol 252**
*1* **fenfluramine 261**
*1* **fluoxetine 273**
*3* guanethidine 295
*3* levodopa 338
*2* **lithium 344**
*1* **meperidine 354**
*1* **metaraminol 356**
*1* **methotrimeprazine 364**
*3* norepinephrine 389
*1* **phenylephrine 400**
*1* **phenylpropanolamine 401**
*1* **pseudoephedrine 402**
*1* **reserpine 402**
*2* **tramadol 453**
*1* **tyramine 454**

Matulane
Also see Antineoplastics
*1* **ethanol 254\***
*3* prochlorperazine 424*

Maxaquin
Also see Quinolones
*3* aluminum 35*

Maxaquin *(Continued)*
*3* antacids 30, 34*, 35, 36
*3* Maalox 35*
*3* magnesium 35*

Maxolon
*3* cyclosporine 176*
*3* ethanol 251*

Measles vaccine
*1* **methotrexate 362**

Mebendazole
*3* carbamazepine 74*
*2* **phenytoin 351***

Meclofenamate
Also see Nonsteroidal anti-
inflammatory drugs
*2* **warfarin 352***

Meclomen
Also see Nonsteroidal anti-
inflammatory drugs
*2* **warfarin 352***

Medihaler Ergotamine
*3* dopamine 229*

Medrol
Also see Corticosteroids
*3* aminoglutethimide 15
*3* clarithromycin 366
*3* cyclosporine 181
*3* erythromycin 366
*3* ketoconazole 327*
*3* oral contraceptives 395
*3* phenobarbital 403
*3* troleandomycin 366*

Medroxyprogesterone
Also see Progestins
*3* aminoglutethimide 15*

Mefenamic acid
Also see Nonsteroidal anti-
inflammatory drugs
*3* cyclosporine 175*
*3* lithium 342*
*2* **warfarin 352***

Mefoxin
Also see Cephalosporins
*2* **warfarin 379**

Mellaril
Also see Neuroleptics
*3* bromocriptine 60*
*3* epinephrine 93
*3* lithium 95
*3* phenobarbital 97
*3* phenylpropanolamine
410*
*3* propranolol 97

Melphalan
Also see Antineoplastics
*3* cimetidine 117*
*3* cyclosporine 175*

Meperidine
Also see Narcotic
analgesics
*3* chlorpromazine 96*
*3* cimetidine 117*
*3* ethanol 250*
*1* **isocarboxazid 354**
*1* **phenelzine 354***
*3* phenobarbital 354*
*3* phenytoin 355*
*2* **selegiline 197, 355***
*1* **tranylcypromine 354**

Meprobamate
*3* ethanol 250*

Mercaptopurine
Also see Antineoplastics
*3* allopurinol 10, 11*
*3* captopril 54
*3* warfarin 54, 355*

Meruvax
*1* **methotrexate 36**

Mestinon
Also see Cholinergics
*3* tacrine 56

Mestranol
*3* ampicillin 28*
*3* carbamazepine 76*, 394
*1* **cigarette smoking 107***
*3* cyclosporine 165, 179*
*3* dexamethasone 395
*2* **dicumarol 397**
*3* doxycycline 397
*3* griseofulvin 292*
*3* hydrocortisone 395
*3* methylprednisolone 395
*3* phenobarbital 394*
*2* **phenprocoumon 397**
*3* phenytoin 394*
*3* prednisolone 395*
*3* prednisone 395
*3* primidone 394
*3* rifabutin 396
*3* rifampin 395*
*3* tetracycline 397*
*2* **warfarin 397***

Metandren
*3* cyclosporine 165
*2* **warfarin 398**

Metaraminol
*1* **isocarboxazid 356**
*1* **pargyline 356***
*1* **phenelzine 356**
*1* **tranylcypromine 356**

Methacycline
Also see Tetracyclines
*3* iron 316

Methadone
Also see Narcotic
analgesics
*3* carbamazepine 75*, 357
*3* phenobarbital 356*
*2* **phenytoin 75, 357***
*3* primidone 357
*3* rifampin 357*

Methandrostenolone
Also see Anabolic steroids
*3* insulin 358
*3* tolbutamide 358*
*2* **warfarin 398**

Methenamine
*3* acetazolamide 358
*3* aluminum 358
*3* magnesium 358
*3* sodium bicarbonate 358*
*3* sulfadiazine 359*
*3* sulfamethizole 359
*3* sulfathiazole 359

Methimazole
*3* theophylline 434

Methionine
*3* levodopa 337*

Methotrexate
Also see Antineoplastics
*2* **aspirin 43*, 299**
*2* **azapropazone 52***
*1* **BCG vaccine 362**
*3* carbenicillin 82*
*3* chloroquine 91*
*3* cholestyramine 103*
*3* colestipol 103
*3* cyclosporine 176*
*2* **diclofenac 204***
*1* **ethanol 251***
*2* **etretinate 258***
*3* flurbiprofen 275*
*3* ibuprofen 299*
*2* **indomethacin 305***
*2* **ketoprofen 334***
*1* **measles vaccine 362**

*3* mezlocillin 82
*1* mumps vaccine 362
*2* naproxen 359*
*1* neomycin 360*
*3* omeprazole 361*
*2* oxyphenbutazone 361
*2* phenylbutazone 361*
*1* polio vaccine 362*
*2* probenecid 363*
*1* rubella vaccine 362
*1* smallpox vaccine 362
*2* sulfinpyrazone 363
*3* thiazides 363*
*3* trimethoprim-sul-
   famethoxazole 363*
*1* typhoid vaccine 362
*1* yellow fever vaccine 362
Methotrimeprazine
   *1* isocarboxazid 364
   *1* pargyline 364*
   *1* phenelzine 364
   *1* tranylcypromine 364
Methoxyflurane
   *3* gentamicin 365
   *3* secobarbital 365*
   *2* tetracycline 365*
Methyldopa
   *3* iron 314*
   *3* lithium 343*
   *3* norepinephrine 366*
Methylphenidate
   *3* guanadrel 294
   *3* guanethidine 294*
   *1* tranylcypromine 193
Methylprednisolone
   Also see Corticosteroids
   *3* aminoglutethimide 15
   *3* clarithromycin 366
   *3* cyclosporine 181
   *3* erythromycin 366
   *3* ketoconazole 327*
   *3* oral contraceptives 395
   *3* phenobarbital 403
   *3* troleandomycin 366*
Methyltestosterone
   *3* cyclosporine 165
   *2* warfarin 398
Metoclopramide
   *3* cyclosporine 176*
   *3* ethanol 251*
Metolazone
   Also see Diuretics;
   Thiazides
   *3* digoxin 211

Metoprolol
   Also see Beta-adrenergic
   blockers
   *3* amiodarone 20*, 23
   *3* bromazepam 202
   *3* cimetidine 125
   *3* ciprofloxacin 132*
   *3* diazepam 202*
   *3* diltiazem 223
   *3* dipyridamole 50
   *3* enoxacin 132
   *3* fluoxetine 272
   *3* lidocaine 341
   *3* nicardipine 384
   *3* nifedipine 386
   *3* norfloxacin 132
   *3* oxazepam 202
   *3* pefloxacin 132
   *3* pipemidic acid 132
   *3* propafenone 366*
   *3* propoxyphene 367*
   *3* quinidine 367*, 427, 431
   *3* rifampin 368*
   *2* terbutaline 369*
   *3* tetracaine 428
   *3* theophylline 429
   *3* verapamil 430
Metronidazole
   *3* carbamazepine 75*
   *3* cholestyramine 103*
   *3* colestipol 103
   *3* diazepam 252, 370
   *3* disulfiram 227*
   *3* ethanol 252*
   *2* fluorouracil 268*
   *3* nitroglycerin 252, 370
   *3* phenytoin 252, 369*, 370
   *3* trimethoprim-sul-
      famethoxazole 252, 370*
   *2* warfarin 370*
Mevacor
   Also see HMG-CoA reductase inhibitors
   *3* cholestyramine 104
   *3* clarithromycin 242
   *2* clofibrate 284
   *3* danazol 185*
   *3* diltiazem 220*
   *3* erythromycin 51, 242*
   *2* fluconazole 321, 326
   *2* gemfibrozil 284*, 285
   *3* isradipine 221, 321*
   *2* itraconazole 231*, 326

   *2* ketoconazole 321, 326*
   *2* mibefradil 220, 373
   *2* miconazole 321, 326
   *2* nefazodone 382
   *3* nicotinic acid 349*
   *3* pectin 350*
   *3* terbinafine 321, 326
   *3* troleandomycin 242
   *3* verapamil 220
   *3* warfarin 148, 286, 350*
Mexate
   Also see Antineoplastics
   *2* aspirin 43*, 299
   *2* azapropazone 52*
   *1* BCG vaccine 362
   *3* carbenicillin 82*
   *3* chloroquine 91*
   *3* cholestyramine 103*
   *3* colestipol 103
   *3* cyclosporine 176*
   *2* diclofenac 204*
   *1* ethanol 251*
   *2* etretinate 258*
   *3* flurbiprofen 275*
   *3* ibuprofen 299*
   *2* indomethacin 305*
   *2* ketoprofen 334*
   *1* measles vaccine 362
   *3* mezlocillin 82
   *1* mumps vaccine 362
   *2* naproxen 359*
   *1* neomycin 360*
   *3* omeprazole 361*
   *2* oxyphenbutazone 361
   *2* phenylbutazone 361*
   *1* polio vaccine 362*
   *2* probenecid 363*
   *1* rubella vaccine 362
   *1* smallpox vaccine 362
   *2* sulfinpyrazone 363
   *3* thiazides 363*
   *3* trimethoprim-sul-
      famethoxazole 363*
   *1* typhoid vaccine 362
   *1* yellow fever vaccine 362
Mexiletine
   Also see Antiarrhythmics
   *3* acetazolamide 372
   *3* phenytoin 371*
   *3* quinidine 371*
   *3* rifampin 372*
   *3* sodium bicarbonate 372*
   *2* theophylline 373*

Mexitil
Also see Antiarrhythmics
*3* acetazolamide 372
*3* phenytoin 371*
*3* quinidine 371*
*3* rifampin 372*
*3* sodium bicarbonate 372*
*2* **theophylline 373***

Mezlin
Also see Penicillins
*3* methotrexate 82

Mezlocillin
Also see Penicillins
*3* methotrexate 82

Mibefradil
Also see Calcium Channel
Blockers
*3* alfentanil 8
*2* **astemizole 49*, 374**
*2* **atorvastatin 373**
*2* **cerivastatin 373**
*2* **cisapride 138***
*3* digoxin 214*
*2* **lovastatin 220, 373**
*3* midazolam 221
*2* **simvastatin 373***
*2* **terfenadine 49, 138, 374***

Micatin
Also see Antifungals;
Imidazoles
*1* **astemizole 49**
*2* **cisapride 137, 138, 139***
*3* cyclosporine 170, 173, 174, 177*
*3* felodipine 260
*3* loratadine 326
*2* **lovastatin 321, 326**
*3* midazolam 327
*3* quinidine 329
*3* tacrolimus 177
*3* tolbutamide 267
*3* triazolam 333
*3* warfarin 324, 333, 374*

Miconazole
Also see Antifungals;
Imidazoles
*1* **astemizole 49**
*2* **cisapride 137, 138, 139***
*3* cyclosporine 170, 173, 174, 177*

*3* felodipine 260
*3* loratadine 326
*2* **lovastatin 321, 326**
*3* midazolam 327
*3* quinidine 329
*3* tacrolimus 177
*3* tolbutamide 267
*3* triazolam 333
*3* warfarin 324, 333, 374*

Micronase
Also see Antidiabetics;
Sulfonylureas
*3* aluminum 32*
*3* antacids 32*
*3* aspirin 41
*3* cimetidine 32, 128
*3* famotidine 32
*3* gemfibrozil 283*
*3* lansoprazole 32
*3* Maalox 32*
*3* magnesium 32*
*3* nizatidine 32
*3* omeprazole 32
*3* rifampin 437
*3* trimethoprim-sul-
famethoxazole 451
*3* warfarin 289*

Micronor
*3* ampicillin 28*
*3* carbamazepine 76*, 394
*1* **cigarette smoking 107***
*3* cyclosporine 165, 179*
*3* dexamethasone 395
*2* **dicumarol 397**
*3* doxycycline 397
*3* griseofulvin 292*
*3* hydrocortisone 395
*3* methylprednisolone 395
*3* phenobarbital 394*
*2* **phenprocoumon 397**
*3* phenytoin 394*
*3* prednisolone 395*
*3* prednisone 395
*3* primidone 394
*3* rifabutin 396
*3* rifampin 395*
*3* tetracycline 397*
*2* **warfarin 397***

Midamor
Also see Diuretics;
Potassium-sparing
diuretics
*2* **potassium 419, 420**

Midazolam
Also see Benzodiazepines
*3* carbamazepine 76*, 375
*2* **clarithromycin 145*, 243**
*3* diltiazem 221*
*3* erythromycin 13, 62, 145, 243*
*3* fluconazole 264*, 267, 322, 327
*3* grapefruit juice 291
*3* itraconazole 63, 201, 264, 322*, 324, 327
*3* ketoconazole 90, 264, 327*, 333
*3* mibefradil 221
*3* miconazole 327
*3* phenytoin 375*
*3* rifampin 438
*2* **roxithromycin 145**
*3* troleandomycin 243, 454
*3* verapamil 221

Midrin
*1* **bromocriptine 59*, 60**

Milk of Magnesia
Also see Antacids
*3* allopurinol 9
*3* aspirin 29*
*3* cefpodoxime 29*
*3* ciprofloxacin 30*, 130
*3* glipizide 32*
*3* glyburide 32*
*3* iron 33*
*3* isoniazid 34*
*3* ketoconazole 34
*3* lomefloxacin 35*
*3* methenamine 358
*3* nifedipine 351
*3* norfloxacin 35*
*3* ofloxacin 36*
*3* penicillamine 37*
*3* pseudoephedrine 37
*3* quinidine 38*
*3* sodium polystyrene sulfonate resin 38*
*3* tetracycline 39*

Miltown
**3** ethanol 250*
Minipress
Also see Alpha blockers
**3** enalapril 62
**3** ibuprofen 306
**3** indomethacin 306*
**3** propranolol 420*
**3** verapamil 421*
Mintezol
**3** carbamazepine 74
**3** theophylline 447*
Misoprostol
**3** phenylbutazone 375*
Mitomycin
Also see Antineoplastics
**2** vinblastine 376*
Mitotane
**1** spironolactone 377*
**3** warfarin 377*
Mobidin
Also see Antacids
**3** allopurinol 9
**3** aspirin 29*
**3** cefpodoxime 29*
**3** ciprofloxacin 30*, 130
**3** glipizide 32*
**3** glyburide 32*
**3** iron 33*
**3** isoniazid 34*
**3** ketoconazole 34
**3** lomefloxacin 35*
**3** methenamine 358
**3** nifedipine 351
**3** norfloxacin 35*
**3** ofloxacin 36*
**3** penicillamine 37*
**3** pseudoephedrine 37
**3** quinidine 38*
**3** sodium polystyrene sulfonate resin 38*
**3** tetracycline 39*
Moclobemide
**2** amitriptyline 149
**2** citalopram 142*
**2** clomipramine 149*
**1** dextromethorphan 195*
**2** ephedrine 239*
**2** imipramine 149

**3** levodopa 338*
**2** phenylpropanolamine 239
**2** pseudoephedrine 239
**3** selegiline 377*
**2** trazodone 149
**3** tyramine 378*, 453
Modicon
Also see Estrogens
**3** ampicillin 28*
**3** carbamazepine 76*, 394
**1** cigarette smoking 107*
**3** cyclosporine 165, 179*
**3** dexamethasone 395
**2** dicumarol 397
**3** doxycycline 397
**3** griseofulvin 292*
**3** hydrocortisone 395
**3** methylprednisolone 395
**3** phenobarbital 394*
**2** phenprocoumon 397
**3** phenytoin 394*
**3** prednisolone 395*
**3** prednisone 395
**3** primidone 394*
**3** rifabutin 396
**3** rifampin 395*
**3** ritonavir 396*
**3** tetracycline 397*
**2** warfarin 397*
Mogadon
Also see Benzodiazepines
**3** ethanol 199
**3** rifampin 203
Monistat
Also see Antifungals; Imidazoles
**1** astemizole 49
**2** cisapride 137, 138, 139*
**3** cyclosporine 170, 173, 174, 177*
**3** felodipine 260
**3** loratadine 326
**2** lovastatin 321, 326
**3** midazolam 327
**3** quinidine 329
**3** tacrolimus 177
**3** tolbutamide 267
**3** triazolam 333
**3** warfarin 324, 333, 374*

Monoamine oxidase inhibitors
Also see Isocarboxazid; Pargyline; Phenelzine; Selegiline; Tranylcypromine
**2** amitriptyline 150, 301
**3** chlorpropamide 312
**1** clomipramine 150*, 301
**2** desipramine 301
**1** dexfenfluramine 191*
**2** dexfenfluramine 191
**1** dextroamphetamine 193*
**2** dextroamphetamine 193
**1** dextromethorphan 195*, 196*
**2** dextromethorphan 197*
**3** disulfiram 228*
**1** ethanol 252
**1** fenfluramine 191, 261*
**2** fenfluramine 261
**1** fluoxetine 273*
**2** fluoxetine 272*
**1** fluvoxamine 273
**2** fluvoxamine 272
**1** food 454
**3** guanadrel 295
**3** guanethidine 295
**2** imipramine 150, 301*
**3** insulin 312*
**3** levodopa 338
**2** lithium 344
**1** meperidine 354
**2** meperidine 197, 355*
**1** metaraminol 356*
**1** methotrimeprazine 364*
**1** methylphenidate 193
**3** moclobemide 377*
**3** morphine 355
**3** norepinephrine 389
**1** paroxetine 273
**2** paroxetine 272
**1** phenylephrine 400
**1** phenylpropanolamine 401
**1** pseudoephedrine 402
**1** reserpine 402
**3** reserpine 402
**1** sertraline 273
**2** sertraline 272

*3* norfloxacin 35*, 36, 390
*3* ofloxacin 30, 35, 36*, 392
*3* penicillamine 37*
*3* phenylpropanolamine 37
*3* pseudoephedrine 37
*3* quinidine 6, 38*, 431*
*3* sodium polystyrene sulfonate resin 38*
*3* tetracycline 39*
*3* thiazides 64*
*3* tocainide 40*

Mysoline
Also see Anticonvulsants; Barbiturates
*3* acetaminophen 3
*3* acetazolamide 6*
*3* clozapine 65
*3* cyclosporine 66
*3* methadone 357
*3* oral contraceptives 394
*3* phenobarbital 404*
*3* phenytoin 410*
*3* tacrolimus 413
*3* valproic acid 422*
*2* **warfarin 408**

Mytelase
*3* tacrine 56

Nabumetone
Also see Nonsteroidal anti-inflammatory drugs
*2* **warfarin 379***

Nadolol
Also see Beta-adrenergic blockers
*3* epinephrine 240
*3* insulin 311
*3* lidocaine 341
*3* neostigmine 384
*3* tacrine 428
*3* theophylline 429

Nafcillin
Also see Penicillins
*3* cyclosporine 177*
*3* tacrolimus 177
*3* warfarin 380*

Nalfon
Also see Nonsteroidal anti-inflammatory drugs
*2* **warfarin 262***

Nalidixic acid
*3* warfarin 381*

Naprosyn
Also see Nonsteroidal anti-inflammatory drugs
*3* cyclosporine 178*, 183
*3* furosemide 281
*3* lithium 343*
*2* **methotrexate 359***
*3* propranolol 307
*2* **warfarin 53, 208, 262, 309, 335, 352, 353, 381*, 409, 418, 444**

Naproxen
Also see Nonsteroidal anti-inflammatory drugs
*3* cyclosporine 178*, 183
*3* furosemide 281
*3* lithium 343*
*2* **methotrexate 359***
*3* propranolol 307
*2* **warfarin 53, 208, 262, 309, 335, 352, 353, 381*, 409, 418, 444**

Narcotic analgesics
Also see Codeine; Dihydrocodeine; Fentanyl; Hydrocodone; Meperidine; Methadone; Morphine; Pentazocine; Propoxyphene
*3* aspirin 44*
*2* **carbamazepine 78*, 231**
*3* carbamazepine 75*, 357
*3* chlorpromazine 96*
*3* cimetidine 117*
*3* diltiazem 8
*3* doxepin 230*
*3* ethanol 250*, 254*
*1* **isocarboxazid 354**
*3* metoprolol 367*
*1* **phenelzine 354***
*3* phenobarbital 354*, 356*
*2* **phenytoin 75, 357***
*3* phenytoin 355*
*3* primidone 357
*2* **quinidine 158***
*3* quinidine 158
*3* rifampin 357*
*2* **selegiline 197, 355***
*3* selegiline 355
*1* **tranylcypromine 354**
*3* warfarin 427*

Nardil
Also see Monoamine oxidase inhibitors
*2* **amitriptyline 150, 301**

*1* **clomipramine 150*, 301**
*2* **desipramine 301**
*1* **dexfenfluramine 191***
*1* **dextroamphetamine 193**
*1* **dextromethorphan 195***
*1* **ethanol 252**
*1* **fenfluramine 191, 261***
*1* **fluoxetine 273**
*3* guanadrel 295
*3* guanethidine 295
*2* **imipramine 150, 301***
*3* levodopa 338
*2* **lithium 344**
*1* **meperidine 354**
*1* **metaraminol 356**
*1* **methotrimeprazine 364**
*3* norepinephrine 389
*1* **phenylephrine 400**
*1* **phenylpropanolamine 401**
*1* **pseudoephedrine 402**
*3* reserpine 402
*2* **tramadol 453**
*1* **trazodone 150, 301**
*1* **tyramine 454**

Navane
Also see Neuroleptics
*3* bromocriptine 61
*3* guanethidine 295*
*3* propranolol 97

Nebcin
Also see Aminoglycosides
*3* atracurium 51
*3* carboplatin 82

Nefazodone
*3* atorvastatin 382
*3* fluvastatin 382
*2* **lovastatin 382**
*3* pravastatin 382
*2* **simvastatin 382***

NegGram
*3* warfarin 381*

Nelfinavir
Also see Antivirals; Protease inhibitors
*3* erythromycin 244
*2* **rifabutin 383, 435**
*2* **rifampin 383*, 435, 436**
*3* ritonavir 440
*3* saquinavir 440

Nelova
Also see Estrogens
*3* ampicillin 28*

Nelova *(Continued)*
  *3* carbamazepine 76*, 394
  *1* **cigarette smoking 107***
  *3* cyclosporine 165, 179*
  *3* dexamethasone 395
  *2* **dicumarol 397**
  *3* doxycycline 397
  *3* griseofulvin 292*
  *3* hydrocortisone 395
  *3* methylprednisolone 395
  *3* phenobarbital 394*
  *2* **phenprocoumon 397**
  *3* phenytoin 394*
  *3* prednisolone 395*
  *3* prednisone 395
  *3* primidone 394
  *3* rifabutin 396
  *3* rifampin 395*
  *3* ritonavir 396*
  *3* tetracycline 397*
  *2* **warfarin 397***
Nembutal
  Also see Barbiturates
  *3* ethanol 253
  *3* theophylline 406
  *2* **warfarin 408**
Neomycin
  Also see Aminoglycosides
  *2* **ethacrynic acid 248**
  *1* **methotrexate 360***
  *3* warfarin 383*
Neoral
  *3* allopurinol 11*
  *3* amiodarone 18*
  *3* amphotericin B 26*
  *3* carbamazepine 66*
  *3* chloroquine 91*
  *3* cisapride 176
  *3* clarithromycin 143*, 145, 168
  *3* clonidine 151*
  *3* clotrimazole 155
  *3* colchicine 159*
  *2* **danazol 165***
  *3* diclofenac 166*, 173, 174, 175
  *3* digoxin 166*
  *3* diltiazem 167*, 178, 184
  *3* doxorubicin 167*
  *3* enalapril 168*
  *3* erythromycin 143, 168*, 244

  *3* felodipine 169*
  *3* fluconazole 170*, 173, 174, 177, 265
  *3* gentamicin 170*
  *3* glipizide 171*
  *3* grapefruit juice 171*
  *3* griseofulvin 172*
  *3* imipenem 172*
  *3* indomethacin 166, 173*
  *3* itraconazole 170, 173*, 174, 177
  *3* ketoconazole 170, 172, 173, 174*, 177, 332
  *3* ketoprofen 166, 174*
  *3* mefenamic acid 175*
  *3* melphalan 175*
  *3* methotrexate 176*
  *3* methylprednisolone 181
  *3* methyltestosterone 165
  *3* metoclopramide 176*
  *3* miconazole 170, 173, 174, 177*
  *3* nafcillin 177*
  *3* naproxen 178*, 183
  *3* nicardipine 167, 178*, 184
  *3* nitrendipine 167, 169, 179, 184
  *3* norethindrone 165
  *3* oral contraceptives 179*
  *3* phenobarbital 66, 180*
  *3* phenytoin 66, 180*
  *3* prednisolone 181*
  *3* primidone 66
  *3* probucol 182*
  *2* **rifampin 182***
  *3* sulindac 166, 173, 174, 175, 178, 183*
  *3* sulphadimidine 183*
  *3* ticlopidine 184*
  *3* troleandomycin 168
  *3* valproic acid 66
  *3* verapamil 167, 178, 184*
Neosar
  Also see Antineoplastics
  *3* allopurinol 11*
  *3* digoxin 163*
  *3* succinylcholine 164*
  *3* warfarin 164*
Neostigmine
  Also see Cholinergics
  *3* atenolol 384
  *3* nadolol 384

  *3* procainamide 384*
  *3* propranolol 384*
  *3* tacrine 56
Neo-Synephrine
  *3* guanethidine 295*
  *3* imipramine 302*
  *1* **isocarboxazid 400**
  *1* **phenelzine 400***
  *1* **tranylcypromine 400**
Neothylline
  *3* probenecid 233*
Netilmicin
  Also see Aminoglycosides
  *3* carboplatin 82
Netromycin
  Also see Aminoglycosides
  *3* carboplatin 82
Neuroleptics
  Also see Chlorpromazine; Chlorprothixene; Fluphenazine; Haloperidol; Loxapine; Perphenazine; Pimozide; Prochlorperazine; Risperidone; Thioridazine; Thiothixene; Trifluoperazine
  *3* amodiaquine 91
  *3* benztropine 54*
  *3* bromocriptine 60*, 61
  *3* carbamazepine 71*
  *3* chloroquine 91*
  *3* cigarette smoking 92*
  *3* clonidine 93*
  *3* desipramine 275
  *3* epinephrine 93*
  *3* fluoxetine 270*
  *3* guanadrel 94
  *3* guanethidine 94*, 293*, 295*
  *3* imipramine 275*
  *2* **levodopa 95***
  *3* lithium 95*, 296*
  *3* lorazepam 348*
  *3* meperidine 96*
  *3* nortriptyline 275
  *3* orphenadrine 55, 96*
  *3* paroxetine 270
  *3* phenobarbital 97*
  *3* phenylpropanolamine 410*
  *3* procarbazine 424*
  *3* propranolol 97*
  *3* quinidine 297*

# Managing Clinically Important Drug Interactions

**519**

*3* sulfadoxine
pyrimethamine 91
*3* trazodone 98*
*3* trihexyphenidyl 55
Neuromuscular blockers
Also see Atracurium;
Diazepam; Orphenadrine;
Pancuronium;
Succinylcholine;
Tubocurarine;
Vecuronium
*3* amphotericin B 27*
*3* carbamazepine 76
*3* chlorpromazine 96*
*3* cimetidine 111*
*3* ciprofloxacin 130*
*2* **clarithromycin 145**
*3* clozapine 155*, 157
*3* cyclophosphamide 164*
*3* diltiazem 456
*3* disulfiram 198*
*2* **echothiophate iodide
234***
*3* ethanol 199*
*3* fluconazole 201, 264, 267
*3* fluoxetine 200*
*3* fluphenazine 96
*3* fluvoxamine 200
*2* **gentamicin 51***
*3* haloperidol 55
*3* isoniazid 200*, 319
*3* itraconazole 201*, 324
*3* ketoconazole 201
*3* labetalol 202
*3* levodopa 201*
*3* metoprolol 202*
*3* metronidazole 252, 370
*3* nicardipine 456
*3* omeprazole 203*
*3* phenytoin 375
*2* **polymyxin 398***
*3* quinidine 432*
*3* rifampin 203*, 438
*3* tobramycin 51
*3* troleandomycin 454
*3* verapamil 456*
Niacin
*3* lovastatin 349*
Nialamide
*3* levodopa 338
Nicardipine
Also see Calcium channel
blockers
*3* cyclosporine 167, 178*,
184

*3* metoprolol 384
*3* propranolol 384*
*3* tacrolimus 178
*3* vecuronium 456
Nicoderm
*3* cimetidine 118*
Nicolar
*3* lovastatin 349*
Nicorette
*3* cimetidine 118*
Nicotine
*3* cimetidine 118*
Nicotinic acid
*3* lovastatin 349*
Nicotrol
*3* cimetidine 118*
Nifedipine
Also see Calcium channel
blockers; Dihydropyri-
dine calcium channel
blockers
*3* atenolol 386
*3* cimetidine 112, 119*,
120, 128
*3* diltiazem 222*
*3* doxazosin 230*
*2* **ethanol 256**
*3* famotidine 119
*3* grapefruit juice 289*
*3* lansoprazole 119
*3* magnesium 351*
*3* metoprolol 386
*3* phenobarbital 385*, 407
*3* phenytoin 386*
*3* propranolol 385, 386*
*3* quinidine 387*, 433
*3* ranitidine 119
*3* rifabutin 388
*3* rifampin 387*
*3* vincristine 388*
Nimodipine
Also see Calcium channel
blockers
*3* cimetidine 120*
*3* omeprazole 120
*3* valproic acid 388*
Nimotop
Also see Calcium channel
blockers
*3* cimetidine 120*
*3* omeprazole 120
*3* valproic acid 388*

Nipride
*3* clonidine 153*
*3* diltiazem 222*
*3* guanabenz 153
*3* guanfacine 153
Nisoldipine
Also see Calcium channel
blockers; Dihydropyri-
dine calcium channel
blockers
*3* cimetidine 112, 120*, 128
*3* famotidine 120
*3* grapefruit juice 290
*3* nizatidine 120
*3* omeprazole 120
*3* propranolol 385, 386
*3* ranitidine 120
Nitrazepam
Also see Benzodiazepines
*3* ethanol 199
*3* rifampin 203
Nitrendipine
Also see Calcium channel
blockers
*3* cimetidine 112, 119,
120*, 128
*3* cyclosporine 167, 169,
179, 184
*3* famotidine 120
*3* grapefruit juice 290
*3* nizatidine 120
*3* omeprazole 120
*3* ranitidine 120
Nitroglycerin
*2* **ergotamine 241***
*3* metronidazole 252, 370
Nitropress
*3* clonidine 153*
*3* diltiazem 222*
*3* guanabenz 153
*3* guanfacine 153
Nitroprusside
*3* clonidine 153*
*3* diltiazem 222*
*3* guanabenz 153
*3* guanfacine 153
Nizatidine
Also see H$_2$-receptor antagonists
*3* cefpodoxime 29, 84
*3* cefuroxime 85
*3* enoxacin 31, 236
*3* glipizide 32, 287

© Copyright Applied Therapeutics, Inc. 1998

Nizatidine *(Contitnued)*
*3* glyburide 32
*3* ketoconazole 115, 329
*3* nisoldipine 120
*3* nitrendipine 120
*3* tolbutamide 128
Nizoral
Also see Antifungals;
 Imidazoles
*3* alprazolam 90, 327, 333
*3* aluminum 34
*3* antacids 34*
*1* **astemizole 48, 49*, 332**
*2* **atorvastatin 326**
*3* buspirone 63
*3* calcium 34
*3* cetirizine 49
*3* chlordiazepoxide 90*
*3* cimetidine 115*, 328, 329
*2* **cisapride 136, 137, 138*, 139**
*3* cyclosporine 170, 172, 173, 174*, 177, 332
*3* diazepam 201
*3* didanosine 207*
*3* ethanol 250*
*3* famotidine 115, 329
*3* felodipine 260
*3* fluvastatin 326
*3* indinavir 303*, 330
*3* lansoprazole 328, 329
*3* loratadine 49, 326*
*2* **lovastatin 321, 326***
*3* magnesium 34
*3* methylprednisolone 327*
*3* midazolam 90, 264, 327*, 333
*3* nizatidine 115, 329
*3* omeprazole 328*, 329
*3* pravastatin 326
*3* quinidine 329*
*3* ranitidine 115, 328, 329*
*3* rifampin 265, 323, 330*
*3* ritonavir 303
*3* saquinavir 303, 330*
*2* **simvastatin 326**
*3* sodium bicarbonate 34*
*3* sucralfate 331*
*3* tacrolimus 174, 265, 331*
*1* **terfenadine 49, 266, 323, 332***
*3* tolbutamide 267

*3* triazolam 90, 324, 327, 333*
*3* warfarin 268, 324, 333*
Noctec
*3* ethanol 86*
*3* warfarin 86*
Nolvadex
Also see Antineoplastics
*2* **aminoglutethimide 16***
Nonsteroidal anti-inflammatory drugs
Also see Bromfenac;
 Diclofenac; Fenoprofen;
 Flurbiprofen; Ibuprofen;
 Indomethacin; Ketoprofen; Kctorolac; Meclofenamate; Mefenamic
 acid; Nabumetone;
 Naproxen; Piroxicam;
 Sulindac; Tolmetin
*2* **acenocoumarol 418**
*3* amikacin 286
*3* atenolol 307
*3* bromfenac 57*, 58
*3* bumetanide 61*
*3* captopril 41
*3* cholestyramine 100*, 104*, 160
*3* colestipol 100, 104, 160*
*3* cyclosporine 166*, 172*, 173, 174*, 175*, 178*, 183*
*3* digoxin 212*
*3* doxazosin 306
*3* furosemide 61, 281*, 308
*3* gentamicin 286*
*3* hydralazine 298*
*3* labetalol 307
*3* lithium 204*, 298*, 304*, 336*, 342*, 343*, 345*
*2* **methotrexate 204*, 305*, 334*, 359***
*3* methotrexate 275*, 299*
*3* oxprenolol 307
*2* **phenprocoumon 276*, 299, 309**
*3* phenylpropanolamine 306*
*3* phenytoin 58*
*3* pindolol 307
*3* prazosin 306*
*3* prednisone 307*
*3* propranolol 307*
*3* sulindac 57
*3* terazosin 306

*3* triamterene 308*
*3* vancomycin 309*
*3* verapamil 205*
*2* **warfarin 53, 58*, 206*, 208, 262*, 276, 299*, 309*, 335*, 352*, 353, 363, 379*, 381*, 409, 418*, 443*, 444, 452***
Norcuron
Also see Muscle relaxants;
 Neuromuscular blockers
*3* amphotericin B 27
*3* diltiazem 456
*2* **gentamicin 51**
*3* nicardipine 456
*3* verapamil 456*
Nordette
Also see Estrogens
*3* ampicillin 28*
*3* carbamazepine 76*, 394
*1* **cigarette smoking 107***
*3* cyclosporine 165, 179*
*3* dexamethasone 395
*2* **dicumarol 397**
*3* doxycycline 397
*3* griseofulvin 292*
*3* hydrocortisone 395
*3* methylprednisolone 395
*3* phenobarbital 394*
*2* **phenprocoumon 397**
*3* phenytoin 394*
*3* prednisolone 395*
*3* prednisone 395
*3* primidone 394
*3* rifabutin 396
*3* rifampin 395*
*3* ritonavir 396*
*3* tetracycline 397*
*2* **warfarin 397***
Norepinephrine
*2* **amitriptyline 301**
*2* **desipramine 301**
*3* guanadrel 294
*3* guanethidine 294*
*2* **imipramine 300***
*3* isocarboxazid 389
*3* methyldopa 366*
*3* phenelzine 389*
*2* **protriptyline 301**
*3* tranylcypromine 389
Norethandrolone
*2* **warfarin 398**

Norethindrone
*3* ampicillin 28*
*3* carbamazepine 76*, 394
*1* **cigarette smoking 107***
*3* cyclosporine 165, 179*
*3* dexamethasone 395
*2* **dicumarol 397**
*3* doxycycline 397
*3* griseofulvin 292*
*3* hydrocortisone 395
*3* methylprednisolone 395
*3* phenobarbital 394*
*2* **phenprocoumon 397**
*3* phenytoin 394*
*3* prednisolone 395*
*3* prednisone 395
*3* primidone 394
*3* rifabutin 396
*3* rifampin 395*
*3* tetracycline 397*
*2* **warfarin 397***

Norethin
Also see Estrogens
*3* ampicillin 28*
*3* carbamazepine 76*, 394
*1* **cigarette smoking 107***
*3* cyclosporine 165, 179*
*3* dexamethasone 395
*2* **dicumarol 397**
*3* doxycycline 397
*3* griseofulvin 292*
*3* hydrocortisone 395
*3* methylprednisolone 395
*3* phenobarbital 394*
*2* **phenprocoumon 397**
*3* phenytoin 394*
*3* prednisolone 395*
*3* prednisone 395
*3* primidone 394
*3* rifabutin 396
*3* rifampin 395*
*3* ritonavir 396*
*3* tetracycline 397*
*2* **warfarin 397***

Norflex
Also see Muscle relaxants;
Neuromuscular blockers
*3* chlorpromazine 96*
*3* fluphenazine 96
*3* haloperidol 55

Norfloxacin
Also see Quinolones
*3* aluminum 35*, 390

*3* antacids 35*, 36
*3* iron 132, 315*
*3* Maalox 35*
*3* magnesium 35*
*3* metoprolol 132
*3* pentoxifylline 133
*3* phenytoin 133
*3* sucralfate 134, 390*, 392
*3* theophylline 134, 238, 390*
*3* warfarin 135, 391*, 393
*3* zinc 135

Norgestimate
*3* ampicillin 28*
*3* carbamazepine 76*, 394
*1* **cigarette smoking 107***
*3* cyclosporine 165, 179*
*3* dexamethasone 395
*2* **dicumarol 397**
*3* doxycycline 397
*3* griseofulvin 292*
*3* hydrocortisone 395
*3* methylprednisolone 395
*3* phenobarbital 394*
*2* **phenprocoumon 397**
*3* phenytoin 394*
*3* prednisolone 395*
*3* prednisone 395
*3* primidone 394
*3* rifabutin 396
*3* rifampin 395*
*3* tetracycline 397*
*2* **warfarin 397***

Norgestrel
*3* ampicillin 28*
*3* carbamazepine 76*, 394
*1* **cigarette smoking 107***
*3* cyclosporine 165, 179*
*3* dexamethasone 395
*2* **dicumarol 397**
*3* doxycycline 397
*3* griseofulvin 292*
*3* hydrocortisone 395
*3* methylprednisolone 395
*3* phenobarbital 394*
*2* **phenprocoumon 397**
*3* phenytoin 394*
*3* prednisolone 395*
*3* prednisone 395
*3* primidone 394
*3* rifabutin 396
*3* rifampin 395*

*3* tetracycline 397*
*2* **warfarin 397***

Norinyl
Also see Estrogens
*3* ampicillin 28*
*3* carbamazepine 76*, 394
*1* **cigarette smoking 107***
*3* cyclosporine 165, 179*
*3* dexamethasone 395
*2* **dicumarol 397**
*3* doxycycline 397
*3* griseofulvin 292*
*3* hydrocortisone 395
*3* methylprednisolone 395
*3* phenobarbital 394*
*2* **phenprocoumon 397**
*3* phenytoin 394*
*3* prednisolone 395*
*3* prednisone 395
*3* primidone 394
*3* rifabutin 396
*3* rifampin 395*
*3* ritonavir 396*
*3* tetracycline 397*
*2* **warfarin 397***

Normodyne
Also see Alpha blockers;
Beta-adrenergic blockers
*3* cimetidine 125
*3* diazepam 202
*3* epinephrine 240
*3* indomethacin 307

Noroxin
Also see Quinolones
*3* aluminum 35*, 390
*3* antacids 35*, 36
*3* iron 132, 315*
*3* Maalox 35*
*3* magnesium 35*
*3* metoprolol 132
*3* pentoxifylline 133
*3* phenytoin 133
*3* sucralfate 134, 390*, 392
*3* theophylline 134, 238, 390*
*3* warfarin 135, 391*, 393
*3* zinc 135

Norpace
Also see Antiarrhythmics
*3* clarithromycin 224
*3* erythromycin 224*
*3* lidocaine 224*

*3* enoxacin 31, 236
*3* glipizide 287
*3* glyburide 32
*3* ketoconazole 328*, 329
*3* methotrexate 361*
*3* nimodipine 120
*3* nisoldipine 120
*3* nitrendipine 120
*3* phenytoin 393*

Oncovin
Also see Antineoplastics
*3* nifedipine 388*

Oral anticoagulants
Also see Acenocoumarol; Dicumarol; Phenindione; Phenprocoumon; Warfarin
*3* acetaminophen 4*
*3* allopurinol 13*
*3* aminoglutethimide 17*
*3* amiodarone 23*
*2* **amobarbital 408**
*2* **aspirin 4, 46***
*2* **azapropazone 53***
*3* azathioprine 54*, 356
*2* **bromfenac 58***
*2* **butabarbital 408**
*3* carbamazepine 81*
*2* **cefamandole 379**
*2* **cefazolin 379**
*2* **cefmetazole 379**
*2* **cefoperazone 379**
*2* **cefotetan 379**
*2* **cefoxitin 379**
*2* **ceftriaxone 379**
*3* chloral hydrate 87*
*2* **chloramphenicol 88***
*3* cholestyramine 106*, 148, 286, 350
*2* **cimetidine 129***
*3* ciprofloxacin 135*, 391, 393
*3* clarithromycin 247
*2* **clofibrate 148*, 286, 350**
*3* colestipol 106, 148, 286, 350
*3* cyclophosphamide 164*
*2* **danazol 186***
*2* **dextrothyroxine 197***
*2* **diclofenac 53, 206*, 208, 262, 309, 335, 352, 353, 409, 418, 444**
*2* **diflunisal 208***

*2* **disulfiram 229***
*3* doxycycline 233*
*3* erythromycin 247*
*3* ethanol 256*
*2* **etodolac 257***
*2* **fenoprofen 262***
*3* fluconazole 268*, 324, 333
*3* fluorouracil 269*
*3* fluoxetine 274*, 441
*2* **flurbiprofen 276***
*3* fluvastatin 350
*3* fluvoxamine 279*
*2* **gemfibrozil 148, 285*, 350**
*3* glucagon 288*
*2* **glutethimide 288***
*3* glyburide 289*
*3* griseofulvin 293*
*3* heparin 297*
*2* **heptabarbital 408**
*2* **ibuprofen 53, 208, 262, 276, 299*, 309, 335, 352, 353, 409, 418, 444**
*2* **indomethacin 309***
*3* isoniazid 320*
*3* itraconazole 268, 324*,333
*3* ketoconazole 268, 324, 333*
*2* **ketoprofen 335***
*3* lovastatin 148, 286, 350*
*2* **meclofenamate 352***
*2* **mefenamic acid 352***
*3* mercaptopurine 54, 356*
*2* **methandrostenolone 398**
*2* **methyltestosterone 398**
*2* **metronidazole 370***
*3* miconazole 324, 333, 374*
*3* mitotane 377*
*2* **moxalactam 379***
*2* **nabumetone 379***
*3* nafcillin 380*
*3* nalidixic acid 381*
*2* **naproxen 53, 208, 262, 309, 335, 352, 353, 381*, 409, 418, 444**
*3* neomycin 383*
*3* nonacetylated salicylates 46
*2* **norethandrolone 398**
*3* norfloxacin 135, 391*, 393

*3* ofloxacin 135, 391, 392*
*2* **oral contraceptives 397***
*2* **oxymetholone 398***
*1* **oxyphenbutazone 409**
*3* paroxetine 399*, 441
*2* **pentobarbital 408**
*2* **phenobarbital 407*, 408**
*1* **phenylbutazone 53, 409***
*3* phenytoin 418*
*2* **piroxicam 418***
*2* **primidone 408**
*3* propafenone 426*
*3* propoxyphene 427*
*3* quinidine 433*
*2* **rifampin 439***
*2* **secobarbital 408**
*3* sertraline 441*
*2* **stanozolol 398**
*3* sucralfate 442*
*3* sulfamethizole 455
*3* sulfamethoxazole 455
*3* sulfaphenazole 455
*2* **sulfinpyrazone 443***
*2* **sulindac 443***
*2* **testosterone 398**
*3* thyroid 451*
*2* **tolmetin 452***
*3* triclofos 455*
*3* trimethoprim-sulfamethoxazole 455*
*3* troleandomycin 247
*3* vitamin E 456*
*3* vitamin K 457*
*3* zafirlukast 457*

Oral contraceptives
*3* ampicillin 28*
*3* carbamazepine 76*, 394
*1* **cigarette smoking 107***
*3* cyclosporine 165, 179*
*3* dexamethasone 395
*2* **dicumarol 397**
*3* doxycycline 397
*3* griseofulvin 292*
*3* hydrocortisone 395
*3* methylprednisolone 395
*3* phenobarbital 394*
*2* **phenprocoumon 397**
*3* phenytoin 394*
*3* prednisolone 395*
*3* prednisone 395
*3* primidone 394
*3* rifabutin 396

Oral contraceptives
*(Continued)*
*3* rifampin 395*
*3* tetracycline 397*
*2* **warfarin 397***
Orap
  Also see Neuroleptics
*3* bromocriptine 61
Orasone
  Also see Corticosteroids
*3* aminoglutethimide 15
*3* aspirin 45*
*3* indomethacin 307*
*3* insulin 310*
*3* oral contraceptives 395
*3* phenobarbital 403*
Orimune
*1* **methotrexate 362***
Orinase
  Also see Antidiabetics;
   Sulfonylureas
*3* aspirin 41
*3* chloramphenicol 88
*3* cimetidine 127*
*1* **ethanol 99, 255***
*3* famotidine 128
*3* fluconazole 266*
*3* itraconazole 267
*3* ketoconazole 267
*3* methandrostenolone 358*
*3* miconazole 267
*3* nizatidine 128
*2* **oxyphenbutazone 409**
*2* **phenylbutazone 408***
*3* phenytoin 415*
*3* rifabutin 437
*3* rifampin 437*
*3* sulfamethizole 451
*3* sulfaphenazole 451
*3* sulfinpyrazone 442*
*3* sulfisoxazole 451
*3* tranylcypromine 312
*3* trimethoprim-sul-
   famethoxazole 451*
Orphenadrine
  Also see Muscle relaxants;
   Neuromuscular blockers
*3* chlorpromazine 96*
*3* fluphenazine 96
*3* haloperidol 55
Ortho-Cept
  Also see Estrogens
*3* ampicillin 28*

*3* carbamazepine 76*, 394
*1* **cigarette smoking 107***
*3* cyclosporine 165, 179*
*3* dexamethasone 395
*2* **dicumarol 397**
*3* doxycycline 397
*3* griseofulvin 292*
*3* hydrocortisone 395
*3* methylprednisolone 395
*3* phenobarbital 394*
*2* **phenprocoumon 397**
*3* phenytoin 394*
*3* prednisolone 395*
*3* prednisone 395
*3* primidone 394
*3* rifabutin 396
*3* rifampin 395*
*3* ritonavir 396*
*3* tetracycline 397*
*2* **warfarin 397***
Ortho-Cyclen
  Also see Estrogens
*3* ampicillin 28*
*3* carbamazepine 76*, 394
*1* **cigarette smoking 107***
*3* cyclosporine 165, 179*
*3* dexamethasone 395
*2* **dicumarol 397**
*3* doxycycline 397
*3* griseofulvin 292*
*3* hydrocortisone 395
*3* methylprednisolone 395
*3* phenobarbital 394*
*2* **phenprocoumon 397**
*3* phenytoin 394*
*3* prednisolone 395*
*3* prednisone 395
*3* primidone 394
*3* rifabutin 396
*3* rifampin 395*
*3* ritonavir 396*
*3* tetracycline 397*
*2* **warfarin 397***
Ortho-Novum
  Also see Estrogens
*3* ampicillin 28*
*3* carbamazepine 76*, 394
*1* **cigarette smoking 107***
*3* cyclosporine 165, 179*
*3* dexamethasone 395
*2* **dicumarol 397**
*3* doxycycline 397

*3* griseofulvin 292*
*3* hydrocortisone 395
*3* methylprednisolone 395
*3* phenobarbital 394*
*2* **phenprocoumon 397**
*3* phenytoin 394*
*3* prednisolone 395*
*3* prednisone 395
*3* primidone 394
*3* rifabutin 396
*3* rifampin 395*
*3* ritonavir 396*
*3* tetracycline 397*
*2* **warfarin 397***
Ortho Tri-Cyclen
  Also see Estrogens
*3* ampicillin 28*
*3* carbamazepine 76*, 394
*1* **cigarette smoking 107***
*3* cyclosporine 165, 179*
*3* dexamethasone 395
*2* **dicumarol 397**
*3* doxycycline 397
*3* griseofulvin 292*
*3* hydrocortisone 395
*3* methylprednisolone 395
*3* phenobarbital 394*
*2* **phenprocoumon 397**
*3* phenytoin 394*
*3* prednisolone 395*
*3* prednisone 395
*3* primidone 394
*3* rifabutin 396
*3* rifampin 395*
*3* ritonavir 396*
*3* tetracycline 397*
*2* **warfarin 397***
Orudis
  Also see Nonsteroidal anti-
   inflammatory drugs
*3* cyclosporine 166, 174*
*2* **methotrexate 334***
*2* **warfarin 335***
Oruvail
  Also see Nonsteroidal anti-
   inflammatory drugs
*3* cyclosporine 166, 174*
*2* **methotrexate 334***
*2* **warfarin 335***
Ovcon
  Also see Estrogens
*3* ampicillin 28*
*3* carbamazepine 76*, 394

Potassium iodide
**3** lithium 346*
Potassium-sparing diuretics
Also see Amiloride;
Spironolactone;
Triamterene
**3** digoxin 218*
**3** diclofenac 308
**3** ibuprofen 308
**3** indomethacin 308*
**1 mitotane 377***
**2 potassium 419*, 420***
Pravachol
Also see HMG-CoA reductase inhibitors
**3** cholestyramine 104*
**3** clofibrate 285
**3** colestipol 104
**3** gemfibrozil 285*
**3** itraconazole 321
**3** ketoconazole 326
**3** nefazodone 382
Pravastatin
Also see HMG-CoA reductase inhibitors
**3** cholestyramine 104*
**3** clofibrate 285
**3** colestipol 104
**3** gemfibrozil 285*
**3** itraconazole 321
**3** ketoconazole 326
**3** nefazodone 382
Prazepam
Also see Benzodiazepines
**3** cimetidine 111
**3** disulfiram 198
**3** rifampin 203
Praziquantel
**3** chloroquine 92*
**3** cimetidine 123*
**3** hydroxychloroquine 92
Prazosin
Also see Alpha blockers
**3** enalapril 62
**3** ibuprofen 306
**3** indomethacin 306*
**3** propranolol 420*
**3** verapamil 421*
Prednisolone
Also see Corticosteroids
**3** aminoglutethimide 15
**3** cyclosporine 181*

**3** isoniazid 318*
**3** oral contraceptives 395*
**3** phenobarbital 403
**3** rifampin 422*
**3** tacrolimus 181
Prednisone
Also see Corticosteroids
**3** aminoglutethimide 15
**3** aspirin 45*
**3** indomethacin 307*
**3** insulin 310*
**3** oral contraceptives 395
**3** phenobarbital 403*
Prelone
Also see Corticosteroids
**3** aminoglutethimide 15
**3** cyclosporine 181*
**3** isoniazid 318*
**3** oral contraceptives 395*
**3** phenobarbital 403
**3** rifampin 422*
**3** tacrolimus 181
Prevacid
Also see Proton pump inhibitors
**3** cefpodoxime 29, 84
**3** cefuroxime 85
**3** digoxin 214
**3** enoxacin 31, 236
**3** glipizide 287
**3** glyburide 32
**3** ketoconazole 328, 329
**3** nifedipine 119
Prilosec
Also see Proton pump inhibitors
**3** cefpodoxime 29, 84
**3** cefuroxime 85
**3** diazepam 203*
**3** digoxin 214*
**3** enoxacin 31, 236
**3** glipizide 287
**3** glyburide 32
**3** ketoconazole 328*, 329
**3** methotrexate 361*
**3** nimodipine 120
**3** nisoldipine 120
**3** nitrendipine 120
**3** phenytoin 393*
Primatene Mist
Also see Sympathomimetics
**3** alprenolol 240

**3** chlorpromazine 93*
**3** clozapine 93
**2 imipramine 240***
**3** labetalol 240
**3** nadolol 240
**3** pindolol 240
**3** propranolol 240*, 429
**2 protriptyline 240**
**3** thioridazine 93
**3** timolol 240
Primaxin
**3** cyclosporine 172*
**3** tacrolimus 172
**3** theophylline 300*
Primidone
Also see Anticonvulsants; Barbiturates
**3** acetaminophen 3
**3** acetazolamide 6*
**3** clozapine 65
**3** cyclosporine 66
**3** methadone 357
**3** oral contraceptives 394
**3** phenobarbital 404*
**3** phenytoin 410*
**3** tacrolimus 413
**3** valproic acid 422*
**2 warfarin 408**
Prinivil
Also see Angiotensin-converting enzyme inhibitors
**3** bunazosin 62
**3** lithium 341*
Probenecid
**3** aspirin 45*
**3** dapsone 187*
**3** dyphylline 233*
**2 methotrexate 363***
**3** thiopental 423*
**3** zidovudine 423*
Probucol
**3** cyclosporine 182*
Procainamide
Also see Antiarrhythmics
**3** amiodarone 22*
**3** cimetidine 124*
**3** edrophonium 384
**3** lomefloxacin 392
**3** neostigmine 384*
**3** ofloxacin 391*
**3** quinidine 423*
**3** trimethoprim 424*

Propranolol
Also see Antiarrhythmics;
Beta-adrenergic blockers
*3* amiodarone 21, 23
*3* bupivacaine 428
*3* chlorpromazine 97*
*3* cimetidine 125*
*3* ciprofloxacin 133
*3* clonidine 154*
*3* cocaine 158*
*3* contrast media 162*
*3* digitoxin 216
*3* digoxin 216*
*3* diltiazem 223*, 430
*3* epinephrine 240*, 429
*3* felodipine 386
*3* flecainide 262*, 263
*3* fluoxetine 271*
*3* guanabenz 154
*3* guanfacine 154
*3* indomethacin 307*
*3* insulin 311*
*3* isradipine 385, 386
*3* lidocaine 341*, 428
*3* local anesthetic 429
*3* naproxen 307
*3* neostigmine 384*
*3* nicardipine 384*
*3* nifedipine 385, 386*
*3* nisoldipine 385, 386
*3* physostigmine 384
*3* piroxicam 307
*3* prazosin 420*
*3* propafenone 367
*3* propoxyphene 367
*3* quinidine 367, 427*, 431
*3* rifampin 368
*3* sulfinpyrazone 307
*3* tacrine 428*
*3* terazosin 421
*3* terbutaline 369
*3* tetracaine 428*
*2* **theophylline 429***
*3* thioridazine 97
*3* verapamil 223, 430*
Propulsid
*3* cimetidine 109*
*2* **clarithromycin 136*, 139**
*3* cyclosporine 176
*2* **erythromycin 136*, 139**
*2* **fluconazole 137, 138, 139**

*2* **itraconazole 137*, 138, 139**
*2* **ketoconazole 136, 137, 138*, 139**
*2* **mibefradil 138***
*2* **miconazole 137, 138, 139***
*2* **troleandomycin 136, 139***
Propylthiouracil
*3* theophylline 434
Prostaglandins
Also see Enprostil
*3* ethanol 238*
Prostigmin
Also see Cholinergics
*3* atenolol 384
*3* nadolol 384
*3* procainamide 384*
*3* propranolol 384*
*3* tacrine 56
Protease inhibitors
Also see Indinavir;
Nelfinavir; Ritonavir;
Saquinavir
*3* azithromycin 144
*3* clarithromycin 144*
*3* desipramine 190*
*3* dirithromycin 144
*3* erythromycin 144, 244*
*3* indinavir 440
*3* ketoconazole 303*, 330*
*3* nelfinavir 440
*3* oral contraceptives 396*
*2* **rifabutin 304*, 434*, 436**
*3* rifabutin 304,*, 383, 434*, 435
*2* **rifampin 383*, 435*, 436***
*3* rifampin 304, 383, 435, 436
*3* ritonavir 440*
*3* saquinavir 440*
*3* theophylline 440*
*3* troleandomycin 144, 244
Proton pump inhibitors
Also see Lansoprazole;
Omeprazole
*3* cefpodoxime 29, 84
*3* cefuroxime 85
*3* diazepam 203*
*3* digoxin 214*

*3* enoxacin 31, 236
*3* glipizide 287
*3* glyburide 32
*3* ketoconazole 328*, 329
*3* methotrexate 361*
*3* nifedipine 119
*3* nimodipine 120
*3* nisoldipine 120
*3* nitrendipine 120
*3* phenytoin 393*
Protostat
*3* carbamazepine 75*
*3* cholestyramine 103*
*3* colestipol 103
*3* diazepam 252, 370
*3* disulfiram 227*
*3* ethanol 252*
*2* **fluorouracil 268***
*3* nitroglycerin 252, 370
*3* phenytoin 252, 369*, 370
*3* trimethoprim-sul-
famethoxazole 252, 370*
*2* **warfarin 370***
Protriptyline
Also see Cyclic antidepressants; Tricyclic antide-
pressants
*3* cimetidine 111, 113, 121
*2* **epinephrine 240**
*2* **norepinephrine 301**
*3* phenobarbital 405*
Provera
Also see Progestins
*3* aminoglutethimide 15*
Prozac
Also see Selective sero-
tonin reuptake inhibitors
*3* alprazolam 14*, 200
*3* amitriptyline 24*
*2* **astemizole 272**
*3* bumetanide 269
*3* buspirone 63*
*3* carbamazepine 70*
*3* cyproheptadine 185*
*3* desipramine 188*
*2* **dexfenfluramine 191*, 260**
*3* dextromethorphan 194*
*3* diazepam 200*
*3* doxepin 189
*2* **fenfluramine 191, 260***
*3* furosemide 269*

*3* haloperidol 270*
*3* imipramine 189
*1* **isocarboxazid 273**
*3* lithium 270*
*3* metoprolol 271
*3* nortriptyline 189
*1* **phenelzine 273**
*3* phenytoin 271*
*3* propranolol 271*
*2* **selegiline 272***
*2* **simvastatin 382**
*3* tacrine 277
*2* **terfenadine 272***
*3* torsemide 269
*1* **tranylcypromine 273***
*3* trazodone 189
*2* **tryptophan 274***
*3* warfarin 274*, 441
Pseudoephedrine
Also see
Sympathomimetics
*3* aluminum 37*
*3* antacids 37*
*1* **isocarboxazid 402**
*3* magnesium 37*
*2* **moclobemide 239**
*1* **phenelzine 402***
*3* sodium bicarbonate 37*
*1* **tranylcypromine 402**
Purinethol
Also see Antineoplastics
*3* allopurinol 10, 11*
*3* captopril 54
*3* warfarin 54, 355*
Pyridostigmine
Also see Cholinergics
*3* tacrine 56
Pyridoxine
*3* levodopa 339*
*3* phenytoin 411*
Pyrimethamine
*2* **folic acid 280***
Quelicin
Also see Neuromuscular
blockers
*3* amphotericin B 27*
*3* cyclophosphamide 164*
*2* **echothiophate iodide
234***
*2* **gentamicin 51**
*3* quinidine 432
Questran
Also see Bile acid-binding
resins

*3* acetaminophen 1*
*3* amiodarone 17*
*3* diclofenac 100*, 160
*3* digitoxin 101
*3* digoxin 100*
*3* fluvastatin 104
*3* furosemide 101*, 161
*3* gemfibrozil 161
*3* hydrocortisone 101*
*3* imipramine 102*
*3* lovastatin 104
*3* methotrexate 103*
*3* metronidazole 103*
*3* phenprocoumon 106
*3* piroxicam 104*
*3* pravastatin 104*
*3* simvastatin 104
*3* tenoxicam 104
*3* tetracycline 162
*3* thiazides 162
*3* thyroid 105*
*3* valproic acid 106*
*3* warfarin 106*, 148, 286,
350
Quinidine
Also see Antiarrhythmics
*3* acetazolamide 6*, 431
*3* amiodarone 22*
*3* antacids 38*, 431
*3* calcium 38*
*3* cimetidine 38, 126*
*3* clarithromycin 243
*2* **codeine 158***
*3* desipramine 302
*3* dextromethorphan 196*
*3* digoxin 216*
*3* encainide 236*
*3* erythromycin 243*
*3* fluconazole 329
*3* haloperidol 297*
*3* hydrocodone 158
*3* imipramine 302*
*3* itraconazole 329
*3* kaolin-pectin 325*
*3* ketoconazole 329*
*3* Maalox 38*
*3* magnesium 38*
*3* metoprolol 367*, 427,
431
*3* mexiletine 371*
*3* miconazole 329

*3* Milk of Magnesia 38*
*3* Mylanta 38*
*3* nifedipine 387*, 433
*3* nortriptyline 302
*3* phenobarbital 405*
*3* phenytoin 405, 411*
*3* procainamide 423*
*3* propafenone 425*
*3* propranolol 367, 427*,
431
*3* rifabutin 431
*3* rifampin 430*
*3* sodium bicarbonate 6,
431*
*3* succinylcholine 432
*3* timolol 367, 427, 431*
*3* Titralac 38*
*3* troleandomycin 243
*3* tubocurarine 432*
*3* verapamil 387, 433*
*3* warfarin 433*
Quinine
*3* cigarette smoking 108*
*3* digitoxin 217
*3* digoxin 217*
Quinolones
Also see Ciprofloxacin;
Clinafloxacin; Enoxacin;
Lomefloxacin; Norflox-
acin; Ofloxacin; Peflox-
acin; Pipemidic acid
*3* aluminum 30*, 35*, 36*,
130, 134, 390, 392
*3* antacids 30*, 31*, 34*,
35*, 36*
*3* cimetidine 31
*3* diazepam 130*
*3* didanosine 130*
*3* famotidine 236
*3* food 131*
*3* foscarnet 131*
*3* iron 132*, 315*
*3* Maalox 30*, 35*, 36*
*3* magnesium 30*, 35*, 130
*3* metoprolol 132*
*3* nizatidine 31, 236
*3* omeprazole 31, 236
*3* pentoxifylline 133*
*3* phenytoin 133*
*3* procainamide 391*
*3* propranolol 132
*3* ranitidine 31, 236*
*3* sucralfate 30, 134*, 389,
390*, 392*

Simvastatin *(Continued)*
**2 mibefradil 373\***
**2 nefazodone 382\***
3 verapamil 374

Sinemet
3 chlordiazepoxide 202
**2 chlorpromazine 95\***
3 diazepam 201\*
**2 haloperidol 95**
3 iron 314\*
3 isocarboxazid 338
3 methionine 337\*
3 moclobemide 338\*
3 nialamide 338
3 phenelzine 338\*
3 phenytoin 339\*
3 pyridoxine 339\*
3 spiramycin 340\*
3 tacrine 340\*
3 tranylcypromine 338

Sinequan
Also see Cyclic antidepressants; Tricyclic antidepressants
3 chlorpropamide 231
3 cimetidine 113\*, 115, 121
3 fluoxetine 189
3 propoxyphene 230\*
3 tolazamide 231\*

Sinex
3 guanethidine 295\*
3 imipramine 302\*
**1 isocarboxazid 400**
**1 phenelzine 400\***
**1 tranylcypromine 400**

Sintrom
Also see Anticoagulants; Oral anticoagulants
3 acetaminophen 4
3 aminoglutethimide 17
3 amiodarone 23
**2 cimetidine 129**
**2 diflunisal 208**
3 glucagon 288
**2 phenobarbital 408**
**2 piroxicam 418**
**2 rifampin 439**
**2 sulfinpyrazone 443**

Slo-Phyllin
3 adenosine 7\*
3 allopurinol 12\*
3 aminoglutethimide 16\*

3 amiodarone 23\*
3 atenolol 429
3 carbamazepine 78\*
3 cigarette smoking 108\*
3 cimetidine 127\*
3 ciprofloxacin 134\*, 238, 390
3 disulfiram 228\*
**2 enoxacin 134, 238\*, 390**
3 erythromycin 245\*, 449
**2 fluvoxamine 278\***
3 imipenem 300\*
3 interferon 313\*
3 isoniazid 319\*
3 lithium 347\*
3 methimazole 434
3 metoprolol 429
**2 mexiletine 373\***
3 moricizine 378\*
3 nadolol 429
3 norfloxacin 134, 238, 390\*
3 pefloxacin 134, 238, 390, 390
3 pentobarbital 406
3 pentoxifylline 400\*
3 phenobarbital 406\*
3 phenytoin 414\*
3 pipemidic acid 134, 238, 390
3 propafenone 426\*
**2 propranolol 429\***
3 propylthiouracil 434
3 radioactive iodine 434\*
3 rifampin 436\*
3 ritonavir 440\*
3 secobarbital 406
3 tacrine 444\*
3 thiabendazole 447\*
3 thyroid 448\*
3 ticlopidine 448\*
**2 troleandomycin 246, 448\***
3 verapamil 449\*
3 zafirlukast 450\*

Smallpox vaccine
**1 methotrexate 362**

Smoking
3 chlorpromazine 92\*
3 insulin 107\*
**1 oral contraceptives 107\***
3 quinine 108\*
3 tacrine 108\*
3 theophylline 108\*

Sodium bicarbonate
Also see Antacids
3 cefuroxime 85
3 ephedrine 31\*
3 glipizide 32\*
3 iron 33\*
3 ketoconazole 34\*
3 lithium 346\*
3 methenamine 358\*
3 mexiletine 372\*
3 pseudoephedrine 37\*
3 quinidine 6, 431\*

Sodium chloride
3 lithium 347\*

Sodium polystyrene sulfonate resin
3 antacids 38\*
3 calcium 38\*
3 Maalox 38\*
3 magnesium 38\*
3 Milk of Magnesia 38\*

Sofarin
Also see Anticoagulants; Oral anticoagulants
3 acetaminophen 4\*
3 allopurinol 13\*
3 aminoglutethimide 17\*
3 amiodarone 23\*
**2 amobarbital 408**
**2 aspirin 4, 46\***
**2 azapropazone 53\***
3 azathioprine 54\*, 356
**2 bromfenac 58\***
**2 butabarbital 408**
3 carbamazepine 81\*
**2 cefamandole 379**
**2 cefazolin 379**
**2 cefmetazole 379**
**2 cefoperazone 379**
**2 cefotetan 379**
**2 cefoxitin 379**
**2 ceftriaxone 379**
3 chloral hydrate 87\*
**2 chloramphenicol 88**
3 cholestyramine 106\*, 148, 286, 350
**2 cimetidine 129\***
3 ciprofloxacin 135\*, 391, 393
3 clarithromycin 247
**2 clofibrate 148\*, 286, 350**
3 colestipol 106, 148, 286, 350

*3* famotidine 120
*3* grapefruit juice 290
*3* nizatidine 120
*3* omeprazole 120
*3* propranolol 385, 386
*3* ranitidine 120
Sulfadiazine
Also see Sulfonamides
*3* methenamine 359*

Sulfadoxine pyrimethamine
*3* chlorpromazine 91
Sulfaethidole
Also see Sulfonamides
Sulfamethizole
Also see Sulfonamides
*3* methenamine 359
*3* phenytoin 413
*3* tolbutamide 451
*3* warfarin 455
Sulfamethoxazole
Also see Sulfonamides
*2* **para-aminobenzoic acid 399***
*3* phenytoin 413, 416
*3* warfarin 455
Sulfamezathine
*3* cyclosporine 183*
*3* tacrolimus 183
Sulfaphenazole
*3* phenytoin 413*
*3* tolbutamide 451
*3* warfarin 455
Sulfasalazine
Also see Sulfonamides
*3* digoxin 218*
Sulfathiazole
*3* methenamine 359
Sulfinpyrazone
*2* **acenocoumarol 443**
*3* aspirin 46*
*2* **methotrexate 363**
*3* propranolol 307
*3* tolbutamide 442*
*2* **warfarin 443***
Sulfisoxazole
Also see Sulfonamides
*3* tolbutamide 451
Sulfonamides
Also see Sulfadiazine;
Sulfaethidole;

Sulfamethizole;
Sulfamethoxazole;
Sulfasalazine;
Sulfisoxazole
*3* methenamine 359*
*2* **para-aminobenzoic acid 399***
*3* phenytoin 413, 416
*3* tolbutamide 451
*3* warfarin 455
Sulfonylureas
Also see Acetohexamide;
Chlorpropamide;
Glipizide; Glyburide;
Tolazamide; Tolbutamide
*3* aluminum 32*
*3* amitriptyline 231
*3* antacids 32*
*3* aspirin 41
*3* chloramphenicol 88*
*3* cimetidine 32, 127*, 128, 287
*3* clofibrate 98*
*3* cyclosporine 170*
*3* doxepin 231*
*3* erythromycin 99*
*1* **ethanol 99*, 255***
*3* famotidine 32, 128, 287
*3* fluconazole 266*
*3* gemfibrozil 283*
*3* imipramine 231
*3* itraconazole 267
*3* ketoconazole 267
*3* lansoprazole 32, 287
*3* Maalox 32*
*3* magnesium 32*
*3* maprotiline 231
*3* methandrostenolone 358*
*3* miconazole 267
*3* nizatidine 32, 128, 287
*3* nortriptyline 231
*3* omeprazole 32, 287
*2* **oxyphenbutazone 409**
*2* **phenylbutazone 408*, 409**
*3* phenytoin 415*
*3* ranitidine 32, 287*
*3* rifabutin 437
*3* rifampin 437*
*3* sodium bicarbonate 32*
*3* sulfamethizole 451

*3* sulfaphenazole 451
*3* sulfinpyrazone 442*
*3* sulfisoxazole 451
*3* tacrolimus 170
*3* thiazides 312
*3* tranylcypromine 312
*3* trimethoprim-sulfamethoxazole 451*
*3* warfarin 289*
Sulindac
Also see Nonsteroidal antiinflammatory drugs
*3* bromfenac 58
*3* captopril 41
*3* cyclosporine 166, 173, 174, 175, 178, 183*
*3* furosemide 281
*2* **warfarin 443***
Sulphadimidine
*3* cyclosporine 183*
*3* tacrolimus 183
Sumycin
Also see Tetracyclines
*3* aluminum 39*
*3* antacids 39*
*2* **bismuth 56, 57***
*3* calcium 39*
*3* cholestyramine 162
*3* colestipol 161*
*3* digoxin 219*
*3* iron 316*
*3* magnesium 39*
*2* **methoxyflurane 365***
*3* oral contraceptives 397*
*3* zinc 447*
Surmontil
Also see Cyclic antidepressants; Tricyclic antidepressants
*3* cimetidine 111, 113
Sympathomimetics
Also see Ephedrine;
Epinephrine;
Isoproterenol;
Phenylpropanolamine;
Pseudoephidrine
*3* alprenolol 240
*3* aluminum 37*
*3* amitriptyline 25*
*3* antacids 31*, 37*
*1* **bromocriptine 59, 60***

Sympathomimetics
*(Continued)*
*3* chlorpromazine 93*
*3* clozapine 93
*3* furazolidone 192
*3* guanadrel 239
*3* guanethidine 239*
*2* imipramine 240*
*3* indomethacin 306*
*1* isocarboxazid 401, 402
*3* labetalol 240
*3* magnesium 37*
*2* moclobemide 239*
*3* nadolol 240
*1* phenelzine 401*, 402*
*3* pindolol 240
*3* propranolol 240*, 429
*2* protriptyline 240
*3* sodium bicarbonate 31*, 37*
*3* thioridazine 93, 410*
*3* timolol 240
*1* tranylcypromine 401, 402

Synalogos-DC
Also see Narcotic analgesics
*3* quinidine 158

Synthyroid
*3* carbamazepine 79*
*3* cholestyramine 105*
*3* colestipol 105
*3* phenytoin 79, 415*
*3* rifampin 79
*3* theophylline 448*
*3* warfarin 451

Tacrine
*3* ambenonium 56
*3* atenolol 428
*3* bethanechol 56*
*3* cigarette smoking 108*
*3* cimetidine 126*
*3* edrophonium 56
*3* enoxacin 237*
*3* fluoxetine 277
*2* fluvoxamine 277*
*3* levodopa 340*
*3* nadolol 428
*3* neostigmine 56
*3* paroxetine 277
*3* propranolol 428*
*3* pyridostigmine 56

*3* sertraline 277
*3* theophylline 444*
*3* trihexyphenidyl 445*

Tacrolimus
*3* allopurinol 11
*3* aminoglutethimide 413
*3* amiodarone 18
*3* carbamazepine 66, 413
*3* chloroquine 91
*3* clarithromycin 143, 145*, 244
*3* clonidine 151
*3* clotrimazole 155*
*3* colchicine 159
*3* danazol 165
*3* digoxin 166
*3* diltiazem 167
*3* doxorubicin 168
*3* erythromycin 145, 168, 244*
*3* fluconazole 155, 170, 265*, 332
*3* glipizide 171
*3* glutethimide 413
*3* grapefruit juice 171
*3* griseofulvin 172
*3* imipenem 172
*3* itraconazole 173, 265, 332
*3* ketoconazole 174, 265, 331*
*3* miconazole 177
*3* nafcillin 177
*3* nicardipine 178
*3* phenytoin 180, 413*
*3* prednisolone 181
*3* primidone 413
*3* rifabutin 413
*2* rifampin 182, 413
*3* sulphadimidine 183
*3* troleandomycin 145, 244
*3* verapamil 184

Tagamet
Also see H$_2$-receptor antagonists
*2* acenocoumarol 129
*3* alfentanil 7*
*3* alprazolam 111
*3* amiodarone 18*
*3* amitriptyline 111, 113
*3* amoxapine 111, 113
*3* carmustine 83*
*3* cefpodoxime 29, 84

*3* cefuroxime 85
*3* chloramphenicol 83
*3* chlordiazepoxide 111
*3* cisapride 109*
*3* citalopram 109*
*3* clorazepate 111
*3* clozapine 110*
*3* desipramine 110*, 113, 115, 121
*3* desmethyldiazepam 111
*3* diazepam 111*
*3* dilevalol 125
*3* diltiazem 112*, 119, 120, 128
*3* doxepin 113*, 115, 121
*3* femoxetine 113*
*3* flecainide 114*
*3* glipizide 32, 128, 287
*3* glyburide 32, 128
*3* halazepam 111
*3* imipramine 113, 115*, 121
*3* ketoconazole 115*, 328, 329
*3* labetalol 125
*3* lidocaine 116*
*3* lomustine 83
*3* maprotiline 111, 113
*3* melphalan 117*
*3* meperidine 117*
*3* metoprolol 125
*3* moricizine 118*
*3* nicotine 118*
*3* nifedipine 112, 119*, 120, 128
*3* nimodipine 119*
*3* nisoldipine 112, 119, 120*, 128
*3* nitrendipine 112, 119, 120*, 128
*3* nortriptyline 113, 115, 121*
*3* paroxetine 122*
*3* phenytoin 83, 122*
*3* pindolol 125
*3* prazepam 111
*3* praziquantel 123*
*3* procainamide 124*
*3* propafenone 124*
*3* propranolol 125*
*3* protriptyline 111, 113, 121
*3* quinidine 38, 126*

*3* tacrine 126*
*3* theophylline 127*
*3* tolbutamide 127*
*3* trazodone 111, 113
*3* triazolam 111
*3* trimipramine 111, 113
*3* verapamil 112, 119, 120, 128*
*2* **warfarin 129***

Talwin
Also see Narcotic analgesics
*3* aspirin 44*

Tambocor
Also see Antiarrhythmics
*3* amiodarone 20*
*3* cimetidine 114*
*3* propranolol 262*, 263
*3* sotalol 263*

Tamoxifen
Also see Antineoplastics
*2* **aminoglutethimide 16***

TAO
Also see Macrolides
*3* alfentanil 8
*3* alprazolam 13, 454
*1* **astemizole 48, 446**
*3* atorvastatin 51
*3* buspirone 62
*3* carbamazepine 65, 68, 79*
*2* **cisapride 136, 139***
*3* clozapine 156
*3* colchicine 160
*3* cyclosporine 168
*3* diazepam 454
*3* disopyramide 224
*3* felodipine 242
*3* indinavir 144
*3* lovastatin 242
*3* methylprednisolone 366*
*3* midazolam 243, 454
*3* quinidine 243
*3* ritonavir 244
*3* tacrolimus 145, 244
*2* **terfenadine 146, 245, 446***
*2* **theophylline 246, 448***
*3* triazolam 246, 454*
*3* valproic acid 247
*3* warfarin 247

Tapazole
*3* theophylline 434

Taractan
Also see Neuroleptics
*3* bromocriptine 61

TCAs
Also see Amitriptyline; Clomipramine; Desipramine; Doxepin; Imipramine; Maprotiline; Nortriptyline; Protriptyline; Trazodone; Trimipramine
*3* altretamine 14*
*3* butaperazine 275
*3* carbamazepine 71*, 72
*3* chlorpromazine 98*, 275
*3* chlorpropamide 231
*3* cholestyramine 102*
*3* cimetidine 110*, 111, 113*, 115*, 121*
*2* **clonidine 25, 152***
*3* clonidine 152
*3* colestipol 102
*3* dextroamphetamine 193*
*3* diltiazem 303
*2* **epinephrine 240***
*3* fluoxetine 24*, 188*, 189
*3* fluphenazine 275*
*3* fluvoxamine 148*
*3* grapefruit juice 149*
*2* **guanabenz 152**
*3* guanabenz 25
*2* **guanadrel 190**
*3* guanethidine 190*
*2* **guanfacine 152**
*3* guanfacine 25*
*3* indinavir 190
*1* **isocarboxazid 150**
*3* isoproterenol 25*
*3* lithium 26*
*2* **moclobemide 149***
*2* **norepinephrine 300*, 301**
*3* paroxetine 24, 189
*3* perphenazine 275
*2* **phenelzine 150*, 301***
*3* phenobarbital 405*
*3* phenylephrine 302*
*3* propoxyphene 230*
*3* quinidine 302*
*3* rifampin 391*
*3* ritonavir 190*
*3* tolazamide 231*

*1* **tranylcypromine 150**
*3* trifluoperazine 98, 275
*3* verapamil 303*

Tegison
*2* **methotrexate 258***

Tegretol
Also see Anticonvulsants
*3* acetaminophen 3
*3* alprazolam 76
*3* amitriptyline 71
*3* clarithromycin 65*, 68, 79
*3* clozapine 65*
*3* cyclosporine 66*
*2* **danazol 66***
*3* desipramine 72
*3* diazepam 76
*2* **diltiazem 67***
*3* doxycycline 67*
*3* erythromycin 65, 68*, 79
*3* felbamate 69*
*2* **felodipine 69***
*3* fluoxetine 70*
*3* fluvoxamine 70*
*3* haloperidol 71*
*3* imipramine 71*
*3* isoniazid 72*
*3* isotretinoin 73*
*3* lamotrigine 73*
*3* lithium 74*
*3* mebendazole 74*
*3* methadone 75*, 357
*3* metronidazole 75*
*3* midazolam 76*, 375
*3* nortriptyline 71
*3* oral contraceptives 76*, 394
*3* phenytoin 75, 77*
*2* **propoxyphene 78*, 231**
*3* tacrolimus 66, 413
*3* theophylline 78*
*3* thiabendazole 74
*3* thyroid 79*
*3* triazolam 76
*3* troleandomycin 65, 68, 79*
*3* valproic acid 80*
*2* **verapamil 81***
*3* warfarin 81*

Tenex
Also see Alpha agonists
*3* amitriptyline 25*

*3* doxepin 231*
*3* imipramine 231
*3* maprotiline 231
*3* nortriptyline 231
Tolmetin
Also see Nonsteroidal anti-
inflammatory drugs
*2* warfarin 452*
Toloxatone
*3* tyramine 452*
Tonocard
Also see Antiarrhythmics
*3* antacids 40*
*3* Mylanta 40*
*3* rifampin 437*
Toradol
Also see Nonsteroidal anti-
inflammatory drugs
*3* lithium 336*
Torsemide
Also see Diuretics; Loop
diuretics
*3* digoxin 211
*3* enalapril 235
*3* fluoxetine 269
Tracrium
Also see Muscle relaxants;
Neuromuscular blockers
*3* amphotericin B 27
*2* gentamicin 51*
*3* tobramycin 51
Tramadol
*2* isocarboxazid 453
*2* phenelzine 453
*2* tranylcypromine 453*
Trandate
Also see Alpha blockers;
Beta-adrenergic blockers
*3* cimetidine 125
*3* diazepam 202
*3* epinephrine 240
*3* indomethacin 307
Tranxene
Also see Anticonvulsants;
Benzodiazepines
*3* cimetidine 111
*3* disulfiram 198
*3* rifampin 203
Tranylcypromine
Also see Monoamine oxi-
dase inhibitors
*3* chlorpropamide 312

*1* clomipramine 150
*1* dexfenfluramine 191
*1* dextroamphetamine 193*
*1* dextromethorphan 196
*3* disulfiram 228*
*1* ethanol 252
*1* fenfluramine 261
*1* fluoxetine 273*
*1* fluvoxamine 273
*1* food 454
*3* guanethidine 295
*3* insulin 312*
*3* levodopa 338
*2* lithium 344
*1* meperidine 354
*1* metaraminol 356
*1* methotrimeprazine 364
*1* methylphenidate 193
*3* norepinephrine 389
*1* paroxetine 273
*1* phenylephrine 400
*1* phenylpropanolamine 401
*1* pseudoephedrine 402
*1* reserpine 402
*1* sertraline 273
*3* tolbutamide 312
*2* tramadol 453*
*1* tyramine 454*
Trazodone
Also see Tricyclic antidepressants
*3* chlorpromazine 98*
*3* cimetidine 111, 113
*3* clonidine 152
*3* fluoxetine 189
*2* moclobemide 149
*1* phenelzine 150, 301
*3* trifluoperazine 98
Trental
*3* ciprofloxacin 133*
*3* enoxacin 133
*3* norfloxacin 133
*3* pefloxacin 133
*3* pipemidic acid 133
*3* theophylline 400*
Triamterene
Also see Diuretics; Potassium-sparing diuretics
*3* diclofenac 308
*3* ibuprofen 308

*3* indomethacin 308*
*2* potassium 420*
Triazolam
Also see Benzodiazepines
*3* carbamazepine 76
*3* cimetidine 111
*3* clarithromycin 246, 454
*3* disulfiram 198
*3* erythromycin 13, 62, 243, 246*, 454
*2* fluconazole 264, 267*, 324, 333
*3* grapefruit juice 291*
*3* isoniazid 201, 319*
*2* itraconazole 63, 201, 322, 324*, 333
*3* ketoconazole 90, 324, 333*
*3* miconazole 333
*3* phenytoin 375
*3* rifabutin 438
*3* rifampin 438*
*3* troleandomycin 246, 454*
Triclofos
*3* warfarin 455*
Tricyclic antidepressants
Also see Amitriptyline;
Clomipramine; Desi-
pramine; Doxepin; Imi-
pramine; Maprotiline;
Nortriptyline; Protrip-
tyline; Trazodone;
Trimipramine
*3* altretamine 14*
*3* butaperazine 275
*3* carbamazepine 71*, 72
*3* chlorpromazine 98*, 275
*3* chlorpropamide 231
*3* cholestyramine 102*
*3* cimetidine 110*, 111, 113*, 115*, 121*
*2* clonidine 25, 152*
*3* clonidine 152
*3* colestipol 102
*3* dextroamphetamine 193*
*3* diltiazem 303
*2* epinephrine 240*
*3* fluoxetine 24*, 188*, 189
*3* fluphenazine 275*
*3* fluvoxamine 148*
*3* grapefruit juice 149*
*2* guanabenz 152

Tricyclic antidepressants
*(Continued)*
**3** guanabenz 25
**2 guanadrel 190**
**3** guanethidine 190*
**2 guanfacine 152**
**3** guanfacine 25*
**3** indinavir 190
**1 isocarboxazid 150**
**3** isoproterenol 25*
**3** lithium 26*
**2 moclobemide 149***
**2 norepinephrine 300*,
301**
**3** paroxetine 24, 189
**3** perphenazine 275
**2 phenelzine 150*, 301***
**3** phenobarbital 405*
**3** phenylephrine 302*
**3** propoxyphene 230*
**3** quinidine 302*
**3** rifampin 391*
**3** ritonavir 190*
**3** tolazamide 231*
**1 tranylcypromine 150**
**3** trifluoperazine 98, 275
**3** verapamil 303*

Trifluoperazine
Also see Neuroleptics
**3** imipramine 275
**3** trazodone 98

Trihexyphenidyl
Also see Anticholinergics
**3** haloperidol 55
**3** tacrine 445*

Trilafon
Also see Neuroleptics
**3** imipramine 275

Tri-Levlen
Also see Estrogens
**3** ampicillin 28*
**3** carbamazepine 76*, 394
**1 cigarette smoking 107***
**3** cyclosporine 165, 179*
**3** dexamethasone 395
**2 dicumarol 397**
**3** doxycycline 397
**3** griseofulvin 292*
**3** hydrocortisone 395
**3** methylprednisolone 395
**3** phenobarbital 394*

**2 phenprocoumon 397**
**3** phenytoin 394*
**3** prednisolone 395*
**3** prednisone 395
**3** primidone 394
**3** rifabutin 396
**3** rifampin 395*
**3** ritonavir 396*
**3** tetracycline 397*
**2 warfarin 397***

Trimazosin
Also see Alpha blockers
**3** enalapril 62

Trimethoprim
**3** dapsone 188*
**3** phenytoin 416*
**3** procainamide 424*

Trimethoprim-sulfamethox-
azole
**3** chlorpropamide 451
**3** dapsone 188
**3** disulfiram 370
**3** glipizide 451
**3** glyburide 451
**3** methotrexate 363*
**3** metronidazole 252, 370*
**3** phenindione 455
**3** phenytoin 416
**3** tolbutamide 451*
**3** warfarin 455*

Trimipramine
Also see Cyclic antidepressants; Tricyclic antide-
pressants
**3** cimetidine 111, 113

Trimpex
**3** dapsone 188*
**3** phenytoin 416*
**3** procainamide 424*

Tri-Norinyl
Also see Estrogens
**3** ampicillin 28*
**3** carbamazepine 76*, 394
**1 cigarette smoking 107***
**3** cyclosporine 165, 179*
**3** dexamethasone 395
**2 dicumarol 397**
**3** doxycycline 397
**3** griseofulvin 292*
**3** hydrocortisone 395
**3** methylprednisolone 395
**3** phenobarbital 394*

**2 phenprocoumon 397**
**3** phenytoin 394*
**3** prednisolone 395*
**3** prednisone 395
**3** primidone 394
**3** rifabutin 396
**3** rifampin 395*
**3** ritonavir 396*
**3** tetracycline 397*
**2 warfarin 397***

Triphasil
Also see Estrogens
**3** ampicillin 28*
**3** carbamazepine 76*, 394
**1 cigarette smoking 107***
**3** cyclosporine 165, 179*
**3** dexamethasone 395
**2 dicumarol 397**
**3** doxycycline 397
**3** griseofulvin 292*
**3** hydrocortisone 395
**3** methylprednisolone 395
**2 phenprocoumon 397**
**3** phenytoin 394*
**3** prednisolone 395*
**3** prednisone 395
**3** primidone 394
**3** rifabutin 396
**3** rifampin 395*
**3** ritonavir 396*
**3** tetracycline 397*
**2 warfarin 397***

Troleandomycin
Also see Macrolides
**3** alfentanil 8
**3** alprazolam 13, 454
**1 astemizole 48, 446**
**3** atorvastatin 51
**3** buspirone 62
**3** carbamazepine 65, 68,
79*
**2 cisapride 136, 139***
**3** clozapine 156
**3** colchicine 160
**3** cyclosporine 168
**3** diazepam 454
**3** disopyramide 224
**3** felodipine 242
**3** indinavir 144
**3** lovastatin 242
**3** methylprednisolone 366*

Vibramycin
  Also see Tetracyclines
  *3* antacids 39
  *3* bismuth 56*, 57
  *3* carbamazepine 67*
  *3* iron 316
  *3* oral contraceptives 397
  *3* phenobarbital 232*
  *3* phenytoin 232*
  *3* warfarin 233*
Vicks Formula 44
  *3* fluoxetine 194*
  *1* isocarboxazid 196
  *1* moclobemide 195*
  *3* paroxetine 194
  *1* phenelzine 195*
  *3* quinidine 196*
  *2* selegiline 197*
  *1* tranylcypromine 196
Vicodin
  Also see Narcotic
    analgesics
  *3* quinidine 158
Vidarabine
  *3* allopurinol 13*
Videx
  Also see Antivirals
  *3* ciprofloxacin 130*
  *3* dapsone 186*
  *3* ganciclovir 206*
  *3* itraconazole 207*
  *3* ketoconazole 207*
Vigabatrin
  *3* phenytoin 417*
Vinblastine
  Also see Antineoplastics
  *2* mitomycin 376*
Vincasar
  Also see Antineoplastics
  *3* nifedipine 388*
Vincristine
  Also see Antineoplastics
  *3* nifedipine 388*
Vira-A
  *3* allopurinol 13*
Virilon
  *3* cyclosporine 165
  *2* warfarin 398

Visken
  Also see Beta-adrenergic
    blockers
  *3* cimetidine 125
  *3* epinephrine 240
  *3* indomethacin 307
Vitamin B_6
  *3* levodopa 339*
  *3* phenytoin 411*
Vitamin E
  *3* dicumarol 456
  *3* iron 317*
  *3* warfarin 456*
Vitamin K
  *3* warfarin 457*
Vivactil
  Also see Cyclic antidepres-
    sants; Tricyclic antide-
    pressants
  *3* cimetidine 111, 113, 121
  *2* epinephrine 240
  *2* norepinephrine 301
  *3* phenobarbital 405*
Voltaren
  Also see Nonsteroidal anti-
    inflammatory drugs
  *3* cholestyramine 100*, 160
  *3* colestipol 100, 160*
  *3* cyclosporine 166*, 173,
    174, 175
  *3* lithium 204*
  *2* methotrexate 204*
  *3* triamterene 308
  *3* verapamil 205*
  *2* warfarin 53, 206*, 208,
    262, 309, 335, 352, 353,
    409, 418, 444
Vumon
  Also see Antineoplastics
  *3* phenytoin 414*
Warfarin
  Also see Anticoagulants;
    Oral anticoagulants
  *3* acetaminophen 4*
  *3* allopurinol 13*
  *3* aminoglutethimide 17*
  *3* amiodarone 23*
  *2* amobarbital 408
  *2* aspirin 4, 46*
  *2* azapropazone 53*
  *3* azathioprine 54*, 356

*2* bromfenac 58*
*2* butabarbital 408
*3* carbamazepine 81*
*2* cefamandole 379
*2* cefazolin 379
*2* cefmetazole 379
*2* cefoperazone 379
*2* cefotetan 379
*2* cefoxitin 379
*2* ceftriaxone 379
*3* chloral hydrate 87*
*2* chloramphenicol 88
*3* cholestyramine 106*,
  148, 286, 350
*2* cimetidine 129*
*3* ciprofloxacin 135*, 391,
  393
*3* clarithromycin 247
*2* clofibrate 148*, 286, 350
*3* colestipol 106, 148, 286,
  350
*3* cyclophosphamide 164*
*2* danazol 186*
*2* dextrothyroxine 197*
*2* diclofenac 53, 206*, 208,
  262, 309, 335, 352, 353,
  409, 418, 444
*2* diflunisal 208*
*3* disulfiram 229*
*3* doxycycline 233*
*3* erythromycin 247*
*3* ethanol 256*
*2* etodolac 257*
*2* fenoprofen 262*
*3* fluconazole 268*, 324,
  333
*3* fluorouracil 269*
*3* fluoxetine 274*, 441
*2* flurbiprofen 276
*3* fluvastatin 350
*3* fluvoxamine 279*
*2* gemfibrozil 148, 285*,
  350
*3* glucagon 288*
*2* glutethimide 288*
*3* glyburide 289*
*3* griseofulvin 293*
*3* heparin 297*
*2* heptabarbital 408
*2* ibuprofen 53, 208, 262,
  299*, 309, 335, 352, 353,
  409, 418, 444